EPILEPSY
Diagnosis and Management

EPILEPSY
Diagnosis and Management

Edited by

Thomas R. Browne, M.D.
Associate Professor of Neurology and Pharmacology, Boston
University School of Medicine; Assistant Chief, Neurology
Service, Veterans Administration Medical Center, Boston,
Massachusetts

Robert G. Feldman, M.D.
Professor of Neurology and Pharmacology and Chairman,
Department of Neurology, Boston University School of Medi-
cine; Chief, Neurology Services, University Hospital and
Veterans Administration Medical Center, Boston, Massachusetts

Little, Brown and Company
Boston/Toronto

Library of Congress Catalog Card No. 82-83677

ISBN 0-316-11114-7

Printed in the United States of America

MV

TO J. KIFFIN PENRY, M.D.

Our major motivation in writing this book was to make available the large body of useful new information on the diagnosis and management of epilepsy that has been produced in the past decade. Dr. Penry has been a pivotal figure in the generation of this body of information. His tireless efforts as physician, investigator, administrator, teacher, and listener have significantly advanced the frontiers of epilepsy and have been an inspiration to all who work in the field.

CONTENTS

CONTRIBUTING AUTHORS

Thomas R. Browne, M.D.
Associate Professor of Neurology and Pharmacology, Boston University School of Medicine; Assistant Chief, Neurology Service, Veterans Administration Medical Center, Boston, Massachusetts

Joyce A. Cramer, B.S.
Research Biologist, Veterans Administration Medical Center, West Haven, Connecticut

Giuscppe Erba, M.D.
Associate Professor of Neurology, Harvard Medical School; Associate in Neurology, Seizure Unit and Division of Clinical Neurophysiology, The Children's Hospital Medical Center, Boston, Massachusetts

Robert G. Feldman, M.D.
Professor of Neurology and Pharmacology and Chairman, Department of Neurology, Boston University School of Medicine; Chief, Neurology Services, University Hospital and Veterans Administration Medical Center, Boston, Massachusetts

Cesare T. Lombroso, M.D., Ph.D.
Professor of Neurology, Harvard Medical School; Chief, Seizure Unit and Division of Clinical Neurophysiology, The Children's Hospita! Medical Center, Boston, Massachusetts

Richard H. Mattson, M.D.
Clinical Professor of Neurology, Yale University School of Medicine, New Haven; Chief, Neurology Service, Veterans Administration Medical Center, West Haven, Connecticut

Allan F. Mirsky, Ph.D.
Chief, Laboratory of Psychology and Psychopathology, National Institute of Mental Health, National Institutes of Health, Bethesda, Maryland

Susan E. Norman, R.N., M.S.N.
Nurse Specialist, Department of Neurology, Beth Israel Hospital, Boston, Massachusetts

Merle M. Orren, Ph.D.
Instructor of Neurology and Psychiatry, Boston University School of Medicine, Boston, Massachusetts

Eileen M. Ouellette, M.D.
Assistant Professor of Neurology, Harvard Medical School; Assistant Neurologist and Pediatrician, Massachusetts General Hospital, Boston

Jonathan H. Pincus, M.D.
Professor of Neurology, Yale University School of Medicine; Assistant Chief, Department of Neurology, Yale-New Haven Hospital, New Haven, Connecticut

Roger J. Porter, M.D.
Chief, Epilepsy Branch, Neurological Disorders Program,
National Institute of Neurological and Communicative
Disorders and Stroke, National Institutes of Health,
Bethesda, Maryland

Nancy L. Ricks, Ed.D.
Assistant to the President, Wilson College, Chambersburg,
Pennsylvania

Terrence L. Riley, M.D.
Associate Professor of Neurology, Boston University School
of Medicine; Director, EEG and Sleep Laboratories, University
Hospital, Boston, Massachusetts

Ernst A. Rodin, M.D.
Clinical Professor of Neurology, The University of Michigan
Medical School, Ann Arbor; Medical Director, Epilepsy Center
of Michigan, Detroit

Edward B. Shaw, B.S.
Administrative Officer, Neurology Service, Veterans
Administration Medical Center, Boston, Massachusetts

Michael C. Trachtenberg, Ph.D.
Associate Professor, Department of Surgery, Division of
Neurosurgery, The University of Texas Medical School at
Galveston, Galveston

Arthur A. Ward, Jr., M.D.
Professor and Chairman Emeritus, Department of
Neurological Surgery, University of Washington School of
Medicine; Program Director, Regional Epilepsy Center,
University of Washington, Seattle

PREFACE

A large volume of useful new information on the diagnosis and management of epilepsy has been published in the past decade. Full-time "epileptologists" have been applying this information and have substantially improved the care they can deliver to patients with epilepsy. We have observed that physicians other than full-time epileptologists often are not aware of much of the new information about the diagnosis and management of epilepsy. This unfortunate state of affairs has arisen because much of the information the clinician needs is published in symposium volumes, clinical pharmacology journals, foreign journals, and subspecialty journals. Few practicing physicians, including neurologists, have the time to keep abreast of the information in these sources, which are somewhat out of the mainstream of the reading done by practicing physicians.

The purpose of this book is to present concise, up-to-date, and clinically oriented reviews of each of the major areas in the diagnosis and management of epilepsy. Because of the depth and complexity of the current knowledge of epilepsy, we chose to follow a "textbook of medicine" format, in which the subject was subdivided into a number of chapters, and recognized experts were invited to write chapters in their areas of expertise. A standard format is followed in many of the chapters so that the reader, once familiar with the format, can quickly locate information on a specific topic.

To effectively manage patients with epilepsy it is necessary to have a clear understanding of the differential diagnosis of the various types of epilepsy (and nonepilepsy), the spectrum and uses of available antiepileptic drugs, the clinical pharmacology of antiepileptic drugs, the uses and limitations of antiepileptic drug serum concentration determinations, and the spectrum and uses of nonpharmacologic therapy. All of the basic information on these topics is contained in this book. The physician who masters this information will improve considerably the quality of care he provides for patients with epilepsy and will find managing such patients more scientifically based and more rewarding than in the past.

T. R. B.
R. G. F.

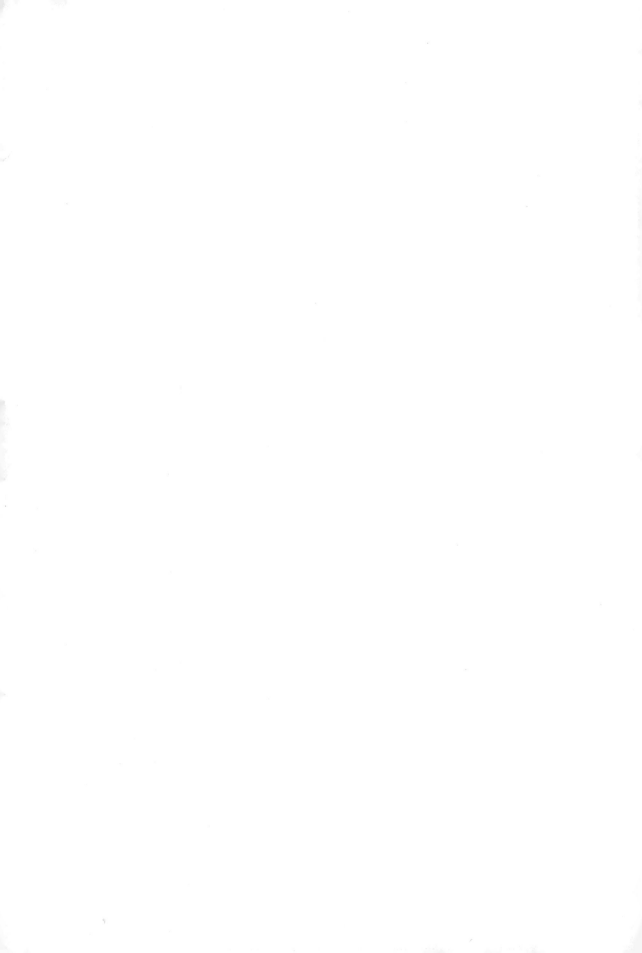

EPILEPSY
Diagnosis and Management

EPILEPSY: AN OVERVIEW

1

Thomas R. Browne
Robert G. Feldman

Definition of Epilepsy

Hippocrates recognized epilepsy as an organic process of the brain. However, many ancient writers considered seizures the work of supernatural forces. In fact, the word *epilepsy* comes from a Greek word meaning "to be seized by forces from without."

Jackson [18] gave direction to the understanding of epilepsy in the late nineteenth century by carefully analyzing individual cases. From his observations, Jackson formulated the modern definition of epilepsy: "*an occasional, excessive, and disorderly discharge of nerve tissue.*" Jackson further concluded: "This discharge occurs in all degrees; it occurs with all sorts of conditions of ill health at all ages, and under innumerable circumstances." His emphasis on the clinical description of a seizure, beginning with the mode of onset, led to the concept of focal epilepsy with subsequent spread of discharging cells.

Epilepsy is a complex symptom caused by a variety of pathologic processes in the brain. It is characterized by occasional (paroxysmal), excessive, and disorderly discharging of neurons, which can be detected by clinical manifestations, electroencephalographic (EEG) recording or both. Paroxysmal discharges of neurons occur when the threshold for firing of the neuronal membranes is reduced beyond the capability of intrinsic membrane-threshold-stabilizing mechanisms to prevent firing (see Chap. 2). The attack may be localized and remain restricted in its focus, or it can spread to other areas of the brain. When the size of the discharging area is sufficient, a clinical seizure occurs; otherwise, it may be limited to localized electrical disturbances. The particular site of the brain affected determines the clinical expression of the seizure. When the synchronized discharges of a neuronal population are recorded by an EEG from the scalp, the paroxysms appear as spikes, slow waves, and spike-wave potentials.

For the patient with epilepsy, the disorder is defined in more personal terms. Among the factors that define epilepsy for the individual are: what he experiences or recalls about the experience; what others around him observe and describe to him; the frequency and duration of attacks; and the impact on his self-image and social adjustment.

Parts of a Seizure

The period during which the seizure actually occurs is defined as the ictus or *ictal* period. The *aura* is the earliest portion of a seizure recognized and the only part remembered by the patient; it may act as a "warn-

1

ing." The time immediately following a seizure is referred to as the *postictal* period; the interval between seizures is the *interictal* period.

INTERICTAL PERIOD

The period between attacks is usually clinically normal in most patients with epilepsy, although their EEGs may show paroxysmal activity consistent with the diagnosis of epilepsy. A seizure disorder may influence the overall performance and adjustment of the patient if subclinical seizures not readily detectable by observation are occurring (such as absence attacks).

In clinical practice, the use of EEG in the diagnosis of epilepsy is based largely on the interictal patterns (see Chap. 11), since clinical seizures are rarely recorded during a routine EEG. Such interictal EEG patterns include focal and generalized spike or spike-wave discharges. The diagnostic significance of these patterns generally increases with increasing voltage, wider distribution, and increasing incidence during the "sampling" of the EEG recording session [23]. Analysis of surface interictal potentials does not always give accurate information about the site of origin of the epileptic activity. In some patients, the recording may be normal [1]. Clinical assesment is necessary to determine the significance of any EEG disturbances found during the interictal period. The physician must ultimately treat the patient, not the EEG.

AURA

The first manifestation of the seizure perceived by the patient is the aura. The aura is the actual beginning of the attack and represents paroxysmal neuronal firing in or near the focus of cerebral origin of the seizure. The aura is thus actually an "ictal" event and not a "preictal" event. An aura may occur but not progress beyond simple symptomatology, or it may progress to a more extensive seizure with alteration of consciousness. Ajmone-Marsan and Goldhammer [2] studied the auras of 187 patients. These auras were divided into seven categories: somatosensory sensations, cephalic sensations, general body sensations, specific sensory sensations, visceral sensations, psychic auras, and "various feelings." Many patients reported seizures in which the aura was the only manifestation; others experienced the aura followed by loss of consciousness with or without motor and "automatic" phenomena. Fifty-seven percent of the patients experienced more than one type of aura. Complex (47%) and visceral (41%) sensations were the most common subjective phenomena reported. Olfactory (8%) and gustatory (5%) auras, although relatively infrequent, were often the most prominent and consistent features of the pa-

tient's seizures when present. A careful history of the events (especially of the initial events) during a patient's aura often can point out the focus of origin of a patient's seizures [2] (see Chaps. 4 and 5). Throughout the entire episode, the relationship between cellular events, clinical phenomena, and EEG manifestations remains very close [3]. The clinical and EEG characteristics of seizures form the basis for their classification.

ICTAL PERIOD

An ictus occurs if epileptic discharging of neurons is sufficient to produce a measurable physiologic effect, evident clinically or as events on an EEG. Unlike interictal paroxysmal discharges, which are brief and intermittent, ictal discharges build up and persist for longer periods. Clinical ictal phenomena depend on the specific cerebral structures involved in the epileptic discharging. Activity confined to silent areas may remain asymptomatic. Activity involving motor, sensory, or limbic structures may produce clinical behavior that can be attributed to discharging of neurons in those particular foci. Generalized activity leads to loss of consciousness that may be accompanied only by staring or by tonic and clonic motor activity of the extremities.

POSTICTAL PERIOD

The postictal period corresponds to the period of neuronal, behavioral, and electroencephalographic return to normal after a paroxysmal discharge of neurons. The clinical manifestations of the postictal period vary with the seizure type.

After a tonic-clonic attack, the immediate postictal period is characterized by altered consciousness and incomplete muscle relaxation. Micturition occurs during the early postictal period owing to relaxation of sphincters. Autonomic functions return progressively to preseizure levels. Respirations return after ictal apnea. Consciousness slowly returns as the patient passes through intermediate levels of increasing vigilance [9] (see Chap. 6).

The postictal phase after a complex partial seizure is highly variable in length and consists of partial impairment of consciousness during which the patient may react to environmental stimuli (see Chap. 5). The reactions to environmental stimuli are often inappropriate and may include violent behavior if the patient is directed to do something he does not wish to do. There are few, if any, postictal symptoms after simple partial seizures and absence seizures (see Chaps. 4 and 7).

Types of Epileptic Seizures and Types of Epilepsy

CLASSIFICATIONS

There are two types of classifications of epilepsy: (1) classifications of the *epileptic seizures* and (2) classifications of *the epilepsies*. Classifications of epileptic seizures are concerned with classifying each individual seizure as a single event. Classifications of the epilepsies are designed to classify syndromes in which the type or types of seizure(s) are one, but not the only, feature of the syndrome. Other features such as etiology, age of onset, and evidence of brain pathology are also included in classifications of the epilepsies.

The classification of epileptic seizures used throughout this book is the Clinical and Electroencephalographic Classification of Epileptic Seizures of the International League Against Epilepsy ("International Classification of Epileptic Seizures") [8]. The classification of the epilepsies used is the International Classification of Epilepsies [22]. The reasons for using these two systems are discussed in Chapter 3. Because accurate diagnosis of the type of epileptic seizure a patient is having is the key to proper management, this book will use the International Classification of Epileptic Seizures in most discussions.

INTERNATIONAL CLASSIFICATION OF EPILEPTIC SEIZURES

The International Classification of Epileptic Seizures is summarized in Table 1-1 and presented in its entirety in Table 3-1. Seizures are first classified into two broad categories: (1) partial seizures (seizures beginning in a relatively small location in the brain) and (2) generalized seizures (seizures that are bilaterally symmetrical and without local onset). Seizures are then further classified depending on the exact clinical and EEG manifestations of the seizure. A summary of the clinical manifestations of the principal types of epileptic seizures recognized by the International Classification of Epileptic Seizures is presented below. For a complete description of the clinical and EEG features of each seizure type, see Chapters 4 through 10 and Table 3-1.

Simple Partial (Focal) Seizures

Simple partial seizures are caused by a local cortical discharge, which results in seizure symptoms appropriate to the function of the discharging area of the brain without loss of consciousness. Simple partial seizures may consist of motor, sensory, autonomic, or psychic signs or symptoms, or combinations of these. Motor symptoms include localized focal jerks, focal jerks that progressively involve a greater number of muscles ("Jacksonian march"), turning of the head and

Table 1-1. Summary of International Classification of Epileptic Seizures

I. Partial (Focal, Local) Seizures
  A. Simple partial seizures (consciousness not impaired)
    1. With motor signs
    2. With sensory symptoms
    3. With autonomic symptoms or signs
    4. With psychic symptoms
  B. Complex partial seizures (temporal lobe or psychomotor seizures; consciousness impaired)
    1. Simple partial onset, followed by impairment of consciousness
      a. With simple partial features (A.1–A.4), followed by impaired consciousness
      b. With automatisms
    2. With impairment of consciousness at onset
      a. With impairment of consciousness only
      b. With automatisms
  C. Partial seizures, evolving to secondarily generalized seizures (tonic-clonic, tonic, or clonic)
    1. Simple partial seizures (A.), evolving to generalized seizures
    2. Complex partial seizures (B.), evolving to generalized seizures
    3. Simple partial seizures, evolving to complex partial seizures, evolving to generalized seizures

II. Generalized Seizures (Convulsive or Nonconvulsive)
  A. Absence (petit mal) seizures
  B. Myoclonic seizures
  C. Clonic seizures
  D. Tonic seizures
  E. Tonic-clonic (grand mal) seizures
  F. Atonic seizures

III. Unclassified Epileptic Seizures (due to incomplete data)

Source: Modified from Dreifus [8].

eyes (versive seizure), change in posture, and vocalization or arrest of speech. Sensory symptoms include simple hallucinations (subjective perceptions of sensory stimuli that do not exist in the environment) of the somatosensory, visual, auditory, olfactory, gustatory, or labyrinthine senses. Autonomic symptoms and signs include epigastric sensations, pallor, sweating, flushing, piloerection, and papillary dilatation. Psychic symptoms may be dysphasic, dysmenic (e.g., déjà vu), cognitive (e.g., dreamy states, distortions of time sense), affective (fear, anger, and so on), illusions (distortions of sensory perception of real environmental stimuli, such as macropsia), or structural hallucinations (e.g., music, visual scenes).

Complex Partial (Psychomotor, Temporal Lobe) Seizures

The crucial distinction between simple partial seizures and complex partial seizures is that consciousness is

4

impaired in the latter and not in the former [8]. Impaired consciousness is defined as the inability to respond normally to exogenous stimuli owing to altered awareness or responsiveness [8].

At the onset of a complex partial seizure, any of the symptoms or signs (motor, sensory, autonomic, or psychic) of a simple partial seizure may occur without impairment of consciousness, providing an aura. The central feature of the complex partial seizure is impairment of consciousness, which may occur with or without a preceding simple partial aura. There may be no other symptoms or signs during the period of impaired consciousness, or there may be automatisms (i.e., unconscious acts that are "automatic" and of which the patient has no recollection). The attack characteristically ends gradually, with a period of postictal drowsiness or confusion.

Absence (Petit Mal) Seizures
Absence seizures consist of sudden onset and cessation of responsiveness. There is no aura and little or no postictal symptomatology. The majority of absence seizures last 10 seconds or less and may be accompanied by mild clonic components, atonic or tonic components, automatisms, or autonomic components. Absence seizures usually begin between the ages of 5 and 12 years and often stop spontaneously in the teens.

Myoclonic Seizures
Myoclonic seizures consist of brief, sudden muscle contractions that may be generalized or localized, symmetric or asymmetric, synchronous or asynchronous. There is usually no detectable loss of consciousness.

Infantile Spasms
The most common form of infantile spasm consists of flexion of the trunk, extension of the arms, and drawing up of the legs ("salaam" posture). Other forms include (1) nodding of the head only, (2) extension of the arms, legs, and trunk and nodding of the head, and (3) a single, momentary shocklike contraction of the entire body ("lightning attack"). Crying, laughing, giggling, flushing, pallor, cyanosis, or brief clonic movements may accompany an attack. Infantile spasms most commonly begin between 3 and 9 months of age.

Clonic Seizures
Clonic seizures occur almost exclusively in early childhood. The attack begins with loss or impairment of consciousness associated with sudden hypotonia or a brief generalized tonic spasm. This is followed by one to several minutes of bilateral jerks, which are often asymmetric and may predominate in one limb. During the attack there may be great variability in the amplitude, frequency, and spatial distribution of these jerks from moment to moment. In other children, particularly those aged 1 to 3 years, the jerks remain bilateral and synchronous throughout the attack. Postictally there may be rapid recovery or a prolonged period of confusion or coma.

Tonic Seizures
Tonic seizures consist of a sudden increase in muscle tone in the axial or extremity muscles, or both, producing a number of characteristic postures. Consciousness is usually partially or completely lost. Prominent autonomic phenomena occur. Postictal alteration of consciousness is usually brief but may last several minutes. Tonic seizures are relatively rare and usually begin between 1 and 7 years of age.

Tonic-Clonic (Grand Mal) Seizures
Before the tonic phase there may be bilateral jerks of the extremities or focal seizure activity. The onset of the seizure is marked by loss of consciousness and increased muscle tone (tonic phase), which usually results in a rigid flexed posture at first and then a rigid extended posture. This is followed by bilateral rhythmic jerks that become further apart (clonic phase). Prominent autonomic phenomena are observable during the tonic and clonic phases. In the postictal phase increased muscle tone occurs first, followed by flaccidity. Incontinence may occur. The patient awakens by passing through stages of coma, confusional state, and drowsiness.

Atonic Seizures
Atonic seizures consist of loss of body tone. This may be manifested as nodding of the head, sagging at the knees, or total loss of body tone associated with falling and injuries. There is usually no detectable loss of consciousness.

Epidemiology of Epilepsy

INCIDENCE

Overall
Woodbury [27] reviewed the available data on the incidence of patients with epilepsy in the United States and concluded that the best minimum estimate was 46.7 per 100,000 population per year. Applying this figure to the 1980 United States population of 226.5 million yields a minimum expected number of 105,800 new cases per year in the United States. An accurate maximum estimate is not available.

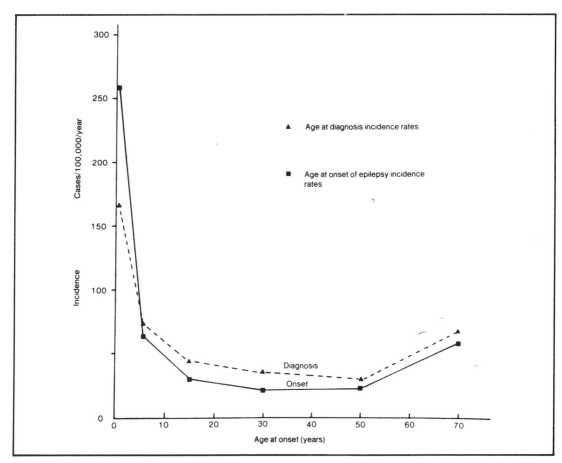

*Figure 1-1. Mean annual epilepsy incidence rates in Roches-
ter, Minnesota, by age, 1935–1964. (Based on data from
W. A. Hauser and L. T. Kurland [15], modified by L. A.
Woodbury [27].)*

By Seizure Type

The most complete and careful study of the epidemiology of epilepsy in the United States was carried out
in Rochester, Minnesota during the period 1935
through 1967 and was reported by Hauser and Kurland [15]. The incidence of various types of epilepsy
by seizure type found in this study is shown in Table
1-2. Tonic-clonic, simple partial, and complex partial
seizures had similar incidences, whereas the incidence
of absence seizures was somewhat less.

By Age

The overall incidence of epilepsy is high in the first
year of life, drops rapidly to a minimum around 30 to
40 years of age, and then rises again (Fig. 1-1). The
incidence of each type of epileptic seizure by age is

Table 1-2. Incidence of Epilepsy by Seizure Type*

Simple partial	12.8
Complex partial	10.4
Multiple or unclassified partial	7.2
Tonic-clonic only	12.5
Incompletely generalized with or without associated tonic-clonic	6.1
Absence with or without associated tonic-clonic	3.4
Other	4.5

*Mean annual rate per 100,000 population. Calculated for Rochester,
Minnesota, 1945–1964.
Source: Modified from Hauser and Kurland [15].

6

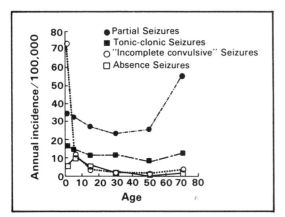

Figure 1-2. Mean annual epilepsy incidence rates, by type of initial epileptic seizure and by age, diagnosed in Rochester, Minnesota, 1935–1964. (Modified from W. A. Hauser and L. T. Kurland [15].)

*Table 1-3. Prevalence of Epilepsy by Type of Initial Seizure**

Simple partial	1.3
Complex partial	1.7
Multiple or unclassified partial	1.0
Tonic-clonic only	1.3
Incompletely generalized with or without associated tonic-clonic	0.4
Absence with or without associated tonic-clonic	0.4
Other	0.2

*Per 1,000 population. Calculated for Rochester, Minnesota, January 1, 1960.
Source: Modified from Hauser and Kurland [15].

*Table 1-4. Prevalence of Epilepsy by Age**

Age (yr)	Rate
0–9	2.8
10–19	4.1
20–39	5.6
40–59	7.0
60+	10.2

*Per 1,000 population. Calculated for Rochester, Minnesota, January 1, 1965.
Source: Modified from Hauser and Kurland [15].

shown in Figure 1-2. Partial seizures occur frequently in the first years of life, somewhat less often in persons aged 20 to 50, and much more often in older people. The incidence of tonic-clonic seizures does not vary much with age. Absence seizures rarely occur after 20 years of age. The incidence of "incomplete convulsions" is high during the first year of life and low thereafter, probably reflecting the immaturity of the infant nervous system.

PREVALENCE

Overall
The only study of the prevalence of epilepsy in the United States that covers all ages is that of Hauser and Kurland [15]. An age-adjusted prevalence of 6.25 per 1,000 population was obtained [15, 27]. Applying this figure to the 1980 population of about 226.5 million gives an estimated number of 1,416,000 patients with epilepsy.

The criteria used by Hauser and Kurland [15] for including epilepsy cases in their study were conservative. Studies conducted in different areas with narrower age groups and more inclusive definitions of epilepsy generally result in higher estimates of prevalence [27]. The higher values range from 9.3 to 33.7 per 1,000 population [27]. These higher prevalence values are due in part to inclusion of single convulsions or febrile convulsions, or both, which were not included in the study of Hauser and Kurland [15].

By Seizure Type
The prevalence of epilepsy by type of initial seizure is shown in Table 1-3. Complex partial, simple partial, and tonic-clonic seizures are the most prevalent types.

By Age
The prevalence of epilepsy by age is shown in Table 1-4. The prevalence increases in a linear fashion through all age groups.

FREQUENCY OF SEIZURE TYPES SEEN IN PRACTICE
The frequency with which patients with various types of epileptic seizures are seen in practice is often different from the prevalence of epileptic seizure types in the general population. This difference is a result of (1) differences in degree of difficulty in diagnosing or treating different types of epileptic seizures; (2) differences in the need for complete control among different types of epileptic seizures; and (3) differences in the age of patients seen and referral patterns among practices. The frequency with which patients with various types of epileptic seizures are seen at several centers is summarized in Table 1-5.

FURTHER READING
Several excellent detailed reviews of the epidemiology of epilepsy have been published [4, 13, 14, 15, 27].

Table 1-5. Frequency With Which Patients With Various Types of Epileptic Seizure Were Seen at Various Centers

Type of Seizure	Boston VA Medical Center*	Michigan Epilepsy Center*	Boston Children's Hospital*
Tonic-clonic only	69	59	48
Tonic-clonic and complex partial	12	17	13
Tonic-clonic and other (including absence)	5	11	20
Complex partial only	7	10	6
Minor and focal	7	0	8
Absence only	0	3	5

*Percent of patients.
Sources: Goodglass et al. [12]; Dennerll et al. [6]; and Lennox and Lennox [19].

Approach to the Patient with Epilepsy

DETERMINE TYPE OF EPILEPSY

The first step in managing a patient who may have epilepsy is to establish definitively whether or not he has epilepsy. If a patient is given a mistaken diagnosis of epilepsy, he is unnecessarily subjected to many inconveniences, including medication with serious side effects, expensive laboratory tests, loss of driver's license, and possible loss of employment.

If a patient has epilepsy, it is extremely important to determine precisely which type(s) of epileptic seizure(s) the patient has in order to determine the correct therapy. An incorrect seizure diagnosis will often result in medication being prescribed that will not control the seizure disorder and that may cause serious side effects.

The best way to diagnose the type of seizure a patient has is to actually observe a seizure, although the physician usually does not have the opportunity to do so. Often the most important differential diagnostic information is a history obtained from the patient and/or reliable observers. The physician must carefully question the patient and observers about the exact details of the aura, the ictus, and the postictal period of the patient's seizures.

The EEG is useful in corroborating the diagnosis of certain types of epilepsy or in differentiating which of several possible types of epilepsy the patient has (see Chap. 11). However, a significant percentage of patients with seizure disorders have normal interictal EEGs. In such cases the physician must treat the patient's seizure disorder according to information obtained from the history, if this information is reliable and clearly points to the diagnosis of a certain type of seizure disorder.

When it is not certain if the patient has epilepsy or which type of seizure a patient has despite a careful history, physical examination, and routine waking and

sleep EEGs, the diagnosis can often be established by means of prolonged monitoring with videotape recording of the patient and his EEG (see Chaps. 11 and 31). This procedure is expensive and requires specialized facilities. However, the consequences of an improper diagnosis can be so catastrophic that it is usually worth the trouble and expense to obtain a definitive diagnosis.

TREAT UNDERLYING CAUSES AND PRECIPITATING FACTORS

Epilepsy is a symptom, not a disease. A seizure can be a symptom of a brain tumor, a brain abscess, encephalitis, meningitis, a metabolic disturbance, drug intoxication, drug withdrawal, and many other disease processes (see Chap. 12). It is imperative that the underlying cause of a patient's seizures be identified and treated to avoid overlooking a reversible cerebral disease process and to facilitate seizure control.

Determining the cause of a patient's seizure disorder involves a combination of history taking, physical examination, and laboratory tests. The history should include questions about family history of epilepsy, birth complications, febrile convulsions (which may precede complex partial seizures; see Chap. 27), middle ear and sinus infections (which may erode through bone and cause cerebral focus), head trauma, alcohol or drug abuse, and symptoms of malignancy. The physical examination should look for evidence of past or recent head trauma, infections of the ears and sinuses, congenital abnormalities (e.g., hemiatrophy, stigmata of tuberous sclerosis), focal or diffuse neurologic abnormalities, stigmata of alcohol or drug abuse, and signs of malignancy. Usually the following laboratory tests should be performed in evaluating the cause of a newly diagnosed seizure disorder: metabolic screening test, EEG recording in waking and sleep states, skull roentgenograms (including views of the sinuses or mastoids if the history

8

indicates possible infection), lumbar puncture (for opening pressure, cell counts, protein and glucose determinations, culture, and serologic examination), and CT scan (if not available, a technetium or other conventional brain scan should be performed).

In addition to determining the underlying cause(s) of a patient's seizure disorder, it is also important to identify and manage factors that precipitate seizures in a given individual, such as anxiety, sleep deprivation, and alcohol withdrawal (see Chap. 12). Management of such precipitating factors will reduce the frequency of seizures and the patient's need for medication.

IDENTIFY AND DEAL WITH PSYCHOLOGIC AND SOCIAL PROBLEMS

Seizures are a relatively rare phenomenon for most patients. However, the psychosocial consequences of epilepsy are present all the time. Loss of a driver's license, of employment, of independence, of self-esteem, and of position in peer groups are all potential problems for the patient with epilepsy and in many cases cause more suffering than the seizures themselves. Furthermore, the anxiety associated with these psychosocial consequences of epilepsy may precipitate seizures in some patients. The physician must anticipate that the patient will experience psychosocial problems as a consequence of having epilepsy and must be prepared to assist him by carefully explaining the nature of his medical problems and the effect these problems will have on driving and employment, by providing emotional support, by giving the patient an opportunity to "talk through" problems, and by referring the patient to various resources available to assist the person with epilepsy (see Chap. 13).

PHARMACOLOGIC THERAPY

The pharmacologic principles of antiepileptic drug administration are reviewed in detail in Chapter 14. These principles may be briefly summarized as follows:

1. Begin therapy with the least toxic antiepileptic drug known to be consistently effective against the patient's type(s) of seizure.
2. Adjust the dosage of the first drug tried until seizures are controlled or toxicity precludes further dosage increase.
3. Add additional drugs only after it has been documented that maximum tolerated dosages of the first drug will not control the patient's seizures.

4. Eliminate unnecessary drugs and strive for monotherapy whenever possible.

SURGICAL THERAPY

The well-established surgical procedures performed for epilepsy involve resection of a seizure focus in the temporal lobe for patients with uncontrolled complex partial seizures or resection of a focus in another area for patients with uncontrolled simple partial seizures (see Chap. 25). Such procedures will significantly reduce partial seizure frequency in 60 to 80 percent of properly selected patients and have a very low morbidity (5–10%) and mortality (less than 1%).

The following criteria must be met before considering a cortical resection procedure: (1) seizure disorder refractory to adequate medical therapy; (2) epileptogenic focus identified and confirmed by several lines of evidence; (3) epileptogenic focus subject to surgical removal without major neurologic deficit; and (4) epileptogenic focus located in cortex that is surgically accessible. An adequate trial of conventional antiepileptic drugs for simple and complex partial seizures would document that seizures are not sufficiently controlled with maximum tolerated doses of phenytoin *and* a barbiturate (phenobarbital or primidone) *and* carbamazepine. These are the safest, most efficacious agents in the three major groups of FDA-approved drugs for the treatment of these types of seizures. The maximum tolerated dose of each drug must be established because high therapeutic serum concentrations of a drug may control seizures when low therapeutic levels do not [20, 26]. All three drugs should be given together because there is evidence that these drugs in combination may control seizures in some patients when the drugs given individually do not [5, 7, 25, 28]. There is no point in referring a patient for cortical resection until he has had an adequate trial of conventional antiepileptic drug therapy. On the other hand, once it is established that seizures are not controlled by conventional antiepileptic drugs, delaying referral for possible surgical therapy may result in unnecessary physical and psychosocial morbidity.

Other surgical procedures for management of epilepsy include hemispherectomy for patients with extensive unilateral cerebral damage and uncontrolled simple partial seizures and stereotactic lesions of various deep structures for uncontrolled complex partial and tonic-clonic seizures (see Chap. 25). The safety and efficacy of these newer procedures are not as well established as they are for cortical resection. Hemispherectomy and stereotactic surgery should be considered along with other possible therapies for patients with intractable epilepsy.

INTRACTABLE EPILEPSY

Many cases of "intractable" epilepsy are due to improper seizure diagnosis, resulting in the use of improper antiepileptic drugs, failure to "push" the drugs used to maximal dosage, or failure to use all available antiepileptic drugs. However, there are some patients who will continue to have seizures despite a proper seizure diagnosis and maximal therapy with all conventional antiepileptic drugs. Patients with simple and complex partial seizures should be considered for cortical resection procedures. For patients whose seizures are not controlled with conventional drugs and who are not candidates for cortical resection procedures, there are three therapeutic options: (1) experimental drugs, (2) experimental surgical procedures, and (3) behavioral therapies (see Chaps. 24, 25, and 31). Such therapies are usually only available at specialized epilepsy centers. The choice of which therapy to give a particular patient will depend on the type of seizure disorder and psychosocial situation the patient has and on which therapies are available at the time of referral.

References

1. Abraham, K., and Ajmone-Marsan, C. Patterns of cortical discharges and their relation to routine scalp electroencephalography. *Electroencephalogr. Clin. Neurophysiol.* 10:447, 1958.
2. Ajmone-Marsan, C., and Goldhammer, L. Clinical Ictal Patterns and Electrographic Data in Cases of Partial Seizures of Frontal-Central-Parietal Origin. In M. A. B. Brazier (Ed.), *Epilepsy: Its Phenomena in Man.* New York: Academic, 1973.
3. Ajmone-Marsan, C., and Gumnit, R. J. Neurophysiological Aspects of Epilepsy. In P. J. Vinken, and G. W. Bruyn (Eds.), *Handbook of Clinical Neurology,* Vol. 15, *The Epilepsies.* Amsterdam: Elsevier, 1974.
4. *Basic Statistics on the Epilepsies.* Philadelphia: Davis, 1975.
5. Cereghino, J. J. et al. The efficacy of carbamazepine combinations in epilepsy. *Clin. Pharmacol. Ther.* 18:733, 1975.
6. Dennerll, P. D., et al. Neurological and psychological factors related to employability of persons with epilepsy. *Epilepsia* 7:318, 1966.
7. Diamond, W. D., and Buchanan, R. A. Clinical studies of the effect of phenobarbital on di-phenylhydantoin plasma levels. *J. Clin. Pharmacol.* 10:306, 1970.
8. Dreifuss, F. E. Proposal for revised clinical and electroencephalographic classification of epileptic seizures. *Epilepsia* 22:489, 1981.
9. Gastaut, H., et al. Generalized Convulsive Seizures Without Local Onset. In P. J. Vinken, and G. W. Bruyn (Eds.), *Handbook of Clinical Neurology,* Vol. 15, *The Epilepsies.* Amsterdam: Elsevier, 1974.
10. Gastaut, H., and Tassinari, C. A. Triggering mechanisms in epilepsy. The electroclinical point of view. *Epilepsia* 7:85, 1966.
11. Geiger, L. R., and Harner, R. N. EEG patterns at the time of focal seizure onset. *Arch. Neurol.* 35:276, 1978.
12. Goodglass, H., et al. Epileptic seizures: Psychological factors and occupational adjustment. *Epilepsia* 4:322, 1963.
13. Hauser, W. A. Epidemiology, Morbidity, and Mortality of Status Epilepticus. In A. V. Delgado-Escueta et al. (Eds.), *Status Epilepticus: Mechanisms of Brain Damage and Treatment.* New York: Raven Press, 1982.
14. Hauser, W. A. Epidemiology of epilepsy. *Adv. Neurol.* 19:313, 1978.
15. Hauser, W. A., and Kurland, L. T. The epidemiology of epilepsy in Rochester, Minnesota, 1935 through 1967. *Epilepsia* 16:1, 1975.
16. Hauser, W. A., Annegeres, J. F., and Elveback, L. R. Remission of seizures and relapse in patients with epilepsy. *Epilepsia* 20:729, 1979.
17. Hess, R. Electroencephalography. In P. J. Vinken, and G. W. Bruyn (Eds.), *Handbook of Clinical Neurology,* Vol. 15, *The Epilepsies.* Amsterdam: Elsevier, 1974.
18. Jackson, J. H. Lectures on the Diagnosis of Epilepsy. In J. Taylor (Ed.), *Selected Writings of John Hughlings Jackson,* Vol. 1. New York: Basic Books, 1931.
19. Lennox, W. G., and Lennox, M. A. *Epilepsy and Related Disorders.* Boston: Little, Brown, 1960.
20. Lund, L. Anticonvulsant effect of diphenylhydantoin relative to plasma levels. *Arch. Neurol.* 31:289, 1974.
21. Masland, R. L. The Classification of the Epilepsies: A Historical Review. In P. J. Vinken, and G. W. Bruyn (Eds.), *Handbook of Clinical Neurology,* Vol. 15, *The Epilepsies.* Amsterdam: Elsevier, 1974.
22. Merlis, J. K. Proposal for international classification of the epilepsies. *Epilepsia* 11:114, 1970.
23. Penfield, W., and Jasper, H. H. *Epilepsy and the*

Functional Anatomy of the Human Brain. Boston: Little, Brown, 1954.

24. *Plan for Nationwide Action on Epilepsy: Report of the Commission for the Control of Epilepsy and its Consequences.* Washington, D.C.: U.S. Dept. of Health, Education, and Welfare, 1978.

25. Rodin, E. A., Rim, C. S., and Rennick, P. M. The effects of carbamazepine on patients with psychomotor epilepsy: Results of a double-blind study. *Epilepsia* 15:547, 1974.

26. Sherwin, A. L., Robb, J. P., and Lechter, M. Improved control of epilepsy by monitoring plasma ethosuximide. *Arch. Neurol.* 28:171, 1973.

27. Woodbury, L. A. Incidence and Prevalence of Seizure Disorders Including Epilepsies in the United States of America: A Review and Analysis of the Literature. In *Plan for Nationwide Action on Epilepsy,* Vol. 4. Washington, D.C.: U.S. Dept. of Health, Education, and Welfare, 1978.

28. Yahr, M. D. et al. Evaluation of standard anticonvulsant therapy in 319 patients. *J.A.M.A.* 150:663, 1952.

BASIC MECHANISMS OF EPILEPSY

2

Michael C. Trachtenberg

The basic mechanisms underlying convulsive disorders are so diverse that to seek a single cause for epilepsy would be a gross oversimplification. Rather, a number of different disorders, singly or in combination, may result in seizure discharge. The clinical appearance of a seizure depends more on the anatomic site at which the disorder occurs than on the basic mechanisms involved in its production.

Several biophysical and biochemical dysfunctions can cause neurons to undergo periods of intense prolonged excitation. Although this excitation is represented by characteristic electrical changes within single cells, the primary defect may or may not be due to changes of that individual cell membrane, because changes in the synaptic input to the cell or changes in the ionic environment of the cell can also result in similar electrical behavior. The limited space available in this chapter permits only an overview of the pertinent mechanisms. Several reviews and symposia, however, can provide more information [11, 13, 23, 29, 40, 44, 59, 60].

Electrical Activity of Neurons During Seizure

The features of neuronal excitation that occur during seizures are seen in Figure 2-1. The EEG appears normal during the interictal period except for a periodic spike, which is followed by a slow negative wave and a silent period. During this EEG spike, as well as during a seizure, a normally quiet extracellular record will show bursts of spikes (unit discharges) corresponding to similar action potential bursts that appear on an intracellular record. The intracellular record also reveals a sustained depolarization that triggers bursts of action potentials (Fig. 2-1). This characteristic depolarization is referred to as the paroxysmal depolarizing shift (PDS) [12, 35].

The appearance of the PDS in several different experimental models of epilepsy—cold lesion [12], penicillin [1], and alumina cream [45] foci, for example—suggests that the PDS, functionally acting as an excessive, prolonged excitatory postsynaptic potential (EPSP), is the final common pathway of the several mechanisms capable of triggering seizures.

Three conceptual frameworks historically have been developed to account for ictal events. The first, the *epileptic neuron* model, holds that alterations in the membrane or metabolic properties of individual neurons make them pathologically hyperexcitable. The second, the *epileptic environment* theory, holds that regulation of the extracellular concentrations of

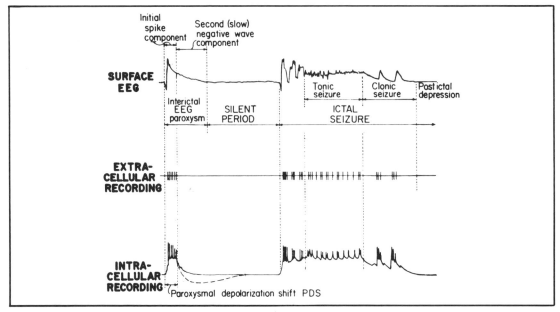

Figure 2-1. Diagram of the relationship between EEG activity, extracellular unit activity (through a high pass filter), and intracellular potentials. Note the sustained depolarization (PDS) of the intracellular record corresponding to the EEG spike. (From G. F. Ayala et al. [1].)

ions or transmitter agents, or both, is suboptimal, resulting in an imbalance whose effect is enhanced neuronal excitation. The third, the *epileptic aggregate or population* theory, maintaining that collective anatomic or physiologic alterations produce a progressive, network-dependent facilitation of excitability, perhaps coupled with a decrease of inhibition. There is evidence to support a combination of these concepts. *All the physiologic, anatomic, and biochemical processes accommodated within these concepts interact* during specific ictal episodes and in interictal periods to further the structural and functional alterations characteristic of epileptic foci. *Each focus is unique in its admixture of neuronal, environmental, and aggregate disorders.* This differential contribution of defects may well account for the differences in clinical efficacy of antiepileptic drugs.

The Epileptic Neuron Model

The cause of the PDS has been the subject of considerable speculation ever since its central role in seizure discharge was ascertained.

Negative Resistance

In the late 1970s, evidence was developed indicating that functional and perhaps structural changes occur in the postsynaptic membrane that alter the character of receptor protein-conductance channels, thereby favoring development of the PDS and enhanced excitability. Cells exhibiting PDSs have a slowly inactivated,

voltage-sensitive inward (depolarizing) current [53, 54]. When the "steady state" current-voltage relation of these cells is plotted, a region of negative slope appears that has been termed negative resistance. An area of negative resistance is inherently electrically unstable and can best be perceived as a step, trigger, or switch zone that allows the cell membrane to change rapidly from one excitability state to another. All neurons and muscle cells have a region of their current-voltage curve that exhibits a negative resistance. This region corresponds to the well known Na^+ conductance action potential zone. The negative resistance discussed here corresponds to a Ca^{2+} conductance and appears later on the current vs. time graph following the inactivation of the Na^+ currents. This can best be understood by regarding epileptic and other bursting neurons as similar to heart cells that have both Na^+ and Ca^{2+} conductances. A negative resistance zone is not unique to cells in epileptic foci but can be seen in many nonspiking neurons of the normal cat spinal cord [54]. These cells, as epileptic neurons, possess a second characteristic supporting their burst activity, namely, a specific voltage at which inward depolarizing currents predominate. When the inward current overcomes the outward currents (to produce a net inward current) the cell depolarizes until a stronger outward (repolarizing) current is activated. This repolarizing current sends the cell back to a voltage where the inward current again predominates and thus produces another depolarization. The result is an oscillation of the membrane potential that is responsible for bursting activity.

A major difference between bursting and epileptic neurons is the regular periodicity of the former, whereas the latter are intermittent and require a trigger to manifest an ictal discharge. It is this need for a trigger that necessitates consideration of problems in regulation of the microenvironment and of neuronal populations.

CALCIUM CONDUCTANCE
In considering the ionic carriers that might underlie the PDS, one finds two candidates that could carry an inward current, Na^+ and Ca^{2+}. The fact that the inward currents are blocked by manganese or cobalt but enhanced by calcium or barium [53] suggests that the inward current is an activated Ca^{2+} conductance. When extracellular potassium concentrations are above normal (7 to 12 mM), as during intense seizure activity, the potassium equilibrium potential across the neuronal membrane is reduced, and therefore any outward K^+ currents are reduced. If the outward currents are decreased sufficiently, the net current will become inward and depolarizing to the extent that Ca^{2+} currents will be triggered, resulting in a PDS and a burst of spikes. The exact steps by which these events proceed is unclear, although it is known that Ca^{2+} concentrations in the extracellular space begin to decline slightly before K^+ concentrations rise [14]. This finding has been taken to suggest that K^+ sustains but does not trigger seizures. However, in Heinemann's study [15] intense stimulation resulted in elevated K^+, and in the penicillin model, potassium must be raised from 3 to 6 mM to evoke Ca^{2+} spikes [41]. In addition, superfusion of the hippocampus with potassium will elicit seizures [62]. Together, these data do not allow a cause-and-effect relationship to be developed at present.

Epileptic neurons appear to have increased Ca^{2+} conductance. It may be that latent calcium channels are utilized, that the efficacy of the calcium channels is increased, or that the number of such channels is elevated chronically. Cyclic AMP, for example, is thought to elicit Ca^{2+} currents in snail neurons [24], and agents that would tend to increase cAMP in the brain will lower the seizure threshold [57] (see also Table 2-1). Factors that might enhance cAMP levels include excess transmitter release, prolonged depolari-

zation by K^+, and activators of adenyl cyclase (e.g., adenosine).

Since development of burst activity depends not on the absolute magnitude of the inward current but on that of the net inward current (inward minus outward), reducing the outward current, which is primarily carried by K^+ or Cl^-, could also produce a PDS. Increasing the extracellular concentration of K^+ has this effect, as does decreasing inhibitory postsynaptic potential (IPSP) chloride conductances. Penicillin acts, in part, on the chloride conductance mechanisms [19].

Finally, it is conceivable that Ca^{2+} entry not only generates the PDS but also terminates the PDS. Calcium may indirectly repolarize the membrane by activating outward potassium currents of the sort described in snail neurons [36]. This current would repolarize the cell membrane and stop the voltage-sensitive calcium influx and therefore the PDS.

Disorders of the Neuronal Microenvironment
In contrast to the recent emphasis on, and the consequent increased number of papers dealing with, the epileptic neuron model, our knowledge about the microenvironment contains more facts but less organization. The cause-and-effect relationship between any of these changes is unknown, as are the cascades that lead to dynamic instability. Both functional and structural alterations occur in epileptic foci. The functional changes involve concentrations of cations and anions, metabolic alterations, and changes in transmitter levels. The structural changes involve both neurons and glia. These, along with yet undefined microanatomic changes, probably form the basis of the functional abnormalities.

FUNCTIONAL ALTERATIONS

Cationic Concomitants of Seizures
It has long been known that excessive extracellular potassium depolarizes neurons and leads to spike discharge. It was presumed, therefore, that extracellular potassium might be elevated in seizures. With the advent of ion-specific electrodes, it was unequivocally shown that extracellular potassium concentrations increased to 8 to 12 mM during seizures [41] (Fig. 2-2A)—ion-specific electrodes actually measure activity, not concentration. Subsequent development of ion-specific microelectrode capabilities revealed that extracellular calcium concentrations decreased by about 85% [14]. Changes in extracellular calcium concentration preceded those of extracellular potassium by milliseconds, and calcium levels returned to normal more quickly than did those of potassium,

14

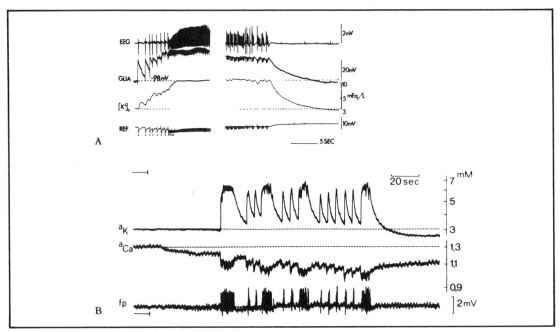

Figure 2-2. A. Relationship of EEG activity, glial membrane potential, extracellular potassium activity, and extracellular field potential in a penicillin focus. B. Relationship of potassium activity (a_K), calcium activity (a_{Ca}), and field potential in pentylenetetrazol focus. Note incremental decrease of a_{Ca} associated with each transient increase of a_K. Also note undershoot of a_K associated with the silent period of the field potential (fp). (From R. Heinemann, H. D. Lux, and M. J. Gutnick [14].)

which could even show an undershoot for some time [9, 14] (Fig. 2-2B). These differences suggest first, that the calcium level changes initially, whereas the change in potassium level is a secondary event. Second, these differences suggest that these cations may be cleared to different pools and perhaps to different cells.

Potassium regulation and glial cell function have long been associated [26, 43, 55]. As potassium rises, glia depolarize, although the glial potential declines more slowly than the potassium changes (Fig. 2-2A). Glia are believed to redistribute K^+ both by passive spatial buffering [55] and by $Na^+ + K^+$ ATPase-based active uptake and redistribution [15]. Redistribution of K^+ would help prevent spread of the seizure. Failure of the spatial buffering system might result in focal accumulation of K^+, which in turn depolarizes neurons, reduces K^+ currents responsible for repolarization, and unmasks Ca^{2+} conductances.

Glia are not the only source of $Na^+ + K^+$ ATPase for K^+ redistribution. This enzyme is also found in all parts of neurons. In synaptosomes, the level of this enzyme in the membrane derived from a freeze-lesion focus is reduced to one-half normal [8]. Although this decrease does not appear to alter the basal level of intra- or extracellular potassium, it would lead to a reduced capability of the synaptic elements to reclaim lost K^+, particularly under stress conditions.

The cellular disposition of calcium is less clear, although it is known that elevation of extracellular K^+ results in a calcium uptake by glia [27]. Mitochondria are a significant and labile store of Ca^{2+} and plasmalemmal events alter the mitochondrial stores.

Metabolic Changes and Anions

Occurring simultaneously with the seizure and ionic changes is a metabolic stimulation that is tightly linked to the level of K^+ accumulation [30]. In particular, the levels of reduced NADH and cytochrome a_3 decrease. Much of this metabolic alteration may be presumed to be glial, in that isolated glia are much more stimulated by excess K^+ than are neurons [16, 17]. This metabolic activation of neurons and glia is accompanied by CO_2 generation. In addition to buffering K^+, glia appear able to buffer CO_2 increases through conversion to bicarbonate through the glial-specific enzyme, carbonic anhydrase. Since mammalian glial cells also contain an HCO_3^-/Cl^- exchange carrier [25], glia may then attempt to remove the HCO_3^-/Cl^- by taking up Cl^- in an equimolar exchange. Should sufficient Cl^- be removed from the extracellular space by glia, then a decrease in neuronal Cl^--mediated IPSPs could follow. Metabolic stimulation of glia then might lead to disinhibition of synapses. Blockade of the glial stimulation by barbiturates [17] may be a partial explanation of their therapeutic efficacy. Although such changes of Cl^- or HCO_3^- have not been measured in mammalian extracellular space, a K^+-stimulated uptake of Cl^- has been shown in glial cells in tissue culture [10] and in amphibian glia [46]. The involvement of carbonic anhydrase in this pathway may help to explain the mechanism of antiepileptic activity of carbonic anhydrase inhibitors.

Glial Transmitter Clearance
The finding that astrocytes have high-affinity uptake systems for many putative transmitters [52] suggests that this cell type normally helps to clear transmitters from the extracellular space. In addition to taking up amino acids (thus removing them from the synaptic cleft), glia can synthesize some transmitters and modify others. For example, glia possess the enzyme glutamine synthetase, which allows conversion of the putative excitatory transmitter glutamate to the putative inhibitory transmitter glutamine. Among the amino acids with presumed transmitter or neuromodulator functions that are synthesized by glia are gamma-aminobutyric acid (GABA) and possibly taurine. Glial production of amino acids, including the putative transmitters and modulators, can be stimulated by K^+. On the basis of brain-slice data [5, 38], elevated K^+ can result in release of both GABA and glycine.

DISORDERS OF GABA METABOLISM. Biochemical lesions interrupting the synthesis, storage, release, or postsynaptic actions of inhibitory neurotransmitters will lead to disinhibition of neurons. The best-described neurotransmitter is GABA, which tends to be an inhibitory neurotransmitter in the mammalian brain.
Synthesis of GABA is achieved by decarboxylation of glutamate through the enzyme glutamic acid decarboxylase (GAD), and this enzyme is rate-limiting [47]. The importance of this pyridoxal-dependent enzyme is illustrated by a patient suffering from seizures who was found at autopsy to have reduced levels of pyridoxal as well as reduced levels of both GAD activity and GABA in the occipital cortex, which exhibited gliosis [31]. Several compounds that have been found to lower the threshold for seizures or frankly elicit seizures also have been found to inhibit GAD (Table 2-1). Hence, reducing available GABA levels appears to have potential as an epileptogenic mechanism.
Many convulsive agents have been found to affect

Table 2-1. Convulsant Agents

I. Convulsants Affecting Inhibition
   A. Convulsants affecting glycine: Competitors for glycine receptors
      Strychnine [39]*
   B. Convulsants affecting GABA metabolism
      1. Competitors for GABA receptors postsynaptically
         Picrotoxin [33, 37]
         Bicuculline [33, 37]
         Penicillin (low concentration) [19, 33]
         Pentylenetetrazole (low concentration) [33]
      2. GAD inhibitors (decreased binding of pyridoxal phosphate) (Vitamin B_6)
         Isoniazid [37]
         Thiosemicarbazide [37]
         4-Deoxypyridoxine [20]
         Vitamin B_6–deficiency [31]
      3. GAD inhibitors (not competitive with pyridoxal)
         Allylglycine [20]
         3-Mercaptopropionic acid [20]

II. Convulsants Affecting cAMP Metabolism
   A. Potentiation of excitatory inputs to cell
      Cyclic AMP [57]
      Dibutyl cyclic AMP [57]
   B. Stimulation of adenyl cyclase
      Adenosine [57]
      Norepinephrine [57]
      Histamine [57]
      Fluoride ion [57]
   C. Inhibitors of phosphodiesterase
      Papaverine [57]
      Aminophylline [57]
      Tolazoline [57]
      Phentolamine [57]
      Caffeine [57]

III. Convulsants Affecting Ion Movements
   A. Blockers of chloride conductance (and IPSPs)
      Penicillin (high concentration) [19, 33]
      Pentylenetetrazole (high concentration) [42]
      Ammonium ion [32]
   B. Blockers of ATPase-mediated potassium clearance
      Ouabain [6]
      Zinc ion [7]
   C. High pCO_2 (presumably affecting chloride and bicarbonate movements)
      Severe hypercapnia [61]

*Bracketed number refers to reference cited.

generation of IPSPs in response to GABA release. Inhibition of GABA binding to postsynaptic receptors is achieved by the convulsants picrotoxin and bicuculline, among many others (Table 2-1). In addition to affecting the postsynaptic receptor, penicillin and pentylenetetrazol also appear to block the Cl^- channel, which normally would carry the ionic current responsible for GABA inhibition. The disinhibition, by allowing excess neuronal discharge, could in turn alter the

Table 2-2. Antiepileptic Agents

I. Antiepileptic Agents Potentiating GABA Effects
  A. Metabolized to GABA in vivo
    2-Pyrrolidone [37]*
  B. Enhanced activity of postsynaptic GABA receptors
    (see Chaps. 17 and 21)
    Benzodiazepines [34, 40]
    Barbiturates [34, 40]
  C. Possible agonists at GABA receptors
    β-p Chlorophenyl-GABA (PCPG) [37]
    1-Hydroxy-3-amino-2-pyrrolidone [3]
    5-Ethyl-5-phenyl-2-pyrrolidone [4]
  D. Inhibitors of GABA uptake
    Chlorpromazine [37]
    Imipramine [37]
    Haloperidol [37]
    2-Hydroxy-GABA [37]
    2-Chloro-GABA [37]
    Benzodiazepines [40]
    Amino-oxyacetic acid [22]
  E. GABA-Transaminase inhibitors
    Amino-oxyacetic acid [37]
    Cycloserine [37]
    di-n-Propylacetate [37]
    Hydroxylamine [37]
    5-Ethyl-5-phenyl-2-pyrrolidone [37]

II. Antiepileptic Agents Affecting Ion Movement
  A. Agents that decrease K^+ permeability
    Trimethadione [59]
    Ethosuximide [59]
    Diazepam [59]
  B. Agents that affect Na^+ movements
    Phenytoin (diphenylhydantoin) [59]
  C. Carbonic anhydrase inhibitors
    Acetazolamide [59]
    Sulthiame [59]

*Bracketed number refers to reference cited.

ionic environment and possibly elicit changes in the membrane proteins, which form the macromolecular substrate for negative resistance and PDS.

Table 2-2 lists several agents related to GABA metabolism and its receptors that have been found to possess some degree of antiepileptic activity. Specific benzodiazepine and barbiturate receptors have been identified in the postsynaptic membrane, which, when activated by a benzodiazepine or barbiturate, enhance binding of GABA to postsynaptic GABA receptors, resulting in prolonged chloride conductance and increased inhibition [34, 40, 51] (see Chaps. 17 and 21). Certain GABA analogs, which will either block GABA uptake or inhibit the catabolic enzyme GABA-transaminase, will enhance the inhibition caused by normally released GABA [37]. Interestingly, 2-pyrrolidone, which is converted to GABA in the brain, also has antiepileptic properties.

MORPHOLOGIC CHANGES IN EPILEPTIC FOCI
Anatomic, degenerative, and regenerative alterations occur in both neurons and glia within the focus. These changes may well provide a basis for sustaining the epileptic activity of the focus.

Neuronal Changes
The gross changes that occur in advanced stages of epilepsy have been known for a long time and have been reviewed recently [50]. It was shown that many patients exhibited extensive loss of neurons and pronounced gliosis. More recent studies of human tissue [50] indicate that the neuronal loss is progressive; that is, a single cell probably undergoes a series of degenerative changes before cell death. A normal healthy cell is particularly marked by its extensive dendritic branching and spines, whereas the diseased cell progressively loses its spines, and the extent of dendritic branching diminishes. We have no reason to presume that the degeneration would lead to selective loss of inputs, although it is possible that more inhibitory synapses could be lost than excitatory ones. The loss of trophic factors associated with synaptic transmission also could lead to the biophysical changes discussed. Alternatively, since Ca^{2+} spikes have been recognized in the dendrites of Purkinje cells [28, 53] and in growth cones, it is also conceivable that the loss of membrane may leave the calcium channels in relatively greater density. It is extremely difficult at present to correlate such biophysical changes with the morphologic alterations.

Also, the cause-and-effect relationship in neuronal degeneration may not support the idea that degeneration leads to the essential biophysical changes. Rather, excessive leaks of Ca^{2+} into cells have been found to cause ultrastructural damage, and the degeneration may therefore be secondary to elevated Ca^{2+} due to the PDS Ca^{2+} currents.

GLIOSIS. Alzheimer [50] showed that epileptic foci have a proliferation of glia. The glia form what is essentially scar tissue made of fibrous astrocytes that may have an intense meshwork of glial processes and a very high content of glial fibrillary acidic protein [2, 50]. When the staining is sufficiently low to reveal a single glial cell, it exhibits the unusual finding of nodules along its slender processes.

What effect these glial changes might have on neuronal membrane conductances is not immediately obvious, but gliosis will affect the ability of the glia to remove excess extracellular potassium and hence may contribute to seizure generation [43].

The Epileptic Cell Population

In attempting to account for seizure activity, researchers developed two theories about the epileptic cell. The first proposed that the cell manifests increased excitation; the second suggested that the cell was subject to a decrease in inhibition.

INCREASED EXCITATION

The idea of increased excitation gained much support during the period when investigators were unable to discover the specific physiologic or biophysical alterations of single cells. It appeared unlikely that a single cell could create the intense activity necessary for a seizure. Rather, it was presumed that many cells exhibit direct or elicitable epileptiform properties and that these cells would be brought into synchrony, thus producing giant EPSPs. To accomplish this, the notion of reverbatory circuits (positive feedback loops) was developed. Little evidence has developed in support of this idea.

LOSS OF SYNAPTIC INHIBITION

Two classes of mechanisms exist whereby inhibitory influences could be diminished. One depends on the selective loss of inhibitory neurons, particularly short axon, local, and inhibitory feedback interneurons. Experiments [49] in undercutting the cortex suggest that this selective anatomic pruning may be a potent contributor to the generation of seizure foci. Some of the consequences of this anatomic loss are described in the discussion of neuronal changes.

Besides potential loss of inhibitory synapses, neurons may become disinhibited through more specific biophysical and biochemical mechanisms. Reduction in inhibitory currents carried by either K^+ or Cl^- could be achieved by elevating extracellular K^+, decreasing extracellular Cl^-, or directly interfering with the conductance channels for these ions.

References

1. Ayala, G. F. et al. Genesis of epileptic interictal spikes. New knowledge of cortical feedback systems suggests a neurophysiological explanation of brief paroxysms. *Brain Res.* 52:1, 1973.
2. Bignami, A., Forno, L., and Dahl, D. The neuroglial response to injury following spinal cord transection in the goldfish. *Exp. Neurol.* 44:60, 1974.
3. Bonta, I. L. et al. 1-hydroxy-3-amino-pyrrolidone-2 (HA-966): A new GABA-like compound, with potential use in extrapyramidal diseases. *Br. J. Pharmacol.* 43:514, 1971.
4. Carvajal, G. et al. Anticonvulsive action of substances designed as inhibitors of γ-aminobutyric acid—α-ketoglutaric acid transaminase. *Biochem. Pharmacol.* 13:1059, 1964.
5. Davies, L. P., Johnston, G. A. R., and Stephanson, A. L. Postnatal changes in the potassium stimulated, calcium-dependent release of radioactive GABA and glycine from slices of rat central nervous tissue. *J. Neurochem.* 25:387, 1975.
6. Donaldson, J., Minnich, J., and Barbeau, A. Ouabain-induced seizures in rats: Regional and subcellular localization of ^{3}H-ouabain associated with $Na^+ + K^+$-ATPase in brain. *Can. J. Biochem.* 50:888, 1972.
7. Donaldson, J. et al. Determination of Na^+, K^+, Mg^{2+}, Cu^{2+}, Zn^{2+}, and Mn^{2+} in rat brain regions. *Can. J. Biochem.* 51:87, 1973.
8. Escueta, A. V. et al. The freezing lesion. II. Potassium transport within nerve terminals isolated from epileptogenic foci. *Brain Res.* 78:223, 1974.
9. Futamachi, K. J., and Pedley, T. A. Glial cells and extracellular potassium: Their relationship in mammalian cortex. *Brain Res.* 109:311, 1976.
10. Gill, T. H., Young, O. M., and Tower, D. B. The uptake of ^{36}Cl into astrocytes in tissue culture by a potassium-dependent saturable process. *J. Neurochem.* 23:1011, 1974.
11. Glaser, G. H., Penry, J. K., and Woodbury, D. M. (Eds.). *Antiepileptic Drugs: Mechanisms of Action.* New York: Raven Press, 1980.
12. Goldensohn, E. S., and Purpura, D. P. Intracellular potentials of cortical neurons during focal epileptogenic discharges. *Science* 139:840, 1963.
13. Harris, P., and Mawdsley, C. (Eds.). *Epilepsy.* New York: Livingstone, 1974.
14. Heinemann, R., Lux, H. D., and Gutnick, M. J. Extracellular free calcium and potassium during paroxysmal activity in the cerebral cortex of the cat. *Exp. Brain Res.* 27:237, 1977.
15. Henn, F. A., Haljamae, H., and Hamberger, A. Glial cell function: Active control of extracellular K^+ concentration. *Brain Res.* 43:437, 1972.
16. Hertz, L. Neuroglial localization of potassium and sodium effects on respiration in brain. *J. Neurochem.* 13:1373, 1966.
17. Hertz, L., Mukerji, S., and Boechler, N. Phenobarbital effect on glial cell respiration in the presence of a high concentration of potassium. *Biochem. Pharmacol.* 27:903, 1978.

18. Hertz, L., and Schousboe, A. Ion and energy metabolism of the brain at the cellular level. *Int. Rev. Neurobiol.* 18:141, 1975.

19. Hochner, B., Spira, M. E., and Werman, R. Penicillin decreases chloride conductance in crustacean muscle: A model for the epileptic neuron. *Brain Res.* 107:85, 1976.

20. Horton, R. W., and Meldrum, B. S. Seizures induced by allyglycine, 3-mercaptopropionic acid and 4-deoxypyridoxine in mice and photosensitive baboons, and different modes of inhibition of cerebral glutamic acid decarboxylase. *Br. J. Pharmacol.* 49:52, 1973.

21. Hotson, J. R., and Prince, D. A. A calcium-activated hyperpolarization follows repetitive firing in hippocampal neurons. *J. Neurophysiol.* 43:409, 1980.

22. Hutchinson, H. T. et al. Uptake of neurotransmitters by clonal lines of astrocytoma and neuroblastoma in culture: I. Transport of γ-aminobutyric acid. *Brain Res.* 66:265, 1974.

23. Jasper, H. H., Ward, A. A., and Pope, A. (Eds.). *Basic Mechanisms of The Epilepsies.* Boston: Little, Brown, 1969.

24. Kandel, E. R. et al. A common presynaptic locus for the synaptic changes underlying short-term habituation and sensitization of the gill-withdrawal reflex in aplysia. *Cold Spring Harbor Symp. Quant. Biol.* 40:465, 1975.

25. Kimelberg, H. K. Glial Enzymes and Ion Transport in Brain Swelling. In A. J. Popp et al. (Eds.), *Neural Trauma: Seminars in Neurological Surgery.* New York: Raven Press, 1979.

26. Kuffler, S. W., and Nicholls, J. G. The physiology of neuroglial cells. *Ergeb. Physiol.* 57:1, 1966.

27. Lazarewicz, J. W. et al. Calcium fluxes in cultured and bulk isolated neuronal and glial cells. *J. Neurochem.* 29:495, 1977.

28. Llinas, R., and Hess, R. Tetrodoxin-resistant dendritic spikes in avian Purkinje cells. *Soc. Neurosci. Abstr.* 2:112, 1976.

29. Lockard, J. S., and Ward, A. A., Jr. *Epilepsy: A Window to Brain Mechanisms.* New York: Raven Press, 1980.

30. Lothman, E. et al. Responses of electrical potential, potassium levels, and oxidative metabolic activity of the cerebral neocortex of cats. *Brain Res.* 88:15, 1975.

31. Lott, I. T. et al. Vitamin B_6-dependent seizures: Pathology and chemical findings in brain. *Neurology* 28:47, 1978.

32. Lux, H. D., Loracher, C., and Neher, E. The action of ammonium on postsynaptic inhibition of cat spinal motoneurons. *Brain Res.* 11:431, 1970.

33. Macdonald, R. L., and Barker, J. L. Specific antagonism of GABA-mediated postsynaptic inhibition in cultured mammalian spinal cord neurons: A common mode of convulsant action. *Neurology* 28:325, 1978.

34. Macdonald, R. L., and Barker, J. L. Enhancement of GABA-mediated postsynaptic inhibition in cultured mammalian spinal cord neurons: A common mode of anticonvulsant action. *Brain Res.* 167:323, 1978.

35. Matsumoto, H., and Ajmone-Marsan, C. Cortical cellular phenomena in experimental epilepsy: Interictal manifestations. *Exp. Neurol.* 9:286, 1964.

36. Meech, R. W., and Standen, N. B. Potassium activation in Helix aspersa neurons under voltage clamp: A component mediated by calcium influx. *J. Physiol.* 249:211, 1975.

37. Meldrum, B. S., and Horton, R. S. Neuronal Inhibition Mediated by GABA and Patterns of Convulsions in Baboons with Photosensitive Epilepsy (Papio Papio). In P. Harris, and C. Mawdsley (Eds.), *Epilepsy.* New York: Livingstone, 1974. Pp. 55–64.

38. Morrel, F. Cellular pathophysiology of focal epilepsy. *Epilepsia* 10:495, 1969.

39. Muller, W. E., and Snyder, S. H. Strychnine binding associated with synaptic glycine receptors in rat spinal cord membranes: Ionic influences. *Brain Res.* 147:107, 1978.

40. Paul, S. et al. (Eds.). *The Pharmacology of Benzodiazepines.* London: Macmillan Press. In press, 1983.

41. Pedley, T. A. et al. Regulation of extracellular potassium concentration in epileptogenesis. *Fed. Proc.* 35:1254, 1976.

42. Pellmar, T. C., and Wilson, W. A. Synaptic mechanism of pentylenetrazole: Selectivity for chloride conductance. *Science* 197:912, 1977.

43. Pollen, D. A., and Trachtenberg, M. C. Neuroglia: Gliosis and focal epilepsy. *Science* 167:1252, 1970.

44. Prince, D. A. Neurophysiology of epilepsy. *Ann. Rev. Neurosci.* 1:395, 1978.

45. Prince, D. A., and Futamachi, K. J. Intracellular recordings from chronic epileptogenic foci in the monkey. *Electroencephalogr. Clin. Neurophysiol.* 29:496, 1970.

46. Ritchie, T. L. et al. K^+-induced ion and water movements in the frog spinal cord and filum terminale. *Exp. Neurol.* 71:356, 1981.

47. Roberts, E., and Hammerschlag, R. Amino Acid Transmitters. In G. J. Seigel et al. (Eds.), *Basic Neurochemistry* (3rd ed.). Boston: Little, Brown, 1981. Pp. 218–245.

48. Rutledge, L. T. Effect of Stimulation on Isolated Cortex. In H. H. Jasper, A. A. Ward, Jr., and A. Pope (Eds.), *Basic Mechanisms of the Epilepsies.* Boston: Little, Brown, 1969. Pp. 349–355.

49. Rutledge, L. T. The effects of denervation and stimulation upon synaptic ultrastructure. *J. Comp. Neurol.* 178:117, 1978.

50. Scheibel, A. B. Morphological correlates of epilepsy: Cells in the hippocampus. *Adv. Neurol.* 27:49, 1980.

51. Scholfield, C. N. Potentiation of inhibition by general anaesthetics in neurones of the olfactory cortex, in vitro. *Pfluegers Arch.* 383:249, 1980.

52. Schrier, B. K., and Thompson, E. J. On the role of glial cells in the mammalian nervous system. Uptake, excretion and metabolism of putative neurotransmitters by cultured glial tumor cells. *J. Biol. Chem.* 249:1769, 1974.

53. Schwartzkroin, P. A., and Slawsky, M. Probable calcium spikes in hippocampal neurons. *Brain Res.* 135:157, 1977.

54. Schwindt, P., and Crill, W. E. Role of a persistent inward current in motoneuron bursting during spinal seizures. *J. Neurophysiol.* 43:1296, 1980.

55. Trachtenberg, M. C., and Pollen, D. A. Neuroglia: Biophysical properties and physiologic function. *Science* 167:1248, 1970.

56. Traub, R. D., and Wong, R. Cellular mechanism of neuronal synchronization in epilepsy. *Science* 216:745, 1982.

57. Walker, J. E., Lewin, E., and Moffitt, B. C. Production of Epileptiform Discharges by Application of Agents Which Increase Cyclic AMP Levels in Rat Cortex. In P. Harris, and C. Mawdsley (Eds.), *Epilepsy.* New York: Livingstone, 1974. Pp. 30–36.

58. Wilson, W. A., and Wachtel, H. Negative resistance characteristics essential for the maintenance of slow oscillations in bursting neurons. *Science* 186:932, 1974.

59. Woodbury, D. M. Antiepileptic Drugs: Pharmacology and Mechanisms of Action. In P. Harris and C. Mawdsley (Eds.), *Epilepsy.* New York: Livingstone, 1974. Pp. 78–95.

60. Woodbury, D. M., and Kemp, J. W. Basic Mechanisms of Seizures: Neurophysiological and Biochemical Etiology. In C. Shagass, S. Gershon, and A. J. Friedhoff (Eds.), *Psychopathology and Brain Dysfunction.* New York: Raven Press, 1977. Pp. 149–182.

61. Woodbury, D. M. et al. Effects of carbon dioxide on brain excitability and electrolytes. *Am. J. Physiol.* 192:79, 1958.

62. Zuckerman, E. C., and Glaser, G. H. Hippocampal epileptic activity induced by localized ventricular perfusion with high-potassium cerebrospinal fluid. *Exp. Neurol.* 20:87, 1968.

CLASSIFICATION OF EPILEPTIC SEIZURES AND OF THE EPILEPSIES

3

Thomas R. Browne

There are two types of classifications of epilepsy: (1) classifications of *the epileptic seizures,* and (2) classifications of *the epilepsies.* Classifications of the epileptic seizures are concerned with classifying each individual *seizure* as a single event. Classifications of the epilepsies are concerned with classifying *syndromes* in which the type or types of seizures are one, but not the only, feature of the syndrome. Other features such as etiology, age of onset, and evidence of brain pathology are included in syndromic classifications of the epilepsies.

Modern classifications of the epileptic seizures and of the epilepsies are based on varying combinations of the following factors: clinical seizure morphology, abnormalities on the electroencephalogram (EEG) during seizures, interictal EEG abnormalities, anatomic substrate of the seizure, etiology, age of onset, and response to drugs. A great deal of confusion arose in the 1950s and 1960s because (1) different systems of classification were proposed, based on some, but not all, of the factors just listed; (2) different terms were used by different classifications to describe the same type of epileptic seizure or epilepsy; and (3) the same term was used by different classifications to describe different types of epileptic seizure or epilepsy. To help resolve this confusion, the International League Against Epilepsy has organized several commissions on terminology to create uniform classifications of epileptic seizures and of the epilepsies. These commissions formulated the Clinical and Electroencephalographical Classification of Epileptic Seizures of the Commission on Terminology of the International League Against Epilepsy [1] (International Classification of Epileptic Seizures) and the International Classification of the Epilepsies [8]. These are the classifications of epileptic seizures and of the epilepsies that are most widely used throughout the world and that will be used throughout this book.

Clinical and Electroencephalographic Classification of Epileptic Seizures of the International League Against Epilepsy

HISTORY
For reasons outlined in the previous paragraph, the International League Against Epilepsy appointed a

This work was supported in part by the Veterans Administration. Jerome K. Merlis, M.D., assisted in the preparation of this chapter.

Commission on Terminology in 1964 to produce a uniform classification of epileptic seizures. Comments were solicited, and the final product of this effort was the first version of the International Classification of Epileptic Seizures published in 1970 [2].

In 1981 a revised version [1] of the International Classification of Epileptic Seizures was adopted by the International League Against Epilepsy. This revised version incorporates advances in knowledge of the clinical neurophysiology of seizures obtained between 1970 and 1981 as well as the comments of a wide range of individual physicians and national and international societies. The 1981 revision is the version that will be used throughout this book.

DETAILS OF CLASSIFICATION
The International Classification of Epileptic Seizures is summarized in Table 1-1 and presented in its entirety in Table 3-1. The classification is based on a combination of three factors: (1) clinical seizure type, (2) electroencephalographic seizure type, and (3) electroencephalographic interictal expression. Each term defines a unique clinical EEG entity, and there is little overlapping of categories. Seizures are first subdivided into two broad categories: (1) partial seizures (seizures beginning locally), and (2) generalized seizures (seizures that are bilaterally symmetrical and without local onset). Seizures are then further classified depending on their exact clinical and EEG manifestations.

ADVANTAGES

Emphasizes Clinical and EEG Information
In systems of classification based on more than one factor the final system of classification will vary according to the weighting of importance assigned to the various factors. The International Classification of Epileptic Seizures emphasizes clinical seizure morphology and ictal and interictal EEG findings. This emphasis is useful and proper in the usual clinical setting because these factors are the information which, in the majority of cases, is most helpful in deciding which antiepileptic drug to give a patient.

Written by Experts
The International Classification of Epileptic Seizures was drafted by an international commission of experts in the field. It was then widely distributed to other experts and agencies with an interest in the classification of epilepsy. Their comments were solicited and incorporated into the final draft. Although no classification of epileptic seizures is universally accepted, the International Classification of Epileptic Seizures

probably represents the best consensus of modern thought.

Widely Recognized
The International Classification of Epileptic Seizures is endorsed by the Commission for the Control of Epilepsy and Its Consequences of the U.S. Public Health Service, the International League Against Epilepsy, the World Federation of Neurology, the World Federation of Neurological Societies, and the International Federation of Societies for Electroencephalography and Clinical Neurophysiology [1, 9]. A modification of the International Classification of Epileptic Seizures is used by the World Health Organization [4].

Provides a Uniform Standard
Any classification of epileptic seizures is, to a certain extent, arbitrary. However, widespread use of a single system of classification facilitates communication among physicians and facilitates understanding and comparison of published reports on the neurophysiology, therapy, and epidemiology of epilepsy.

DISADVANTAGES

*Preferred Terms Are Different
from Those Used by Many Clinicians*
The preferred terms in the International Classification of Epileptic Seizures are different from those used by many clinicians in this country. *Tonic-clonic* is used instead of *grand mal. Absence* is used instead of *petit mal, complex partial* instead of *psychomotor* or *temporal lobe,* and *simple partial* instead of *focal* or *Jacksonian.* Nevertheless, the International Classification of Epileptic Seizures is preferred because of its greater precision of terminology. Each term defines a unique clinical-EEG seizure type, whereas the older terms used in this country tend to be imprecise and ambiguous. For instance, *petit mal* is used by some physicians to refer only to typical absence seizures with 3-Hz spike-wave on the EEG and by other physicians to refer to all seizures other than grand mal (e.g., absence, atypical absence, myoclonic, atonic). *Grand mal* is used by some physicians to refer only to tonic-clonic seizures and by others to describe all seizures with large motor movements (e.g., tonic-clonic, tonic, clonic, hemiclonic). The terms *psychomotor seizure* and *temporal lobe seizure* are less precise than *complex partial seizures* combined with one of the modifiers of the International Classification of Epileptic Seizures because (1) not all complex partial seizures have psychic or motor components; (2) not all complex partial seizures begin in the temporal lobe; and

Table 3-1. International Classification of Epileptic Seizures

I. Partial (Focal, Local) Seizures

Partial seizures are those in which, in general, the first clinical and electroencephalographic changes indicate initial activation of a system of neurons limited to part of one cerebral hemisphere. A partial seizure is classified primarily on the basis of whether or not consciousness is impaired during the attack. When consciousness is not impaired, the seizure is classified as a simple partial seizure. When consciousness is impaired, the seizure is classified as a complex partial seizure. Impairment of consciousness may be the first clinical sign, or simple partial seizures may evolve into complex partial seizures. In patients with impaired consciousness, aberrations of behavior (automatisms) may occur. A partial seizure may not terminate, but instead progress to a generalized motor seizure. Impaired consciousness is defined as the inability to respond normally to exogenous stimuli by virtue of altered awareness and/or responsiveness.

There is considerable evidence that simple partial seizures usually have unilateral hemispheric involvement and only rarely have bilateral hemispheric involvement; complex partial seizures, however, frequently have bilateral hemispheric involvement.

Partial seizures can be classified into one of the following three fundamental groups:

A. Simple partial seizures
B. Complex partial seizures
1. With impairment of consciousness at onset
2. Simple partial onset followed by impairment of consciousness
C. Partial seizures evolving to generalized tonic-clonic convulsions (GTC)
1. Simple evolving to GTC
2. Complex evolving to GTC (including those with simple partial onset)

Clinical Seizure Type	EEG Seizure Type	EEG Interictal Expression
A. *Simple partial seizures* (consciousness not impaired)	Local contralateral discharge starting over the corresponding area of cortical representation (not always recorded on the scalp)	Local contralateral discharge
1. With motor signs (a) Focal motor without march (b) Focal motor with march (Jacksonian) (c) Versive (d) Postural (e) Phonatory (vocalization or arrest of speech)		
2. With somatosensory or special-sensory symptoms (simple hallucinations, e.g., tingling, light flashes, buzzing) (a) Somatosensory (b) Visual (c) Auditory (d) Olfactory (e) Gustatory (f) Vertiginous		
3. With autonomic symptoms or signs (including epigastric sensation, pallor, sweating, flushing, piloerection and pupillary dilatation)		
4. With psychic symptoms (disturbance of higher cerebral function). These symptoms rarely occur without impairment of consciousness and are much more commonly experienced as complex partial seizures (a) Dysphasic (b) Dysmnesic (e.g., déjà-vu) (c) Cognitive (e.g., dreamy states, distortions of time sense) (d) Affective (fear, anger, etc.) (e) Illusions (e.g., macropsia) (f) Structured hallucinations (e.g., music, scenes)		
B. *Complex partial seizures* (with impairment of consciousness; may sometimes begin with simple symptomatology) 1. Simple partial onset followed by impairment of consciousness (a) With simple partial features (A.1.–A.4.) followed by impaired consciousness (b) With automatisms	Unilateral or, frequently bilateral discharge, diffuse or focal in temporal or frontotemporal regions	Unilateral or bilateral generally asynchronous focus; usually in the temporal or frontal regions

Table 3-1 (Continued)

Clinical Seizure Type	EEG Seizure Type	EEG Interictal Expression

2. With impairment of consciousness at onset
  (a) With impairment of conscious-ness only
  (b) With automatisms		

C. *Partial seizures evolving to secondarily generalized seizures* (This may be generalized tonic-clonic, tonic, or clonic) 1. Simple partial seizures (A) evolving to generalized seizures 2. Complex partial seizures (B) evolving to generalized seizures 3. Simple partial seizures evolving to complex partial seizures evolving to generalized seizures	Above discharges become secondarily and rapidly generalized	

II. Generalized Seizures (Convulsive or Nonconvulsive)

Generalized seizures are those in which the first clinical changes indicate initial involvement of both hemispheres. Consciousness may be impaired and this impairment may be the initial manifestation. Motor manifestations are bilateral. The ictal electro-encephalographic patterns initially are bilateral, and presumably reflect neuronal discharge which is widespread in both hemispheres.

Clinical Seizure Type	EEG Seizure Type	EEG Interictal Expression
A. 1. *Absence seizures*	Usually regular and symmetrical 3 Hz but may be 2–4 Hz spike-and-slow-wave complexes and may have multiple spike-and-slow-wave complexes. Abnormalities are bilateral	Background activity usually normal although paroxysmal activity (such as spikes or spike-and-slow-wave complexes) may occur. This activity is usually regular and symmetrical

(a) Impairment of consciousness only
  (b) With mild clonic components
  (c) With atonic components
  (d) With tonic components
  (e) With automatisms
  (f) With autonomic components
  (b through f may be used alone or in combination)		

2. *Atypical absence*	EEG more heterogeneous; may include irregular spike-and-slow-wave complexes, fast activity or other paroxysmal activity. Abnormalities are bilateral but often irregular and asymmetrical	Background usually abnormal; paroxysmal activity (such as spikes or spike-and-slow-wave complexes) frequently irregular and asymmetrical

May have:
  (a) Changes in tone that are more pronounced than in A.1
  (b) Onset and/or cessation that is not abrupt		

B. *Myoclonic seizures* Myoclonic jerks (single or multiple)	Polyspike and wave, or sometimes spike and wave or sharp and slow waves	Same as ictal
C. *Clonic seizures*	Fast activity (10 c/sec or more) and slow waves; occasional spike-and-wave patterns	Spike-and-wave or polyspike-and-wave discharges

Table 3-1 (Continued)

Clinical Seizure Type	EEG Seizure Type	EEG Interictal Expression
D. *Tonic seizures*	Low voltage, fast activity or a fast rhythm of 9–10 c/sec or more decreasing in frequency and increasing in amplitude	More or less rhythmic discharges of sharp and slow waves, sometimes asymmetrical. Background is often abnormal for age
E. *Tonic-clonic seizures*	Rhythm at 10 or more c/sec decreasing in frequency and increasing in amplitude during tonic phase, interrupted by slow waves during clonic phase	Polyspike and waves or spike and wave, or, sometimes, sharp and slow wave discharges
F. *Atonic seizures* (astatic seizures) (combinations of the above may occur, e.g., B and F, B and D)	Polyspikes and wave or flattening or low-voltage fast activity	Polyspikes and slow wave

III. Unclassified Epileptic Seizures

Includes all seizures that cannot be classified because of inadequate or incomplete data and some that defy classification in hitherto described categories. This includes some neonatal seizures, e.g., rhythmic eye movements, chewing, and swimming movements.

IV. Addendum

Repeated epileptic seizures occur under a variety of circumstances:

(1) As fortuitous attacks, coming unexpectedly and without any apparent provocation; (2) as cyclic attacks, at more or less regular intervals (e.g., in relation to the menstrual cycle, or the sleep-waking cycle); (3) as attacks provoked by: (a) nonsensory factors (fatigue, alcohol, emotion, etc.), or (b) sensory factors, sometimes referred to as "reflex seizures."

Prolonged or repetitive seizures (status epilepticus). The term *status epilepticus* is used whenever a seizure persists for a sufficient length of time or is repeated frequently enough that recovery between attacks does not occur. Status epilepticus may be divided into partial (e.g., Jacksonian), or generalized (e.g., absence status or tonic-clonic status). When very localized motor status occurs, it is referred to as epilepsia partialis continua.

Source: Dreifuss [1].

(3) some seizures arising in the temporal lobe are not manifested clinically as complex partial seizures.

Failure to Specify Anatomic Substrate, Etiology, Age of Onset, Seizure Frequency, Modifying and Precipitating Factors, Interictal Neurophysiologic Changes, or Response to Drugs

The International Classification of Epileptic Seizures is based chiefly on clinical and EEG data. The classification precisely describes *the epileptic seizures* but does not completely describe *the epilepsies*. Seizures in the young child with benign febrile convulsions, the teenager with primarily generalized tonic-clonic seizures, and the adult with alcohol withdrawal seizures would all be classified as tonic-clonic seizures by the International Classification of Epileptic Seizures, but the epilepsy suffered by each of these patients differs significantly in management, in prognosis, and in its impact on the patient's life style.

Requires Detailed Seizure Description and EEG Data That Are Not Always Available

Lavy et al. [5] attempted to apply the "clinical seizure type" and EEG portions of the International Classifi- cation of Epileptic Seizures to 450 patients to evaluate how well the classifications worked in a busy neurologic practice. Their major criticism was that the detailed and complete seizure descriptions and EEG evaluations required to classify seizures by the International Classification are not always available to the practitioner. The patient and his relatives may not be able to provide a reliable complete description of the patient's seizures. Several routine EEGs may show either no abnormality or some but not all abnormalities present in a given patient.

The problems pointed out by Lavy et al. [5] are real, but usually can and should be overcome. Patients and relatives can often be instructed to observe certain features of seizures that will aid in the differential diagnosis. Prolonged monitoring of the patient and his EEG with videotape recording is increasingly available and can often provide the information necessary for a precise seizure diagnosis (see Chap. 11). Because of the catastrophic consequences of an improper seizure diagnosis, it is usually worth the effort to follow these guidelines to obtain a definitive seizure diagnosis when the diagnosis is uncertain.

International Classification of the Epilepsies

History

In 1968 the Commission on Terminology of the International League Against Epilepsy set out to produce an International Classification of the Epilepsies to supplement its International Classification of Epileptic Seizures. A workshop was organized consisting of individual experts and international societies with an interest in classification of the epilepsies. The resulting classification was published in 1970 [8].

DETAILS OF CLASSIFICATION

The International Classification of the Epilepsies is presented in its entirety in Table 3-2. This system of classification categorizes patients into one of five broad groups or subgroups based on (1) seizure form, (2) presence of neurologic or psychologic evidence of brain pathology, (3) age of onset, (4) etiology, (5) ictal EEG, and (6) interictal EEG. Again, this system relies most heavily on clinical seizure morphology and on ictal and interictal EEG phenomena.

ADVANTAGES

The International Classification of the Epilepsies represents a "state of the art" consensus on a broad classification of epilepsy syndromes. The classification is modern, is based on expert opinion, and provides a uniform standard for national and international communication.

DISADVANTAGES

Within each of the five broad groups or subgroups of epilepsy of this system of classification there are several types of epileptic seizures. Thus a patient with "primarily generalized epilepsy" may have any combination of absence, myoclonic, or tonic-clonic seizures. Because management of epilepsy depends upon precise seizure diagnosis, the diagnostic categories of the International Classification of the Epilepsies do not convey all the information needed by a physician to treat patients or to evaluate reports of treatment given to patients.

INTERNATIONAL CLASSIFICATION OF EPILEPTIC SEIZURES VERSUS INTERNATIONAL CLASSIFICATION OF THE EPILEPSIES FOR ROUTINE USE

Management of epilepsy depends on precise seizure diagnosis. The International Classification of Epileptic Seizures precisely classifies seizure types with little ambiguity or overlap of terms. The International Classification of the Epilepsies has rather broad categories with several seizure types within each category.

In most situations in routine practice and in published communications, it is preferable to use the International Classification of Epileptic Seizures to be as precise as possible in describing seizure type. To provide a complete description of a patient's condition, it may be necessary to furnish information on the etiology, age of onset, brain pathology, or precipitating or modifying factors in addition to the seizure type.

Other Systems of Classification

CLASSIFICATION OF MASLAND

To deal with the problem of completely defining the epilepsy syndrome suffered by a given patient, Masland developed a system of classification of the epilepsies involving four criteria: (1) etiology, (2) seizure patterns and EEG, (3) anatomy, and (4) age or circumstances of occurrence [6, 7]. To define a given patient's epilepsy, it is necessary to specify the appropriate terms from each of the four criteria. The terms in the Masland classification are derived from the glossary of the World Health Organization (WHO). The "seizure pattern and EEG" criteria of the Masland classification and the WHO glossary are derived chiefly from the International Classification of Epileptic Seizures. Although it is not widely used or endorsed and although it is slightly cumbersome because each patient is assigned diagnostic terms from four different categories, the Masland classification represents probably the best attempt at a systematic classification of all the many facets of epilepsy present in a given patient and uses precise, modern, internationally accepted terminology to describe them [6, 7].

INTERNATIONAL CLASSIFICATION OF DISEASES

The International Classification of Diseases (ICD) [4] of the World Health Organization has been modified for use in the United States by the U.S. National Center for Health Statistics. The WHO version and the United States version of the ICD are based on a simplified modification of the International Classification of Epileptic Seizures. Both versions have serious deficiencies. First, the categories of epilepsy are broad, and patients with several types of epileptic seizure could be assigned to one diagnostic group. Second, because the ICD contains many overlapping synonyms, a patient with only one type of clinical and electroencephalographic epileptic seizure could be classified in one of several types of epilepsy. Third, the ICD is based primarily on clinical seizure type and fails to include information on EEG features, mode of onset, anatomic localization, and etiology.

Table 3-2. International Classification of the Epilepsies

I. Generalized Epilepsies

1. Primary Generalized Epilepsies
   A. *Clinical criteria*
      (1) Seizures. Seizures that are generalized from the onset in the form of absences, bilateral myoclonus, and tonic-clonic seizures. One or more of these types of seizures can occur in the same patient.
      (2) Neurologic status. The usual absence of neurologic or psychologic evidence of cerebral abnormality.
      (3) Age of onset. Onset in childhood and adolescence, although they are liable to persist to, and may even begin at, any age.
      (4) Etiology. Lack of any clear etiology.
   B. *Electroencephalographic criteria*
      (1) Interictal EEG. The presence (usually) of bilaterally synchronous spikes, polyspikes, spike-and-wave, or polyspike-wave complexes. These may occur singly or rhythmically, at about 3/s. They are spontaneous or are induced by hyperventilation, intermittent photic stimulation, or sleep.
      (2) Ictal EEG. The occurrence (usually) of synchronous and symmetrical discharges with a given type[a] of seizure (rhythmic at about 3/s spike-and-wave complexes during absences; polyspike-wave complexes during bilateral myoclonus; "recruiting" rhythms at about 10/s, followed by rhythmic polyspike-waves during tonic-clonic seizures).
2. Secondary Generalized Epilepsies
   A. *Clinical criteria*
      (1) Seizures. Seizures that are generalized *from the onset* in the form of absences, bilateral myoclonus, tonic or atonic seizures, or tonic-clonic seizures. One or more of these seizures can occur in a single patient.
      (2) Neurologic status. The presence (usually) of neurologic or psychologic signs (i.e., mental deficiency or deterioration), or both, which indicates diffuse cerebral pathology.
      (3) Age of onset. Onset at any age; most frequent in childhood.
      (4) Etiology. May be ascribed (usually) to diffuse or multifocal cerebral lesions.
   B. *Electroencephalographic criteria*
      (1) Interictal EEG. Slow background activity with sharp and slow wave complexes usually symmetrical and synchronous, or asymmetrical, or even asynchronous. These are less frequently induced by hyperventilation and photic stimulation. Sleep may be effective.
      (2) Ictal EEG. Ictal patterns that may contain diminution in amplitude of background EEG activities, a low voltage rapid discharge, a "recruiting" rhythm at about 10/s, sharp and slow wave discharges at about 2/s, and spike-and-wave or polyspike-wave discharges. The sharp and slow wave discharges are less synchronous and symmetrical, and are more variable in topographic distribution than the other discharge types and than those in primary generalized epilepsy. The correlation between these ictal EEG patterns and the seizure types is not as good as in primary generalized epilepsy.[b]
3. Undetermined Generalized Epilepsies
   Using the criteria above may mean that the information available concerning a given patient with a generalized epilepsy may not be adequate to determine whether it is primary or secondary. The patient's condition will then be classified as generalized epilepsy, undetermined.

II. Partial (Focal, Local) Epilepsies

   A. *Clinical criteria*
      (1) Seizures. Partial seizures (of local onset) with or without generalization, whose manifestations (chiefly initial) are of many forms as detailed in the International Classification of Epileptic Seizures. Postictal focal neurologic deficit may be present.
      (2) Neurologic status. The presence (frequently) of neurological signs related to the epileptogenic lesion.
      (3) Age of onset. Onset at any age.
      (4) Etiology. Associated (usually) with brain damage.
   B. *Electroencephalographic criteria*
      (1) Interictal EEG. Occurrence of local spikes or spike-and-wave complexes (usually). Sleep, hyperventilation, and photic stimulation are less effective activators than in other types of epilepsies. The site of the epileptogenic focus should correspond to the clinical symptoms of the seizures.
      (2) Ictal EEG. Local discharges related to the lesion. In many cases, these may be diffuse; they may even be absent. Postictal focal abnormalities may be present.

iII. Unclassifiable Epilepsies

This group comprises all those epilepsies that cannot be classified in one of the above mentioned generalized or partial groups, either because they are atypical or because data are insufficient. The epilepsy with "erratic seizures" in the newborn and the unilateral seizures of childhood may have to be included in this category.

The above groups may differ significantly in cyclic characteristics, response to medication, prognosis, and so forth. As our understanding of the basic mechanisms of the epilepsies increases, modification of this classification will undoubtedly be necessary.

[a]The precise ictal patterns of the various types of epileptic seizures are described in detail in the International Classification of Epileptic Seizures [1].
[b]The most usual correlates are described in the International Classification of Epileptic Seizures [1].
Source: Merlis [8].

28

OLDER CLASSIFICATIONS OF EPILEPSY

Classifications of epilepsy have been in use since the days of Hippocrates (400 B.C.) [7]. Early classifications are interesting because they reflect the scientific knowledge and philosophic views of their time. The history of the classifications of epilepsy has been reviewed by Masland [7].

References

1. Dreifuss, F. E. Proposal for revised clinical and electroencephalographic classification of epileptic seizures. *Epilepsia* 22:489, 1981.
2. Gastaut, H. Clinical and electroencephalographical classification of epileptic seizures. *Epilepsia* 11:102, 1970.
3. Gastaut, H. Comments on "clinical and EEG classification of epilepsy." *Epilepsia* 13:506, 1972.
4. *International Classification of Diseases: 9th Revision, Clinical Modification.* Washington, D.C.: U.S. Department of Health and Human Services, 1980.
5. Lavy, S., Carmon, A., and Yahr, I. Assessment of clinical and electroencephalographic classification of epileptic patients in everyday neurological practice: A survey of 450 cases. *Epilepsia* 13:498, 1972.
6. Masland, R. L. Comments on the classification of epilepsy. *Epilepsia* 10:S22, 1969.
7. Masland, R. L. The Classification of the Epilepsies: A Historical Review. In O. Magnus, and A. M. Lorentz de Haas (Eds.), *Handbook of Clinical Neurology,* Vol. 15, *The Epilepsies.* Amsterdam: Elsevier, 1974.
8. Merlis, J. K. Proposal for an international classification of the epilepsies. *Epilepsia* 11:114, 1970.
9. *Plan for Nationwide Action on Epilepsy: Report of The Commission for the Control of Epilepsy and Its Consequences,* Vol. 1. Washington, D.C.: U.S. Dept. of Health, Education and Welfare, 1978.

SIMPLE PARTIAL SEIZURES (FOCAL SEIZURES)

4

Thomas R. Browne
Giuseppe Erba

Definitions

Simple partial seizures are caused by a local cortical discharge that results in seizure symptoms appropriate to the function of the discharging area of brain without impairment of consciousness. Simple partial seizures may consist of motor, sensory, autonomic, or psychic symptoms and signs. The same symptoms and signs may occur in both simple partial and complex partial seizures. The crucial distinction is that impairment of consciousness occurs in the latter but not in the former [5]. Impaired consciousness is defined as the inability to respond normally to exogenous stimuli by virtue of altered awareness or responsiveness [5]. Responsiveness refers to the ability of the patient to carry out simple commands or willed movements, and awareness refers to the patient's contact with events during the period in question and its recall [5].

Etiology

By definition, partial seizures are *symptomatic* of a hemispheric lesion. Abnormal CT scans are found in approximately 50 percent of patients with partial seizures [48]. The types of lesions found in a large series of patients operated on for partial seizures are summarized in Table 4-1. Lesions may be static or progressive in nature. Most partial seizures in infancy and childhood represent the consequence of perinatal encephalopathies, and the seizures are the manifestations of static gliotic lesions. Partial seizures of "late onset" may indicate a new focal process, and in such cases a brain lesion (neoplasm, cerebrovascular accident, or inflammatory process) must be ruled out.

BRAIN TUMORS
Brain tumors are found in 10 to 20 percent of all patients with focal seizures [32, 34], and in 30 to 60 percent of patients with focal seizures that begin after 30 years of age [21, 34, 39].

CEREBROVASCULAR DISEASE
Cerebrovascular disease (embolic or occlusive) is more often an etiologic factor in the elderly than in the young [45]. Focal seizures (immediate or delayed) occur in 10 percent of patients who have had a cerebrovascular accident [36]. To produce a partial seizure, the vascular insufficiency caused by embolic or occlusive phenomena must selectively involve major or second-order arterial vessels. Waddington performed

Table 4-1. Etiology of Focal Seizures*

Epileptogenic Lesion	Percent of Patients
Birth complication (e.g., trauma, anoxia, cord compression)	25
Postnatal trauma	20
Tumors	19
Postinflammatory brain scarring	12
Arteriovenous malformation	1
Miscellaneous	5
Unknown	17

*Based on findings at surgery in 1,355 patients at the Montreal Neurological Institute. Includes both simple and complex partial seizures.
Source: Modified from Rasmussen [32].

angiographic studies on patients of all ages with focal motor seizures [43]. Occlusion of small arterial branches to the motor and premotor cortex or abnormally small "vestigial" vessels in the same areas (representing recanalization after occlusion) were found in 20 percent of the group. Particularly at risk are patients with either valvular or cyanotic heart disease who are prone to embolic phenomena and brain abscesses in the watershed areas. In children, simple partial seizures may be due to vascular malformations (e.g., arteriovenous malformations), hyperviscosity syndromes (e.g., sickle cell disease, thalassemia), or occlusion of major cerebral arteries acquired prenatally (porencephaly) or postnatally (acute infantile hemiplegia). Arterial occlusions in the posterior circulation can be the underlying cause of partial seizures with visual manifestations [35].

OTHER ETIOLOGIES
Trauma is a common cause of seizures in all age groups (see Chap. 12). Among the neurocutaneous syndromes, Sturge-Weber disease is almost exclusively associated with simple partial seizures from very early infancy. A subacute localized inflammatory process of the type described by Rasmussen and McCann can lead to extremely frequent and intractable simple partial seizures [33]. Finally, it should be remembered that focal seizures can also occur during transient metabolic encephalopathies (e.g., hypocalcemia in the neonate or hypoglycemia in the elderly).

The many possible structural and metabolic causes of partial seizures are reviewed in more detail in Chapter 12.

GENETICS
A genetic trend has not been definitely established for simple partial seizures [22].

Pathophysiology

Partial seizures represent paroxysmal phenomena within the cortical structures of one hemisphere, due to spread of abnormally synchronous neuronal discharges to the areas surrounding a chronic seizure focus of abnormal neurons and glial cells. A cerebral insult (e.g., anoxic, traumatic, inflammatory) typically results in an area of complete neuronal destruction surrounded by an area of partial neuronal damage. Seizure activity originates at areas of partial neuronal damage, possibly as a result of selective loss of inhibitory inputs [44]. The cellular and subcellular mechanisms of partial seizures are reviewed in more detail in Chapter 2.

Seizure Phenomena

Regardless of etiology and pathophysiology, the nature of the seizure manifestations is strictly dependent on the region of the cortex where they originate and its functions. Electrical stimulation studies of the human cortex confirm that simple partial seizures originate and develop within neuronal populations of the primary motor, premotor, supplementary motor, and primary sensory receptive areas of one hemisphere [25]. A precise, analytical classification of partial seizure types based on their phenomenology is, therefore, of great value in localizing the epileptogenic focus in a given patient. It also provides a useful reference for detecting changes in seizure patterns that may represent the first signal of the progressive nature of the responsible lesion. Following the International Classification of Epileptic Seizures [5], the manifestations of simple partial seizures will be divided into four groups: (1) with motor signs, (2) with somatosensory or special sensory symptoms, (3) with autonomic symptoms or signs, and (4) with psychic symptoms.

SIMPLE PARTIAL SEIZURES WITH MOTOR SIGNS
Owing to the extensive representation of the motor cortex and to the high epileptogenicity of the frontal lobes, focal motor seizures are among the most frequently encountered varieties of simple partial seizure. The symptoms are, at least initially, always strictly contralateral to the hemispheric focus and may represent the expression of excitatory (positive-irritative) phenomena, inhibitory (negative-suppressive or paralytic) phenomena, or a combination of the two.

Focal Motor Seizures With and Without March
The simplest form of simple partial seizure with motor signs is clonus, which consists of rhythmic alternating contraction and relaxation of muscle groups controlled by the part of the motor cortex where hypersynchronous discharges take place (somatomotor

seizure). The episodes may be self-limited (clonic focal seizure), recurrent (focal motor status epilepticus), or continuous (epilepsia partialis continua). Spread of the discharge along contiguous areas of the precentral gyrus gives rise to the characteristic "march" of spreading involvement of muscle groups in "Jacksonian" seizures. Transient paralytic phenomena (Todd's paralysis) are a common postictal manifestation of an excitatory clonic seizure, especially if it is severe or repeated [32].

"Somatic inhibitory" attacks are infrequent as solitary manifestations of a seizure. Usually there is sensory loss or dysesthesia and weakness [32].

Versive Seizures

The premotor cortex contains mechanisms for the elaboration of motor acts of a more complex nature and is concerned with bilateral synergistic movements. It includes the supplementary motor area (parasagittal and mesial aspect of area 6) and the frontal eye field (area 8). Electrical stimulation of area 8 in humans produces contralateral conjugate eye movements and turning of the head to the contralateral side ("versive" seizures) [32]. Because of the anatomic connections of the frontal eye field with parietal regions on both sides, homolateral or contralateral versive seizures can result from spreading of paroxysmal discharges from a parietal focus. Recent work also indicates that homolateral and contralateral versive movements occur with almost equal frequency when the versive movements are caused by seizures originating in the temporal lobe [24].

Postural Seizures

Discharges within the supplementary motor area may cause asymmetrical dystonic posturing of the limbs ("postural" seizures), which may be associated with vocalization or speech arrest [27, 32]. The same phenomena have been observed when the focus is located in the premotor cortex or when the electrical discharges spread to these areas [1].

Phonatory Seizures

"Aphasic" seizures consist primarily of speech arrest and/or inability to verbalize while consciousness is fully retained [29, 32]. They should not be confused with the dysphasic phenomena frequently observed in the context of complex partial seizures, usually in the postictal recovery phase. Classic examples of ictal inability to speak are the "Sylvian" seizures [16a, 17]. They start with a feeling of numbness in the mouth, tongue, and throat and progress to a total paralysis of

speech articulation while understanding of spoken language is intact. This seizure pattern is associated with spike discharges in the central and midtemporal regions on either side. Aphemia (speech arrest) as well as vocalization (phonatory seizures) are unlikely to occur as isolated features but are frequently a component of supplementary motor seizures.

SIMPLE PARTIAL SEIZURES WITH SOMATOSENSORY OR SPECIAL SENSORY SYMPTOMS

Somatosensory Seizures

Seizures arising in or near the central region may begin with either motor or sensory phenomena [32]. Electrical stimulation of the postcentral gyrus elicits motor rather than sensory responses in 25 percent of stimulations [26, 32]. This reflects the intimate intermingling of sensory and motor functions in the pre- and postcentral areas.

Somatosensory seizures are usually described as "numbness," "tingling," "pins and needles," or "like a weak electric shock" [32]. Less frequently, there is a sense of movement, desire to move, or inability to move [32]. The former sensations are more likely with postcentral foci, while the latter sensations are more likely with precentral foci [32]. The initial somatosensory sensation may be the only manifestation of a seizure. The focal discharge may spread to the adjacent sensory cortex, producing a Jacksonian march of sensory phenomena. The focal discharge also may spread to the adjacent motor cortex, producing motor symptoms.

Visual Seizures

Among the "special sensory" seizures, attacks starting with simple visual symptoms are relatively common and are indicative of a focus in the vicinity of the calcarine fissure [32]. Visual simple partial seizures consisting of crude positive symptoms such as flashes of lights or colors in the contralateral hemifield are more frequently described than negative symptoms such as scotomas or hemianopia. These negative manifestations are more often prodromes of migrainous rather than of epileptic attacks (see Differential Diagnosis). Nevertheless, we have observed "amaurotic" seizures consisting of "fading vision" without other manifestations in patients with Sturge-Weber disease. Discharges arising in the occipital lobe may spread to the temporal lobe, producing complex partial seizure phenomena [2, 46], or to the parietal and central lobes, producing somatosensory or somatomotor seizure phenomena [32]. Visual illusions and hallucinations usually represent seizure phenomena arising from the posterior temporal area (see Chap. 5).

Auditory Seizures

Seizures arising near the cortex of Heschel's region of the first temporal gyrus may produce simple auditory phenomena usually described as a "humming," "buzzing," "hissing," "whistling," "knocking," "roaring," or "tapping" [32]. Auditory illusions or hallucinations result from discharges arising in the auditory association areas of the temporal lobe (see Chap. 5).

Simple auditory seizures are rare. More commonly, a "rumbling noise" or a "humming," especially if associated with hyperacusis, represents the prodrome or the only transient manifestation of a migraine attack.

Olfactory and Gustatory Seizures

Olfactory and gustatory sensations may occur, usually in the form of unpleasant odors and tastes [4, 5]. Rasmussen has emphasized that an olfactory or gustatory sensation as the *initial* symptom of a partial seizure often indicates a glioma in or beneath the insula [31]. However, a recent study indicates that there is not an increased risk of brain tumor when the group of patients with olfactory and gustatory sensations at *any time* during a seizure is considered [11a].

Vertiginous Seizures

A vague feeling of "dizziness" or lightheadedness is often described as the initial or the only manifestation of an attack. This sensation is rarely described as true vertigo. Vertiginous sensations without alteration of consciousness are extremely frequent expressions of vestibular irritative phenomena (peripheral or central), although they have been described also as true epileptic manifestations of seizure foci in the middle or posterior portion of the first temporal gyrus ("tornado epilepsy") [14, 32, 38].

Because the olfactory, gustatory, auditory, and equilibrium functions are bilaterally represented, seizure phenomena originating in these centers can be only of the "irritative" type. Unilateral loss of function due to inhibitory phenomena would go unnoticed. Because of the multiple links of these paleocortical structures with the limbic system, hypothalamus, and brain stem centers, they seldom occur as isolated phenomena and are likely to progress to a complex partial seizure or a simple partial seizure with autonomic symptoms.

SIMPLE PARTIAL SEIZURES

WITH AUTONOMIC SYMPTOMS OR SIGNS

Epigastric sensations, flushing or pallor, sweating, pupillary dilatation, diaphoresis, piloerection, nausea, vomiting, borborygmi, incontinence, etc., are usually a component of complex partial seizures or tonic seizures (see Chaps. 5 and 8). Similar ictal phenomena may occur in isolation as manifestations of an epileptogenic focus located in the orbitofrontal cortex [41].

SIMPLE PARTIAL SEIZURES WITH PSYCHIC SYMPTOMS

Psychic symptoms (disturbances of cerebral function) may be dysphasic, dysmnesic (e.g., déjà vu), cognitive (e.g., dreamy states, distortions of time sense), affective (e.g., fear, anger), illusions (e.g., macropsia), or structured hallucinations (e.g., music, scenes) [5]. Such symptoms can occasionally occur without impairment of consciousness as part of a simple partial seizure. More commonly, psychic symptoms occur in association with impaired consciousness as part of a complex partial seizure. Psychic symptoms are discussed in more detail in Chapter 5.

COMPLEX PARTIAL SEIZURES WITH SIMPLE PARTIAL ONSET, AND SIMPLE PARTIAL SEIZURES EVOLVING TO COMPLEX PARTIAL SEIZURES, EVOLVING TO GENERALIZED SEIZURES

Complex partial seizures typically involve large portions of temporal-limbic structures (often bilaterally) and impair consciousness (see Chap. 5). Focal discharges may originate in circumscribed areas of temporal-limbic structures in such a fashion that they produce recognizable symptoms or signs (sensory, autonomic, psychic) of a partial seizure but do not impair consciousness. If the discharge remains circumscribed and if consciousness is never impaired, the seizure is classified as a simple partial seizure regardless of the complexity of the symptoms. If the discharge spreads to involve larger portions of temporal-limbic structures and if consciousness becomes impaired, the seizure is classified in the group of "complex partial seizures with simple partial onset" [5]. Similarly, focal discharges originating in structures outside the temporal-limbic structures (initially presenting as symptoms or signs of a partial seizure without impairment of consciousness) may spread to temporal-limbic structures, producing a complex partial seizure [2, 46]. Such a seizure would also be classified in the group of complex partial seizures with simple partial onset [5]. Regardless of where the focal discharges begin, complex partial seizures with simple partial onset may spread further and become secondarily generalized (tonic-clonic, tonic, or clonic). Such a seizure would be classified in the group of "simple partial seizures evolving to complex partial seizures evolving to generalized seizures" [5].

SIMPLE PARTIAL SEIZURES EVOLVING TO GENERALIZED SEIZURES
Focal hypersynchronous discharges giving rise to any type of simple partial seizure may spread to produce a secondarily generalized seizure (tonic-clonic, tonic, or clonic) without an intervening complex partial phase. Such a seizure would be classified in the group of "simple partial seizures evolving to generalized seizures" [5]. A focus in the central cortex causing elementary clonus may spread *sequentially* along the same gyrus (Jacksonian march) or *centrifugally* over the cortex, disregarding the gyral pattern. This explains why version of the head and eyes may occur following a simple motor, sensory, or visual seizure after spread of the discharges to the premotor cortex. This same mechanism of spread explains the occurrence of all types of compound forms of partial seizures. Likewise, discharges may spread *deeply* through cortical-subcortical pathways, leading to *secondary generalization*. Such spread can occur so rapidly that the initial symptoms referable to the primary focus may go unnoticed, leading to false localization or to an erroneous diagnosis of primary generalized epilepsy.

EEG Phenomena

INTERICTAL EEG
Abnormal interictal EEGs are found in 80 to 90 percent of patients with simple partial seizures if multiple EEGs are performed and all types of abnormalities are considered [9, 15]. Focal spike or sharp discharges are found in interictal EEGs in 40 to 85 percent of patients with simple partial seizures and correspond to the areas of focal cortical epileptogenic activity [1, 8, 9, 15]. There is an absence of focal spikes in 15 to 60 percent of patients for several reasons: (1) spikes are an intermittent phenomenon, (2) spikes originating from small areas of cortex may be markedly attenuated at the scalp, (3) spikes may originate from cortical areas distant from the convexity and be unrecorded at the scalp [8, 10].

Interictal, focal, paroxysmal rhythmic activity (focal hypersynchrony) occurs in the EEGs of approximately 50 percent of patients with focal seizures [8, 11]. Focal hypersynchrony may occur in patients without focal spikes and sharp waves and is a valuable EEG sign in establishing the diagnosis and localization of focal epilepsy [8, 11, 25].

Interictal focal slow-wave activity and/or suppression of normal background rhythms is present in 75% of patients with focal seizures [8] (Fig. 4-1). These abnormalities result from a combination of factors including preexisting parenchymal damage, focal epileptic activity, and postictal phenomena [8]. High-voltage, frontal slow waves may be the only surface EEG phenomenon in orbitofrontal seizures [41]. Following tumor removal, focal sharp waves or slow activity may remain.

The value of sleep and sleep deprivation in demonstrating focal spike- and sharp-wave discharges in the temporal area is reviewed in Chapters 5 and 11. Sleep recordings are also valuable for demonstrating spikes in other areas as well. The frequency of abnormal EEGs is increased by 20 to 25 percent in patients with focal nontemporal lobe seizures if sleep recordings are performed [9]. Central spikes in Sylvian seizures are especially prominent during sleep [16a].

ICTAL EEG

Preictal Changes
Interictal spikes and sharp waves show decreased occurrence or abrupt cessation just before the onset of ictal discharges in 75 percent of patients with focal epilepsy (Fig. 4-2) [8, 30]. Geiger and Harner [8] theorize that this occurs because when the dendritic membranes of epileptogenic aggregate neurons become increasingly depolarized, each subsequent paroxysmal depolarizing shift (see Chap. 2) produces a smaller and smaller net depolarization shift and a smaller and smaller spike discharge when recorded by an AC-coupled amplifier.

Ictal and Postictal EEG Changes
At the time of onset of clinical seizures, 90 percent of patients with focal seizures show a transformation in the scalp EEG from an interictal pattern to a sustained rhythmic pattern (Figs. 4-1 and 4-2) [8]. The initial frequency of rhythmic ictal transformation (RIT) is most often in the range of 13 to 30 Hz but may be slower (see Table 4-2). The RIT shows a progressive increase in amplitude and a decrease in frequency as clinical seizures develop (Figs. 4-1 and 4-2) [8]. Spread to adjacent areas of brain is indicated by the development of RIT in those areas. Termination of rhythmic ictal activity may be associated with the gradual development of slow-wave and spike-slow-wave activity that gradually decreases in frequency and then gives way to postictal slowing or depression of voltage, or both (Fig. 4-2) [8]. Rhythmic ictal activity can also subside abruptly, especially if the seizure has remained focal and mild [8]. In the 10 percent of cases that show no RIT, the interictal pattern of mixed sharp and rhythmic activity persists without observable change during the clinical seizure [8].

Geiger and Harner [8] were unable to correlate the frequency of the RIT with the area of cortex involved or with the acuteness or nature of the pathologic lesion

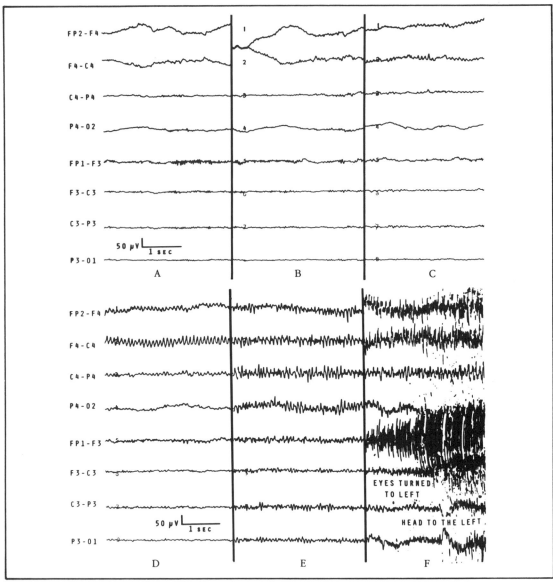

Figure 4-1. EEG pattern in 60-year-old man with adversive seizures. A. Baseline interictal recording shows suppression of beta over right frontal region. B. Twenty sec later, onset of seizure demonstrates low-voltage 18–22 Hz activity in right frontal area. C. At 30 sec rhythmic ictal activity gradually increases in voltage while slowing to 15 Hz. D. At 40 sec 10-Hz activity of the right frontal area spreads to right central area. E. At 55 sec 10-Hz activity spreads to posterior cranial regions and opposite hemisphere. F. At 65 sec there is tonic adversive seizure to left. (From L. R. Geiger and R. N. Harner [8]. Copyright 1978, American Medical Association.)

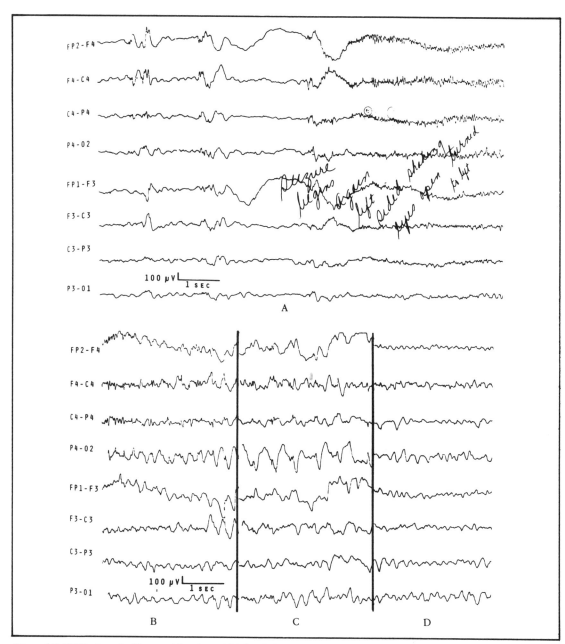

Figure 4-2. EEG pattern in 10-year-old patient with left-sided adversive and clonic seizures. A. Repetitive mixed sharp and slow discharges interictally. Cessation of interictal sharp and slow activity, followed by low-voltage fast rhythmic activity over the right frontal region. B. At 10 sec rhythmic discharges become slower (4 Hz) and higher in voltage. C. At 20 sec mixed high voltage, 1.5–2.5 Hz activity, which is most prominent over the right hemisphere and is associated with sharp and spike discharges and gradual attenuation of ictal rhythmic activity. D. At 30 sec there is postictal slowing. (From L. R. Geiger and R. N. Harner [8]. Copyright 1978, American Medical Association.)

Table 4-2. Ictal EEG Patterns
in 41 Patients With Focal Seizures

Ictal Pattern	Percent of Patients
Rhythmic Ictal Transformation (RIT)	
13–30 Hz	50
8–12 Hz	10
4–7 Hz	20
RIT + persistence of interictal sharp activity	10
No Change From Interictal Pattern	10
Total	100

Source: Geiger and Harner [8]. Copyright 1978, American Medical Association.

causing the RIT. They present evidence that the frequency of the initial RIT is principally dependent upon the distance from the epileptogenic focus at which the recording is made. The closer one is to the source of the RIT, the more rapid is the initial RIT.

Differential Diagnosis

MIGRAINE

The differentiation between migraine and simple partial seizures with sensory-motor, visual, vertiginous, or auditory symptomatology may be difficult. This is particularly true in childhood migraine where an attack may consist of a neurologic prodrome (e.g., scotoma) without headache and may be complicated by true epileptic manifestations (presumably secondary to transient cerebral ischemia). In such cases the EEG may be abnormal for several days after an attack. A positive family history of migraine and a previous history of paroxysmal headaches of vascular type should be actively searched for. Whereas patients with migraine do not describe vividly their symptoms throughout the attack, and bystanders are usually able to document at least partial impairment of consciousness during the seizure. Fear of impending danger may be pronounced and persistent throughout an attack of migraine because of acute awareness of the events. A sensation of fear is not a useful point in the differential diagnosis of migraine versus complex partial seizures.

SYNCOPE

Syncopal attacks may mimic closely partial seizures with autonomic manifestations (see Chap. 10). Syncope is frequent in children, in whom vagal reflexes are particularly easy to elicit, and in predisposed individuals of all ages. A finding of a positive family history for fainting is helpful. The essential point is to establish a cause-and-effect relationship between the triggering events and the attacks and, possibly, to reproduce an attack in the EEG laboratory during electrocardiographic (ECG) monitoring [20].

TRANSIENT ISCHEMIC ATTACK

For a discussion of transient ischemic attacks, see Chapter 5.

Management

ESTABLISHMENT OF DIAGNOSIS AND ETIOLOGY

Since by definition simple partial seizures are secondary to a hemispheric lesion, the presence of a progressive, treatable condition (neoplasm, brain abscess, encephalitis, vasculitis) must be ruled out. Negative findings during early investigations or a history of preceding cerebral insult (e.g., head trauma, perinatal anoxia) do not exclude new pathology. Therefore, possible progression of lesions must be monitored carefully during follow-up examinations by asking about changing patterns in seizure symptomatology and by repeated neurologic examinations, EEGs, and anatomic studies. The advent of the CT scan has revealed an unexpectedly large number of cases of long-standing partial seizures due to slowly growing neoplasms [7].

Identification and correction of the underlying causes and precipitating factors (e.g., metabolic abnormality states, congenital heart defects, infection) represent the first step of rational management. When an anatomically accessible lesion is identified (abscess, hematoma, tumor), surgical intervention should be considered. Meanwhile, symptomatic control and prevention of further seizure activity by pharmacologic means is mandatory.

Videotape recording of ictal events and concomitant EEG allow careful analysis of the clinical manifestations. The ability to follow a rapid sequence of events in slow motion may offer cues to the correct localization of the point of seizure origin and the correct classification of seizure type(s). In appropriate settings, temporary diminution of antiepileptic drugs to increase the chances of observing a seizure during prolonged monitoring is a recommended procedure.

ANTIEPILEPTIC DRUGS

Phenytoin, carbamazepine, phenobarbital, and primidone are the drugs usually employed to treat simple partial seizures. The relative advantages and disadvantages of these four drugs are reviewed in Chapter 14. When migraine and seizure phenomena coexist in the same patient, a combination of antiepileptic drugs and drugs for the prevention of migraine may be the most effective treatment.

ELECTIVE SURGERY

"Elective" surgery for partial seizures should be considered when conservative measures (treatment of underlying causes and antiepileptic drugs) have proven ineffective. Patients with poorly controlled partial seizures due to chronic epileptogenic foci should be recommended for consideration of surgery only in specialized centers because the appropriate selection of patients for such treatment is crucial. Appropriate selection requires performance of sophisticated neurophysiologic, radiologic, and neuropsychologic tests, and interpretation of the test results by persons experienced in the application of such test results to selection of candidates for cortical resection procedures. Surgery for partial seizures is reviewed in more detail in Chapter 25 and elsewhere [28].

Prognosis

Studies on the prognosis of simple partial seizures have produced conflicting results [13]. Some early studies report that focal seizures of nontemporal lobe origin follow the same relatively good course as nonfocal tonic-clonic seizures, that is, good seizure control in 50 to 75 percent of patients [6, 12, 47]. On the other hand, several studies report a less favorable outcome for simple partial seizures, good seizure control being obtained in only 25 to 35 percent of patients [16, 25, 42]. In a study of 19 children with Jacksonian seizures and a good seizure control with antiepileptic drugs, 11 (58%) had a recurrence of seizures when antiepileptic drugs were discontinued [41a]. Simple partial seizures in patients with intracranial tumors or a combination of seizure types are more difficult to control, and some of the variability in the reported studies may be due to these factors [12, 16, 37, 41a].

Age at onset of simple partial seizures is also an important factor. Focal seizures in the newborn are often caused by transient, nonstructural conditions and carry a good prognosis for later spontaneous cessation of seizures (see Chap. 26) [3, 18]. Focal seizures beginning between 6 months and 9 years of age are sometimes followed by spontaneous remission [3, 13], especially the benign childhood Sylvian seizures [16a, 17]. Spontaneous remission is unlikely if simple partial seizures begin after 9 years of age [13]. Appropriate selection requires performance of sophisticated neurophysiologic, radiologic, and neuropsychologic tests, and interpretation of the test results by persons experienced in the application of such test results to selection of candidates for cortical resection procedures.

References

1. Ajmone-Marsan, C., and Ralston, B. *The Epileptic Seizure.* Springfield, Ill.: Thomas, 1957.
2. Babb, T. L. et al. Neuronal firing patterns during the spread of an occipital seizure to the temporal lobes in man. *Electroencephalogr. Clin. Neurophysiol.* 51:104, 1981.
3. Beaussart, M., Beaussart-Boulange, L., and LeSoin, J. J. On 340 cases of infantile convulsions. *Electroencephalogr. Clin. Neurophysiol.* 22:95, 1967.
4. Daly, D. D. Ictal clinical manifestations of complex partial seizures. *Adv. Neurol.* 11:57, 1975.
5. Dreifuss, R. E. Proposal for revised clinical and electroencephalographic classification of epileptic seizures. *Epilepsia* 22:489, 1981.
6. Frantzen, E. An analysis of the results of treatment of epileptics under ambulatory supervision. *Epilepsia* 2:207, 1961.
7. Gastaut, H., and Gastaut, J. L. Computerized Axial Tomography in Epilepsy. In J. K. Penry (Ed.), *Epilepsy: The Eighth International Symposium.* New York: Raven Press, 1977.
8. Geiger, L. R., and Harner, R. N. EEG patterns at the time of focal seizure onset. *Arch. Neurol.* 35:276, 1978.
9. Gibbs, F. A., and Gibbs, E. L. *Atlas of Electroencephalography,* Vol. 2. Cambridge, Mass.: Addison-Wesley, 1952.
10. Goldensohn, E. S., Zablow, L., and Stein, B. Interrelationships of form and latency of spike discharge from small areas of human cortex. *Electroencephalogr. Clin. Neurophysiol.* 29:321, 1970.
11. Harner, R. N. The significance of focal hypersynchrony in clinical EEG. *Electroencephalogr. Clin. Neurophysiol.* 31:293, 1971.
11a. Howe, J. G., and Gibson, J. D. Uncinate seizures and tumors: A myth reexamined. *Ann. Neurol.* 11:227, 1982.
12. Jüül-Jensen, P. *Epilepsy: A Clinical and Social Analysis of 1020 Adult Patients with Epileptic Seizures.* Copenhagen: Munksgaard, 1963.
13. Kiørboe, E. Medical Prognosis of Epilepsy. In P. J. Vinken, and G. W. Bruyn (Eds.), *Handbook of Clinical Neurology,* Vol. 15, *The Epilepsies.* Amsterdam: Elsevier, 1974.
14. Kogeorgos, J., Scott, D. F., and Swash, M. Clinical features and management of vertiginous TLE. *Electroencephalogr. Clin. Neurophysiol.* 51:52P, 1981.
15. Kooi, K. A., Tucker, R. P., and Marshall, R. E. *Fundamentals of Electroencephalography.* Hagerstown, Md.: Harper & Row, 1978.

38

16. Kuhl, V., Kiørboe, E., and Lund, M. The prognosis of epilepsy with special reference to traffic security. *Epilepsia* 8:195, 1967.

16a. Lerman, P., and Kivity, S. Benign focal epilepsy of childhood: A follow up study of 100 recovered patients. *Arch. Neurol.* 32:261, 1975.

17. Lombroso, C. T. Sylvian seizures and mid temporal spike foci in children. *Arch. Neurol.* 17:52, 1967.

18. Lombroso, C. T. Convulsive Disorders in Newborns. In R. Thompson (Ed.), *Pediatric Neurology and Neurosurgery.* New York: S. P. Medical and Scientific Books, 1978.

19. Lombroso, C. T., and Erba, G. Primary and secondary bilateral synchrony in epilepsy: A clinical and electroencephalographic study. *Arch. Neurol.* 22:321, 1970.

20. Lombroso, C. T., and Lerman, P. Breath holding spells (cyanotic and pallid infantile syncope). *Pediatrics* 38:563, 1967.

21. Martin, H. L., and McDowell, F. Evaluation of seizures in the adult. *Arch. Neurol. Psychiat.* 71:101, 1954.

22. Newmark, M. E., and Penry, J. K. *Genetics of Epilepsy: A Review.* New York: Raven Press, 1980.

23. Niedermeyer, E., Zobniw, A. M., and Yarworth, S. Depth electroencephalography. *J. Electrophys. Techn.* 1:215, 1976.

24. Ochs, R. F., Gloor, P., and Ives, J. P. The diagnostic value of head turning in the localization of seizures. *Neurology* 32:92a, 1982.

25. Penfield, W., and Jasper, H. *Epilepsy and the Functional Anatomy of the Human Brain.* Boston: Little, Brown, 1954.

26. Penfield, W., and Rasmussen, T. *The Cerebral Cortex of Man.* London: Macmillan, 1950.

27. Penfield, W., and Welch, K. The supplementary motor area of the cerebral cortex: A clinical and experimental study. *Arch. Neurol. Psychiat.* 66:289, 1961.

28. Purpura, D. P., Penry, J. K., and Walter, R. D. (Eds.). *Neurosurgical Management of the Epilepsies.* New York: Raven Press, 1975.

29. Racy, A. et al. Epileptic aphasia: First onset of prolonged monosymptomatic status epilepticus in adults. *Arch. Neurol.* 37:418, 1980.

30. Ralston, B. L., and Papatheodorou, C. A. The mechanism of transition of interictal spiking foci into ictal seizure discharges: Observations in man. *Electroencephalogr. Clin. Neurophysiol.* 12:297, 1960.

31. Rasmussen, T. Surgical treatment of patients with complex partial seizures. *Adv. Neurol.* 11:415, 1975.

32. Rasmussen, T. Seizures With Local Onset and Elementary Symptomatology. In P. J. Vinken, and G. W. Bruyn (Eds.), *Handbook of Clinical Neurology,* Vol. 15, *The Epilepsies.* Amsterdam: Elsevier, 1974.

33. Rasmussen, T., and McCann, W. Epilepsy due to chronic encephalitis. Its course and results of surgical therapy. *Trans. Am. Neurol. Assoc.* 93:89, 1968.

34. Raynor, R. B., Paine, R. S., and Carmichael, E. A. Epilepsy of late onset. *Neurology* 9:111, 1959.

35. Remillard, G. M., Ethier, R., and Anderman, F. Temporal lobe epilepsy and perinatal occlusion of the posterior cerebral artery: A syndrome analogous to infantile hemiplegia and demonstrable etiology in some patients. *Neurology* 24:1001, 1974.

36. Richardson, E. P., and Dodge, P. R. Epilepsy in cerebral vascular disease. *Epilepsia* 3:49, 1954.

37. Rodin, E. A. *The Prognosis of Patients with Epilepsy.* Springfield, Ill.: Thomas, 1968.

38. Smith, B. H. Vestibular disturbances in epilepsy. *Neurology* 10:465, 1960.

39. Sumi, S. M., and Teasdale, R. D. Focal seizures: A review of 150 cases. *Neurology* 13:582, 1963.

40. Taylor, J. (Ed.). *Selected Writings of John Hughlings Jackson.* London: Hodder & Stoughton, 1931.

41. Tharp, B. R. Orbital frontal seizures: A unique electroencephalographic and clinical syndrome. *Epilepsia* 13:627, 1972.

41a. Thurston, J. H. et al. Prognosis in childhood epilepsy: Additional follow-up of 148 children 15 to 23 years after withdrawal of anticonvulsant therapy. *N. Engl. J. Med.* 306:831, 1982.

42. Trolle, E. Drug therapy of epilepsy. *Acta Psychiat. Scand.* 36 (Suppl. 150):187, 1961.

43. Waddington, M. M. Angiographic changes in focal motor epilepsy. *Neurology* 20:879, 1970.

44. Ward, A. A. Basic Mechanisms of the Epilepsies. In M. Critchley, J. L. O'Leary, and B. Jennett (Eds.), *Scientific Foundations of Neurology.* Philadelphia: Davis, 1972.

45. White, P. T., Bailey, A. A., and Bickford, R. G. Epileptic disorders in the aged. *Neurology* (Minneap.) 3:674, 1953.

46. Williamson, P. D. et al. Complex partial seizures with occipital lobe onset. *Epilepsia* 22:247, 1981.

47. Yahr, M. D., and Merritt, H. H. The drug therapy of convulsive seizures. *Int. J. Neurol.* (Montevideo) 1:76, 1959.

48. Yang, P. J. et al. Computed tomography and childhood seizure disorders. *Neurology* 29:1084, 1979.

COMPLEX PARTIAL SEIZURES (PSYCHOMOTOR OR TEMPORAL LOBE SEIZURES)

Robert G. Feldman

Definitions

The central feature of complex partial seizures (CPS) is impairment of consciousness. Impairment of consciousness is defined as the inability to respond normally to exogenous stimuli by virtue of altered awareness or responsiveness [10]. Responsiveness refers to the ability of the patient to carry out simple commands or willed movement, and awareness refers to the patient's contact with events during the period in question and its recall [10].

The period of impairment of consciousness may or may not be preceded by symptoms or signs of a simple partial seizure. There may be no other manifestations during the period of impaired consciousness, or there may be automatisms (that is, nonreflex actions performed "automatically," without conscious volition and for which the patient has no recollection).

CPS in its various forms, constitutes 42% of the partial seizure category and 20% of all types of epilepsy [23]. The common overlap of psychogenic behavioral manifestations and clinical phenomena associated with CPS makes diagnosis and management difficult and challenging.

Etiology

NEUROPATHOLOGIC FINDINGS

Several groups have studied the neuropathology of specimens taken from patients undergoing temporal lobe resection for CPS and have reported similar results [12, 26a, 37]. Approximately 50 percent of the specimens examined showed mesial temporal sclerosis, with loss of nerve cells in the hippocampus accompanied by fibrosis, gliosis, and atrophy. The possible role of febrile seizures in producing mesial temporal sclerosis is discussed in Chapter 27. Another 20 percent of the specimens showed circumscribed foci of abnormal tissue ("hamartomas"). Ten percent of specimens had miscellaneous lesions such as tumors, posttraumatic scars, infections, vascular lesions, and tuberous sclerosis. Approximately 20 percent of the specimens showed no lesions.

CT SCANS

The CT scan is abnormal in 30 to 50 percent of patients with CPS [47, 48, 63]. Focal CT scan abnormalities are found in approximately 25 percent of patients with

Table 5-1. Observed Responses to Stimulation of Temporal Lobe Structures in Humans

Structure Stimulated	Observed Response
Temporal neocortex	
Primary auditory area (anterior temporal gyrus of Heschel, either side)	Unformed auditory sensation (e.g., buzz, whistle)
Auditory association areas (superior temporal convulution, either side)	Formed auditory hallucination or illusion
Visual association area (posterior temporal cortex, nondominant side)*	Formed visual hallucination or illusion
Other structures	Reproduction of experiences, déjà vu, jamais vu, affective changes
Insula	Visceral sensations
Amygdaloid and periamygdaloid area	Psychoparetic reactions, vague emotional sensations of anxiety or fear, decreased awareness, elaborate functional behavior including learned acts, activation of secretions, masticatory movements, vocalization, shifting, arrest of motor activity, contraversive conjugate deviation of head and eyes, ipsilateral face twitching, complex visual hallucinations
Hippocampus	Memory disturbances, fear, grooming and pleasure reactions (including penile erection), inhibition of secretions, complex visual hallucinations

*Stimulation of primary visual area in occipital lobe produces unformed visual sensations, such as colored lights, stars, or colored flashes.
Source: Data from Gloor et al. [21a], Kaada [28], Penfield and Jasper [44], Penfield and Perot [45], and Van Buren [60].

CPS [47]. A CT scan is more likely to be abnormal in CPS patients whose age of onset of CPS was over 30 years or who have mesiobasal EEG discharges [47].

GENETICS

A genetic tendency has not been definitely established for patients with CPS [43].

Pathophysiology

The basic mechanisms underlying focal seizure discharges are reviewed in Chapter 2. The pathophysiology of simple partial seizures and simple partial seizures evolving to CPS, generalized seizures, or both is reviewed in Chapter 4. This section will review the pathophysiology of discharges in temporal-limbic structures thought to be responsible for CPS.

Functional connections of the limbic system produce the behaviors and experiences that occur during a CPS. An elaborate system of association pathways from the hippocampal formation provides the means for the spread of seizure activity from one focus to other areas. Using depth electrode recording techniques during CPS, one routinely finds seizure activity in several limbic system sites: cingulate gyrus, amygdala, hippocampus, hippocampal gyrus, and selected thalamic nuclei [5]. The actual focus of origin of the seizure activity in a given patient usually is determined by finding the site where seizure activity

is first recorded by the depth electrodes. Electrical stimulation of temporal lobe structures during neurosurgical procedures with local anesthesia also has led to elucidation of the pathophysiology of CPS in humans. The results of this work are summarized in Table 5-1. Analysis of the anatomic substrata of CPS offers an explanation for the various clinical manifestations and electroclinical relationships of this disorder [17, 31].

Seizure Phenomena

CLASSIFICATION

The central feature of CPS is impairment of consciousness. The period of impaired consciousness may or may not be preceded by symptoms or signs (motor, sensory, autonomic, or psychic) of a simple partial seizure. There may be no other symptoms or signs during the period of impaired consciousness, or automatisms may be present. The International Classification of Epileptic Seizures [10] divides CPS into four groups: (1) CPS with simple partial onset followed by impairment of consciousness only, (2) CPS with simple partial onset followed by impaired consciousness and automatisms, (3) CPS with impairment of consciousness at onset with impairment of consciousness only, and (4) CPS with impairment of consciousness at onset with automatisms.

Three major areas describe seizure phenomena during CPS: (1) impairment of consciousness; (2) types of simple partial onset; and (3) automatisms.

IMPAIRMENT OF CONSCIOUSNESS

Impairment of consciousness is defined above. During the period of impaired consciousness a patient may look "vacant" or "frightened." Although sometimes able to recount vague sensations, the patient does not realize that anything more has occurred.

TYPES OF SIMPLE PARTIAL ONSET

Simple Partial Onset with Motor Signs,
with Somatosensory or Special Sensory Symptoms,
with Autonomic Symptoms or Signs
See Chapter 4.

Simple Partial Onset with Psychic Symptoms
Psychic symptoms (disturbances of cerebral function) occasionally can occur without impairment of consciousness as part of a simple partial seizure. More commonly, psychic symptoms occur in association with impaired consciousness as part of a CPS. This association presumably exists because focal discharges responsible for psychic symptoms often arise in or near temporal-limbic structures (see Table 5-1) and frequently trigger discharge sufficient to impair consciousness. The frequent association of psychic symptoms and motor automatisms with CPS is responsible for the old term *psychomotor seizure.*

The psychic symptoms that occur during a CPS may be: (1) dysphasic, (2) dysmnesic, (3) cognitive, (4) affective, (5) illusions, or (6) structured hallucinations.

Dysphasic symptoms may take the form of speech arrest, vocalization, or palilalia (involuntary repetition of a syllable or phrase) [10].

Dysmnesic symptoms, distortions of memory, may take the form of a temporal disorientation, a dreamy state, a flashback, a sensation as if an experience had occurred before (déjà vu, if visual; déjà entendu, if auditory), or a sensation as if a previously experienced sensation had not been experienced (jamais vu, if visual; jamais entendu, if auditory) [10, 22, 24]. Occasionally a patient may experience a rapid recollection of episodes from the past (panoramic vision) [10, 24].

Jackson [24] reported a patient who spoke of a "peculiar train of ideas as reminiscence of a former life," and another who said, "It seems as if I went back to all that occurred in my childhood." After a seizure one of our patients recounts the sensation of being in a "deep, dark tunnel" from which he cannot get out; he had been trapped in a coal bin as a child.

Cognitive symptoms may include dreamy states, distortions of time sense, and sensations of unreality,

detachment, or depersonalization [10]. Prolonged episodes of confusion and inability to function cognitively for as long as 2 days, during which the EEG showed continuous, semirhythmic, 4- to 6-Hz spike activity over both frontotemporal regions, have been reported [38].

Affective symptoms may include fear, pleasure, displeasure, depression, rage, anger, irritability, elation, and eroticism [7, 10]. Some individuals may have inappropriate affective reactions to environmental stimuli, possibly because of misinterpretation of cues during the clouded consciousness of a seizure [9]. Fear is the most frequent affective symptom and may be accompanied by objective signs of autonomic activity such as pupil dilation, pallor, flushing, piloerection, palpitation, and hypertension [10].

Unlike the affective symptoms of psychiatric disease, those of CPS occur in attacks lasting a few minutes, tend to be unprovoked by environmental stimuli, and usually abate rapidly [10]. An eight-year-old patient of ours clings to her mother during a CPS lasting 2 minutes or less. After "holding on" during the seizure, the patient "snaps out of it" and states that she has had a "feeling that something terrible will happen."

Less commonly, patients describe exhilaration, elation, serenity, satisfaction, and pleasure (ecstatic seizures, Dostoyevsky epilepsy) [4, 62]. The enjoyable sensation may be similar to or different from sexual pleasure [4]. Sexual pleasure during an aura may consist of either sexual arousal or orgasm [6, 7, 49]. Sexual affect must be differentiated from nonsexual sensory hallucinations of the genital areas [46, 49].

Violent affect and behavior during CPS are discussed below.

Illusions are distorted perceptions in which objects are perceived as deformed [10]. Polyoptic illusions such as monocular diplopia, macropsia, micropsia, or distortions of distance may occur. Distortions of sound, including microacusia and macroacusia, may be experienced. Depersonalization, a feeling that the person is outside the body, may occur. The patient may experience altered perception of the size or weight of a limb.

Structured hallucinations are perceptions without corresponding external stimuli and may affect somatosensory, visual, auditory, olfactory, or gustatory senses [10]. Seizures arising from primary receptive areas tend to give rather primitive hallucinations, whereas seizures arising from association areas tend to give more elaborate symptoms (see Chap. 4 and Table 5-1) [10].

AUTOMATISMS

Definition

The International Classification of Epileptic Seizures [10] has adopted Gastaut's [15] definition of automatisms:

More or less coordinated…involuntary motor activity occurring during the state of clouding of consciousness either in the course of, or after, an epileptic seizure, usually followed by amnesia of the event.

The automatism may be simply a continuation of an activity that was going on when the seizure occurred, or it may be a new activity developed in association with the ictal impairment of consciousness. Usually the activity is commonplace in nature, often provoked by the subject's environment or by sensations during the seizure; fragmentary, primitive, infantile, or antisocial behavior is occasionally seen. Automatisms can be detected in more than 90 percent of CPS recorded on videotape and reviewed in detail later [11, 59].

Gastaut and Broughton [16] distinguish five types of phenomena that may occur during an automatism: alimentary, mimetic, gestural, ambulatory, and verbal.

Alimentary. Automatic chewing movements, increased salivation, or borborygmus may occur as a CPS automatism.

Mimetic. Movements of the face resulting in expressions of fear, bewilderment, discomfort, or vacant tranquillity are components of mimetic automatisms. Mimetic automatisms may also be associated with laughing (gelastic seizures) or crying (lacrimonic seizures).

Gestural. Repetitive movements of the hands and fingers noted during gestural seizures may resemble purposeful behavior. Patients may appear to be carrying out an elaborate task or simply patting their hands in a particular fashion. Sexual gestures such as masturbating activity or pelvic thrusting, which may occur as part of a CPS, are associated chiefly with CPS that originate in the frontal area of the brain [52].

Ambulatory. Wandering or running (cursive seizures) are dangerous forms of CPS, because consciousness is impaired during the automatism, and the patient may unknowingly run out into traffic or into obstacles.

Verbal. Sometimes shrill cries occur with the onset of a tonic-clonic seizure, and humming may occur during an absence seizure. However, audible verbal expressions are almost exclusively a feature of automatic behavior in CPS. Short phrases, expletives, or swearing commonly are repeated in an automatic fashion. The spontaneous vocalization of words may reflect a previous experience. For example, a patient

Table 5-2. Automatisms During Complex Partial Seizures in 79 Patients

Automatism	No. of Patients
Chewing, swallowing, pursing lips	74
Looking around, smiling, grimacing or crying	43
Attempting to sit up	39
Examining or fumbling with objects	28
Tonic adversive head turning	11
Bilateral arm movements	11
Bilateral leg movements	11
Fighting restraint	7
Unilateral tonic extremity motion	7
Verbalization	6
Standing up	6
Walking or running away	6

Source: Modified from Escueta et al. [11].

of ours has seizures characterized by vocal repetition of "Myer, you're killing me!" These episodes, which began at age 64 after a small cerebral infarction in the temporal lobe, were misdiagnosed as paranoid ideation until an EEG confirmed a paroxysmal disorder. The statement referred to his old friend Myer, with whom he had played cards more than 25 years earlier.

One should be aware that the patient may recognize the onset of a CPS during the aura and produce volitional verbal expressions. This prescience commonly causes outcries such as "Here it comes!" or "No, no, no!"

Relative Frequency of Automatisms.

The relative frequency with which various types of automatisms were observed in 79 patients with CPS is shown in Table 5-2.

COMPOUND FORMS OF CPS

Most complex partial seizures exhibit a combination of the symptoms listed above. Escueta et al. [11] studied 691 CPS occurring in 79 patients and found that most CPS were compound forms of two types.

Type I CPS accounted for 405 of the 691 attacks and had three clinical phases. During phase I, the patient was essentially motionless and totally unresponsive to superficial and deep pain. After approximately 10 seconds, a phase II of 10 to 60 seconds' duration was observed. During this time the patient remained unresponsive and showed automatisms such as repeated chewing, blinking, and swallowing. During phase III, the longest phase of type I (0.5 to 12 minutes), impairment of consciousness of a less profound nature was observed. Automatisms could be interrupted, and the patient sometimes reacted to environmental cues. This phase is best described as a "cloudy state." Type II CPS accounted for 286 of the 691 attacks and consisted of reactive automatisms during impaired consciousness; a motionless staring state was not observed, although stereotyped movements occurred. Automatisms occurring during the cloudy states of type II or during phase III of type I attacks were considered reactive because the behavior appeared purposeful. Amnesia for the entire attack ensued. Motor responses were coordinated and were sufficient to carry out the patient's intended actions; they appeared both appropriate and inappropriate.

AURA

The aura of a CPS is that portion of the seizure that occurs before consciousness is lost and for which memory is retained after the seizure [10]. In practice, the aura is usually the simple partial onset of a "CPS with simple partial onset." The aura is truly part of the seizure and is not a preictal phenomenon. The aura, however, may warn that consciousness will soon be lost. Auras occur in approximately 50 percent of patients with CPS and most commonly take the form of fear, rising epigastric sensation, unilateral "funny feeling" or "numbness," or visual disturbances [11].

DURATION OF CPS

Clinical complex partial seizures (including time elapsed until recovery of normal consciousness) may last 11 seconds to 28 minutes [11, 59]. The average total duration of a CPS is 1 to 3 minutes [11, 59]. In one study [59], the actual seizures lasted 3 to 241 seconds (mean, 49 seconds), and the postictal phase lasted 3 to 433 seconds (mean, 69 seconds).

CPS EVOLVING TO GENERALIZED SEIZURES

The seizure discharges of a CPS may become secondarily generalized, producing a generalized seizure (tonic-clonic, tonic, or clonic).

SIMPLE PARTIAL SEIZURES EVOLVING TO CPS, EVOLVING TO GENERALIZED SEIZURES

See Chapter 4.

CPS STATUS EPILEPTICUS

See Chapter 30.

EEG Phenomena

INTERICTAL EEG

Almost 50 percent of the patients studied during the interictal period by Gibbs and Gibbs [20] had normal EEG tracings during wakefulness. But when supplementary electrodes and activation procedures were used, this number dropped to 10 percent. Gibbs et al. [19] identified a "psychomotor type of discharge" in 300 epileptic subjects. These were spikes arising from the anterior temporal region in 90 percent of patients who had a history of CPS. Although most spike activity in patients with CPS was located over the anterior temporal area (73%) [19, 20], Gastaut et al. [17] found that interictal discharges were located outside the temporal region in 8% of the patients. About 25 to 30 percent of patients have bitemporal discharging [20]. Clinical manifestations of seizures were correlated with EEG findings in the study of King and Ajmone-Marsan [29]. Primary visual auras occurred in 32 percent of patients with EEG abnormalities located posteriorly, whereas visual auras occurred in only 5 percent of patients with anterior foci. A sensation of fear was more common in patients with unilateral than bilateral temporal spikes. Automatic behavior was seen in 95 percent of patients with temporal spike activity, 53 percent of patients with frontocentral foci, and 61 percent of those with central disturbances. Auras of déjà vu were present exclusively in patients with anterior temporal abnormalities.

The paroxysms may not be limited to a site localized over one temporal region. When they arise from temporal areas bilaterally, they may be independent of one another, synchronous, or transmitted from one side to the other by commissural pathways. Bilateral discharges independent of one another were found in 80 percent of patients with CPS [17]. Jasper et al. [26] found epileptic discharges confined to one temporal lobe in 34 percent, transmitted from one temporal lobe to the opposite in 24 percent, synchronous on both sides in 19 percent, and independent on both sides in 23 percent. Focal discharges arising in the mesial surface of the frontal lobe may trigger generalized bisynchronous paroxysmal discharges [26].

ICTAL EEG

During a clinical CPS, any of the following can be recorded from scalp EEG electrodes: (1) sustained rhythm of spikes or sharp waves and rhythmic slowing, (2) attenuation of amplitude (suppression), (3) rhythmic slow waves, (4) 10- to 30-Hz fast activity, (5) spike-wave complexes, (6) other changes or variants of the above, or (7) no change (10 to 30% of patients) [1, 11, 31]. These patterns may be focal, lateralized, bilateral or diffuse. The relative frequency with which these patterns are recorded during CPS is shown in Table 5-3.

Table 5-3. EEG Patterns Recorded During Complex Partial Seizures in 79 Patients

Pattern	No. of Patients	
Focal	30	
Initial low-voltage 18 to 30 Hz or 10 to 12 Hz in one NP electrode		19
Bimedial temporal 20 to 30 Hz rhythms with phase reversals in one NP electrode		6
Frontotemporal 2 Hz spike waves with phase reversals in one NP electrode		2
Initial 3 to 6 Hz waves in NP and lateral temporal electrode on one side		3
Lateralizing	9	
Diffuse onset on one hemisphere with 12 Hz spikes		7
Diffuse bilateral 6 Hz waves prominent in the temporal lobe and occipital area of one side		2
Bimedial temporal	15	
20 to 30 Hz in both NP electrodes without focal features		15
Diffuse and bilateral	25	
4 to 6 Hz sharp waves or low-voltage slow waves		18
Diffuse low-voltage 18 to 30 Hz		3
10 to 20 Hz discharges lateralized to different sides during different attacks		4
Total	79	

Source: Modified from Escueta et al. [11].

POSTICTAL EEG

The postictal EEG usually consists of generalized or localized delta activity. Postictal changes may provide information about lateralization or localization of the site of origin of a CPS. Localized or asymmetrical delta activity is evident after about 40 percent of CPS. If interictal paroxysmal abnormalities in the EEG had been present before the seizure, they usually are absent in the immediate postictal period and reappear gradually as the postictal delta activity diminishes. When a CPS becomes a generalized seizure and terminates with a tonic-clonic attack, the postictal EEG abnormality is characterized by diffuse slowing [1] (see Chap. 6).

SPECIAL TECHNIQUES

Sleep EEG (see Chap. 11)

Sleep activates anterior temporal spike discharging [20]. Sleep studies are critical for demonstrating EEG abnormalities in 10 percent or more of seizure patients. The use of sleep to bring out evidence of focal epileptic activity in a patient suspected of having CPS requires a recording that includes stages 1 to 3 of non-REM sleep [32]. Most interictal epileptiform abnormalities, including focal spikes and sharp waves in patients with CPS, emerge or increase in number during non-REM sleep but decrease or disappear during REM sleep. Sleep deprivation has value in activating seizure discharges. Mattson et al. [39] found that after being deprived of sleep for 26 to 28 hours, 34 percent of seizure patients whose EEGs previously had been normal showed activation of focal or generalized epileptiform disturbances, and abnormalities that had been present previously increased in 56 percent of seizure patients.

Extra Scalp Electrodes

Extra scalp electrodes, in addition to electrodes in the standard positions of the International 10–20 System, in regions selected for the individual patient may help localize an abnormality.

Nasopharyngeal and Sphenoidal Electrodes (see Chap. 11)

Nasopharyngeal and sphenoidal electrodes detect abnormalities (usually mesial temporal spikes) that could not be detected by surface electrodes in 7 percent or more of the EEGs of patients with CPS. Nasopharyngeal and sphenoidal electrodes are equally good for detection of the presence of mesial temporal spikes, although sphenoidal electrodes provide more reliable information on the lateralization of mesial temporal spikes. Nasopharyngeal and sphenoidal leads also have been used to assess asymmetry of beta activity induced by administration of barbiturate compounds. Unilateral reduction of beta activity in recordings made with sphenoidal leads has been correlated with mesial temporal sclerosis and unilateral temporal lobe damage.

Hyperventilation

Hyperventilation can precipitate focal EEG discharges, clinical seizures, or both in some patients with CPS (see Chap. 11).

Depth Electrodes (see Chap. 25)

Intracerebral depth electrodes have provided information about the precise site(s) of origin of CPS not otherwise obtainable by scalp electrodes [5]. The combination of scalp electrodes, depth electrodes, and computer analysis of EEGs during seizures may improve accuracy in predicting the site of origin of seizure activity [5, 34].

Differential Diagnosis

The recognition of a CPS is difficult in some instances because the clinical expression may resemble absence seizures, migraine, syncope, transient ischemic attacks, or affective psychosis. Furthermore, hysterical seizures may resemble CPS, and some patients have both CPS and hysterical seizures. It is imperative that CPS be differentiated from these other entities because therapy for each is different.

The setting in which the episode occurs, the associated findings, the mode of onset, and the mode of recovery may be useful indicators of etiology. Therefore, a careful history and time profile of events must be obtained in each case.

CPS VS. ABSENCE SEIZURE
See Chapter 7.

CPS VS. MIGRAINE, SYNCOPE, AND MOTIVATIONALLY
DETERMINED EPISODIC BEHAVIOR
(HYSTERICAL SEIZURES, PSEUDOSEIZURES)
See Chapter 10.

CPS VS. TRANSIENT ISCHEMIC ATTACK (TIA)
Transient weakness, sensory loss, paresthesias, speech arrest, or amnesia may be due to a CPS or a TIA. A CPS is more likely if the patient is young, loses consciousness, or has psychic symptoms or automatisms. A TIA is more likely if the patient is middle aged, has cardiovascular disease, or has symptoms (transient monocular blindness) or signs (carotid bruit, decreased carotid pulse) typically associated with the TIA syndrome. These clinical criteria do not definitively differentiate a CPS from a TIA because consciousness may be lost during a TIA, because most middle aged patients will have evidence of vascular disease if examined carefully, and because cerebrovascular accidents not infrequently result in seizures (see Chap. 12). The EEG between attacks may be normal or show focal slowing in both a CPS and a TIA. The presence of focal spikes on the EEG strongly suggests a partial seizure disorder.

CPS VS. AFFECTIVE PSYCHOSIS
When ideational disturbances, hallucinations, or inappropriate affects occur during a seizure, they develop suddenly and do not build up over several days or weeks as they do in an affective psychosis.

MISCELLANEOUS
Hypoglycemia, drugs, alcohol, or even the effects of industrial toxins such as carbon dioxide or solvents may induce cognitive nor sensory phenomena similar to CPS.

Neurobehavioral and Psychosocial Aspects of CPS

EMOTIONAL ACTIVATION OF CPS
Patients with CPS are vulnerable to emotional activation of seizure activity because the anatomic structures involved during CPS are those that subserve normal emotional responses [13]. Stevens [54] found that EEG abnormalities were activated by emotional stress in 75 percent of patients with CPS, in fewer than 50 percent of patients with tonic-clonic seizures, and in none of her control subjects. Conversely, reducing emotional stress (which may happen during hospitalization) may decrease the occurrence of CPS.

INTERICTAL PERSONALITY
Several authors [2, 3, 21] have described an "interictal personality" of patients with CPS, characterized by such features as "stickiness," humorlessness, dependence, obsessionalism, circumstantiality, philosophic interests, religiosity, anger, personalized significance attached to trivial events, hypergraphia, altered sexual interest, and emotionality. There is no doubt that some patients with CPS do exhibit these personality traits, but serious questions still exist about how specific these traits are for CPS and what proportion of all patients with CPS have these traits. The psychosocial effects of having any form of epilepsy or any chronic disease and patient referral patterns must be determined before any study of a specific interictal personality for CPS can be evaluated.

*Psychosocial Effects of All Forms
of Epilepsy and Chronic Disease*
Standardized personality tests or profiles have been employed in many studies that have tried to differentiate the interictal personality of individuals with CPS from those with other types of epilepsy or other chronic disease or those with primarily psychiatric disorders. Standage and Fenton [53] found high-current psychiatric morbidity among patients with epilepsy as indicated by raised "previous neurotic illness" scores and raised "neuroticism" scores on the Eysenck Personality Inventory. The authors considered the difference from the control patients, who had chronic musculoskeletal disorders, to be insignificant, however. Selection factors were considered important in this study; thus, the development of psychiatric disturbances in patients with epilepsy made referral to neurologic referral centers more likely. On the present state examinations, a difference was not seen between patients with CPS and patients with other types of epilepsy. Each group of patients with epilepsy showed high scores on depression and accompanying somatic symptoms, irritability, low self-opinion, symp-

toms of anxiety, subjectively impaired memory and concentration, and disturbed interpersonal relationships. These traits were attributed to chronicity of the disability and the possible instability of family structures rather than to specific effects of CPS. Lindsay et al. [35] prospectively studied 100 children with CPS. Eighty-five percent of the subjects had psychologic problems in childhood. Yet 75 percent of the group had no psychiatric disorder in later life. It was concluded that preserved intelligence, controlled epilepsy, and a positive attitude in the family were potent predictors of a good outcome.

Some patients with CPS have a stereotyped way of conducting themselves in stressful situations, and their maneuvers may resemble those in sociopathic personality disorders. Nevertheless, such sociopathic and manipulative acts are seen in other chronic illnesses in which the patient perceives a somatic disturbance as a constant threat to existence. Personality traits that have been considered unique in persons with temporal lobe epilepsy may simply reflect a person's accumulation of learned responses to the feeling of having no control over his environment or his behavior. Parents, teachers, and medical personnel contribute to the patient's self-view by their behavior and reactions [14]. The personality of the individual with epilepsy does not occur in a vacuum but is affected by his relationship with the immediate environment.

Effects of Referral Patterns
The incidence of psychopathology in patients with all types of epilepsy referred to university hospital clinics in the United States reflects the fact that such patients are a select group who, because of seizure intractability, indigence, or psychologic or social failure, tend to gravitate toward publicly supported facilities. The incidence of psychiatric hospitalization among private patients with epilepsy is only one half that of the university clinic population [56].

Prevalence of Interictal Personality or Psychopathology
The prevalence of the interictal personality of CPS, psychopathology, or both among patients with CPS has been variously reported as very high [2, 3], intermediate [35, 58, 61], and low [53, 55]. These discrepancies arise because of differences in control for the effect of chronic disease, in referral patterns, and in study techniques.

Conclusion
Some patients with CPS do exhibit traits of the interictal personality of CPS. More studies are needed, however, to determine the prevalence of these traits in nonselected patients, their specificity for CPS, and the pathophysiology and psychodynamics of the trait.

VIOLENT BEHAVIOR
Attempts to restrain a patient who has clouded sensorium after a tonic-clonic or complex partial seizure may result in defensive and aggressive behavior [8]. Well organized or unprovoked, directed acts of violence are very rarely a manifestation of epilepsy, however.

A distinguished international panel recently has reviewed all available videotaped instances of violence purported to have occurred during a seizure [8]. From an estimated population of 5,400 patients with epilepsy, the authors found only 6 patients with non-directed aggressive motions and 7 patients exhibiting actual or threatened directed violence toward property or persons during seizures. All episodes of directed violence occurred during CPS. The aggressive behavior usually was followed by or mixed with more common types of CPS automatisms (e.g., lip smacking, swallowing, blinking). All aggressive acts appeared suddenly, without evidence of planning, and lasted an average of 29 seconds. All violent automatisms were stereotyped, simple, short-lived, fragmentary, and unsustained, and they never resulted in a consecutive series of purposeful movements. On the basis of these data, the panel concluded that it would be nearly impossible to commit murder or manslaughter during the random, unsustained automatisms of CPS. The violent automatisms were followed by a period of postictal confusion. The patients had no recollection of their violent actions after the seizure.

The panel suggested five relevant criteria for determining whether, in a specific instance, a violent crime was the result of an epileptic seizure. First, the diagnosis of epilepsy in such a person should be established by at least one neurologist with special competence in epilepsy. Second, the presence of epileptic automatisms should be documented by the history and by closed-circuit television and electroencephalographic biotelemetry. Third, the presence of aggression during epileptic automatisms should be verified in a videotape-recorded seizure in which ictal epileptiform patterns are also recorded on the EEG. Fourth, the aggressive or violent act should be characteristic of the patient's habitual seizures, as elicited in the history. Finally, a clinical judgment should be made by the neurologist, attesting to the possibility that the act (the alleged crime) was part of a seizure.

Although serious directed violence rarely, if ever, occurs during a CPS, evidence exists that interictal violent behavior is more common in patients with seizures than in the general population [57]. Stevens and Hermann [57], in reviewing the many variables involved in this association, have concluded that interictal psychopathology and violence occur when bilateral, deep, or diffuse cerebral pathology is present. They regard both the psychopathology and the seizures as epiphenomena of cerebral damage, and they dispute the concept that CPS "cause" psychopathology.

When aggressive behavior or other socially significant episodic disturbances are expressed, it is essential that the possibility of psychogenic, nonepileptic bases for this behavior (emotionally determined episodic behaviors) be ruled out [42]. This topic is reviewed in Chapter 10.

MEMORY LOSS

Poor memory and memory loss are frequent complaints of the patient with CPS. Mayeux et al. [41] formally studied intelligence, auditory and visual memory, and language in three groups of patients: (1) CPS with left temporal EEG focus; (2) CPS with right temporal EEG focus; and (3) generalized seizures. The major abnormality found was poor performance on confrontation-naming tests in patients with CPS and a left temporal EEG focus. This anomia in turn resulted in impairment on many verbal subtests of intelligence and memory.

PSYCHOSIS

A psychosis resembling paranoid schizophrenia has been noted in some patients with CPS [55, 56]. Some have reported, and some have denied, that the psychosis of CPS can be differentiated from schizophrenia because patients with CPS retain more affect and are less socially isolated than are patients with schizophrenia. It is not clear at present whether the psychosis of CPS represents the chance coexistence of CPS and schizophrenia (both common diseases), a psychosocial reaction to epilepsy, or the manifestation of a structural lesion in the limbic system. The psychosis of CPS usually is not improved following temporal lobectomy (see Chap. 25).

EPISODES OF AIMLESS WANDERING (PORIOMANIA)

Patients with CPS may experience prolonged episodes of aimless wandering followed by retrograde amnesia for this behavior. Using three patients and a review of the literature, Mayeux et al. [40] postulated that this behavior is a prolonged postictal automatism and is not psychogenic. Adjustment of antiepileptic drug therapy eliminated this behavior in all three patients.

Management

DRUG THERAPY

Phenytoin, carbamazepine, phenobarbital, and primidone are the standard medications used for treating CPS. The general advantages and disadvantages of these drugs are reviewed in Chapter 14, and specific details of their pharmacology and administration are reviewed in Chapters 16, 17, and 18. The barbiturates (phenobarbital and primidone) have both sedating and disinhibiting properties. Patients with CPS who have irritable, volatile personalities (common after head injuries) may experience a worsening of behavior with barbiturates because of their disinhibiting effect. On the other hand, CPS patients with anxious personalities may experience a decrease in anxiety and emotionally precipitated seizures with barbiturates because of their sedating properties.

NEUROSURGICAL THERAPY

Neurosurgical therapy should be considered only when conventional antiepileptic drugs given together in maximum tolerated doses have failed to control a patient's CPS. However, once it has been established that antiepileptic drugs have failed, one should quickly consider neurosurgical therapy. For both neurophysiologic and psychosocial reasons, a patient with poorly controlled CPS is more likely to have a good response to neurosurgical intervention if the operation is performed early rather than late in the course of the illness.

Temporal lobectomy, the usual neurosurgical procedure for control of CPS, has been performed for over 50 years and produces excellent results in properly selected patients. Complex partial seizures are markedly reduced or abolished in 60 to 70 percent of patients after temporal lobectomy. The morbidity rate is 5 to 10 percent, and the mortality is under 1 percent. Neurosurgical therapy of epilepsy is reviewed in detail in Chapter 25.

BEHAVIORAL THERAPY

Behavioral methods of seizure control, whether drawn from learning theory, conditioning, psychodynamic processes, or various biofeedback techniques, usually have been used as adjuncts to pharmacologic treatment. Accumulating evidence suggests that some behavioral methods may be useful in treating selected patients who have seizure disorders.

Behavioral therapies have three theoretical targets: (1) the seizure as a response to specific environmental triggers (internal and external), (2) the seizure as a reinforced behavior, and (3) the seizure as a symptom of the emotional state of the patient. Treatment programs can be directed toward antecedent events, stimuli, or postictal behavior response. Details of the various forms of behavioral therapy are reviewed in Chapter 24.

Prognosis

Investigations of the relationship between prognosis and seizure type emphasize the relatively poor prognosis of CPS compared with that of a purely generalized disorder [27, 33, 50]. For example, in Jüül-Jensen's [27] study, 36 percent of all patients with seizures involving the temporal lobe became free of seizures, or nearly so, for at least 2 years. If additional signs indicated a temporal lobe disorder (temporal focus in the EEG), only 20 percent had a favorable course compared with 64 percent of patients with tonic-clonic seizures only. Patients exhibiting a combination of various types of seizures generally have a poorer prognosis than do those with a single type [27, 50].

Although strong evidence is lacking, it appears that proper use of modern antiepileptic drugs, aided by the monitoring of blood levels, has decreased the number of seizures among patients with epilepsy. In a comparative study of therapeutic results in patients from the Johns Hopkins Hospital in 1946 and 1963, Livingston [36] showed that in 1946, 17 percent of patients were seizure-free for 5 years. In 1963, however, complete seizure control was obtained in approximately 60 percent of patients, whereas in another 25 percent, seizures were so reduced that they did not cause any significant handicaps. Other factors reported to affect the prognosis of CPS [27, 50] favorably include a low seizure frequency and no sign of mental deterioration prior to therapy, late age at onset of seizures, and relatively short duration of illness prior to therapy.

References

1. Ajmone-Marsan, C., and Ralston, B. L. *The Epileptic Seizure: Its Functional Morphology and Diagnostic Significance.* Springfield, Ill.: Thomas, 1957.
2. Bear, D. M. The Temporal Lobes: An Approach to the Study of Organic Behavioral Changes. In M. S. Gazzaniga (Ed.), *Handbook of Behavioral Neurobiology,* Vol. 2. New York: Plenum, 1979.
3. Bear, D., and Fedio, P. Quantitative analysis of interictal behavior in temporal lobe epilepsy. *Arch. Neurol.* 34:454, 1977.
4. Cirrgnotta, F., Todesco, C. V., and Layares, E. Temporal lobe epilepsy with ecstatic seizures (so-called Dostoyevsky Epilepsy). *Epilepsia* 21: 705, 1980.
5. Crandall, P. H., Walter, R. D., and Dymond, A. The ictal electroencephalographic signal identifying limbic system seizure foci. *Proc. Am. Assoc. Neurol. Surg.* 1:1, 1971.
6. Currier, R. D. et al. Sexual seizures. *Arch. Neurol.* 25:260, 1971.
7. Daly, D. D. Ictal clinical manifestations of complex partial seizures. *Adv. Neurol.* 11:57, 1975.
8. Delgado-Escueta, A. V. et al. The nature of aggression during epileptic seizures. *N. Engl. J. Med.* 305:711, 1981.
9. Detre, T. P., and Feldman, R. G. Behavior Disorder Associated with Seizure States: Pharmacological and Psychosocial Management. In G. H. Glaser (Ed.), *EEG and Behavior.* New York: Basic Books, 1963.
10. Dreifuss, F. E. Proposal for revised clinical and electroencephalographic classification of epileptic seizures. *Epilepsia* 22:489, 1981.
11. Escueta, A. V. D. et al. Complex partial seizures on closed-circuit television and EEG: A study of 691 attacks in 79 patients. *Ann. Neurol.* 11:292, 1982.
12. Falconer, M. A., and Cavanaugh, J. B. Clinicopathological considerations of temporal lobe epilepsy due to small focal lesions: A study of cases submitted to operation. *Brain* 82:483, 1959.
13. Feldman, R. G., and Paul, N. L. Identity of emotional triggers in epilepsy. *J. Nerv. Ment. Dis.* 162:343, 1976.
14. Feldman, R. G., and Ricks, N. L. Non-pharmacologic and Behavioral Methods. In G. S. Ferris (Ed.), *Treatment of Epilepsy Today.* Oradell, N.J.: Medical Economics Co., Book Division, 1978.
15. Gastaut, H. Definitions. In *Dictionary of Epilepsy,* Part 1. Geneva: World Health Organization, 1973.
16. Gastaut, H., and Broughton, R. *Epileptic Seizures.* Springfield, Ill.: Thomas, 1972.
17. Gastaut, H. et al. Etude electrographique chez l'homme et l'animal des descharges epileptiques dites "psychometrices." *Dev. Neurol.* 88:310, 1953.
18. Gastaut, H., and Tassinari, C. A. IV. The Ictal and Interictal EEG in Different Types of Epilepsy. In A. Remond (Ed.), *Handbook of Electroencephalography and Clinical Neuroradiology,* Vol. 13A, *The Epilepsies.* Amsterdam: Elsevier, 1975.
19. Gibbs, E. L., Gibbs, F. A., and Fuster, B. Psychomotor epilepsy. *Arch. Neurol. Psychiatry* 60:331, 1948.
20. Gibbs, F. A., and Gibbs, E. L. *Atlas of Electroencephalography.* Vol. 3, *Epilepsy* (2nd ed.). Reading, Mass.: Addison-Wesley, 1960.

21. Glaser, G. H., Newman, R. J., and Schafer, R. Interictal Psychosis in Psychomotor Temporal Lobe Epilepsy. In G. H. Glaser (Ed.), *EEG and Behavior*. New York: Basic Books, 1963.

21a. Gloor, P. et al. The role of the limbic system in experiential phenomena of temporal lobe epilepsy. *Ann. Neurol.* 12:129, 1982.

22. Gowers, W. R. The Hughlings Jackson lecture on special sense discharges from organic disease. *Brain* 32:303, 1910.

23. Hauser, W. A., and Kurland, L. T. The epidemiology of epilepsy in Rochester, Minnesota, 1935 through 1967. *Epilepsia* 16:1, 1975.

24. Jackson, J. H. Lectures on the Diagnosis of Epilepsy. In J. Taylor (Ed.), *Selected Writings of John Hughlings Jackson*, Vol. 1. London: Hodder and Stoughton, 1931.

25. Jackson, J. H. On Right- or Left-Sided Spasm at the Onset of Epileptic Paroxysms and on Crude Sensation Warnings and Elaborate Mental States. In J. Taylor (Ed.), *Selected Writings of John Hughlings Jackson*, Vol. 1. London: Hodder and Stoughton, 1931.

26. Jasper, H., Pertuisset, B., and Flanigan, H. EEG and cortical electrograms in patients with temporal lobe seizures. *Arch. Neurol. Psychiatry* 65:272, 1951.

26a. Jensen, I., and Klinken, L. Temporal lobe epilepsy and neuropathology. *Acta Neurol. Scand.* 54:391, 1976.

27. Jüül-Jensen, P. *Epilepsy. A Clinical and Social Analysis of 1020 Adult Patients with Epileptic Seizures*. Copenhagen: Munksgaard, 1963.

28. Kaada, B. R. Somato-motor autonomic and electrocorticographic responses to electrical stimulation of "rhinecephalic" and other structures in primates, cat, and dog. *Acta Physiol. Scand.* 24: (Suppl. 83):1, 1951.

29. King, D. W., and Ajmone-Marsan, C. Clinical features and ictal patterns in epileptic patients with EEG temporal lobe foci. *Ann. Neurol.* 2:138, 1977.

30. Klass, D. W. The electroencephalogram in the evaluation of seizures: Current clinical applications. *Med. Clin. N. Am.* 52:949, 1968.

31. Klass, D. W. Ictal Clinical Manifestations of Complex Partial Seizures. In J. K. Penry, and D. D. Daly (Eds.), *Complex Partial Seizures and Their Treatment*. New York: Raven Press, 1975.

32. Klass, D. W., and Fischer-Williams, M. Activation and Provocation Methods in Clinical Neurophysiology. I. Sensory Stimulation. II. Sleep and Sleep Deprivation. In A. Remond (Ed.), *Hand-book of Electroencephalography and Clinical Neurophysiology*. Amsterdam: Elsevier, 1975.

33. Lennox, W. G. *Epilepsy and Related Disorders*. 2 Vols. Boston: Little, Brown, 1960.

34. Lieb, J. P. et al. A comparison of EEG seizure patterns recorded with surface and depth electrodes in patients with temporal lobe epilepsy. *Epilepsia* 17:137, 1976.

35. Lindsay, J., Ounstead, C., and Richards, P. Long-term outcome in children with temporal lobe seizures. *Dev. Med. Child. Neurol.* 21:285, 1979.

36. Livingston, S. *Living with Epileptic Seizures*. Springfield, Ill.: Thomas, 1963.

37. Margerison, J. H., and Corsellis, J. A. N. Epilepsy and the temporal lobes: A clinical electroencephalographic and neuropathological study of the brain in epilepsy with particular reference to the temporal lobes. *Brain* 89:499, 1966.

38. Markand, O. N., Wheeler, G. L., and Pollack, S. L. Complex partial status epilepticus (psychomotor status). *Neurology* (Minneap.) 28:189, 1978.

39. Mattson, R. H., Pratt, K. L., and Calverly, J. R. Electroencephalograms of epileptics following sleep deprivation. *Arch. Neurol.* 13:310, 1965.

40. Mayeux, R. et al. Poriomania. *Neurology* (Minneap.) 24:1616, 1979.

41. Mayeux, R. et al. Interictal memory and language impairment in temporal lobe epilepsy. *Neurology* (Minneap.) 30:120, 1980.

42. Monroe, R. R. *Episodic Behavioral Disorder*. Cambridge, Mass.: Harvard University Press, 1970.

43. Newmark, M. E., and Penry, J. K. *Genetics of Epilepsy: A Review*. New York: Raven Press, 1980.

44. Penfield, W., and Jasper, H. *Epilepsy and the Functional Anatomy of the Human Brain*. Boston: Little, Brown, 1954.

45. Penfield, W., and Perot, P. The brain's record of auditory and visual experience: A final summary and discussion. *Brain* 86:595, 1963.

46. Penfield, W., and Rasmussen, T. *The Cerebral Cortex of Man*. New York: Macmillan, 1950.

47. Pritchard, P. B., and Hungerford, G. D. Computerized tomography in temporal lobe epilepsy: Electroanatomical correlates. *Electroencephalogr. Clin. Neurophysiol.* 50:185P, 1980.

48. Ratzka, M. et al. CT-Ergebnisse bei Patienten mit Epilepsie: Ein prospektive Studie. *Neuroradiology* 16:332, 1978.

49. Remillard, G. et al. Predominance of sexual aura in females with temporal lobe epilepsy: A finding suggesting sexual dimorphism in the human. *Epilepsia*. In press, 1982.

50. Rodin, E. A. *The Prognosis of Patients with Epilepsy*. Springfield, Ill.: Thomas, 1968.

51. Serafetinides, E. A. Behavioral automatism: Epileptic or non-epileptic? *Curr. Concepts Psychiatry* 5:14, 1979.

52. Spencer, S. S. et al. Sexual automatisms in complex partial seizures. *Epilepsia.* In press, 1982.

53. Standage, K. F., and Fenton, G. W. Psychiatric symptom profiles of patients with epilepsy: A controlled investigation. *Psychol. Med.* 5:152, 1975.

54. Stevens, J. R. Emotional activation of the electroencephalogram in patients with convulsive disorders. *J. Nerv. Ment. Dis.* 128:339, 1959.

55. Stevens, J. R. Interictal clinical manifestations of complex partial seizures. *Adv. Neurol.* 11:85, 1975.

56. Stevens, J. R. Psychiatric implications of psychomotor epilepsy. *Arch. Gen. Psychiatry* 14:461, 1966.

57. Stevens, J. R., and Hermann, B. P. Temporal lobe epilepsy, psychopathology, and violence: The state of the evidence. *Neurology* 31:1127, 1981.

58. Taylor, D. C., and Falconer, M. A. Clinical, socioeconomic, and psychological changes after temporal lobectomy for epilepsy. *Br. J. Psychiatry* 114:1247, 1968.

59. Theodore, W. H., Porter, R. J., and Penry, J. K. Complex partial seizures: A videotape analysis of 108 seizures in 25 patients. *Neurology* 31:108, 1981.

60. Van Buren, J. M. Some autonomic concomitants of ictal automatism. A study of temporal lobe attacks. *Brain* 81:505, 1958.

61. Van Buren, J. M. et al. Surgery of Temporal Lobe Epilepsy. In D. Purpura, J. K. Penry, and R. D. Walter (Eds.), *Advances in Neurophysiology,* Vol. 8. New York: Raven Press, 1975.

62. Williams, D. The structure of emotions reflected in epileptic experiences. *Brain* 79:29, 1956.

63. Yang, P. J. et al. Computed tomography and childhood seizure disorders. *Neurology* 29:1084, 1979.

TONIC-CLONIC (GRAND MAL) SEIZURES

6

Thomas R. Browne

Definitions

Tonic seizures consist of increased tone in the axial or extremity muscles, or both, producing characteristic postures and accompanied by characteristic autonomic phenomena. Tonic seizures are relatively rare, occur chiefly in childhood, and are discussed in detail in Chapter 8.

Clonic seizures consist of bilateral jerks of the face and extremities that may be symmetrical or asymmetrical, rhythmic or arrhythmic. Clonic seizures are relatively rare, occur chiefly in early childhood, and are discussed briefly in Chapter 1 and in more detail in the review of Gastaut et al. [10].

Tonic-clonic seizures consist of an initial increase in tone of certain muscles (tonic phase) followed by bilateral symmetrical jerking of the extremities (clonic phase). Tonic-clonic seizures can occur at any age and are the most frequent type of seizure disorder seen in most practices (see Chap. 1).

Primarily generalized tonic-clonic seizures are bilaterally symmetrical and without focal features at onset. There is no clinical or EEG evidence of focal brain lesions.

Secondarily generalized tonic-clonic seizures begin with focal seizure activity and/or occur in patients with clinical or EEG evidence of a focal brain lesion.

Etiology

STRUCTURAL LESIONS

A presumptive etiology can be found in 20 to 25 percent of patients with tonic-clonic seizures [11, 17]. The most common presumptive etiologies are trauma, encephalitis, birth injury, brain tumor, and cerebrovascular accident [11]. Focal paroxysmal activity is found in the EEGs of 20 to 40 percent of patients with tonic-clonic seizures [11, 16], suggesting that these seizures are secondary to a focal lesion that produces so-called secondarily generalized tonic-clonic seizure activity. However, the majority of patients with tonic-clonic seizures do not have historical evidence of a structural brain abnormality or focal EEG abnormalities [11, 16, 17] and are said to have primarily generalized tonic-clonic seizures.

GENETICS

A higher than expected prevalence of nonfebrile seizures has been reported in the offspring (4.7%),

This work was supported in part by the Veterans Administration.

close relatives (siblings or parents, 5.2%), and relatives (7 to 10%) of patients with primarily generalized tonic-clonic seizures [19]. A similar increase has not been demonstrated in the relatives of patients with secondarily generalized tonic-clonic seizures [19].

Pathophysiology

CLINICAL AND EEG PHENOMENA

The clinical and EEG phenomena occurring during tonic-clonic seizures in humans are reviewed in detail later in this chapter. In the present section we will discuss the pathophysiologic mechanisms thought to be responsible for these phenomena.

ANIMAL MODELS

The pathophysiology of tonic-clonic seizures has been studied in animals by precipitating seizures with cerebral anoxia, strychnine, pentylenetetrazol (Metrazol), beta-ethyl-beta-methylglutarimide (Megimide), a combination of Metrazol and strychnine, and a combination of anoxia and strychnine [9]. Only Metrazol and Megimide produce the exact sequence of events seen in human tonic-clonic seizures (a few clonic jerks followed by a tonic phase and loss of consciousness followed by a clonic phase) [9, 22]. The results of these animal experiments may be summarized as follows: (1) the motor phenomena of tonic-clonic seizures result from relative hyperactivity of the brain stem reticular formation; (2) relative hyperactivity of the brain stem reticular formation can be produced either by hypersynchronous firing of the brain stem reticular formation or by suppression of the normal inhibitory effects of the diencephalon and telencephalon upon the brain stem reticular formation; and (3) unconsciousness results from hypersynchronous discharge of the thalamocortical pathways, leading to cerebral inhibition.

MODE OF ONSET AND PROPAGATION

Based on the animal studies just described, three possible modes of onset for primarily generalized tonic-clonic seizures were postulated: (1) hypersynchronous activity begins in the brain stem reticular formation and then spreads to involve the thalamocortical pathways; (2) hypersynchronous activity begins in the thalamocortical pathways, inactivates the diencephalic and telencephalic structures, and then results in loss of inhibition of the brain stem reticular formation; or (3) hypersynchronous activity begins simultaneously in the brain stem reticular formation and in the thalamocortical pathways [9, 22]. Rodin et al. [22] resolved this debate by recording high-frequency activity from many sites in the brains of cats

given Megimide. They found that early myoclonic jerks were associated with brief bursts of high-voltage, extremely fast activity in the midbrain reticular formation and that the onset of tonic-clonic seizure activity coincided with sustained high-voltage firing of the midbrain reticular formation. The thalamus, cortex, and limbic structures became involved in the seizure discharges only after the reticular formation had been firing for several seconds. Maximal reticular discharge occurred during the clinical tonic phase and then gradually waned. During the clinical clonic phase, brief bursts of high-frequency activity were recorded in the reticular formation. The periods of "electrical silence" seen on the surface EEG during the clonic phase were characterized by low-voltage reticular formation activity. Clinical behavior correlated with the downward discharge from the reticular formation to the spinal cord. The upward discharges caused the changes seen in the EEG but did not seem relevant to the observed clinical seizures.

These data were obtained from Megimide-induced tonic-clonic seizures in cats, not spontaneous tonic-clonic seizures in humans. However, the lack of consistent correlation between surface EEG activity and clinical seizure activity in humans during spontaneous tonic-clonic seizures suggests that similar mechanisms are operative [22].

The mechanism that produces spontaneous hypersynchronous discharge in the brain stem reticular formation or thalamocortical pathways, or both in humans is unknown. There is no clinical or EEG evidence of focal structural lesions in the majority of patients with tonic-clonic seizures [11, 16]. No consistent areas of brain involvement are found in autopsy studies of patients with tonic-clonic seizures. A hereditary-genetic biochemical or structural abnormality might be postulated, but a family history of epilepsy is present in only 8 percent of patients with only tonic-clonic seizures [11].

In patients with secondarily generalized tonic-clonic seizures paroxysmal activity in a focal cortical area may cause generalized tonic-clonic seizures when it spreads to the thalamocortical pathways or to the brain stem reticular formation. There is no definitive evidence to establish if one of these two proposed mechanisms, or some other mechanism, is responsible for the onset of secondarily generalized tonic-clonic seizures.

MODE OF TERMINATION

Experimental evidence indicates that both neuronal fatigue and activation of a thalamocaudate system of active inhibition play a role in the termination of tonic-clonic seizures [9, 22], but disagreement exists about the relative importance of these two factors [9, 22].

Seizure Phenomena

The material on seizure and EEG phenomena of tonic-clonic seizures in this and the following sections is based on the work of Gastaut et al. [10], unless otherwise indicated.

AURA

Only 15 percent of patients with tonic-clonic seizures report an aura [11]. Patients with secondarily generalized seizures may show signs of focal seizure phenomena appropriate to the focus of origin, whereas patients with primarily generalized seizures may experience a succession of bilateral jerks (usually in flexion) lasting several seconds and sometimes resulting in falls or jerky cries (see Figs. 6-1 and 6-2).

TONIC PHASE

Flexion Phase

The tonic phase usually consists of a brief phase in flexion followed by a longer one in extension. Consciousness is lost during the tonic phase in over 95 percent of patients [17]. The flexion phase usually begins in the face (eyes open, ocular globes rotated upward, mouth held rigidly half open), neck (held rigid in semiflexion), and trunk (chest bent forward on pelvis). The flexion phase then spreads to the extremities, involving the arms more than the legs and the proximal muscles more than the distal muscles. The arms are elevated, adducted, and externally rotated, and the legs and thighs are flexed, adducted, and externally rotated.

Extension Phase

The extension phase begins in the axial musculature with extension of the back and neck. The mouth snaps shut (the tongue may be bitten). The thoracic and abdominal muscles then contract, sometimes producing a "tonic cry" as air is forced over the vocal cords. The arms are lowered and adducted. The forearm may remain flexed or may be extended and pronated. Fingers may be clenched upon the extended wrists or extended upon flexed wrists. The legs are extended, adducted, and externally rotated.

Vibratory Tonic Period

During the period of transition from the tonic to the clonic phase ("vibratory tonic period"), tetanus becomes less complete. Tonic rigidity is replaced by a fine tremor, which increases in amplitude and decreases in frequency from 8 to 4 Hz. The tremor is due to intermittent decreases in tone. The tremor begins in the extremities and spreads proximally.

CLONIC PHASE

During the clonic phase, muscle relaxation completely interrupts tonic contraction. The rhythmic return of muscle tone causes the appearance of rhythmic jerks, which become farther and farther apart until the seizure ends. The tongue may be bitten owing to clonic masseter movements. Each jerk may be accompanied by a cry.

AUTONOMIC PHENOMENA

Autonomic phenomena begin in the preictal phase, are maximal at the end of the tonic phase, and decrease abruptly at the onset of the clonic phase. Autonomic phenomena that may be observed during a tonic-clonic seizure include increased blood pressure, increased heart rate, increased bladder pressure, increased sphincter tone, flushing, cyanosis, piloerection, perspiration, increased salivation, and increased bronchial secretion (see Figs. 6-1 and 6-2).

Apnea begins with violent expiration at the onset of the tonic phase and persists during the tonic and clonic phases (except for violent forced expirations with clonic jerks) and often into the early postictal period. Apnea cannot be explained entirely on the basis of muscular contractions; a central mechanism is probably involved in maintaining it.

IMMEDIATE POSTICTAL PHASE

Complete muscular relaxation does not occur immediately. About 5 seconds after the last clonic jerk, there is a new period of tonic contraction lasting from several seconds to 4 minutes. Muscle tone is most increased in the cephalic muscles, and the tongue may be bitten. The trunk and arms may be extended but not as violently as during the tonic phase.

Between the last clonic jerk and the immediate postictal tonic phase, the bladder sphincter muscles relax; at this point incontinence occurs (Fig. 6-2). Incontinence is reported by 35 percent of patients with tonic-clonic seizures [17]. It does not occur during the tonic or clonic phase because of increased sphincter tone.

Respirations return during the immediate postictal phase. The combination of a clenched jaw and increased secretions results in partial obstruction of respiration. Respirations are stertorous, and accessory muscles of respirations are activated. Blood pressure and skin resistance return to normal, but tachycardia persists. Cyanosis changes to pallor. Loss of conscious-

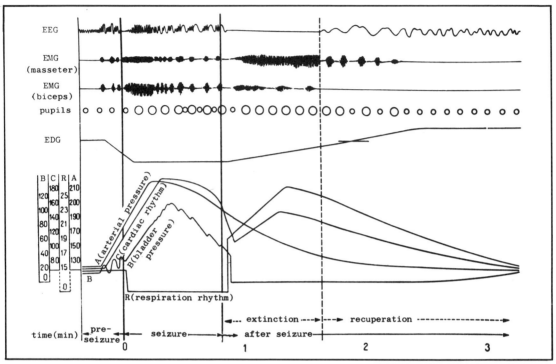

EEG

EMG
(masseter)

EMG
(biceps)

pupils

EDG

A(arterial pressure)

C(cardiac rhythm)

B(bladder pressure)

R(respiration rhythm)

extinction   recuperation

time(min)   pre-   seizure   after seizure
seizure

0   1   2   3

Figure 6-1. Schematic representation of a generalized tonic-clonic seizure. The preseizure period is characterized by generalized jerks (EMG) and multiple spike discharges (EEG), a sudden fall in skin resistance (EDG= electrodermogram), increase in arterial pressure (A), bladder pressure (B), and tachycardia (C).

The seizure proper lasts an average of a little less than a minute and is expressed in the EEG and EMG by tonic and clonic sequences accompanied by marked vegetative phenomena: apnea, arterial hypertension, intravesicular hypertension, tachycardia, drop in skin resistance, and mydriasis, which disappears rhythmically with the muscle relaxation of the clonic phase, producing hippus. Except for the apnea, which persists during the entire convulsion, all autonomic changes attain their maximum expression at the end of the tonic phase and then progressively decrease during the clonic phase.

The immediate postictal period begins with complete electroencephalographic silence; followed by a second tonic phase of variable intensity predominating in the head muscles, recurrence of mydriasis, second tachycardia, and acceleration of respiration, which reappears after the last myoclonus. Note that it is after this last jerk and before the reappearance of tonic spasm that the subject is in complete muscular relaxation. It lasts only several seconds, during which urinary incontinence may occur owing to the lack of sphincter muscle tone.

The period of recuperation contains a return to normal of all of the previously disturbed vegetative phenomena. Note the new episode of hippus, corresponding to rhythmic interruption of mydriasis during the intervals of muscle relaxation that interrupt the end of the postictal hypertonic spasm. The spasm lasts longer in the muscles of mastication than in those of the limbs. The EEG shows slow-wave activity that later progressively accelerates until recuperation of normal cerebral rhythms is attained. (From H. Gastaut et al. [10].)

ness remains complete, and pupillary and cutaneous reflexes are absent. Deep tendon reflexes are variably modified.

LATER POSTICTAL PHASE
In the later postictal phase there is more or less complete flaccidity. The cardiac rate returns to normal. Deep tendon reflexes are usually diminished, and the plantar response is sometimes extensor. The patient may awaken by passing through successive stages of coma, confusional state, and drowsiness or may pass directly into sleep without awakening.

Postictal Pulmonary Edema
Postictal pulmonary edema is a rare complication of tonic-clonic seizures manifested by dyspnea, cough, blood-stained sputum, and abnormal chest roentgenogram (see Chap. 30) [1, 23]. It may occur immediately or several hours after a tonic-clonic seizure and is more common in young patients and in those with expanding cerebral mass lesions [23]. Postictal pulmonary edema may be caused by increased intracranial pressure during the seizure ("neurogenic pulmonary edema") [23]. Usually self-limited, postictal pulmonary edema usually requires only oxygen as therapy [23]. It must be distinguished from the more dangerous complication of aspiration pneumonia, however.

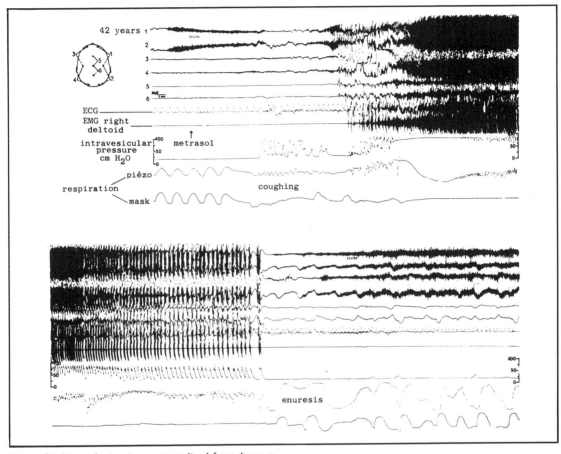

Figure 6-2. Tonic-clonic seizure, generalized from the start (Metrazol-induced). Polygraphic study including DC recording of bladder pressure. The Metrazol produced a series of coughs, each of which caused an abrupt increase in bladder pressure. The seizure then starts with a number of massive jerks easily observed on the deltoid EMG recording and present also in scalp muscles. At this time the bladder pressure increases up to 100 mm Hg, the rising phase showing superimposed increases due to compression from the myoclonus. Respiration, as recorded by a face mask thermocouple and thoracic strain gauge (piezo), is arrested. Just following the preictal myoclonic phase, a rhythmic cerebral discharge at 10 Hz is evident in the region of the vertex. The EEG subsequently becomes obscured by muscle artifacts. The bladder pressure reaches a peak during the tonic phase and then progressively decreases during the clonic phase, each jerk producing a new compressive rise in pressure. Following the last jerk, there is a postictal extinction of cerebral activity followed by a second episode of intense contraction of head muscles. Subsequently, respiration is re-established, and postictal tachycardia is evident. All recordings were made at 15 mm/sec paper speed. (From H. Gastaut et al. [10].)

DURATION OF PHASES

The average duration of the various phases of a tonic-clonic seizure are as follows: tonic phase, 10 to 30 seconds; clonic phase, 30 to 50 seconds; immediate

postictal phase, 1 to 5 minutes; later postictal phase, 2 to 10 minutes; total, 5 to 15 minutes [10, 18].

CLONIC-TONIC-CLONIC SEIZURES

Some generalized convulsive seizures commence with a clonic phase passing into tonic and clonic phases similar to those described above.

EEG Phenomena

PREICTAL PHASE

During the preictal phase of a secondarily generalized tonic-clonic seizure the EEG may show focal attenuation, sharp waves, or slow activity. EEG activity during the preictal phase of a primarily generalized tonic-clonic seizure may show bursts of polyspike and wave complexes, each complex associated with myoclonic jerks and sometimes a cry (see Figs. 6-1, 6-2, and 6-3).

TONIC PHASE

The tonic phase begins with a 1- to 3-second period of EEG flattening ("desynchronization") or with low-

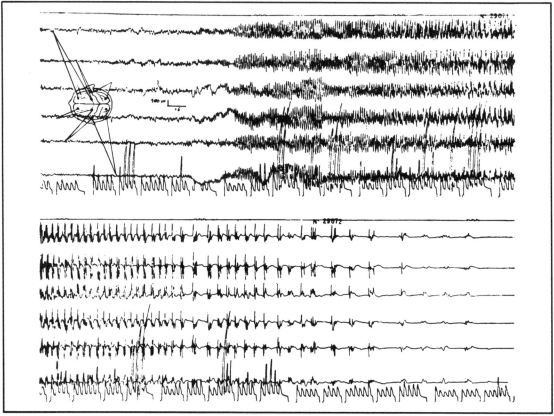

Figure 6-3. EEG recording of a generalized tonic-clonic seizure. On the last line of the recording there is an automatic frequency analysis of the right temporo-occipital region. (From H. Gastaut et al. [10].)

voltage fast activity. Then surface negative waves at about 10 Hz appear and increase rapidly in amplitude ("epileptic recruiting rhythm"). After about 10 seconds the recruiting rhythm becomes combined with an apparently separate rhythm of slow waves increasing in amplitude and decreasing in frequency from 3 Hz to 1 Hz. The slow rhythm becomes progressively more prominent, and the recruiting rhythm becomes progressively less prominent until the recruiting rhythm appears only as brief bursts of rapid activity between surface negative slow waves.

CLONIC PHASE

During the clonic phase bursts of 10-Hz recruiting rhythm alternates with slow waves. Bursts of recruiting rhythm are associated with generalized jerks, and slow waves are associated with relaxation. The slow waves become slower, and the bursts of recruiting rhythm become farther apart.

POSTICTAL PHASE

The EEG is isoelectric for a few seconds to 1 minute after the last clonic jerk ("cortical extinction"). Then low-voltage, very slow delta activity appears. The EEG frequency picks up through the delta range into the theta range and then into the alpha range. Postictal tonic contraction begins during the period of cortical extinction and persists during the early slow-wave phase.

INTERICTAL EEG

Secondarily Generalized Tonic-Clonic Seizures

Focal paroxysmal activity is seen in the interictal EEGs of 20 to 40 percent of patients with tonic-clonic seizures [11, 16], and these patients are assumed to have secondarily generalized tonic-clonic seizures. The focal paroxysmal activity may consist of grouped spike discharges, theta waves, or isolated spikes [16] and is most often recorded over the rolandic area (71%) and less frequently over the temporal area (29%) or the parietal-occipital area (10%) [16].

Table 6-1. Differential Diagnosis of Syncope Versus Tonic-Clonic Seizure

	Syncope	Tonic-Clonic Seizure
Age of onset	Adult or Child	Adult or Child
Sleep	Cardiac causes	During awakening, after deprivation
Variability	Depends on initial condition or posture (usually erect)	Similar patterns regardless of posture
Incontinence	Rarely	Often
Tongue biting or injury	Not likely	Often
Skin color	Pale	Flushed
Respirations	Slow unless syncope due to hyper-ventilation	Apnea, stentorous
Perspiration	Cold, clammy	Hot, sweaty
Duration	Brief unless cardiac recovery with head down	5 to 15 minutes, no recovery with head down
EEG: during event	Nonspecific slow	Specific paroxysms
EEG: between events	Usually normal	May show paroxysmal activity
ECG between events	May be abnormal	Usually normal
Focal abnormality on neurologic examination or EEG	Usually not present	Sometimes present

Primarily Generalized Tonic-Clonic Seizures

Sixty to 80 percent of patients with tonic-clonic seizures do not have focal abnormalities on EEG [11, 16]. These patients are assumed to have primarily generalized tonic-clonic seizures. Thirty to 50 percent of patients with primarily generalized tonic-clonic seizures have normal interictal EEGs [11, 16]. The remainder usually have normal EEG background activity and intermittent bilateral polyspike and wave, spike-wave, or sharp and slow discharges [10]. Bilateral discharges increase during non-REM sleep, and runs of 10-Hz "recruiting rhythms" without clinical seizures ("grand mal discharges" of Gibbs and Gibbs) may occur [10, 11]. EEG discharges seldom occur during REM sleep [10]. Photosensitivity in patients with tonic-clonic seizures is reviewed briefly in Chapters 11 and 12 and in detail by Newmark and Penry [20].

Differential Diagnosis

SYNCOPAL ATTACK (see Chap. 10)
Syncopal attacks consist of brief episodes of impaired consciousness, generalized weakness, and inability to stand owing to impaired circulation to the brain. Consciousness is impaired or lost when (1) blood pressure falls below 60 to 80 mm Hg systolic, (2) cardiac rate is less than 40 per minute or greater than 150 per minute, and (3) asystole of 4 to 15 seconds occurs. Syncope may have many causes, including vasovagal syncope ("ordinary faint"), postural hypertension, hyperventilation syncope, Stokes-Adams attack, carotid

sinus reflex sensitivity, sinus tachycardia, premature ventricular contractions, or paroxysmal atrial tachycardia. In most cases the differential diagnosis of syncope versus seizure can be made fairly easily using the criteria outlined in Table 6-1.

There are at least two situations in which the diagnosis of syncope versus seizure can be confusing. First, myoclonic jerks or a tonic-clonic seizure can be precipitated by a syncopal attack in a person who does not have epilepsy. Animal work has shown that the telencephalon and diencephalon are more sensitive to anoxia and ischemia than the brain stem and that generalized anoxia or ischemia can result in "liberating" the brain stem from higher cortical inhibitory control and in myoclonic or tonic-clonic seizures [9]. Thus, the observation of myoclonic jerks or a true tonic-clonic seizure during a syncopal episode does not necessarily mean that a patient has epilepsy. The second confusing situation is that of hyperventilation syncope, in which tetany and carpopedal spasm may be mistaken for tonic-clonic movements.

CLONIC SEIZURES
Often the initial tonic phase of a tonic-clonic seizure is not observed by the nurse or relative who is brought to the patient's aid by the sounds of the dramatic events that take place during a tonic-clonic seizure. The observer witnesses only the clonic phase. One must then decide whether the patient had a tonic-clonic or a clonic seizure based on incomplete historical informa-

58

tion. Clonic seizures are suggested by occurrence in early childhood, jerks that vary randomly in location and frequency, and absence of cyanosis. Tonic-clonic seizures are suggested by occurrence in older children or adults, jerks that are bilaterally synchronous and become progressively farther apart, and the presence of cyanosis.

TONIC SEIZURES
For a discussion of tonic seizures, see Chapter 8.

HYSTERICAL SEIZURES
For a discussion of hysterical seizures, see Chapter 10.

Management
Phenytoin, carbamazepine, phenobarbital, and primidone are the drugs usually employed to treat tonic-clonic seizures. The relative advantages and disadvantages of these four drugs in the treatment of tonic-clonic seizures are reviewed in Chapter 14.

Prognosis

REMISSION OF TONIC-CLONIC SEIZURES
Fifty-five to 63 percent of patients with only tonic-clonic seizures experience remission of the seizures [8, 14, 15, 25, 26]. Remission rates are lower in patients with other types of seizures (especially complex partial seizures) in addition to tonic-clonic seizures [3, 17, 21].

CONTROL OF TONIC-CLONIC SEIZURES
WITH ANTIEPILEPTIC DRUGS
Most reported studies indicate that complete or nearly complete control of tonic-clonic seizures can be achieved in the majority of patients with single drug therapy with phenytoin, carbamazepine, phenobarbital, and primidone or with varying combinations of these four drugs (see Chaps. 16, 17, and 18). Gibbs and Gibbs [11] state that tonic-clonic seizures can be controlled with antiepileptic drugs in 85 percent of patients.

INTELLIGENCE
Most studies report that the mean intelligence quotient (IQ) of groups of patients with tonic-clonic seizures is 90 to 100, with a wide range of scores by different individuals [5, 6, 7, 12, 27]. Scores tend to be lower in patients with symptomatic epilepsy [27] and in patients with multiple types of epileptic seizures [4, 12]. There is also some evidence that early onset [6, 7] and high frequency of tonic-clonic seizures [5, 12] are associated with lower IQ scores. These lower scores,

however, could be due to the cerebral process that causes early or severe epilepsy or to antiepileptic drugs rather than to the actual seizures.

References
1. Archibald, R. B., and Armstrong, J. D. Case report: Recurrent postictal pulmonary edema. *Postgrad. Med.* 63:210, 1978.
2. Cereghino, J. J. et al. Carbamazepine for epilepsy. *Neurology* (Minneap.) 24:401, 1974.
3. Chao, D. H. C., Druckman, R., and Kellaway, P. *Convulsive Disorders of Children.* Philadelphia: Saunders, 1958.
4. Collins, A. L., and Lennox, W. G. The intelligence of 300 private epileptic patients. *Proc. Assoc. Res. Nerv. Ment. Dis.* 26:586, 1947.
5. Dikmen, S., and Matthews, C. G. Effect of major motor seizure frequency upon cognitive-intellectual functions in adults. *Epilepsia* 18:21, 1977.
6. Dikmen, S., Matthews, C. G., and Harley, J. P. Effect of early versus late onset of major motor epilepsy on cognitive-intellectual performance: Further considerations. *Epilepsia* 18:31, 1977.
7. Folsom, A. Psychological testing in epilepsy: I. Cognitive function. *Epilepsia* 2:15, 1953.
8. Frantzen, E. An analysis of the results of treatment in epileptics under ambulatory supervision. *Epilepsia* 2:207, 1961.
9. Gastaut, H. Pathophysiology of grand mal seizures generalized from the start. *J. Nerv. Ment. Dis.* 127:21, 1958.
10. Gastaut, H. et al. Generalized Convulsive Seizures Without Local Onset. In P. J. Vinken, and G. W. Bruyn (Eds.), *Handbook of Clinical Neurology,* Vol. 15, *The Epilepsies.* Amsterdam: Elsevier, 1974. Pp. 107–129.
11. Gibbs, F. A., and Gibbs, E. L. *Atlas of Electroencephalography,* Vol. 2. Cambridge, Mass.: Addison-Wesley, 1952.
12. Halstead, H. Abilities and behavior of epileptic children. *J. Ment. Sci.* 102:28, 1957.
13. Ives, E. R. Comparison of efficacy of various drugs in treatment of epilepsy. *J.A.M.A.* 147:1332, 1951.
14. Jüül-Jensen, P. *Epilepsy: A Clinical and Social Analysis of 1020 Adult Patients with Epileptic Seizures.* Copenhagen: Munksgaard, 1963.
15. Kiørboe, E. The prognosis of epilepsy. *Acta Psychiat. Scand.* 36:166, 1961.
16. Kreindler, A., and Popescu Tismana, G. D. Interseizure activity in the EEG of patients with grand mal epilepsy. *Electroencephalogr. Clin. Neurophysiol.* 27:655, 1969.

17. Lennox, W. G., and Lennox, M. A. *Epilepsy and Related Disorders,* Vol. 1. Boston: Little, Brown, 1960.

18. Mashur, K. F. Videoanalysis of grand mal seizures. *Epilepsia* 20:179, 1979.

19. Newmark, M. E., and Penry, J. K. *Genetics of Epilepsy: A Review.* New York: Raven Press, 1980.

20. Newmark, M. E., and Penry, J. K. *Photosensitivity and Epilepsy: A Review.* New York: Raven Press, 1979.

21. Rodin, E. A. *The Prognosis of Patients with Epilepsy.* Springfield, Ill.: Thomas, 1968.

22. Rodin, E. et al. Mechanisms involved in grand mal seizures. *Trans. Am. Neurol. Assoc.* 94:333, 1969.

23. Sarkar, T. K., and Munshi, A. T. Postictal pulmonary edema. *Postgrad. Med.* 61:281, 1977.

24. Shorvon, S. D., and Reynolds, E. H. Unnecessary polypharmacy for epilepsy. *Br. Med. J.* 1:1635, 1977.

25. Trolle, E. Drug therapy of epilepsy. *Acta Psychiat. Scand.* [Suppl.] 150:187, 1961.

26. Yahr, M., and Merritt, H. H. The drug therapy of convulsive seizures. *Int. J. Neurol.* 1:76, 1959.

27. Zimmerman, F. T., Burgemeister, B. B., and Putnam, J. J. Intellectual and emotional makeup of the epileptic. *Arch. Neurol. Psychiat.* 65:545, 1951.

ABSENCE (PETIT MAL) SEIZURES

7

Thomas R. Browne
Allan F. Mirsky

Definitions

The essential feature of the absence seizure is a brief episode of decreased responsiveness or altered consciousness without preictal warning or postictal symptoms. Decreased responsiveness may be accompanied by automatisms, mild clonic movements, increased or decreased postural tone, or autonomic phenomena in varying combinations. The absence seizure is a unique seizure type with well-defined clinical and EEG features. According to the International Classification of Epileptic Seizures [12], "petit mal" seizures should be used as a synonym for absence seizures only. Unfortunately, "petit mal" is often used imprecisely as a catch-all term for all types of seizure other than "grand mal." Atypical absence, myoclonic, atonic, complex partial, and simple partial seizures are sometimes improperly called "petit mal" seizures. Most authorities now no longer use the term "petit mal" to avoid the ambiguity often associated with it.

Etiology

There is a long-standing debate about whether absence epilepsy is an "acquired" or a "genetic" condition. Evidence exists for both types of etiology, but the preponderance of evidence favors a genetic etiology.

EVIDENCE FOR ACQUIRED ETIOLOGY
Clinical and experimental evidence indicates that structural lesions in the cerebral cortex, thalamus, and midbrain can produce spike-wave discharges and absencelike behavior in animals. The question then becomes how often such structural lesions can be found in patients with absence seizures.

Only one autopsy on a child with typical absence seizures has been reported, and no abnormality was found [7]. Three groups of investigators report that 0 to 10 percent of patients with absence seizures have abnormal computerized axial tomography (CT) scans [17, 35, 47].

By combining data from the history, neurologic examination, and laboratory tests (other than CT scans), evidence of focal neurologic abnormalities can be found in 5 to 25 percent of patients with absence seizures [8, 19, 22, 23, 25, 26, 46]. These abnormalities are usually mild and nonprogressive. Brain tumors are very rare in patients with absence seizures [1].

This work was supported in part by the Veterans Administration.

61

One possible source of acquired structural lesions that might cause absence seizures is prenatal and perinatal trauma. One of the authors has reviewed the prenatal and perinatal histories of 166 patients with absence seizures and compared them with those of the general population [3]. The only statistically significant findings were increased proportions of precipitate labor and face presentations in patients with absence seizures. However, it would be incorrect to imply that perinatal complications are the major cause of absence seizures, since the incidence of precipitate labor was 39 percent and the incidence of face presentation was 1.8 percent. Furthermore, the data may have been biased because mothers often underestimate the duration of labor.

Overall, it appears that most cases of absence seizures cannot be explained on the basis of an acquired lesion. The preponderance of evidence now favors a genetic etiology for the majority of cases.

EVIDENCE FOR GENETIC ETIOLOGY

The typical age of onset and age of disappearance of absence seizures (see below), the dramatic response of absence seizures to certain drugs, and the lack of evidence of acquired central nervous system disease in most patients are indirect evidence in favor of a genetic cause of absence seizures. Direct evidence based on studies of families with absence seizures also exists.

Lennox and Lennox [25] reported (1) a family history of epilepsy in 34 percent of patients with 3-Hz spike-wave discharges; (2) a concordance rate of 75 percent for absence seizures in monozygotic twins; (3) a concordance rate of 84 percent for 3-Hz spike-wave discharges in monozygotic twins; and (4) a concordance rate of 0 percent for both absence seizures and 3-Hz spike-wave discharges in dizygotic twins. Metrakos and Metrakos [29, 30] studied 211 probands with "centrencephalic" EEG abnormalities (see later discussion, Centrencephalic Theory) and 223 siblings of probands. "Centrencephalic" EEG abnormalities were found in 37 percent of siblings of probands. On the basis of these data they postulated that absence seizures are inherited either as a mendelian dominant trait or by a multifactorial mechanism of inheritance [29, 30].

However, the Metrakos' data may be questioned because they include the following EEG findings in their "centrencephalic abnormality" group: (1) typical 3-Hz spike-waves; (2) atypical 2- to 4-Hz spike-waves; (3) multiple spike-and-wave; and (4) paroxysmal 3- to 6-Hz spike-waves. Only 81 of 211 probands and 5 of 223 siblings of probands had typical 3-Hz spike-waves

on EEG in the Metrakos' study [29, 30]. More recently, Doose et al. [10] studied 252 probands with absence seizures and 3-Hz spike-wave, 242 siblings of probands, and 685 healthy controls. They reported that (1) 7.6 percent of siblings of probands had 3-Hz spike-wave; (2) 20 percent of siblings of probands between the ages of 5 and 6 years had 3-Hz spike-wave; and (3) 1.9 percent of control children had 3-Hz spike-wave.

Pathophysiology

The exact location and nature of the structural and/or biochemical lesion responsible for absence seizures is not known. There is a long-standing debate about whether 3-Hz spike-wave discharges are produced by a mesencephalic or diencephalic ("centrencephalic") mechanism or by some cortical process. Recent work with the generalized penicillin epilepsy model has added new information relevant to this debate.

CENTRENCEPHALIC THEORY

The fact that 3-Hz spike-wave discharges in absence seizures appear simultaneously in virtually all EEG locations led Penfield and Jasper [40] to speculate that the pathophysiologic mechanism must involve cerebral structures with widespread connections to the two hemispheres. They also noted that loss of consciousness was a primary symptom of the "absence" attack and concluded that it resulted from a disturbance of function involving the upper brain stem. These electrographic and behavioral considerations led them to postulate the existence of a centrencephalic system involving brain stem structures and widespread connections to the two hemispheres. This system was postulated to be involved in maintaining consciousness and in producing absence attacks.

CORTICAL THEORY

Other theorists argued that 3-Hz spike-wave activity begins in and generalizes from one or more cortical foci and does not originate in a centrencephalic system [16, 27, 28]. Clinical and experimental data provide some evidence for both the centrencephalic and cortical theories.

During human absence seizures, paroxysmal activity has been recorded from the cerebral cortex (especially the premotor cortex), subcortical white matter, midline thalamic nuclei, and hypothalamus [24, 27, 44]. Generalized spike-wave discharges and/or absencelike behavior has been produced in animals by electrical stimulation of, or epileptogenic foci in, the following areas: the cerebral cortex (especially the premotor cortex), intralaminar thalamic nuclei, midline thalamic nuclei, the hypothalamus, and the mesencephalic reticular formation [24, 27, 44, 51].

INHIBITORY PATHWAY THEORY

Many ascending and descending pathways interconnect the midbrain reticular formation, the hypothalamus, intralaminar thalamic nuclei, and the cerebral cortex (especially the premotor cortex). Some of these pathways are inhibitory, raising the possibility that spike-wave discharges and absence seizures could be due to paroxysmal activation of inhibitory, or largely inhibitory, pathways connecting these and other structures. There is experimental evidence to support this possibility.

Clinical absence seizures are characterized largely by inhibitory phenomena (see next section). The areas of monkey cortex in which epileptogenic foci are most likely to produce bilateral spike-wave discharges and absencelike behavior are the superior frontal and premotor areas, and these areas are believed to have a descending inhibitory function [16, 27]. Finally, there is experimental evidence that drugs effective against absence seizures (ethosuximide, valproic acid, trimethadione) inhibit cortical and subcortical inhibitory pathways, whereas drugs that are not effective against absence seizures (phenytoin, carbamazepine) do not have this action [14, 15, 16].

RECURRENT CORTICAL INHIBITION THEORY

Recent work with the generalized penicillin epilepsy model in cats has helped to expand our knowledge of the pathophysiology of spike-wave discharges. This work was summarized by Gloor [21] as follows: (1) the clinical and EEG manifestations of seizures produced by the model are similar to those of human absence seizures; (2) stimulation of certain thalamic areas (intralaminar nuclei, nucleus lateralis posterior, pulvinar) under normal conditions produces recruiting responses in the awake cat and spindles in the sleeping cat; (3) under the condition of mild generalized increase in excitability of cortical neurons (produced by systemic penicillin), these neurons respond to stimulation of the same thalamic areas by elaborating spike-wave complexes; (4) changes in excitability at the thalamic level are not required to bring about the transformation of cortical response; (5) changes in the brain stem reticular formation are not required to produce spike-wave discharges, but any depression of the ascending, desynchronizing drive of the brain stem greatly facilitates the likelihood of elaboration of spike-wave discharges; (6) the spike component of the spike-wave complex corresponds with excitatory postsynaptic potentials (EPSPs), and the slow wave corresponds with inhibitory postsynaptic potentials (IPSPs); (7) the production of slow waves and interference with higher cortical function occur as the result of the firing of recurrent intracortical inhibitory pathways in response to the action potentials produced by the preceding volley of EPSPs in the hyperexcitable cortical neurons.

The generalized penicillin epilepsy model has been invoked to elucidate the cellular mechanisms of spike-wave discharges; this work has also been summarized by Gloor [21] (Fig. 7-1). Under normal physiologic conditions, surface cortical waves of the ongoing resting EEG correlate with membrane fluctuations of intracortical neurons that often fail to elicit action potentials, because the EPSPs of many cortical neurons (contributing through their summation to the emergence of a surface EEG wave) fail to reach the critical levels of discharge of action potentials. Under these conditions there is little excitation of recurrent intracortical inhibitory pathways, and IPSPs occur infrequently. However, a moderate increase in cortical excitement may lead to rhythmic activation of recurrent intracortical inhibitory neurons because the inhibitory neurons are more frequently and consistently recruited by the increased firing of pyramidal cells. The surface EEG expression of these changes are spikes (corresponding to excitation of neurons) and slow waves (corresponding to the longer period of inhibition of neurons produced by recurrent intracortical inhibitory pathways). The functions of individual neurons during such spike-wave activity are normal in terms of their synaptic responses and membrane potential changes. It is only the recurrent rhythmic sequence of excitation and inhibition that is in some way abnormal. Gloor [21] termed this abnormality *first degree epileptogenesis.* This contrasts with the neuronal function during the classic focal epileptic spike or sharp wave of a focal cortical epileptic lesion. In these instances, the excitatory drive is more potent, leading to paroxysmal depolarizing shifts of the neuronal membrane, with superimposed high-frequency bursts of action potentials (see Chap. 2). Individual neurons thus behave in an abnormal manner. This change represents a further increase in the intensity of neuronal hyperexcitability and has been termed *second degree epileptogenesis* by Gloor [21].

The mechanism responsible for producing first degree epileptogenesis of cortical neurons in patients with absence seizures is unknown. Gloor [21] speculates that an undetermined biochemical lesion with an underlying genetic cause in patients with absence seizures may render some cortical synapses more

64

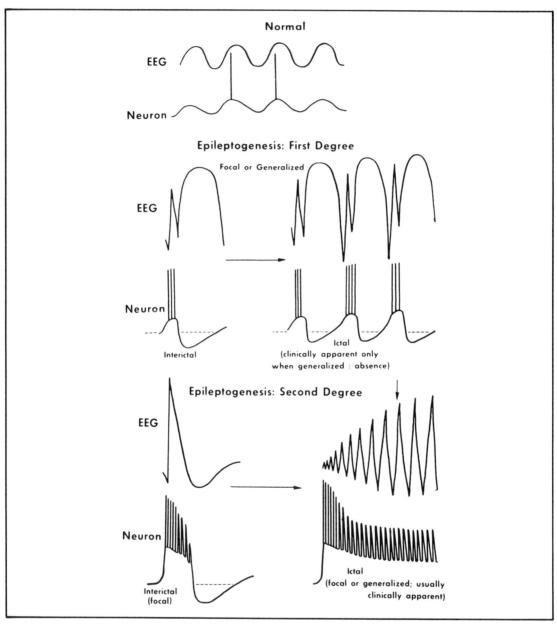

Figure 7-1. Diagrammatic representation of the relationship between surface EEG and intracellularly recorded activity of cortical neurons during normal rhythmic background activity and two types of interictal and ictal epileptic conditions representing two degrees of epileptogenesis. (From P. Gloor [21].)

efficient or that there may be a diffuse pathologic condition of gray matter.

Myslobodsky [36] has produced animal studies related to these investigations. Gloor's theme of disturbed inhibitory functions in cortical regions is also central to Myslobodsky's view of spike-wave seizures. However, he affords the ascending reticular formation (RAF) a more central role. Myslobodsky postulates that failure of the RAF to control normal inhibitory processes results in an excessive amount of cerebral inhibition.

CONCLUSION

Gloor has summarized his view of the pathophysiology of absence seizures as follows [21]:

...bilaterally synchronous spike-and-wave discharge represents an abnormal response pattern of cortical neurons to afferent thalamocortical volleys normally involved in the elicitation of spindles. Such a response occurs under conditions of diffuse mild cortical hyperexcitability that causes cortical neurons to generate an increased number of action potentials per afferent volley. This secondarily leads to powerful activation of the intracortical recurrent inhibitory pathway. The result is an alternation of short periods of increased cortical excitation corresponding to the EEG spike with longer-lasting periods of intense cortical inhibition corresponding to the wave component of the spike-and-wave complex. This pattern of widespread synchronous oscillation between increased excitation and increased inhibition profoundly disrupts the normal pattern of neuronal activity necessary for sustaining higher nervous functions, i.e., such components of mental activity as perception, cognition, memory, and voluntary motor activity. It is the disruption of these components of mental activity that occurs to a variable degree during generalized spike-and-wave discharges, rather than disruption of a more fundamental mechanism of maintenance of consciousness related to...upper brain stem functions, that characterizes the disturbances of higher nervous functions typical for the absence attack.

Although Gloor's hypothesis represents an attractive synthesis of many observations, it cannot be taken as the final answer. There is much evidence for alternative hypotheses. Cats cannot be subjected to neurobehavioral testing to see if the spike-wave discharges produced by systemic penicillin produce behavioral deficits similar to those seen in human absence seizures. Attempts to produce absence seizures in primates with systemic penicillin have so far proved unsuccessful (D. Prince, personal communication). Brain stem functions (auditory evoked potentials) are altered during spontaneous human absence seizures [33], an observation at variance with Gloor's view that altered brain stem function is not a factor in the genesis of spike-wave discharges.

Seizure Phenomena

AGE OF ONSET

Absence seizures begin in the majority of patients between 5 and 10 years of age [25, 46]. In a minority of patients the condition can have its onset between 1 and 4 or after 10 years of age [25, 46]. There are scattered reports of adult-onset absence seizures, although it is difficult to be certain if such patients did not have absence seizures at an earlier age that were overlooked.

THE ABSENCE

The essential feature of the absence seizure is a brief period of cessation of ongoing activities and loss of responsiveness or reduced consciousness (the "absence"). There is no warning, and the onset is very sudden. The patient stops talking, eating, walking, or whatever he is doing. Breathing may continue normally, but if the attack lasts more than 5 to 10 seconds, a brief respiratory arrest may be observed [34]. The eyes may become vacant and usually stare straight ahead, although they may move upward. During an attack the patient is usually unresponsive when spoken to, although occasionally there may be a grunt in response to a question. The attack ends as suddenly as it started, and the patient is back to his usual level of alertness. He may or may not be able to recall what he was doing before the attack. He is often unaware that he had an attack. The majority of absence seizures last less than 10 seconds [42].

ABSENCE SEIZURES WITH IMPAIRMENT
OF CONSCIOUSNESS ONLY

Although the absence is the essential feature of absence seizures, only 9 percent of such seizures occur as absence seizures with impairment of consciousness only ("simple absences"). The only manifestations of these "simple absences" are a cessation of ongoing activities and a loss of responsiveness (Fig. 7-2) [42]. In the remaining 91 percent the following additional phenomena are seen singly or in varying combinations: mild clonic components, atonic components, tonic components, and automatisms (Fig. 7-2) [42]. Autonomic components are also observable in an unknown percentage of patients.

MILD CLONIC COMPONENTS

Mild clonic movements are observable in approximately one half of absence seizures (Fig. 7-2). The most common form of mild clonic movement is rhythmic fluttering of the eyelids; other forms include fine rhythmic movements of the corner of the mouth, fingers, arms, and shoulders [42]. These movements

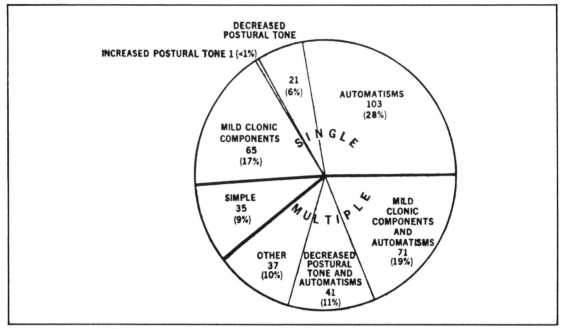

Figure 7-2. Relative frequency of different types of absence seizure as determined by videotape analysis of 374 absence seizures. (From J. K. Penry, R. J. Porter, and F. E. Dreifuss [42].)

usually do not impair posture, although they may cause the patient to lose control of objects in his hand.

ATONIC COMPONENTS

Decreased postural tone occurs in approximately 20 percent of absence seizures [42]. Loss of postural tone may lead to drooping of the head, slumping of the trunk, dropping of the arms and relaxation of grip, or buckling at the knees. More extensive loss of postural tone may be sufficient to cause the head to fall backward and the trunk to arch [42]. Tone is rarely sufficiently diminished to cause the patient to fall [12]. The decrease in postural tone may be symmetrical or asymmetrical.

TONIC COMPONENTS

Increased postural tone occurs in approximately 5 percent of absence seizures [42]. Increased muscle tone may affect the flexor or extensor muscles symmetrically or asymmetrically [12] and may cause the patient to draw the head backward and to arch the trunk [42]. If the patient is standing, increased tone may lead to retropulsion. The head may be drawn tonically to one side [12]. Occasionally, slight clonic activity may interrupt the smooth tonic muscle construction, leading to intermittent postural deviation [42].

AUTOMATISMS

Automatisms are observable in approximately two thirds of absence seizures. Automatisms are apparently purposeful movements occurring without awareness during the absence attack and subdivided into "perseverative" and "de novo" types. Perseverative automatisms represent persistence of activity engaged in before the onset of the seizure such as handling of objects or walking, although these activities may be distorted during the seizure [41, 42]. De novo automatisms are movements initiated after the onset of the seizure, most commonly involving the face, head, or upper extremities [41, 42]. Lip smacking, chewing, and fumbling with the fingers are the most common de novo automatisms [41, 42]. Others include swallowing, lip licking, grimacing, yawning, scratching, rubbing, shuffling the legs, walking, and stepping in place [41, 42]. Formed speech rarely occurs during an absence seizure, but occasionally a patient will hum [41, 42]. Some de novo automatisms appear to be responses to environmental stimuli. If spoken to, the patient may turn toward the spoken voice; when touched or tickled he may touch the site; placing gum in the mouth may result in chewing movements [41, 42]. The probability that an automatism will occur during an absence seizure increases as seizure duration increases, and in absence seizures lasting longer than 18 seconds the probability of an automatism is greater than 95 percent [42].

AUTONOMIC COMPONENTS

The incidence of autonomic phenomena during absence seizures is not precisely known because documentation of such phenomena requires specialized techniques. Autonomic phenomena that have been reported during absence seizures include decreased vasomotor tone, decreased skin resistance, brief respiratory arrest, reduced gastric and esophageal motility, pupil dilatation, pallor, flushing, piloerection, tachycardia, salivation, and urinary incontinence [34, 42]. These changes are not specific for absence seizures and are observable with other types of seizures.

CLASSIFICATION OF ABSENCE SEIZURES

Based on the presence or absence of the phenomena just described, the International Classification of Epileptic Seizures [12] classifies absence seizures as follows: (1) impairment of consciousness only, (2) with mild clonic components, (3) with atonic components, (4) with tonic components, (5) with automatisms, (6) with autonomic components (types 2 through 6 may occur alone or in combination).

ABSENCE STATUS EPILEPTICUS

This topic is reviewed in Chapter 30.

EEG Phenomena

EEG PATTERNS DURING ABSENCE SEIZURES

The classic EEG pattern seen during absence seizures is the 3-Hz spike-wave discharge (Fig. 7-3). The EEG and clinical details of 3-Hz spike-wave discharges are summarized in Table 8-3. The National Institutes of Health group has examined over 600 absence seizures recorded on split-screen videotape with simultaneous recording of the clinical seizure and the EEG [3, 12, 42]. Every absence seizure was accompanied by bilateral spike-wave discharges. The discharges were not always fully generalized and were not always exactly 3 Hz. However, all absence seizures were accompanied by bilateral spike-wave or multiple spike- and slow-wave discharges of 2 to 4 Hz.

CLINICAL SIGNIFICANCE OF SPIKE-WAVE DISCHARGES

These data indicate that all absence seizures are accompanied by spike-wave paroxysms. One can then ask if all spike-wave paroxysms cause absence seizures or at least a measurable impairment in alertness. Several groups have studied the responsiveness of patients before, during, and after 3-Hz spike-wave paroxysms [6, 34, 48, 49, 50]. All agree that responsiveness is decreased during most spike-wave paroxysms, falls with the onset of the 3-Hz EEG pattern, and begins to recover well before the pattern has disappeared from the EEG. There is some disagreement about when behavioral signs begin in relation to the 3-Hz spike-wave EEG abnormality. Mirsky and Van Buren [34], using a visual attention task, reported that a significant impairment of visual attentive capacity

Figure 7-3. Typical 3-Hz spike-wave paroxysm.

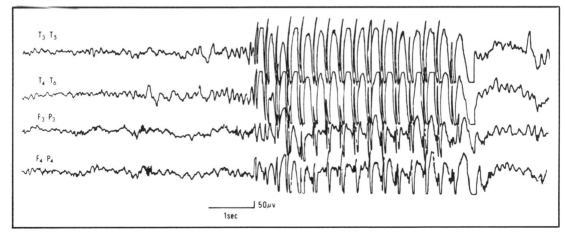

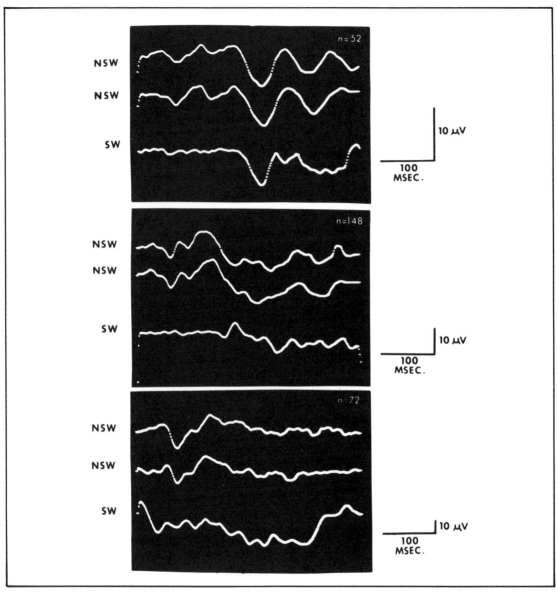

NSW

NSW

SW

n = 52

10 μV

100
MSEC.

NSW

NSW

SW

n=148

10 μV

100
MSEC.

NSW

NSW

SW

n=72

10 μV

100
MSEC.

Figure 7-4. Reduced visually evoked potentials seen in three patients with absence epilepsy. The figure presents averages (n indicated in upper right corner of each graph) to strobe stimuli presented during non-spike-wave (NSW) and spike-wave (SW) periods. The averages were obtained from parietal-occipital (P_3–O_1 or P_4–O_2) recordings. (From Mirsky and Orren [32].)

was evident about 0.5 seconds *before* the onset of 3-Hz seizure paroxysms. Geller and Geller [18] reported similar findings. Orren [39] has described reduced visual evoked potentials in several patients beginning 200 to 500 msec before the onset of a spike-wave paroxysm. (This finding is compatible with the results reported by Mirsky and Orren [32] of reduced visual evoked potentials during spike-wave paroxysms (Fig. 7-4) and the earlier [31] report by Mirsky et al. of similar effects seen in experimental absence seizures in monkeys.)

On the other hand, Browne et al. [6] measured 671 auditory reaction times immediately before, during, and immediately after 310 typical 3-Hz spike-wave paroxysms (Fig. 7-5). All reaction times during the 1 second before a paroxysm were within normal

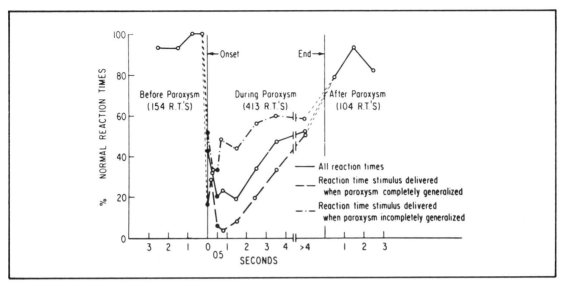

Figure 7-5. Graph of 671 reaction times to auditory stimuli from 26 patients showing percent of normal reaction times before, during, and after 3-Hz spike-wave paroxysm. (From T. R. Browne et al. [5].)

limits. However, only 45 percent of reaction times measured at the onset of a paroxysm were normal. Maximum impairment of responsiveness occurred 0.5 to 1.0 second into the paroxysm, regardless of its duration. At this time, only 4 percent of reaction times were normal when the paroxysm was completely generalized, and only 33 percent of reaction times were normal when the paroxysm was incompletely generalized. Responsiveness then gradually improved during and after the paroxysm.

Differences in the exact temporal profile of altered responsiveness during spike-wave discharges as measured by various groups may be due to differences in the type of task stimulus used (visual vs. auditory), the complexity of the task, or possibly the inclusion of data from spike-wave forms other than "typical" 3-Hz spike-wave forms. Some support for the significance of stimulus modality is provided by Orren [38], who studied the responsiveness of several patients during 3-Hz spike-wave bursts using sustained attention tasks that involved either visual or auditory signals. In several patients she observed greater responsiveness to auditory cues than to visual cues during spike-wave paroxysms.

In addition to these effects on attentiveness, several studies have suggested that the spike-wave paroxysm may have deleterious effects on memory. Retrograde memory deficits for verbal or visual material presented during the period several seconds prior to spike-wave bursts have been reported [18, 34].

Erba and Cavazzuti [13] have reported that during some spike-wave paroxysms significant impairment of the ability to perform complex tasks (e.g., copying complex figures, searching tasks, word fluency) can be documented without any measurable impairment of motor control, vigilance, or memory. Such disruptions are particularly apt to occur in teenagers with a history of absence or tonic-clonic seizures at an earlier age, incompletely generalized 2.5- to 3-Hz spike-waves on EEG, and no obvious clinical absence seizures at the present time. The disruptions can profoundly alter behavioral and learning patterns and yet not appear to parents or teachers to be caused by a seizure problem.

Despite some quantitative differences in some of the results just mentioned, it is the consensus of most studies that 3-Hz spike-wave paroxysms, especially if fully generalized, almost invariably cause a measurable impairment in performance. This conclusion has two clinically significant consequences. First, therapy should be aimed at suppressing all spike-wave bursts. Second, counting spike-wave bursts on prolonged EEG recordings is probably a valid method of evaluating the effectiveness of antiabsence drugs [5].

INTERICTAL EEG PATTERNS
The EEG background is usually normal, although paroxysmal activity may occur (spikes or spike- and slow-wave complexes) [4, 12, 25, 42]. This activity is usually regular and symmetrical. Slowing is seldom present.

Hyperventilation
Spike-wave paroxysms can almost always be precipitated by hyperventilation in untreated patients with absence seizures [4, 5]. Once antiabsence medication is begun, spike-wave paroxysms may disappear.

Photic Stimulation
Spike-wave paroxysms can be provoked by photic stimulation in a minority of patients with absence seizures (see Chap. 11) [37, 42].

Differential Diagnosis
The major differential diagnostic problem in patients with absence seizures is differentiating among absence, atypical absence, myoclonic, atonic, and complex partial seizures. Other conditions that may cause apparent brief lapses of consciousness or impaired attentiveness in children include daydreaming, fatigue, metabolic or lead encephalopathy, and psychosis (e.g., childhood schizophrenia or infantile autism).

ATYPICAL ABSENCE, MYOCLONIC, AND ATONIC SEIZURES
See Chapter 8.

COMPLEX PARTIAL SEIZURES
One of the most common errors in the diagnosis and management of epilepsy is in confusing absence and complex partial seizures. Both seizure types are characterized by altered consciousness and automatisms, and patients with absence seizures are frequently diagnosed as having complex partial seizures

and vice versa. This error in diagnosis initiates an unfortunate sequence of events because the medications prescribed do not control the patient's seizures; the patient is often "pushed" to toxic levels of drugs in a vain attempt to control the seizures, and the patient then becomes demoralized.

The differential diagnostic features of absence versus complex partial seizures are shown in Table 7-1. Absence seizures usually begin between 5 and 10 years of age. Complex partial seizures are relatively rare before 10 years of age but can occur [20]. Auras with psychic and sensory phenomena are common with complex partial seizures (see Chap. 5) but never occur with absence seizures. The majority of absence seizures last less than 10 seconds [42], whereas complex partial seizures typically last a minute or more. Alteration of consciousness and staring occur in both types of seizure. Simple or complex automatisms are seen in both seizure types and are often similar (see Chap. 5). Absence seizures cannot usually be differentiated from complex partial seizures on the basis of morphology of automatisms [11]. Formed speech, sometimes incoherent or dysphasic, may occur during complex partial seizures but never during absence seizures [42]. Incontinence sometimes occurs with complex partial seizures but is extremely rare with absence seizures [11, 42]. It is usually possible to differentiate absence from complex partial seizures if a reliable history covering the points in Table 7-1 can be obtained. In a minority of patients the history can be misleading because some complex partial seizures consist chiefly of loss of consciousness

Table 7-1. Differential Diagnosis of Absence Versus Complex Partial Seizures

	Absence	Complex Partial
Age of onset	Childhood	Any age, although rare in childhood
Aura	None	Common
Seizure		
Duration	Seconds	Minutes
Alertness	Out of contact	Out of contact
Automatisms	Simple or complex	Simple or complex
Staring	Yes	Yes
Speech	Never formed; patient sometimes hums	Incoherent, dysphasic, or none
Postictal confusion	Never	Often
Amnesia for attack	Yes	Yes, some islands of memory
Precipitation by hyperventilation	Often	Rarely
Precipitation by photic stimulation	Sometimes	Very rarely
EEG	3-Hz spike-wave	Temporal slowing or sharp activity

Source: Modified from Dreifuss [11]. By permission of Raven Press.

and automatisms without the other features included in Table 7-1. Histories can also mislead because young children with complex partial seizures may not have all of the clinical features of such seizures seen in adults [20].

The EEG can provide objective information that is often very helpful in differential diagnosis of absence versus complex partial seizures. The EEG background is usually normal in patients with absence seizures. Spontaneous spike-wave paroxysms are sometimes seen, and spike-wave paroxysms can almost always be precipitated by hyperventilation in untreated patients with absence seizures [4, 5]. Once antiabsence medication is begun, spike-wave paroxysms may disappear, and it may not be possible to induce them by hyperventilation or photic stimulation. The interictal EEG in patients with complex partial seizures may be normal or may show unilateral or bilateral temporal slowing and/or sharp activity (see Chap. 5).

Management

ETHOSUXIMIDE
Ethosuximide (see Chap. 19) is the drug of first choice for absence seizures because it is extremely effective, and most patients experience little or no side effects during chronic administration. Ethosuximide is extremely effective in controlling both clinical absence seizures and 3-Hz spike-wave discharges on EEG. The common side effects of ethosuximide, gastrointestinal upset and drowsiness, tend to occur early in therapy and then diminish as tolerance develops. The drug seldom causes behavioral or cognitive disturbances. About 1 to 7 percent of patients taking ethosuximide develop leukopenia, which is reversible if detected early.

VALPROIC ACID
Valproic acid (see Chap. 20) is also extremely effective in controlling clinical absence seizures and 3-Hz spike-wave discharges on EEG. Valproic acid has some activity against tonic-clonic seizures (which ethosuximide does not) and seldom causes leukopenia. Despite the possible advantages of valproic acid, ethosuximide remains the drug of first choice for patients with only absence seizures because (1) the risk of serious or fatal hepatotoxicity as a result of valproic acid administration appears to be greater (50 deaths as of 1981) than the risk of bone marrow depression as a result of ethosuximide administration; (2) the common side effects of valproic acid (gastrointestinal upset and drowsiness) are more severe and persistent than those seen with ethosuximide; (3) the longer elimination half-life of ethosuximide allows for

more constant blood levels with less frequent administration; (4) valproic acid is much more expensive than ethosuximide; (5) valproic acid produces more clinically significant drug interactions with other antiepileptic drugs than ethosuximide; and (6) the onset of antiabsence effect occurs significantly sooner with ethosuximide than with valproic acid. In patients with both absence and tonic-clonic seizures, valproic acid may be the drug of first choice because it has activity against both seizure types.

CLONAZEPAM
Clonazepam's efficacy in controlling absence seizures (see Chap. 21) is approximately equal to that of ethosuximide and valproic acid. However, clonazepam is now the third choice drug for this condition because disabling side effects (drowsiness, ataxia, behavioral disturbances) and development of tolerance to the antiepileptic effect of the drug are more common with clonazepam than with ethosuximide or valproic acid.

ACETAZOLAMIDE
Acetazolamide (see Chap. 22) has some effect against absence seizures and probably causes fewer side effects than the three drugs mentioned above. However, acetozolamide probably does not control absence seizures completely as often as these three drugs, and the antiabsence effect of acetazolamide is often transient.

METHSUXIMIDE
Methsuximide (see Chap. 19) is less effective and more toxic than ethosuximide in most patients with absence seizures. Methsuximide can be tried when less toxic agents fail.

TRIMETHADIONE
Trimethadione (see Chap. 22) is very effective in controlling absence seizures. However, it is seldom used now because of its high incidence of serious side effects (sedation, hemeralopia, neutropenia, rash, nephrotic syndrome, hepatitis, pancytopenia).

PHENSUXIMIDE
Phensuximide (see Chap. 19) is less effective and more toxic than ethosuximide or methsuximide in most patients with absence seizures.

PROPHYLACTIC THERAPY FOR TONIC-CLONIC SEIZURES
One third to one half of all patients with absence seizures also develop tonic-clonic seizures before or after the onset of absence seizures. This has led some physicians to advocate the administration of pro-

phylactic tonic-clonic antiepileptic drugs as well as antiabsence medication to patients with only absence seizures [26]. This practice is of questionable value. The child presenting with absence seizures who has not yet had a tonic-clonic seizure has only a 25 percent chance of developing tonic-clonic seizures in the future [47]. Moreover, there are many real and potential dangers associated with chronic antiepileptic drug administration for tonic-clonic seizures [45]. Not administering prophylactic drugs for tonic-clonic seizures will avoid exposure to the chronic toxicity of unnecessary drugs in the majority of patients with absence seizures and will reduce by several years the cumulative exposure to such drugs in patients who do develop tonic-clonic seizures. Such seizures should be treated vigorously with phenytoin if they do appear. Phenobarbital should be avoided because the drowsiness caused by the drug may make absence seizures worse [43].

Prognosis

ABSENCE SEIZURES

Absence seizures often cease spontaneously, usually in the teenage years. Reported rates of cessation of absence seizures vary from 50 to 70 percent of patients [22, 46]. There is no way of predicting a priori which patients will cease having absence seizures. However, in a prospective follow-up study, Sato et al. [46, 47] found that the following prognostic factors were useful for predicting cessation of absence seizures: normal or above normal intelligence, normal EEG background, negative history for tonic-clonic seizures, and a negative family history of seizure disorders. Nearly 90 percent of patients with all of these prognostic factors ceased having seizures of any type.

TONIC-CLONIC SEIZURES

Tonic-clonic seizures occur in one third to one half of patients with absence seizures [4, 19, 25, 26, 46]. Tonic-clonic seizures precede absence seizures in approximately half of those patients [47]. There is no way to be certain which patients with absence seizures will develop tonic-clonic seizures. In some cases tonic-clonic seizures end spontaneously in the teens. However, in the majority of patients the tonic-clonic seizures persist past the teens [46, 47]. Normal intelligence and a negative family history of seizures are favorable prognostic indicators of spontaneous cessation of tonic-clonic seizures [46, 47].

COMPLEX PARTIAL SEIZURES

There are scattered reports of patients with absence seizures who later develop complex partial seizures.

The preponderance of evidence indicates that this happens very rarely [46, 47].

INTELLIGENCE AND NEUROLOGIC FUNCTION

The majority of patients with absence seizures have average or above average intelligence [4, 25, 46]. However, some reports indicate that as many as 20 to 30 percent of patients with absence seizures have IQs of less than 90 [22, 23, 46].

It is, however, difficult to rule out a possible impairment of intelligence produced by large doses of antiepileptic drugs, especially when these compounds are prescribed in combination. The deleterious effect on cognitive abilities of such medications has been described by a number of authors [9].

References

1. Ajmone Marsan, C., and Lewis, W. R. Pathologic findings in patients with "centrencephalic" electroencephalographic patterns. *Neurology* (Minneap.) 10:992, 1960.
2. Browne, T. R. Clinical pharmacology of antiepileptic drugs. *Drug Therapy Reviews* 2:469, 1979.
3. Browne, T. R. Unpublished data, 1982.
4. Browne, T. R. et al. Ethosuximide in the treatment of absence (petit mal) seizures. *Neurology* (Minneap.) 25:515, 1975.
5. Browne, T. R. et al. Clinical and electroencephalographic estimates of absence seizure frequency. *Arch. Neurol.* In press, 1983.
6. Browne, T. R. et al. Responsiveness before, during, and after spike-wave paroxysms. *Neurology* (Minneap.) 24:654, 1974.
7. Cohen, R. Neuropathological study of a case of petit mal epilepsy. *Electroencephalogr. Clin. Neurophysiol.* 24:282, 1968.
8. Dalby, M. A. Epilepsy and 3 per second spike and wave rhythms: A clinical electroencephalographic and prognostic analysis of 346 patients. *Acta Neurol. Scand.* [Suppl.] 40:45, 1969.
9. Dodrill, C. B., and Wilkus, R. J. Neuropsychological Correlates of Anticonvulsants and Epileptiform Discharges in Adult Epileptics. In W. A. Cobb, and H. Van Juijn (Eds.), *Contemporary Clinical Neurophysiology* (EEG Suppl. No. 34). Amsterdam: Elsevier, 1978.
10. Doose, H. et al. Genetic factors in spike-wave absences. *Epilepsia* 14:57, 1973.
11. Dreifuss, F. E. The Differential Diagnosis of Partial Seizures with Complex Symptomatology. In J. K. Penry, and D. D. Daly (Eds.), *Advances in Neurology*, Vol. 11, *Complex Partial Seizures and Their Treatment.* New York: Raven Press, 1975.

12. Dreifuss, F. E. Proposal for revised clinical and electroencephalographic classification of epileptic seizures. *Epilepsia* 22:489, 1981.

13. Erba, G., and Cavazzuti, V. Incomplete absence: Selective and variable functional loss during spike-wave activity. *Electroencephalogr. Clin. Neurophysiol.* 50:217P, 1980.

14. Fromm, G. H. et al. Antiabsence drugs and inhibitory pathways. *Neurology* (N.Y.) 30:126, 1980.

15. Fromm, G. H. et al. Effect of anticonvulsant drugs on inhibitory and excitatory pathways. *Epilepsia* 22:65, 1981.

16. Fromm, G. H., and Kohli, C. M. The inhibitory pathways in petit mal epilepsy. *Neurology* (Minneap.) 22:1011, 1972.

17. Gastaut, H., and Gastaut, J. L. Computerized transverse axial tomography in epilepsy. *Epilepsia* 17:337, 1976.

18. Geller, M., and Geller, A. Brief amnesic effects of spike-wave discharge. *Neurology* (Minneap.) 20:1089, 1970.

19. Gibbs, F. A., and Gibbs, E. L. *Atlas of Electroencephalography,* Vol. 3, *Epilepsy* (2nd ed.). Reading, Mass.: Addison-Wesley, 1960.

20. Glaser, G. H., and Dixon, M. S. Psychomotor seizures in childhood: A clinical study. *Neurology* (Minneap.) 6:646, 1956.

21. Gloor, P. Generalized epilepsy with spike-wave discharge. A reinterpretation of its electrographic and clinical manifestations. *Epilepsia* 20:571, 1979.

22. Hertott, P. The clinical, electroencephalographic and social prognosis in petit mal epilepsy. *Epilepsia* 4:298, 1963.

23. Holowach, J., Thurston, D. L., and O'Leary, J. Petit mal epilepsy. *Pediatrics* 30:893, 1962.

24. Jasper, H. H. Mechanisms of Propagation: Extracellular Studies. In H. H. Jasper, A. A. Ward, and A. Pope (Eds.), *Basic Mechanisms of the Epilepsies.* Boston: Little, Brown, 1969.

25. Lennox, W. G., and Lennox, M. A. *Epilepsy and Related Disorders.* Vol. 1. Boston: Little, Brown, 1960.

26. Livingston, S. et al. Petit mal epilepsy: Results of a prolonged follow-up study of 117 patients. *J.A.M.A.* 194:113, 1965.

27. Marcus, E. M. Experimental Models of Petit Mal Epilepsy. In D. P. Purpura et al. (Eds.), *Experimental Models of Epilepsy.* New York: Raven Press, 1972.

28. Marcus, E. M., and Watson, C. W. Bilateral synchronous spike-wave electrographic patterns in the cat. Interaction of bilateral cortical foci in the intact, the bilateral cortical-callosal, and adiencephalic preparation. *Arch. Neurol.* 14:601, 1966.

29. Metrakos, J. D., and Metrakos, K. Genetics of convulsive disorders, Part 1 (Introduction, problems, methods, and base lines). *Neurology* 10:228, 1960.

30. Metrakos, K., and Metrakos, J. D. Genetics of convulsive disorders, Part 2 (Genetic and electroencephalographic studies in centrencephalic epilepsy). *Neurology* 11:464, 1961.

31. Mirsky, A. F. et al. Visual evoked potentials during experimentally induced spike-wave activity in monkeys. *Electroencephalogr. Clin. Neurophysiol.* 35:25, 1973.

32. Mirsky, A. F., and Orren, M. M. Attention. In L. H. Miller, A. J. Kastin, and C. A. Sandman (Eds.), *Neuropeptide Influences on the Brain and Behavior.* New York: Raven Press, 1977.

33. Mirsky, A. F. et al. Brainstem Auditory Evoked Potential (BAEP) Alterations During Induced and Spontaneous Generalized Spike-Wave Activity in Animals and Humans. *9th Annual Meeting, Society for Neuroscience Abstracts* 641, 1979.

34. Mirsky, A. F., and Van Buren, J. M. On the nature of the "absence" in centrencephalic epilepsy: A study of some behavioral, electroencephalographic and autonomic factors. *Electroencephalogr. Clin. Neurophysiol.* 18:334, 1965.

35. Moseley, I. F., and Bull, J. W. Computerized Axial Tomography, Carotid Angiography and Orbital Phlebography in the Diagnosis of Space-Occupying Lesions of the Orbit. In G. Salamon (Ed.), *Advances in Cerebral Angiography.* New York: Springer-Verlag, 1975.

36. Myslobodsky, M. *Petit Mal Epilepsy, A Search for the Precursors of Spike-Wave Activity.* New York: Academic, 1976.

37. Newmark, M. E., and Penry, J. K. *Photosensitivity and Epilepsy: A Review.* New York: Raven Press, 1979.

38. Orren, M. M. Visuomotor behavior and visual evoked potentials during petit mal seizures. Ph.D. dissertation, Boston University, 1974.

39. Orren, M. M. Evoked Potential Studies in Petit Mal Epilepsy. In W. A. Cobb, and H. Van Duyn (Eds.), *Contemporary Clinical Neurophysiology* (EEG Suppl. No. 34). Amsterdam: Elsevier, 1978.

40. Penfield, W., and Jasper, H. *Epilepsy and the Functional Anatomy of the Human Brain.* Boston: Little, Brown, 1954.

41. Penry, J. K., and Dreifuss, F. E. Automatisms associated with absence of petit mal epilepsy. *Arch. Neurol.* 21:142, 1969.

42. Penry, J. K., Porter, R. J., and Dreifuss, F. E. Simultaneous recording of absence seizures with video-

tape and electroencephalography: A study of 374 seizures in 48 patients. *Brain* 98:427, 1975.

43. Penry, J. K., and So, E. L. Refractiveness of absence seizures and phenobarbital. *Neurology* 31:158, 1981.

44. Pollen, D. A. Experimental spike and wave responses in petit mal epilepsy. *Epilepsia* 9:221, 1968.

45. Reynolds, E. H. Chronic antiepileptic toxicity: A review. *Epilepsia* 16:319, 1975.

46. Sato, S., Dreifuss, F. E., and Penry, J. K. Prognostic factors in absence seizures. *Neurology* (Minneap.) 26:788, 1976.

47. Sato, S. et al. Prognostic factors in absence seizures: Long-term follow-up study. *Neurology* (N.Y.) 30:329, 1980.

48. Schwab, R. S. Method of measuring consciousness in attacks of petit mal epilepsy. *Arch. Neurol. Psychiatr.* 41:215, 1939.

49. Schwab, R. S. Reaction time in petit mal epilepsy. *Res. Publ. Assoc. Res. Nerv. Ment. Dis.* 26:339, 1947.

50. Shimazono, Y. et al. Disturbance of consciousness in petit mal epilepsy. *Epilepsia* 2:49, 1953.

51. Weir, B. Spike-wave from stimulation of reticular core. *Arch. Neurol.* 11:209, 1964.

ATYPICAL ABSENCE, MYOCLONIC, ATONIC, AND TONIC SEIZURES, AND THE "LENNOX-GASTAUT SYNDROME"

8

Giuseppe Erba
Thomas R. Browne

Introduction and Definitions

Atypical absence, myoclonic, atonic, and tonic seizures are all forms of generalized seizures. They are discussed together because they often occur in the same patient in varying combinations and because they may share common pathophysiologic mechanisms. It is important to recognize from the onset that any of these types of seizures can be an expression of either primarily generalized epilepsy (often associated with normal intelligence, normal interictal EEG, and good response to therapy) or of secondarily generalized epilepsy (often associated with lowered intelligence, abnormal interictal EEG, and poor response to therapy). Thus, although the clinical seizures have common features in many patients, the presence of such seizures can be associated with a wide range of etiologies and outcomes.

The *Lennox-Gastaut syndrome* is a seizure disorder of childhood characterized by: (1) *interictal* slow spike-wave discharges on the EEG; (2) atypical absence, myoclonic, atonic, and tonic seizures in varying combinations in the same patient; and (3) an encephalopathy with mental retardation and neurologic deficits of various etiology (see below and Table 8-1). Although the Lennox-Gastaut syndrome is the context in which these seizures are most commonly observed, the same types of ictal manifestations can be observed in a variety of conditions.

Etiology of Atypical Absence, Myoclonic, Atonic, and Tonic Seizures

PRIMARILY GENERALIZED FORMS

Only a minority of patients with these types of seizures have primarily generalized (idiopathic) epilepsy. In these cases, usually one seizure type predominates and is associated with the more typical expressions of generalized epilepsy (i.e., absence and/or tonic-clonic seizures). An example is the "impulsive petit mal" described by Janz [19, 38], a form of myoclonic seizures starting around puberty associated with generalized tonic-clonic seizures and benign evolution. Although this group has not been extensively studied, anecdotal data [20, 30, 31] suggest a genetic predisposition similar to that documented in more detail for absence and tonic-clonic seizures (see Chaps. 6 and 7).

This work was supported in part by the Veterans Administration.

76

Table 8-1. Clinical Features of Lennox-Gastaut Syndrome

Age at onset of seizures	
Usual age	Infancy–7 years
Range	1 day–13 years
Age at onset of slow spike-wave EEG abnormality	
Usual age	1–7 years
Range	3 months–13 years
Sex	50–61% are males
Typical seizure types	
Atypical absence	17–60%*
Myoclonic	11–28%
Atonic	26–56%
Tonic	17–92%
Other seizure types sometimes seen	
Tonic-clonic	15–56%
Infantile spasms	18–22%
Unilateral	9–22%
Clonic	9%
Complex partial	7–10%
Mental retardation	47–96%
Neurologic deficits	30–75%
Abnormal computerized axial tomographic scan	52–90%
Abnormal pneumoencephalogram	50–66%

*Percentage of patients.

Source: Based on data from J. J. Chevrie and J. Aicardi [11]; H. Gastaut and J. L. Gastaut [28]; H. Gastaut et al. [30, 34]; T. Kurokawa [42]; I. Langenstein et al. [46]; W. G. Lennox and M. A. Lennox [48]; E. Niedermeyer [56]; and L. Sorel [62].

SECONDARILY GENERALIZED FORMS

Most frequently, atypical absence, myoclonic, atonic, and tonic seizures are *symptomatic* of an underlying acquired encephalopathy of a fixed or progressive nature. These seizures can also be manifestations of a number of specific syndromes (metabolic, infectious, degenerative) or a nonspecific response to a wide variety of cerebral insults (which will be discussed later in this chapter).

ETIOLOGY OF LENNOX-GASTAUT SYNDROME

See Lennox-Gastaut Syndrome below.

Atypical Absence Seizures

DEFINITIONS AND SEIZURE PHENOMENA

Lennox and Davis [47] first made the observation that during "slow" or "atypical" spike-wave activity in the EEG the patient could manifest subtle motor manifestations (e.g., twitching) and/or staring but still be responsive. Gastaut et al. [31, 34] have distinguished two varieties of atypical absence seizures. In the first

variety, responsiveness is decreased, but not completely abolished, and the onset and cessation of decreased responsiveness are more gradual than in typical absence seizures. Erba and Cavazzuti [22] have documented that during slow spike-wave activity certain subjects present a very selective and variable impairment of high cortical functions while they are still responsive and able to attend to the assigned task. This variety of incomplete absence seizure may also be accompanied by automatisms, an increase or decrease in postural tone (sometimes more pronounced than in typical absence seizures), or autonomic phenomena [17, 31, 34].

The second variety of atypical absence seizures consists of impaired consciousness accompanied by mild tonic motor phenomena (opening of palpebrae, revulsion of eyes superiorly, rigidity of jaw and neck, increase in axial muscle tone). Both clinically and electroencephalographically this type of seizure has many similarities to tonic seizures (see below) and is probably best regarded as a variant of tonic seizures.

EEG PHENOMENA

Interictal EEG

In the primarily generalized forms and in those secondary to a chronic focus, the interictal EEG may be normal. When there is an underlying encephalopathy, the EEG background is usually abnormal in both varieties of atypical absence seizures and may show the abnormalities typical of the Lennox-Gastaut syndrome or other forms of slowing, spikes, or irregular spike-wave activity. These abnormalities are often asymmetrical.

Ictal EEG

During the first variety of atypical absence seizure, the EEG shows diffuse, but not completely generalized, often asymmetrical slow spike-wave bursts, usually 5 to 15 seconds in duration (Fig. 8-1). However, similar-appearing slow spike-wave paroxysms may fail to produce a measurable alteration of responsiveness (see below).

During the second variety of atypical absence seizure, the ictal EEG may show: (1) flattening of the background activity; (2) low-voltage fast activity, frequently of progressively increasing amplitude; (3) rhythmic discharge of sharp wave activity at 10 Hz; or (4) any combination of these three patterns. These EEG ictal manifestations are similar to those observed during tonic seizures and atonic seizures (see below).

Neither form of atypical absence seizure is usually precipitated by hyperventilation or photic stimulation.

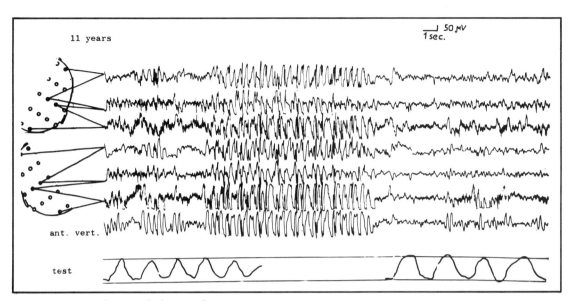

Figure 8-1. Slow spike-wave discharge with accompanying atypical absence seizure. Impairment of consciousness and suspension of ongoing motor activity are demonstrated by loss of ability to perform a simple writing task at the bottom of the EEG paper. (From H. Gastaut et al. In P. J. Vinken and G. W. Bruyn [Eds.], Handbook of Clinical Neurology, Vol. 15, The Epilepsies. *Amsterdam: Elsevier, 1974.)*

PATHOPHYSIOLOGY

The mechanisms responsible for the production of atypical absence seizures are presumably similar to those responsible for the production of absence seizures (see Chap. 7 and Pathophysiology under Tonic Seizures and Lennox-Gastaut Syndrome below).

DIFFERENTIAL DIAGNOSIS

Typical Absence Seizures

Typical absence seizures have sudden onset and cessation, begin at age 5 to 12 years, seldom are associated with serious mental retardation or structural CNS damage, respond well to therapy, are associated with 3-Hz spike-wave discharges during the seizure, and usually have a normal interictal EEG (Table 8-2, Fig. 8-2). Atypical absence seizures usually begin before 5 years of age, often are associated with serious mental retardation or structural CNS damage, respond poorly to therapy, and often have an abnormal interictal EEG. The alteration of responsiveness during atypical absence seizures is often less complete and more gradual in onset and cessation and the EEG usually shows "slow" and/or incompletely generalized spike-waves. Despite these differences, both typical and atypical absence seizures may be accom-

panied by similar-appearing automatisms, increases or decreases in postural tone, or autonomic phenomena. One form may be difficult to distinguish from the other except by the degree of impairment in awareness.

Whereas atypical absence seizures are frequent and easily recognizable in the context of the Lennox-Gastaut syndrome, incomplete absences can also occur in patients who are neurologically and intellectually intact. For instance, patients with absence seizures who have almost outgrown their disorder may have only fleeting and evanescent absences [22] (see Chap. 7).

Complex Partial Seizures

Complex partial seizures can usually be differentiated from typical and atypical absence seizures on the basis of criteria reviewed in Chap. 7.

Other Conditions

"Daydreaming," fatigue, metabolic or lead encephalopathy, and psychosis (e.g., childhood schizophrenia or infantile autism) may cause apparent brief lapses of consciousness or impaired attentiveness in children.

MANAGEMENT AND PROGNOSIS

The management and prognosis of atypical absence seizures are discussed later in this chapter.

Myoclonic Seizures

DEFINITIONS

Myoclonus is a brief, involuntary muscle contraction involving one or several muscles that may or may not

Table 8-2. *Absence, Atypical Absence, Myoclonic, and Atonic Seizures*

Clinical and EEG Features	Absence (Typical Petit Mal)	Atypical Absence (Atypical Petit Mal)	Myoclonic	Atonic (Astatic, Drop Attack)
Clinical				
Seizure	Sudden onset and cessation of loss of responsiveness. May be accompanied by automatisms, mild clonic movements, increased or decreased postural tone, or autonomic phenomena	Brief decrease of responsiveness that is often incomplete and has gradual onset and cessation. May be accompanied by automatisms, increase or decrease in tone, or autonomic phenomena	Myoclonic jerks. Symmetrical or asymmetrical, synchronous or asynchronous. Usually no detectable loss of consciousness	Loss of body tone (atonic) Usually no detectable loss of consciousness
Precipitated by hyperventilation	Often	Seldom	Seldom	Seldom
Age at onset	5–12 yr	1–7 yr	1–7 yr	1–7 yr
Evidence of structural CNS damage	5–25%	More often than typical absence, but not invariably present		
Associated mental retardation	Seldom	More often than typical absence, but not invariably present		
Associated seizures	One third to one half of patients have other types of seizures, usually tonic-clonic	Atypical absence, myoclonic, and atonic seizures tend to occur in various combinations in the same patient. Tonic-clonic and tonic seizures are also frequently present, but typical absence seizures rarely are present		
Prognosis	Seizures end in late childhood. Normal intelligence	Seizures end in late childhood. However, the mental retardation progresses or remains unchanged, and tonic-clonic seizures may develop		
Response to antiepileptic drugs	Usually good	Often refractory to therapy		
EEG				
Ictal	3-Hz spike-wave	Slow spike-wave or other irregular spike-and-slow-wave complexes	Polyspike-and-wave, slow spike-wave, or sharp and slow waves	Slow spike-wave, 3-Hz spike-wave, polyspike-and-wave, a mixture of rhythmic slow waves, or fast recruiting rhythms
Interictal				
Background	Usually normal	Often abnormal (slow)	Often abnormal (slow)	Often abnormal (slow)
Paroxysmal activity	Usually none. Sometimes spike-waves or polyspike-and-waves	Slow spike-wave or polyspike-and-wave	Same as ictal	Slow spike-wave or polyspike-and-wave

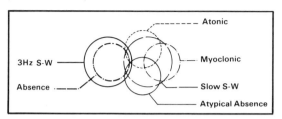

Figure 8-2. Extent of coexistence of absence, atypical absence, myoclonic, and atonic seizures with each other and with 3-Hz spike-wave and slow spike-wave.

produce body movements [30]. Myoclonus, when recorded on an electromyogram (EMG), shows bi- or polyphasic potentials of 20 to 100 msec duration that may be followed by tonic contraction of the muscle or by transient (up to 350 msec) hypotonia [30, 57].

Myoclonus may be either epileptic or nonepileptic in origin. Epileptic myoclonus is distinguished from nonepileptic myoclonus by a concomitant generalized discharge of polyspike-and-wave or spike-wave discharge on the EEG [30, 57]. Gastaut et al. [30, 31] distinguish four principal types of epileptic myoclonus: (1) infantile spasms, (2) myoclonic absences, (3) bilateral massive epileptic myoclonus, and (4) epileptic myoclonus occurring in various specific syndromes (e.g., progressive myoclonic epilepsy, subacute spongioform encephalopathy, subacute sclerosing panencephalitis).

INFANTILE SPASMS
See Chapter 9.

MYOCLONIC ABSENCES

Myoclonus During Typical Absence Seizures
See Chapter 7.

Myoclonus During Atypical Absence Seizures
Atypical absence seizures may contain myoclonus similar to that of typical absences. Myoclonus associated with atypical absence seizures tends to differ from that of typical absence seizures in that it is slower, more irregular, and has a smaller amplitude of movements [31, 51].

BILATERAL MASSIVE EPILEPTIC MYOCLONUS

Seizure Phenomena
The myoclonus is bilateral and symmetrical [30] (Fig. 8-3). Minimally, it may be restricted to the periorbital and palpebral muscles. As it becomes more diffuse it includes the axial and finally the peripheral muscles in a succession of generalized jerks. Massive

myoclonus may be repeated at variable frequencies (1 to 5 Hz) and for a variable period of time (2 seconds to minutes or hours). Myoclonic attacks may terminate in a tonic-clonic seizure. Isolated massive myoclonus is probably not accompanied by any loss of consciousness, but prolonged myoclonic episodes probably do alter consciousness. Autonomic phenomena (tachycardia, bradycardia, sweating) are sometimes present.

Massive myoclonus frequently occurs on awakening and can be facilitated by either eye closure or sleep deprivation. Many cases of sensory-provoked seizures (especially photic-induced) are of the massive myoclonic type [30] (see Chap. 12).

*Etiology, Associated Seizure Types
and Neurologic Deficits*
Myoclonic seizures may be either an expression of primarily or secondarily generalized epilepsy. The clinical features tend to be quite different in the two groups. Patients with primarily generalized myoclonic seizures are frequently subject to spontaneous and isolated jerks, usually in flexion [30]. Ninety percent of patients with primarily generalized myoclonic seizures also have tonic-clonic seizures, and one third of patients with tonic-clonic seizures also have bilateral massive myoclonus [30]. The following features tend to characterize the primarily generalized group: most frequent occurrence in the morning upon awakening; onset after or around puberty (especially the "impulsive petit mal" of Janz [19, 38]); lack of recognizable etiology; no neurologic or intellectual deficits; normal EEG background activity; greater incidence of positive family history for epilepsy; brief duration of seizure phenomena; no association with tonic seizures, although sometimes may be associated with atonic seizures [30, 52].

Patients with secondarily generalized myoclonic seizures tend to show the following characteristics: earlier age of onset; evidence of symptomatic etiology; lack of evidence for genetic factors; neurologic and intellectual deficits; abnormal EEG background; frequent association with myoclonic status epilepticus and/or tonic seizures [52].

Age of Onset
Onset before the age of 4 years is most often associated with symptomatic etiology (Lennox-Gastaut syndrome or other), the clinical features of secondarily generalized myoclonic seizures, and poor prognosis. However, there is a smaller group of patients in the same age range with primarily generalized myoclonic seizures (the cryptogenic group of Aicardi and Chevrie [2]) whose clinical features include no evidence of

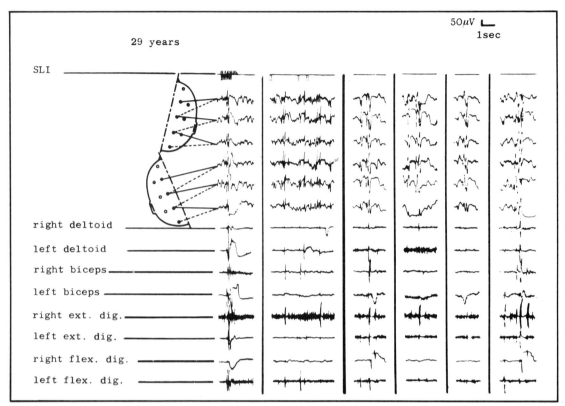

29 years

SLI

right deltoid

left deltoid

right biceps

left biceps

right ext. dig.

left ext. dig.

right flex. dig.

left flex. dig.

50μV

1sec

Figure 8-3. Photically induced and spontaneous bilateral massive epileptic myoclonus. SLI= strobe light indicator. (From H. Gastaut et al. In P. J. Vinken, and G. W. Bruyn [Eds.], Handbook of Clinical Neurology, Vol. 15, The Epilepsies. Amsterdam: Elsevier, 1974.)

neurologic or mental compromise, good response to therapy, and good prognosis. Thus, it is an error to assume that all young children with myoclonic seizures will do poorly.

Primarily generalized myoclonic seizures most often have their onset during adolescence and represent the most common expression of epilepsy in this age group. They also usually carry a good prognosis [19, 20, 21, 38, 52]. However, symptomatic myoclonus and myoclonus due to specific syndromes (e.g., Lafora's disease, subacute sclerosing panencephalitis) can also occur in this age group.

EEG PHENOMENA

Interictal EEG
The interictal EEG is usually normal in the primarily generalized form. Photosensitive epileptic myoclonus usually belongs to this group (see Chap. 12). Other forms of "sensory-induced" myoclonic seizures may either present a normal or very abnormal interictal EEG according to whether they are idiopathic or symptomatic forms.

The interictal EEG of the secondarily generalized forms may show slowing and/or paroxysmal activity

(focal, multifocal, diffuse), including the Lennox-Gastaut syndrome.

Ictal EEG
The isolated, spontaneous massive jerk is associated with a bilaterally synchronous and symmetrical spike-wave, polyspike-and-wave, or, rarely, sharp- and slow-wave discharge [30] (see Fig. 8-3). The spikes or sharp waves usually last 60 to 100 msec. The EMG (see Fig. 8-3) shows that the myoclonus is usually very brief (15 to 40 msec). Multiple spikes or fast waves may precede, be synchronous with, or succeed the jerk. Slow waves, when present, are usually associated with postmyoclonic inhibition of muscle tone (see Fig. 8-3).

PATHOPHYSIOLOGY
See Pathophysiology under Atonic Seizures below.

EPILEPTIC MYOCLONUS OCCURRING IN VARIOUS SPECIFIC SYNDROMES
This topic is reviewed elsewhere [30, 44].

DIFFERENTIAL DIAGNOSIS

Absence Seizures with Mild Clonic Components

Myoclonic seizures can be differentiated from absence seizures with mild clonic components on the following grounds: (1) consciousness is usually not lost during myoclonic seizures; (2) the jerks of myoclonic seizures are usually larger in amplitude and less regular than the mild clonic components of absence seizures; (3) the EEG during myoclonic seizures shows polyspikes, polyspike-and-wave, or slow spike-wave, whereas during typical absence seizures it shows 3-Hz spike-wave discharges.

Infantile Spasms

Infantile spasms begin during the first 6 months of life in 50 percent of the cases and during the first year in 85 percent. Myoclonic seizures can be difficult to differentiate from the flexor type of infantile spasm. However, in myoclonic seizures the EEG tends to show the "fast" variety of spike-wave activity, and the background lacks the characteristic disorganization of hypsarrhythmia. Behavioral-cognitive difficulties associated with myoclonic seizures tend to improve considerably when seizures come under control and spike-wave activity in the EEG disappears [52].

Nonepileptic Myoclonus

Nonepileptic varieties of myoclonus include: physiologic diurnal and hypnagogic myoclonus present in all normal subjects; pathophysiologic states in which reactivity to unexpected sensory stimuli becomes abnormally intensified, "leg jitters"; "restless leg syndrome"; spinal cord disease with myoclonus; dyssynergia cerebellaris myoclonica; subcortical segmental myoclonus; paramyoclonus multiplex; opsoclonus-myoclonus syndrome; and certain intoxications, infections, degenerative disorders, and metabolic diseases [17, 30, 44]. Epileptic myoclonus is distinguished from nonepileptic myoclonus on the basis of a concomitant generalized polyspike-and-wave or spike-wave discharge on the EEG [30, 57].

MANAGEMENT AND PROGNOSIS

The management and prognosis of myoclonic seizures are discussed later in this chapter.

Atonic (Astatic) Seizures or Drop Attacks

DEFINITIONS AND SEIZURE PHENOMENA

Atonic seizures occur in 0.4 [8] to 12 percent [15] of patients with epilepsy. The minimal expression is a brief nodding of the head or a sagging of the body. There may be a sagging at the legs, followed by the patient's "catching himself" before he falls. In the full-blown attack, the patient falls to the floor (if standing)

and may be injured. If the patient is seated, a fall forward occurs that may injure the teeth or nose. Most attacks last 1 to 4 seconds [29, 34, 61]. In more prolonged atonic seizures, the slumping may slowly progress in a rhythmic, step-by-step fashion [18]. There is seldom a detectable alteration of consciousness; nor is there an aura or postictal confusion. The patient usually picks himself up immediately and resumes what he was doing. There is no tongue-biting, change in skin color, or loss of sphincter control. Atonic attacks are frequently preceded or followed by myoclonic jerks [18, 31, 48, 49, 61], which may also occur during an attack [51].

Atonic attacks may occur spontaneously or in response to one of the following sensory stimuli: photic stimulation [29, 31], auditory stimuli [44, 48], startle [44], or light touch or tapping the skin [9]. In some patients starting to walk may precipitate an atonic attack [44, 45].

Atonic seizures usually occur between 6 months and 7 years of age [11, 49], but they may begin in the teens [48]. It is unusual for atonic seizures to begin in adulthood. However, falling attacks, which probably represent atonic seizures, can begin in adults of any age following a cerebral insult (e.g., hypoxia) [43, 45].

Ictal atonia can occur exclusively in association with fever in young children. Such seizures carry a good prognosis, like simple febrile convulsions, and are rarely followed by chronic epilepsy [31].

EEG PHENOMENA

Interictal EEG

The interictal EEG is abnormal in a large percentage of patients with atonic seizures [47, 56]. The most common interictal EEG abnormality is a slow spike-wave pattern [48]. Twenty-six to 56 percent of patients with slow spike-wave patterns in the interictal EEG also have atonic seizures [11, 47, 62]. Many other interictal EEG abnormalities have been described in patients with atonic seizures: excessive background slowing, polyspike-and-wave, frequent generalized spikes and sharp waves, continuous delta waves, parasagittal spikes and slow waves, temporal spikes, frontal spikes, and bilaterally synchronous spikes during sleep [34, 43, 47, 48, 57]. Typical 3-Hz spike-wave discharges rarely are seen. The interictal EEG is often normal in the subgroup of patients with atonic seizures as a manifestation of a primarily generalized seizure disorder.

Ictal EEG

EEGs recorded during atonic seizures have shown the following patterns: slow spike-wave [10, 31, 34, 48, 51]; 3-Hz spike-wave [2, 10, 51]; polyspike-and-wave

82

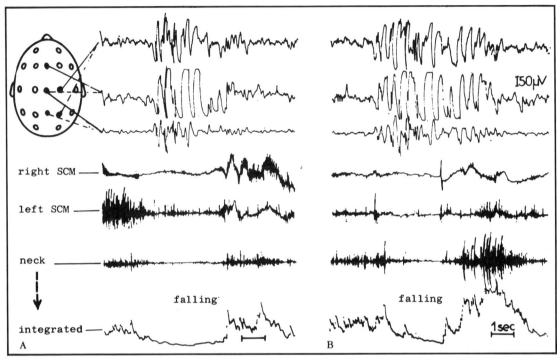

Figure 8-4. Atonic seizure (EEG recording with EMGs of the right and left sternocleidomastoid and posterior cervical muscles, the latter also integrated in the last channel). A. In the first atonic seizure, a rather irregular spike-wave discharge is associated with abrupt and complete loss of postural tone. B. In the second atonic seizure, the loss of tone is preceded by a brief myoclonic jerk, and postural tone returns before the end of the discharge. (From H. Gastaut et al. In P. J. Vinken, and G. W. Bruyn [Eds.], Handbook of Clinical Neurology, Vol. 15, The Epilepsies. Amsterdam: Elsevier, 1974.)

[10, 29, 31, 45]; rhythmic slow waves [5, 51]; and fast recruiting rhythms similar to those occurring in tonic seizures (Fig. 8-4) [10, 12, 18, 27, 51]. In prolonged atonic seizures, the initial drop attack may be associated with a fast recruiting discharge whereas the following period of atonia and akinesia may show concomitant spike and wave in the EEG. Atonic seizures with concomitant generalized spike-wave discharges in the ictal EEG tend to be accompanied by normal interictal EEG activity, whereas atonic seizures with ictal fast-recruiting discharges are more often associated with diffuse abnormalities of interictal EEG (especially the Lennox-Gastaut syndrome).

PATHOPHYSIOLOGY

There has been some controversy in the past as to whether "drop attacks" are due to atonia or to active muscle contraction throwing the patient down. Observations with simultaneous EEG, EMG, and video recording indicate that loss of axial muscle tone is the cause of the drops in most cases [18, 29, 31, 45, 47, 51]. This does not exclude concomitant peripheral myoclonic manifestations (i.e., proximal muscle contractions and abduction of the extremities). However, even in cases where phenomena are mixed, the term "atonic" seizure seems to be the most appropriate when the resulting effect is a drop to the ground.

The mechanism underlying the loss of muscle tone during the slow spike-wave, 3-Hz spike-wave, and rhythmic slow discharges is presumably inhibition of the cortical and subcortical motor systems [36, 47, 51] (see Chap. 7).

Lance and Adams [45] postulate a slightly different mechanism in patients with polyspike-and-wave EEG discharges and myoclonic and atonic seizures after an anoxic event. Such patients have an enhanced sensitivity of specific thalamic sensory nuclei to normal sensory input. This enhanced sensitivity results in an excessive discharge to cortical projection areas of the thalamic nuclei. This excessive discharge first results in excitation of the motor cortex which sometimes manifests itself as polyspikes on the EEG and/or myoclonic jerks. Following the period of cortical excitation, there is a period of inhibition in the motor cortex which sometimes manifests itself as slow waves on the

EEG, a decrease in activity on the EMG, and atonic attacks.

Lombroso and Erba [51] postulate that atonic seizures accompanied by fast recruiting rhythms on the EEG (similar to those recorded during tonic seizures) may be caused by cortical discharges affecting brainstem structures that in turn influence spinal motor function. Motor tone may be decreased (producing an atonic seizure) or increased (producing a tonic seizure).

DIFFERENTIAL DIAGNOSIS

Absence Seizures with Loss of Postural Tone
Atonic seizures can usually be distinguished from absence seizures with loss of postural tone by the following characteristics: (1) there is often no detectable loss of consciousness during atonic seizures; (2) the loss of postural tone in absence seizures is usually gradual and is not associated with injuries, whereas the loss of tone in atonic seizures is usually rapid and is often associated with injuries; (3) the EEG during atonic seizures may show slow spike-wave, polyspike-and-wave, or fast recruiting rhythms, whereas in typical absence seizures it shows 3-Hz spike-wave discharges. There are also some patients who have mild loss of postural tone during slow spike-wave discharges. It can be extremely difficult to distinguish among absence seizures with loss of postural tone, atypical absence seizures with loss of postural tone, and atonic seizures purely on the basis of clinical observation of the seizures.

The following additional features help to differentiate atonic seizures from absence seizures with loss of postural tone: (1) seizures are seldom precipitated by hyperventilation; (2) the age of onset is younger (before 5 years of age); (3) evidence of structural CNS damage and mental retardation is usually present; (4) atonic seizures tend to occur in combination with atypical absence, myoclonic, and tonic seizures; (5) the interictal background EEG activity is usually abnormal, showing an excess of slow and slow spike-wave activity. The differences between 3-Hz spike-wave and slow spike-wave are summarized in Table 8-3.

Infantile Spasms
Infantile spasms, like atonic seizures, may be characterized by nodding of the head and tend to occur in young children with evidence of CNS compromise. However, atonic head-nodding should be apparent only when the patient is in the upright position. A patient with infantile spasms will show the flexor type of infantile spasms during which the neck is forcefully flexed forward and the extremities abducted in any

position. These phenomena are myoclonic or tonic in nature and are quite different from those of an atonic seizure. However, both manifestations can coexist in the same patient both in the infantile spasm group and the older Lennox-Gastaut syndrome group. Infantile spasms tend to occur in a series of rapid, successive seizures. It is rare to have a rapid succession of atonic attacks. Infantile spasms begin during the first 6 months of life in 50 percent of cases and during the first year of life in 85 percent. They seldom begin after age 2. They thus have a different age spectrum than atonic seizures. Finally, the presence of hypsarrhythmic pattern in the EEG and the response to ACTH treatment in the infantile spasms are two additional points of differentiation.

Tonic Seizures
Both atonic and tonic seizures can be associated with violent falls and mental retardation, and the ictal and interictal EEG patterns for both seizure types are often similar. Falls are less common with tonic seizures because the leg muscles are often not involved or may have increased extension tone (holding the patient erect unless asymmetrical). Patients who fall in a rigid posture (like a tree) are having a tonic seizure. Patients who fall by collapsing (like an accordion) may be having an atonic seizure or a global tonic seizure with triple flexion of the lower extremities. Tonic seizures can occur while lying down, whereas atonic seizures cannot be recognized in this position. A definitive distinction between these seizure types sometimes requires simultaneous EEG and EMG recordings.

Cataplexy
Cataplectic attacks usually have an emotional precipitant, whereas atonic seizures do not. Patients with cataplexy almost invariably have narcolepsy as well and may also have attacks of sleep paralysis or hypnagogic hallucinations. None of these associated symptoms are present in patients with atonic seizures. Patients with narcolepsy and cataplexy have characteristic "sleep-onset REM" during sleep EEGs, but this is absent in patients with atonic seizures. Cataplexy characteristically occurs in individuals of normal intelligence, begins in the middle and late teens (less than 5 percent of cases begin before age 10), and persists throughout the patient's lifetime. Atonic seizures tend to occur in mentally retarded children, begin before 10 years of age, and cease in the teens.

Syncope
Patients may slump to the floor during syncopal attacks, but the fall is usually relatively slow and con-

Table 8-3. *3-Hz Spike-Wave Versus Slow Spike-Wave*

EEG and Clinical Features	3-Hz Spike-Wave (Typical Spike-Wave, Fast Spike-Wave; Typical Petit Mal)	Slow Spike-Wave (Atypical Spike-Wave, Petit Mal Variant)
EEG		
Spike	Sharp; same amplitude as wave	Blunted, slow (~150 msec), sometimes triphasic, sometimes missing, often higher in voltage than wave
Wave	Smooth, regular, 3-Hz	Irregular, 1–2 Hz
Bilaterally symmetrical	Almost always	Often not; may be focal
Rhythmic	Yes	Often not
Area of maximum voltage	Frontocentral or fully generalized	Variable (often frontal or temporal)
Spike-wave ratio	1:1	Variable
Interictal EEG	Usually normal	Often abnormal (esp. slowing)
Precipitated by:		
Hyperventilation	Often	Seldom
Photic stimulation	Sometimes	Seldom
Sleep	Often	Often
Clinical		
Seizure type: During spike-wave	Absence	Atypical absence, myoclonic, or atonic
At other times	Usually none. If any, usually tonic-clonic	Tonic-clonic or tonic. Very seldom see typical absence
Association with seizure	Fully generalized 3-Hz spike-wave discharge almost always impairs performance. Incompletely generalized 3-Hz spike-wave discharge usually but not always impairs performance	Clinical seizures not always visible
Age at onset of seizures and EEG abnormality	Usually after 5 yr	Usually before 5 yr (1–7 yr)
Age of cessation	Stops spontaneously in teens	Usually stops in later childhood
Sex	Female > male	Male > female
Evidence of brain damage	Minority (5–15%)	Majority
Mental retardation	Small minority	About 50% severely retarded and an additional 40% mildly or moderately retarded
Response to antiepileptic drugs	Good	Less satisfactory

trolled, and self-injury is unusual. The reverse is true with atonic attacks. Other features distinguishing syncopal attacks from atonic attacks are the occurrence of premonitory symptoms, longer duration of the attack, clouding of consciousness, later age of onset, and relation to posture and exercise (see Chap. 10).

Vagal syncope attacks in children may be quite sudden and are sometimes confused with seizures [53]. Vagal syncope is triggered by emotions such as fear and anger, by unexpected trauma or pain, by tactile stimulation of certain regions (especially the scalp), or by stimuli to which the patient may be particularly sensitized (e.g., the sight of blood). Syncopal attacks of vagal origin are very similar to atonic seizures, but are accompanied by intense pallor and perspiration. If the syncope lasts long enough, the fall to the ground may be accompanied by brief, clonic jerks. Differential diagnosis is established by (1) identification of precipitating factors; (2) normal EEG; (3) reproduction of the attack in the EEG laboratory by delivering an appropriate stimulus (e.g., ocular compression) during concomitant EEG and EKG monitoring [53].

Pseudoseizure
Emotionally-induced seizures do not always mimic convulsive episodes with a great deal of thrashing and dramatic manifestations. Not infrequently, they are

represented by "fainting" episodes during which the patient falls to the ground remaining atonic and unresponsive. A consistent lack of abnormalities in waking and sleep EEGs (especially if recorded during an episode), absence of neurologic deficits, and predisposing emotional or environmental factors are the leading points in the differential diagnosis.

MANAGEMENT AND PROGNOSIS
The management and prognosis of atonic seizures are discussed later in this chapter.

Akinetic Seizures
Gastaut et al. [31] described a type of seizure in which the patient is motionless (akinetic), although postural tone and deep tendon reflexes are preserved, and consciousness does not appear to be impaired. In practice, seizures during which akinesia is the only ictal clinical manifestation are very uncommon. Most seizures with akinesia represent a motor arrest during an incomplete absence or complex partial seizure, or represent the effect of a generalized increase or decrease of muscle tone during tonic or atonic seizures.

Tonic Seizures

DEFINITIONS AND CLINICAL FEATURES
Tonic seizures consist of tonic contraction of certain muscle groups, accompanied by altered consciousness, but there is no progression to a clonic phase. Gastaut et al. [31, 33] have described three varieties of tonic seizures: (1) axial, (2) axorhizomelic, and (3) global. There are, however, certain features common to all tonic seizures.

Features Common to All Types of Tonic Seizures
The *duration* of tonic seizures is brief, usually about 10 seconds. Duration ranges from a few seconds to 1 minute.

There is usually at least partial *abolition of consciousness* during tonic seizures. However, at the onset of the ictal phenomena, there may be an alerting [23], and arousal from light stages of sleep may occur [24]. Postictal alteration of consciousness is usually brief, but may last several minutes. During tonic status epilepticus, the patient may appear extremely lethargic but is still responsive [23, 24].

Ocular phenomena are usually prominent and may include fixation of the eyes, eyelid retraction, superior ocular deviation (rarely, ocular convergence), nastagmoid ocular movements, and mydriasis with loss of pupillary reflexes.

Autonomic phenomena are usually present and may include tachycardia, hypertension, respiratory distress (tachypnea ending in apnea), capillary congestion followed by cyanosis, or glandular hypersecretion (lacrimal, salivary, tracheobronchial, and sweat glands).

Activation by sleep is typical of tonic seizures, and Gastaut et al. [30] reported that tonic seizures during sleep can be recorded in 92 percent of patients with Lennox-Gastaut syndrome if proper recording techniques are employed. Tonic seizures usually are much more frequent during non-REM sleep than during wakefulness but never occur during REM sleep [26]. The clinical manifestations of tonic seizures are often less dramatic in sleep and can be easily overlooked (e.g., they may resemble stretching, yawning, and similar movements). Tonic seizures, if frequent, can disrupt sleep organization owing to a decrease or disappearance of REM sleep and stages III and IV of non-REM sleep [23, 26, 54, 64]. This can produce daytime drowsiness, which in turn will facilitate tonic seizures. A sleep EEG should always be performed on a patient suspected of having tonic seizures.

Axial Tonic Seizures
In axial tonic seizures there is a characteristic sequence of muscle group involvement that produces a characteristic sequence of clinical phenomena: (1) neck muscles (erect position of head); (2) facial muscles (eyes wide open); (3) muscles of mastication (jaw fixed, usually open); and (4) respiratory and abdominal muscles (cry, apnea).

Axorhizomelic (Axial and Proximal Extremities) Tonic Seizures
Axorhizomelic seizures begin with a sequence of events identical to those seen in axial tonic seizures. The tonic activity then spreads to the proximal upper extremities, producing elevation of the shoulders and abduction of the arms. The lower extremities are rarely involved, and hence the patient seldom falls.

Global Tonic Seizures
Global tonic seizures begin in a manner similar to axorhizomelic tonic seizures, but the tonic contractions extend to the periphery of the limbs. The arms are pulled upward and are semiflexed in front of the head with clenched fists, producing a body position similar to that of a child defending himself against a facial blow. The lower limbs are contracted in a triple flexion position or, less often, are in forced extension.

Tonic Status Epilepticus
Tonic seizures may become progressively more frequent, approaching status epilepticus. Progressive diminution of muscular contractions may take place during successive seizures, the seizures changing into

axorhizomelic and subsequently into axial types. However, the autonomic phenomena continue and may even intensify. Eventually, the motor phenomena may become so minimal that the attacks may appear to have ceased. Death, however, may occur owing to accumulating autonomic effects (bronchial secretions and respiratory depression). Such an evolution requires immediate clinical recognition, continuous EEG monitoring, and prompt therapy (intravenous phenytoin).

Variants of Tonic Seizures

In addition to the three typical varieties of tonic seizures, there are many variants. The variant producing the appearance of an atypical absence seizure was discussed above. In some varieties, the autonomic phenomena are so prominent that the attack might be considered a form of autonomic epilepsy. Some authors describe major, minor, and minimal tonic seizures according to the severity and extent of the tonic manifestations. Tonic seizures may be limited to selective muscle groups (those of the eyes, face, larynx, neck, and extremities), and the increase in muscle tone may be asymmetrical or unilateral (dystonic seizures or focal tonic seizures). The most intense global tonic seizures may end in one or several generalized rapid clonic jerks.

EEG PHENOMENA

Interictal EEG

The waking record usually contains slow spike-wave discharges, polyspike-and-wave discharges, and diffuse slowing of the background activity [24, 30]. During periods of remission of clinical symptomatology, the waking EEG may be normal [23]. In most cases however, a sleep EEG will activate paroxysmal abnormalities. During non-REM sleep, EEG discharges similar to those occurring during clinical tonic seizures may occur without obvious clinical manifestations.

Ictal EEG

Three types of generalized, synchronous, and symmetrical EEG patterns may occur during a tonic seizure (Fig. 8-5): (1) simple flattening ("desynchronization") of all activity recorded throughout an attack; (2) very rapid activity (20 ± 5 Hz), initially of low voltage and then progressively increasing in amplitude to 50 to 100 μV; and (3) rhythmic discharge at about 10 Hz, identical to that of the tonic phase of tonic-clonic seizures ("epileptic recruiting rhythm"; see Chap. 6) except that it may be of high amplitude from the onset [7, 27, 30, 33]. Combinations of these three patterns may be seen. There may be a brief burst of slow spike-wave or polyspike-and-wave activity preceding the ictal discharge. Postictally there may be a more or less brief burst of slow waves. Clinically identical tonic seizures may occur in the same patient with any of these three EEG patterns. Furthermore, any of the three EEG patterns may be associated with atonic and other seizure types in a patient who also has tonic seizures [7, 27, 51].

PATHOPHYSIOLOGY

It is assumed that tonic seizures without clonic manifestations represent prematurely interrupted tonic-clonic seizures (see Pathophysiology, Chap. 6). Tonic attacks with forceful expiratory "cry," stiffening of the trunk and extremities in extension posture, and apnea mimic the onset of a tonic-clonic seizure. The mechanism by which the seizure terminates without a clonic phase is unknown. In addition, the tonic phase of a tonic seizure is usually of shorter duration and is followed by a brief relaxation period with minimal or no postictal depression by clinical observation or EEG recording. The lack of clonic and postictal phases may in some way facilitate repetitive attacks and may be related to the strong tendency of these patients to develop tonic status epilepticus. The similarity of tonic seizures with "cerebellar" and "decerebrate" fits, as well as their association with mechanisms of sleep and arousal [23, 24, 26] suggests that ictal discharges may originate in low brain stem structures [33] and that activation of the cortex may be mediated through the mesencephalic reticular activating system. Tonic seizures may represent the expression of secondary generalization from a focal lesion, especially if located within the frontal lobe. Such seizures are probably mediated through the supplementary motor area. Secondary generalization from a unilateral focus may account for the asymmetric and dystonic posturing often observed in tonic seizures. See also "Pathophysiology" in "Atonic Seizures" section above.

DIFFERENTIAL DIAGNOSIS

Tonic-Clonic Seizure

In a tonic seizure, the arms are usually semiflexed, and the legs contracted in triple flexion (less often in extension) [30]. In the tonic phase of a tonic-clonic seizure, the initial posture is usually one of arms flexed and legs extended. Later, both the arms and legs usually are extended [30]. In tonic seizures the jaw is usually lowered, whereas in tonic-clonic seizures the jaw is usually clenched; thus, tongue biting does not occur in tonic seizures. In addition, if tonic seizures occur during a period of light sleep, there may be an arousal and brief periods of stereotyped, com-

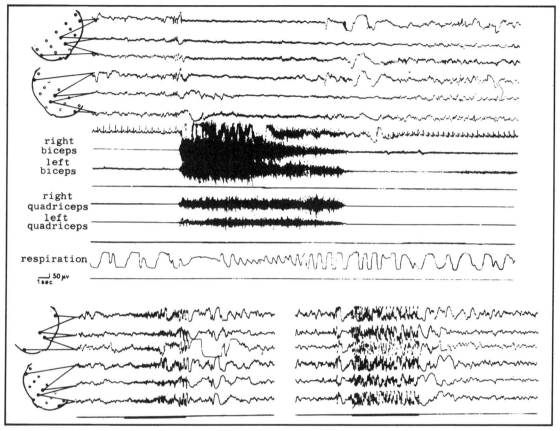

right
biceps
left
biceps

right
quadriceps
left
quadriceps

respiration

50 μv
1 sec.

Figure 8-5. Three common types of ictal EEG discharges recorded during tonic seizures. The polygraphic recording of the first seizure shows a flattening of all EEG channels during tonic muscle contraction. Respiration is highly modified (apnea followed by low amplitude and high frequency), and the cardiac rate is accelerated. The lower left recording shows a rapid low-amplitude discharge followed by postictal slowing. The lower right recording shows an epileptic recruiting rhythm followed by postictal slowing. (From H. Gastaut et al. In P. J. Vinken, and G. W. Bruyn [Eds.], Handbook of Clinical Neurology, Vol. 15, The Epilepsies. Amsterdam: Elsevier, 1974.)

plex automatisms (looking around, smiling) which mark the end of the attack [20]. Other patients will gasp and go back to sleep after a tonic seizure in sleep [23]. These corollary manifestations are most unusual in tonic-clonic seizures. However, when tonic seizures are followed by a brief period of rapid tremor-like contractions, differentiation from a short tonic-clonic attack is difficult. Features of the interictal EEG may be helpful. The interictal EEG is more likely to be normal in patients with idiopathic tonic-clonic seizures, whereas the interictal EEG of patients with

tonic seizures is more likely to show slow spike-wave activity and/or evidence of diffuse encephalopathy.

"Autonomic Epilepsy"

In many instances, the motor manifestations of a tonic seizure may be minimal, and the autonomic manifestations of tonic seizures (mydriasis, piloerection, perspiration, tachycardia, respiratory irregularities, etc.) may occur prominently without motor phenomena. These autonomic manifestations are similar to those observed during the initial tonic phase of a tonic-clonic seizure and during complex partial seizures with prominent autonomic features. In the latter, automatisms, dizziness, nausea and vomiting may be prominent manifestations which are never reported during tonic seizures. Although tonic-clonic and complex partial seizures may be facilitated by fatigue and drowsiness, the relationship between tonic seizures and sleep cycles is even more striking [23, 26, 33, 34].

Psychosis

During periods of tonic status epilepticus, the motor manifestations of tonic seizures may be almost imperceptible. The patient is in a constant state of lethargy. His responsiveness is retained but the ability to reason may be greatly impaired; his motions are slow. Slow responsiveness, slow motion, bizarre behavior and impaired cognitive functions may simulate catatonic psychosis unless EEG monitoring is obtained to document repetitive ictal discharges.

Absence Seizure

Minimal tonic seizures with motor manifestations involving only ocular and facial musculature are difficult to differentiate from absence seizures because the patient may be simply staring straight ahead with an inexpressive look on his face. However, the onset of the fixed stare is more gradual and slower in tonic seizures and more abrupt in absence seizures. Awareness of the environment and ability to respond may be preserved during minor tonic seizures [23]. The concomitant EEG discharges (fast recruiting activity in tonic seizure; generalized 3-per-second spike waves in absence seizure) are totally different in the two types of seizures and represent the best criteria for differentiation.

Decerebrate Rigidity and "Cerebellar Fits"

In a tonic seizure the arms are usually semiflexed and the legs contracted in triple flexion [30]. In decerebrate rigidity and "cerebellar fits," both the arms and legs are extended from the onset [30].

MANAGEMENT AND PROGNOSIS
A discussion of the management and prognosis of tonic seizures appears later in this chapter.

Lennox-Gastaut Syndrome

DEFINITION
Lennox et al. [47, 48] described in detail the symptoms and seizure manifestations (atypical absence, atonic, myoclonic) associated with "slow" spike-wave activity in the EEG. They stressed early age of onset, high association with brain damage, and poor response to antiepileptic drugs. Gastaut et al. [34] redefined the "Lennox syndrome" as a childhood epileptic encephalopathy and stressed the importance of tonic seizures and of atypical absences.

Following these descriptions, the Lennox-Gastaut syndrome gained general acceptance as a nosologic entity. The Lennox-Gastaut syndrome is present in 10 percent of all children with epilepsy [3, 32] and constitutes one of the most difficult management problems in epilepsy.

Patients with Lennox-Gastaut syndrome have the following characteristics: (1) *interictal* slow spike-wave discharges on the EEG; (2) atypical absence, myoclonic, atonic, and tonic seizures in varying combinations; (3) psychomotor retardation and a variety of neurologic deficits (see Table 8-1). The above signs and symptoms are variable and may change in time. The course of the condition may be marked by periods of considerable remission and exacerbation. Thus, the simple label of "Lennox-Gastaut syndrome" does not define precisely the patient's condition at a given time. Information about probable etiology, neurologic and neuropsychologic deficits, seizure type(s), and EEG abnormalities should be given in order to describe completely a patient's condition.

ETIOLOGY

Symptomatic Forms

The Lennox-Gastaut syndrome is accompanied by evidence of pre-existing brain damage by history, neurologic examination, or psychometric testing in 30 to 75 percent of patients [11, 34, 42, 48, 56]. Computerized axial tomography or a pneumoencephalogram reveals abnormalities in 50 percent or more of patients with this syndrome [11, 28, 34, 46]. The etiologic factors usually associated with this syndrome include: birth injury or asphyxia, encephalitis or meningitis, prenatal injury, and trauma [11, 34, 42, 48, 56]. Less common etiologic factors include tumors, tuberous sclerosis, vascular anomalies, dehydration, subdural hematoma, kernicterus, intraventricular hemorrhage, homocystinuria, toxoplasmosis, hypoglycemia, neurolipidosis, and familial encephaloretinal dysplasia [11, 34, 42, 48, 56]. A family history of epilepsy can be found in only 2.5 to 27.2 percent of patients [11, 34, 42, 48]. Thus, most cases of Lennox-Gastaut syndrome appear to be due to acquired brain damage.

The great variety of diseases that may result in Lennox-Gastaut syndrome suggest that the syndrome represents a nonspecific response of the 1- to 7-year-old brain to diffuse damage rather than a specific disease. This situation is analogous to the nonspecific hypsarrhythmic response to diffuse damage in infants. In fact, 15 to 25 percent of patients with Lennox-Gastaut syndrome have a history of preceding hypsarrhythmia or infantile spasms, or both [11, 34, 48, 56], and the slow spike-wave pattern later evolves in approximately one third of patients with infantile spasms [39].

Cryptogenic Forms

Ten to 20 percent of patients with the Lennox-Gastaut syndrome present a history of normal development and no evidence of pre-existing cerebral insults prior to the onset of the epileptic disorder. Often no definable neurologic disease is apparent when the patient exhibits the first epileptic manifestation of the syndrome. At times these early seizures may be accompanied by behavioral and neurologic changes suggestive of a subacute encephalitic process, although CSF and EEG studies are not diagnostic for any specific condition. In other cases, the patient starts with an unexpected tonic-clonic seizure followed by a seizure-free interval before the other signs and symptoms of the full syndrome become apparent. The severity of the epileptic disorder and the alternating course of the condition is not different in cryptogenic forms from the symptomatic forms, suggesting an ongoing encephalopathic process in both.

EEG PHENOMENA

The slow spike-wave EEG pattern was the central feature of the first descriptions of the syndrome by Lennox et al. and Gastaut [34, 47, 48]. Distinction between ictal and interictal EEG is difficult in Lennox-Gastaut syndrome because clinical manifestations are often not obvious during slow spike-wave discharges.

Slow Spike-Wave EEG Pattern
("Petit Mal Variant"): EEG Phenomena
Slow spike-wave discharges consist of runs of spikes which are often blunted, slow (150 msec), triphasic, and higher or lower in voltage than the accompanying slow wave (or sometimes missing entirely) followed by irregular 1- to 2-Hz slow waves (see Table 8-3 and Fig. 8-1) [31, 34, 47, 48]. The runs of spikes and waves are often irregular and/or asymmetrical (may be focal) and have a variable spike/wave ratio [31, 34, 47, 48]. The area of maximum voltage is variable (often frontal or temporal) [31, 34, 47, 48]. Slow spike-wave discharges are seldom precipitated by hyperventilation or photic stimulation but are, as a rule, activated by drowsiness and sleep [26, 34, 47, 48, 56]. During non-REM sleep, slow spike-wave discharges are often replaced by polyspike and polyspike-and-wave discharges [26, 34]. REM sleep is usually associated with a marked decrease in all forms of paroxysmal discharges [26, 34].

Slow Spike-Wave EEG Pattern: Seizure Phenomena
Slow spike-wave discharges may be accompanied by atypical absence, myoclonic, or atonic seizures [30, 31, 34, 47, 48]. These ictal manifestations have been described in detail above. However, often no clinical manifestations are obvious during slow spike-wave discharges. For this reason, such discharges were originally described as an *interictal* EEG abnormality [31, 34, 47, 48]. The clinical features associated with

slow spike-wave discharges are summarized in Table 8-3.

Slow Spike-Wave EEG Pattern:
Effects on Responsiveness
See Altered Responsiveness under Clinical Phenomena below.

Ictal EEG During Atypical Absence,
Myoclonic, Atonic, and Tonic Seizures
The slow spike-wave EEG pattern or any of several other EEG patterns may be recorded during these seizure types (see above).

Interictal EEG
As a rule, there is diffuse slowing of the background activity in many or all areas. The posterior rhythm seldom reaches the expected frequency or rhythmicity for age. Sleep spindles are rare and/or poorly recognizable. Vertex activity and K-complexes are often obscured by the frequent occurrence of generalized paroxysmal discharges. Scoring of all night sleep recordings is particularly difficult, although different sleep stages are usually represented, except during tonic status epilepticus when there may be selective deprivation of slow wave sleep [23, 54].

CLINICAL PHENOMENA

Atypical Absence, Myoclonic, Atonic,
Tonic, and Tonic-Clonic Seizures
These are the seizure types usually seen in association with Lennox-Gastaut syndrome (see Table 8-1). The clinical and EEG features of these types of seizures are reviewed above and in Chapter 6.

Altered Responsiveness
Responsiveness is almost always impaired by fully generalized 3-Hz spike-wave paroxysms and is often impaired by incompletely generalized 3-Hz spike-wave paroxysms (see Chap. 7). The effects of slow spike-wave paroxysms are more variable. Erba et al. [21, 25] studied latency of response to stimuli of various modalities during and between slow spike-wave paroxysms in children and adolescents with cryptogenic forms of Lennox-Gastaut syndrome. Responsiveness was often preserved during slow spike-wave discharges, especially during the initial and final part of the discharge, although the latency for both motor and cognitive functions was greatly increased. Between discharges great variability of performance was observed, with latencies varying from close to normal to a 20-fold increase. The highest values were recorded in periods preceding or following slow spike-waves, especially during bursts of slow wave

activity. However, increased latency was often seen even without apparent concomitant changes in the EEG. A distinctive feature of the Lennox-Gastaut syndrome may be a continuous fluctuation of response latencies to sensory stimuli (simple reaction time, verbal latencies). If sufficient time is allowed to process the information, the ability to produce correct responses may be preserved.

Mental Retardation

Psychomotor retardation is an important aspect of the syndrome, is almost invariably present at some time during the illness, and tends to be more severe in patients with evidence of psychomotor retardation prior to onset of the syndrome [2, 34, 47]. Using conventional IQ measures, evidence of mental retardation is apparent at the onset of the epileptic manifestations in 30 percent of patients with slow spike-waves and in 93 percent of patients 5 years after the onset [2]. Once the seizures and EEG changes are established, there is slowing or arrest of psychomotor development despite lack of evidence of progressive degenerative CNS disease [2, 34]. Progressive diminution of IQ scores may be observed during the course of this condition due to lack of new learning rather than loss of previously acquired skills. The bradykinesia characteristic of these patients (see Altered Responsiveness above) will cause failure in virtually all time-based tasks. IQ scores remain quite constant during remissions and exacerbations of the syndrome [20], whereas studies of simple motor reaction time, verbal latencies, and percent correctness in simple cognitive tasks are much more related to the patient's current clinical status.

PATHOPHYSIOLOGY

The mechanisms responsible for the production of slow spike-wave discharges are presumably similar to those responsible for the production of 3-Hz spike-wave discharges (see Chap. 7). The factor responsible for production of "first degree epileptogenesis" in brains of patients with slow spike-wave may be diffuse gray matter damage, since such patients often have evidence of diffuse cerebral deficits [36] (see Table 8-1). The incomplete alteration of responsiveness often noted during slow spike-wave discharges may be due to the incomplete generalization and/or less regular and less complete excitation and inhibition of structures involved in higher cortical function [22, 36]. Delays in motor and verbal output that fluctuate continuously and unpredictably without interfering with perceptual threshold are also in support of this hypothesis [21]. The poor relationship of these fluctuations with recognizable scalp EEG changes sug-

gests that excess inhibitory activity may take place at subcortical rather than cortical levels.

Management of Atypical Absence, Myoclonic, Atonic, and Tonic Seizures, and the Lennox-Gastaut Syndrome

The first step in seizure management is to determine if tonic seizures are present (Table 8-4). If tonic seizures are present, they should be treated first with phenytoin and then with phenytoin and phenobarbital if phenytoin alone is not successful. If atypical absence, myoclonic, or atonic seizures are present without tonic seizures or persist after phenytoin (with or without phenobarbital) is given for tonic seizures, drugs should be administered in the sequence listed in Table 8-4.

TONIC SEIZURES

Phenytoin

Phenytoin (see Chap. 16) is especially effective against the tonic phase of experimental seizures in animals and is the most consistently effective drug against tonic seizures in humans [33].

Phenobarbital

Phenobarbital (see Chap. 17) is sometimes effective against tonic seizures and should be added to the drug regimen if phenytoin alone does not control them.

Phenytoin with or without phenobarbital may also control the accompanying atypical absence, myoclonic, and atonic seizures in a minority of patients with tonic seizures. If these other seizures are controlled with phenytoin and/or phenobarbital, further drug therapy is not needed. If the other seizures persist, specific medication for them should be given.

Hypnotics

When frequent tonic seizures in sleep prevent progression from light stages to deep stages of non-REM sleep, hypnotics such as chloral hydrate may be beneficial at the beginning of the night [23, 24]. The presumed mechanism is that the drug increases the threshold of arousal by inducing stage III and stage IV sleep. In these stages, although electrical discharges and clinical tonic seizure may still frequently occur, the patient is not aroused and does not become sleep deprived.

ATYPICAL ABSENCE, MYOCLONIC, AND ATONIC SEIZURES

Ethosuximide

Ethosuximide (see Chap. 19) is effective against atypical absence, myoclonic, and atonic seizures in

Table 8-4. Management of Atypical Absence, Myoclonic, Atonic, and Tonic Seizures

Are Tonic Seizures Present?

Yes → Phenytoin (+ Phenobarbital if necessary)

Are Atypical Absence, Myoclonic, and Atonic Seizures Controlled?

Yes → No further therapy needed

No →

No →

1. Ethosuximide
   if not successful:
2. Valproic acid
   if not successful:
3. Clonazepam
   if not successful:
4. Diazepam
   if not successful:
5. Ketogenic diet
   if not successful:
6. Miscellaneous drugs
   (acetazolamide, methsuximide, trimethadione, corticosteroids)

only a minority of patients. However, it is the first drug to try because of its lack of systemic and neurologic toxicity and lack of drug interactions.

Valproic Acid

Valproic acid (see Chap. 20) is effective against atypical absence, myoclonic, and atonic seizures in some patients. Administration of valproic acid requires awareness of the following potential difficulties: (1) hepatic toxicity, (2) sedation and/or nausea; (3) increased phenobarbital level (and sedation) if given together with valproic acid.

Clonazepam

Clonazepam (see Chap. 21) is effective against atypical absence, myoclonic, and atonic seizures in some patients. However, patients with Lennox-Gastaut syndrome often have associated mental slowing, clumsiness, and hyperactivity, and these neurologic deficits are often made worse by the sedation, ataxia, and hyperactivity that may be associated with clonazepam therapy.

Diazepam

For reasons outlined in Chapter 21, clonazepam is usually more effective as a chronic oral antiepileptic drug than diazepam. Gastaut et al. [34] reported a beneficial effect, often transient, in a minority of patients with Lennox-Gastaut syndrome treated with diazepam. A trial of diazepam may be worthwhile in patients who do not tolerate clonazepam. Special care must be taken when giving diazepam intravenously to patients with Lennox-Gastaut syndrome because it may precipitate tonic status epilepticus [60, 63].

Ketogenic Diet

The ketogenic diet is sometimes effective in controlling atypical absence, myoclonic, and atonic seizures when conventional antiepileptic drugs fail, especially in children 6 years of age and under [14, 41, 48, 50]. However, the necessity for severe carbohydrate restriction results in a diet that is so unpalatable and difficult to prepare that only a minority of children and parents are able to maintain it for more than a few weeks. The use of a medium-chain triglyceride diet to produce ketosis offers promise of equally good results with a simpler, more palatable diet [37].

Acetozolomide, Methsuximide, Trimethadione, and Corticosteroids

These drugs are occasionally helpful in controlling Lennox-Gastaut syndrome when other antiepileptic drugs fail [6, 13, 14, 16] (see Chaps. 19 and 22).

Prognosis of Atypical Absence, Myoclonic, Atonic, and Tonic Seizures, and the Lennox-Gastaut Syndrome

PRIMARILY GENERALIZED SEIZURES

The primarily generalized forms of atypical absence, myoclonic, atonic, and tonic seizures are probably due to more than one etiologic syndrome, and their prognosis has not been comprehensively studied. Anecdotal data suggest that this group of seizures is often associated with absence of neurologic deficits, normal intelligence, normal interictal EEG, other forms of primarily generalized seizures occurring in the same patient (especially tonic-clonic seizures in patients with myoclonic seizures), good response to antiepileptic drugs, and a genetic predisposition to epilepsy [2, 19, 20, 30, 31, 38, 52].

LENNOX-GASTAUT SYNDROME

Response to Therapy

All reported series of Lennox-Gastaut syndrome emphasize the refractoriness of the associated seizures to therapy. Less than one third of patients have a good response to antiepileptic drugs [4, 34, 42, 56, 59]. The recent addition of antiepileptic drug-level monitoring, valproic acid, and clonazepam to the therapeutic armamentarium may lead to some improvement in the management of this condition [65] (see Chaps. 20 and 21).

Age of Cessation of Seizures and Slow Spike-Wave Pattern

The slow spike-wave EEG pattern and the atypical absence, myoclonic, atonic, and tonic seizures sometimes cease in late childhood [4], but the exact time and probability of cessation have not been studied in detail. Patients with the characteristic EEG and seizure manifestations of Lennox-Gastaut syndrome who are 20 to 40 years old have been reported [4, 32, 56, 59]. Many patients who cease having atypical absence, myoclonic, atonic, and tonic seizures in late childhood continue to have other types of seizures (tonic-clonic, simple partial, or complex partial seizures).

Intelligence and Neurologic Deficits

Mental retardation and neurologic deficits present prior to the onset of the epileptic encephalopathy of Lennox and Gastaut will persist into adulthood even after disappearance of clinical seizures and slow spike-wave discharges in the EEG. In cryptogenic cases (previously normal neurologically and intellectually), slowness in mental processes persist even after disappearance of clinical seizures and paroxysmal abnormalities in the EEG. Throughout the course of the syndrome, periods of exacerbation of seizure activity are usually associated with worsening of neuropsychologic deficits. The final level of mental development attained tends to be most severely impaired in patients with onset of seizures before 2 years, tonic or atonic seizures, evidence of brain damage, abnormal neuro-ophthalmologic findings, or an EEG with slow spike-wave frequency of less than 1.5 Hz [4, 11]. Although most patients are mentally retarded as adults, a small percentage will have normal or above average intelligence [4, 11, 34].

OTHER SECONDARILY GENERALIZED FORMS

The prognosis of other secondarily generalized forms of atypical absence, myoclonic, atonic, and tonic seizures depends on the disease process responsible for the underlying cerebral insult.

References

1. Aicardi, J. The problem of the Lennox syndrome. *Dev. Med. Child. Neurol.* 15:77, 1973.
2. Aicardi, J., and Chevrie, J. J. Myoclonic epilepsies of childhood. *Neuropaediatrie* 3:177, 1971.
3. Alving, J. Classification of the epilepsies: An investigation of 402 children. *Acta Neurol. Scand.* 60:157, 1979.
4. Blume, W. T., David, R. B., and Gomez, M. R. Generalized sharp and slow wave complexes: Associated clinical features and long-term follow-up. *Brain* 96:289, 1973.
5. Bogan, F. Petit mal and akinetic epilepsy in a 4-year-old boy without spike and wave complexes. *Electroencephalogr. Clin. Neurophysiol.* 25:290, 1968.
6. Brambilla, F., Giardini, M., and Leuti, C. Treatment of different kinds of epilepsy by synthetic ACTH. *Electroencephalogr. Clin. Neurophysiol.* 35:439, 1973.
7. Brenner, R. P., and Atkinson, R. Generalized paroxysmal fast activity: Electroencephalographic and clinical features. *Ann. Neurol.* 11:386, 1982.

8. Bridge, E. M. *Epilepsy and Convulsive Disorders in Children.* New York: McGraw-Hill, 1979.

9. Calderon-Gonzalez, R., Hopkins, J., and McLean, W. T. Tap seizures; A form of sensory precipitation epilepsy. *J.A.M.A.* 198:521, 1966.

10. Chayasirisobhon, S., and Rodin, E. A. Atonic-akinetic seizures. *Electroencephalogr. Clin. Neurophysiol.* 50:225P, 1981.

11. Chevrie, J. J., and Aicardi, J. Childhood epileptic encephalopathy with slow spike-wave: A statistical study of 80 cases. *Epilepsia* 13:259, 1972.

12. Courjon, J., and Favel, P. L'aspect électrographique des crises akinétiques. *Rev. Neurol.* 105:211, 1961.

13. Deisenhammer, L., and Scherrer, H. Treatment of astatic petit mal with ACTH. *Electroencephalogr. Clin. Neurophysiol.* 30:169, 1971.

14. Devivo, D. How to Use Steroids and the Ketogenic Diet. In P. L. Morselli, J. K. Penry, and C. E. Pippenger (Eds.), *Antiepileptic Drug Therapy in Pediatrics.* New York: Raven Press, 1982.

15. Doose, H. et al. Centrencephalic myoclonic-astatic petit mal: Clinical and genetic investigations. *Neuropaediatrie* 2:59, 1970.

16. Dravet, C. et al. Il synacthen nella therapia della sindrome di Lennox-Gastaut. *Riv. Neurol.* 42:327, 1971.

17. Dreifuss, F. E. Proposal for revised clinical and electroencephalographic classification of epileptic seizures. *Epilepsia* 22:489, 1981.

18. Egli, M. et al. Differential diagnosis of epileptic drop attacks. *Electroencephalogr. Clin. Neurophysiol.* 51:70P, 1981.

19. Enrile-Bascal, F. E., and Delgado-Escueta, A. V. Myoclonic, tonic-clonic seizures of adolescence. The syndrome of Janz. *Neurology* 31:113, 1981.

20. Erba, G. Unpublished data, 1982.

21. Erba, G., and Cavazzuti, V. Ictal and interictal response-latency in Lennox-Gastaut syndrome. *Electroencephalogr. Clin. Neurophysiol.* 42:717, 1977.

22. Erba, G., and Cavazzuti, V. Incomplete "absence": Selective and variable functional loss during spike-wave activity. *Electroencephalogr. Clin. Neurophysiol.* 50:217P, 1980.

23. Erba, G., and Cavazzuti, V. Tonic seizures with arousal: Report of a case. *Sleep Res.* 10:245, 1981.

24. Erba, G., Cavazzuti, V., and Lombroso, C. T. A case of pure tonic seizures. *Electroencephalogr. Clin. Neurophysiol.* 46:15P, 1979.

25. Erba, G. et al. The importance of concomitant EEG monitoring and continuous performance test in epileptic patients. *Electroencephalogr. Clin. Neurophysiol.* 43:295, 1977.

26. Erba, G., Moschen, R., and Ferber, R. Sleep-related changes in EEG discharge activity and seizure risk in patients with Lennox-Gastaut syndrome. *Sleep Res.* 10:247, 1981.

27. Fariello, R. G., Doro, J. M., and Forster, F. M. Generalized cortical electrodecremental event: Clinical and neurophysiological observations in patients with dystonic seizures. *Arch. Neurol.* 36:285, 1974.

28. Gastaut, H., and Gastaut, J. L. Computerized Axial Tomography in Epilepsy. In J. K. Penry (Ed.), *Epilepsy: The Eighth International Symposium.* New York: Raven Press, 1977.

29. Gastaut, H., and Regis, H. On the subject of Lennox's "akinetic" petit mal. *Epilepsia* 2:298, 1961.

30. Gastaut, H. et al. Generalized Convulsive Seizures Without Focal Onset. In P. J. Vinken, and G. W. Bruyn (Eds.), *Handbook of Clinical Neurology,* Vol. 15, *The Epilepsies.* Amsterdam: Elsevier, 1974.

31. Gastaut, H. et al. Generalized Nonconvulsive Seizures Without Focal Onset. In P. J. Vinken, and G. W. Bruyn (Eds.), *Handbook of Clinical Neurology,* Vol. 15, *The Epilepsies.* Amsterdam: Elsevier, 1974.

32. Gastaut, H. et al. Relative frequency of different types of epilepsy: A study employing the classification of the International League Against Epilepsy. *Epilepsia* 16:457, 1975.

33. Gastaut, H. et al. An electro-clinical study of generalized epileptic seizures of tonic expression. *Epilepsia* 4:15, 1963.

34. Gastaut, H. et al. Childhood epileptic encephalopathy with diffuse slow spike-waves (otherwise known as "petit mal variant") or Lennox Syndrome. *Epilepsia* 7:139, 1966.

35. Gibbs, F. A. Petit mal variant revisited. *Epilepsia* 12:89, 1971.

36. Gloor, P. Generalized epilepsy with spike-and-wave discharge: A reinterpretation of its electrographic and clinical manifestations. *Epilepsia* 20:571, 1979.

37. Huttenlocher, P. R., Wilbourn, A. J., and Signore, J. M. Medium chain triglycerides as a therapy for intractable childhood epilepsy. *Neurology* 21:1097, 1971.

38. Janz, D. The Natural History of Primarily Generalized Epilepsies with Sporadic Myoclonias of the "Impulsive Petit Mal" Type. In E. Lugaresi, P. Pazzauglia, ad C. A. Tassinari (Eds.), *Evolution*

and Prognosis of Epilepsy. Bologna: Italseber-Avio Gagal, 1973.

39. Jeavons, P. M., and Bower, B. D. Infantile Spasms. In P. J. Vinken, and G. W. Bruyn (Eds.), *Handbook of Clinical Neurology,* Vol. 15, *The Epilepsies.* Amsterdam: Elsevier, 1974.

40. Karbowski, K., Bassells, F., and Schneider, H. Electroencephalographic aspects of Lennox Syndrome. *Europ. Neurol.* 4:301, 1970.

41. Keith, H. *Convulsive Disorders in Children.* Boston: Little, Brown, 1963.

42. Kurokawa, T. et al. West Syndrome and Lennox-Gastaut Syndrome: A survey of natural history. *Pediatrics* 65:81, 1980.

43. Lance, J. W. The falling attacks of myoclonus. *Proc. Aust. Assoc. Neurol.* 1:49, 1963.

44. Lance, J. W. Myoclonic jerks and falls: Aetiology, classification and treatment. *Med. J. Aust.* 55:113, 1968.

45. Lance, J. W., and Adams, R. D. The syndrome of intention or action myoclonus as a sequel to hypoxic encephalopathy. *Brain* 86:111, 1963.

46. Langenstein, I. et al. Computerized cranial transverse axial tomography (CTAT) in 145 patients with primary and secondary generalized epilepsies. *Neuropaediatrie* 11:15, 1979.

47. Lennox, W. G., and Davis, J. P. Clinical correlates of the fast and slow spike-wave electroencephalog. *Pediatrics* 5:626, 1950.

48. Lennox, W. G., and Lennox, M. A. *Epilepsy and Related Disorders,* Vol. 1. Boston: Little, Brown, 1960.

49. Lison, M. P. Crises tônicas axiais e crises acineticas: Estudio clínico longitudinal de pacientes tratadas com derivados benzodiazepínicos. *Arq. Neuro. Psyquiat.* (S. Paulo) 28:347, 1970.

50. Livingston, S. *Comprehensive Management of Epilepsy in Infancy, Childhood, and Adolescence.* Springfield, Ill.: Thomas, 1972. Pp. 69–86.

51. Lombroso, C. T., and Erba, G. Drop epileptic seizures: Atonic, tonic, myoclonic components: Clinical and electrophysiological correlates. *Electroencephalogr. Clin. Neurophysiol.* 46:12P, 1979.

52. Lombroso, C. T., and Erba, G. Myoclonic Seizures: Considerations in Taxonomy. In H. Akimoto, H. Kazamatzuri, and M. Seino (Eds.), *XIIIth Epilepsy International Symposium.* New York: Raven Press, 1982.

53. Lombroso, C. T., and Lerman, P. Breathholding spells (cyanotic and pallid infantile syncope). *Pediatrics* 39:563, 1967.

54. Madsen, J. A., and Matsuo, F. Sleep seizures with arousal: A condition causing sleep deprivation. *Electroencephalogr. Clin. Neurophysiol.* 47:27P, 1979.

55. Newmark, M. E., and Penry, J. K. *Photosensitivity and Epilepsy: A Review.* New York: Raven Press, 1979.

56. Niedermeyer, E. The Lennox-Gastaut syndrome: A severe type of childhood epilepsy. *Dtsch. Zeitscheift für Nervenheilk.* 195:263, 1969.

57. Niedermeyer, E. et al. Myoclonus and the electroencephalogram: A review. *Clinical EEG* 10:75, 1979.

58. Oller-Daurella, L. A special type of attack observed in the Lennox-Gastaut syndrome in adults. *Electroencephalogr. Clin. Neurophysiol.* 29:529, 1970.

59. Osawa, T. et al. Therapy-Resistant Epilepsies with Long-Term History: Slow Spike-and-Wave Syndrome. In J. K. Penry (Ed.), *Epilepsy: The Eighth International Symposium.* New York: Raven Press, 1977.

60. Prior, P. F. et al. Tonic status epilepticus precipitated by intravenous diazepam in a child with petit mal status. *Epilepsia* 13:467, 1972.

61. Schneider, H., Vassella, F., and Karbowski, K. The Lennox Syndrome. *Europ. Neurol.* 4:289, 1970.

62. Sorel, L. L'épilepsie myokinétique grave de la première enfance avec pointe-onde lent (petit mal variant) et son traitement. *Rev. Neurol.* (Paris) 110:215, 1964.

63. Tassinari, C. A. et al. Tonic status epilepticus precipitated by intravenous benzodiazepine in five patients with Lennox-Gastaut Syndrome. *Epilepsia* 13:421, 1972.

64. Tassinari, C. A. et al. Epileptic Seizures During Sleep in Children. In J. K. Penry (Ed.), *Epilepsy: The Eighth International Symposium.* New York: Raven Press, 1977.

65. Viani, F. et al. Long-Term Monitoring of Antiepileptic Drugs in Patients with Lennox-Gastaut Syndrome. In J. K. Penry (Ed.), *Epilepsy: The Eighth International Symposium.* New York: Raven Press, 1977.

66. Vinken, P. J., and Bruyn, G. W. *Handbook of Clinical Neurology,* Vol. 15, *The Epilepsies.* Amsterdam: Elsevier, 1974.

INFANTILE SPASMS

9

Cesare T. Lombroso

The syndrome of infantile spasms (IS) occurs in one child out of every 4,000 to 6,000 [33] and has an overwhelmingly poor prognosis. Its eponym of "West's syndrome" reminds us that the clinical description of the syndrome has hardly improved since West's initial description in 1841 [56]. Our inability to make significant refinements in the clinical description parallels our lack of progress in understanding the underlying factors responsible for this form of epilepsy. No theory has successfully explained why such a broad etiologic range is expressed in a common set of symptoms; why the incidence of psychomotor retardation is so high; whether the psychomotor retardation exists prior to the onset of spasms or appears dramatically with them or shortly after they begin; or why the ictal and interictal EEG patterns are so unusual and distinct.

Definitions

IS is an age-related form of epilepsy, very often complicated by moderate to severe psychomotor retardation, whose anatomic and pathophysiologic substrata are unknown, whose etiology is heterogeneous, and whose clinical manifestations consist basically of brief spasms. The syndrome is usually associated with distinct ictal and interictal EEG features, such as the "decremental" ictal pattern and the "hypsarrhythmic" interictal pattern.

The peripheral ictal manifestations can vary from child to child and at different times in the same child, but in general the use of the term *spasms* seems justified. Many descriptive terms have been used (*massive myoclonic jerks, infantile myoclonic epilepsy, salaam seizures, jackknife convulsions, flexor spasms*), implying, with some justification, that there are somewhat different patterns in the clinical manifestations of this form of epilepsy. However, there is danger in the use of some of these terms as a substitute for the more general term *IS.* By using the term *myoclonic,* for example, one runs the risk of considering infantile spasms as a subgroup of the myoclonic epilepsies, which is itself a heterogeneous category with an unsatisfactory taxonomy (see Chap. 8). The term also overstresses the myoclonic component of infantile spasms at the expense of the tonic, atonic, and clonic components. Other terms still widely used for infantile spasms likewise are misleading. Among these are *minor motor seizures* and *minor motor epilepsy* [6, 37]. These terms create taxonomic, diagnostic, and prognostic confusion. Minor motor epilepsy, for example, may include other seizure patterns such as simple partial and absence seizures, which have nothing in common with IS. Another risk involves the use of the term *minor* with its implicit suggestion that IS represent a relatively benign syndrome.

There is confusion in the literature about the appropriate taxonomic category for IS. The 1970 International Classification of Epileptic Seizures [19] placed infantile spasms in the category of generalized seizures, with EEG characteristics of its own. This classification can be criticized because (1) focal ictal features are not uncommon in IS, (2) focal lesions of the central nervous system (CNS) are often present, (3) the natural evolution of IS is often toward seizures that do not fall within the "generalized" categories, and (4) the EEG correlations are usually different from those associated with generalized epilepsies. A wholly satisfactory definition, and hence valid classification, of IS still eludes us. It is clear that IS should not be classified as a distinct seizure pattern because it exhibits various patterns that are similar to those occurring in other epileptic syndromes [40]. This was the consensus of the Commission on the Classification of Epileptic Seizures, and the term IS was dropped from the 1981 revision of the International Classification of Epileptic Seizures [11].

Etiology

SYMPTOMATIC VERSUS IDIOPATHIC GROUPS

Feré [14] first suggested the subdivision of IS into two groups, symptomatic and idiopathic, based on the presence or absence of etiologic clues. Most authors have adopted these groupings, labeling *idiopathic* those patients in whom there is no evidence of abnormality preceding the onset of spasms or in whom there is some abnormality that cannot be classified etiologically. This group is often subdivided into *cryptogenic* and *doubtful* categories. Cryptogenic patients have normal development before the onset of spasms and provide no etiologic clues to their disease. Doubtful patients have abnormal development preceding onset of spasms but provide no etiologic clues. Patients labeled *symptomatic* have identifiable etiologic factors. Some authors subdivide the symptomatic category according to the developmental stage in which injury occurred, that is, prenatal, perinatal, and postnatal. The inherent difficulties involved in these etiologic classifications are evident by the marked discrepancies among series reported by various authors (see Table 9-1).

Classification of patients into particular categories may be affected by the stage of the disease in which neurologic evaluation is made. It is also possible to

Table 9-1. Etiologic Classification of IS in 10 Reported Series

Etiologic Classification	Median (%)	Range (%)
Idiopathic	38[a]	25–56[a]
Cryptogenic	31[b]	13–80[b]
Doubtful	69[b]	20–87[b]
Symptomatic	64[a]	44–75[a]
Prenatal factors	24[c]	4–38[c]
Perinatal factors	45[c]	18–80[c]
Postnatal factors	38[c]	15–67[c]

[a]Percent of total.
[b]Percent of idiopathic.
[c]Percent of symptomatic.
Source: Modified from J. R. Lacy and J. K. Penry [33].

overlook neurologic factors that, upon closer inspection, are found to have existed long before spasms emerged. Although these categories are primarily descriptive of whether etiologic information is available, they are of some prognostic importance. The outlook is somewhat better for the idiopathic group.

The subdivision of the idiopathic group into cryptogenic and doubtful categories also remains controversial. Although some of the infants classified in the cryptogenic (or idiopathic) group may not have a perfectly normal previous neurologic biography, we feel this further subdivision adds complications to an already difficult taxonomy. Further, the infants that we would classify in the cryptogenic group in spite of some suspicious historical antecedents or some very soft neurologic signs still appear distinct from infants in the symptomatic group in that their development was not affected until the onset of IS.

ETIOLOGIC FACTORS

General

Table 9-2 lists etiologic factors for 165 children (59 percent of our total series) who were placed in the symptomatic group of our prospective study of IS [40]. Among the prenatal factors that affect the symptomatic group, those most frequently mentioned in the literature include uterine hemorrhage, toxemia, hydrocephalus, congenital encephalopathy, congenital toxoplasmosis, congenital syphilis, congenital cytomegalovirus infection, and low birth weight. Perinatal factors include various birth-related injuries and anoxia. Postnatal factors reported most commonly include meningitis, encephalitis, trauma, dehydration with vascular thrombosis, and subdural hematoma [33, 45].

Table 9-2. Etiologic Factors* in 165 Cases of Symptomatic IS

Prenatal (46)	Hypoxic-ischemic encephalopathy, intrauterine infections, maternal toxemia or diabetes, first trimester bleeding, drug addictions, "dysmaturity"
Perinatal (39)	Obstetrical traumas including cesarean section due to abruptio placentae and other complications of labor, hypoxic-ischemic encephalopathy (fetal heart deceleration, persistent acidosis, need for resuscitation after 5–10 minutes, Apgar scores < 5 after 10 minutes or more)
Postnatal (49)	
Metabolic (13)	Primary hypoglycemia, congenital enzymatic defects including "maple syrup" disease, nonketotic or ketotic hyperglycinemia, urea-cycle disorders, PKU, Leigh's syndrome, and miscellaneous others
Hemorrhagic (13)	Subependymal, intraventricular, parenchymal, subarachnoidal, trauma-X
Infections (18)	Bacterial or viral meningoencephalitides, general sepsis, brain abscess
Hypoxic-ischemic (5)	Sudden respiratory-cardiac complications after first few hours or days of life requiring resuscitation and assisted respiration with several pO_2 values < 40 mm Hg
Dysgenetic and/or chromosomal (34)	Tuberous sclerosis (19 cases), megalencephaly with cortical dysplasia, polymicrogyria, schizencephaly; Down's, Marinesco-Sjögren's, Aicardi's, de Lange's, Sturge-Weber syndromes; incontintia pigmenti
CNS Degenerative disease (5)	Lipidoses, Alpers' syndrome
Miscellaneous (10)	Vitamin B_6-dependency, drowning, late trauma, lithium poisoning, lead intoxication

*Multiple factors were present in 18 cases, mostly involving babies with hypoxic-ischemic insult.
Source: C. T. Lombroso [40].

Metabolic Causes
Neonatal hypoglycemia is frequently found in the history of IS patients. Disturbances in the metabolism of amino acids (phenylketonuria, hyperornithinemia, hyperammonemia, homocitrullinuria, histidinemia) have been found in some cases [13, 51].

Tuberous Sclerosis
Tuberous sclerosis is reported in a significant number of IS patients. We found tuberous sclerosis in 20 percent of the babies in our series [40], and Charlton and Mellinger [8] found it in 13 percent of their 195 patients. Lacy and Penry [33] believe that the incidence of tuberous sclerosis in these infants may be much higher than is presently realized and support the proposal that babies with IS be examined for depigmented nevi.

Hypoxic-Ischemic Insults
A higher incidence of prenatal and perinatal hypoxic-ischemic insults as possible main etiologic factors was found in our series (Table 9-2) than in other series.

Hormones and Neurotransmitters
Particular interest has been recently focused on the etiologic significance of disturbances in brain hormone levels. Pyridoxine deficiency and its associated overload of tryptophan, and elevation of serotonin and/or its precursor 5-hydroxytryptophan have been implicated in the pathophysiology of IS [3, 10, 24, 29, 32, 33, 57].

Male-Female Ratio
Nearly all studies that include male-female ratios have found a preponderance of males. In our study [40] the male-female ratio was nearly 2:1. Females who develop IS, however, appear to have a worse developmental prognosis [40, 45].

Genetics
A positive family history of epilepsy among first-, second-, and third degree relatives was found in some studies [15, 17, 45]. These positive family histories appear primarily in the cryptogenic group. Majewska [43] mentions her belief that in children with prior normal development and later onset of spasms genetic factors as well as additional immunologic factors are at work. The genetics of IS is a controversial area that requires further study.

Aicardi Syndrome
Aicardi et al. [2] have described a syndrome in female infants consisting of three principal features—agenesis of the corpus callosum, chorioretinitis, and IS. Other associated features often include hypsarrhythmic and periodic EEG patterns, muscular hypo-

tonia or hypertonia, and anomalies of vertebral bone development.

Immunizations

Several authors have implicated immunization reactions as a causative factor in the onset of IS. The pertussis vaccine is most commonly named [5, 32a, 29, 53a, 58]. A postimmunization encephalomyelitic reaction is implied. Although attractive, this relationship remains highly speculative. No convincing data, in terms of clinical events or signs, CSF findings, or autopsy reports, have been published. On the other hand, the peak age of onset for IS closely overlaps that common for immunization. Charlton [9] reports that in 4 of his cases who developed IS closely following diphtheria-pertussis-tetanus (DPT) immunization, 1 later proved to have tuberous sclerosis. For these reasons, we have not accepted postvaccination reaction as a causative factor in IS. Eleven babies in our series developed IS sometime after vaccination [40]. Ten of them were classified in the cryptogenic group. One belonged to the symptomatic category owing to a history of neonatal distress, hemiparesis, and the presence of porencephaly on CT scan.

Viral Infections

We have noted a curious phenomenon during some viral infections. Although during bacterial infections the frequency and severity of IS may be aggravated, certain viral invasions seem to be accompanied by a temporary abatement of the spells. In addition to anecdotal reporting by parents of such events, we have documented this phenomenon more objectively in a group of 6 infants who, following measles vaccination, experienced an apparent decrease or absence of their otherwise frequent flurries of spasms. This occurred between the sixth and tenth days following the immunization, presumably coinciding with the time of induced viremia. Wider collection of data is required before we can confirm this association.

Pathophysiology

Although the pathophysiologic factors responsible for IS remain obscure, recent interest has focused on serotonin and related neurotransmitters, especially in the pons [10, 32]. In studies of the effects of several different steroid and benzodiazepine drugs on sleep in IS, it has been found that REM-sleep time increased significantly in patients who responded to treatment [18, 27]. This suggests that improvements in REM-sleep and IS may arise at the pontine level. Critical balances of hormones between neurons of the gigantocellular area, the dorsal raphe, and the locus

ceruleus may be upset biochemically or anatomically. Abnormal discharges from these pontine structures would be projected diffusely through the brain and could be responsible for the hypsarrhythmic EEG patterns.

While attractive, these hypotheses require more validation, both at the laboratory and clinical levels. The downplay of cortical dysfunction in IS runs counter to several factors including etiologies, pathologic findings, and developmental delays. These theories, however, merit further investigations in the hope of elucidating how such multiple etiologies may express themselves with such relatively homogenous clinical manifestations.

Seizure Phenomena

CLINICAL SEIZURES

The spasms are typically very brief (usually from a fraction of a second to 5 seconds, although some may last as long as 60 seconds). The spasms generally occur in clusters of up to 10 or more within a single episode. These clusters may repeat themselves up to 60 times a day. The duration, frequency, and intensity of the spasms vary considerably [7, 12, 29, 30, 37].

The spasms are of three main types: flexor, extensor, and a mixture of both. In flexor spasms there is flexion of the neck and at times the trunk, with flexion and usually adduction of the legs. The arms, also in flexion, can be adducted or abducted. Extensor spasms, the least common, consist of extension of the legs while the arms, also extended, tend usually to be abducted and thrust forward. With careful monitoring, it is usually possible to find some extension of the trunk and neck. Such extension spasms raise the possibility that these are primarily tonic seizures, most often encountered in older patients with Lennox-Gastaut syndrome (see Chap. 8). Most frequently one sees mixed forms in which either the arms are flung forward and out and the legs are flexed, or the arms are flexed while the legs are extended.

There are also fragmentary forms, the most common being head nodding, which are myoclonic (due to muscle contraction). Head nodding due to loss of tone may be seen with IS, but is more characteristic of Lennox-Gastaut syndrome and absence seizures. A spasm may be limited to one side only with or without adversive elements. Infantile spasms are very rarely confined to one limb or to the neck and shoulders. The latter partial forms are more common in babies less than 3 months old. They are also seen in newborns, in whom full extensor or flexor spasms are rare.

In our recent prospective study of 286 IS patients,

the frequency of the various types of IS was as follows: mixed flexor-extensor spasms, 50 percent; flexor spasms, 42 percent; extensor spasms, 19 percent; partial spasms, 12 percent; unilateral spasms, 6 percent; atonic spells, 12 percent; atypical absences, 5 percent; and myoclonic jerks, 17 percent [40].

RELATED PHENOMENA

Numerous ictal concomitants of the spasms have been described. Among these, respiratory irregularities, vocalizations such as brief cries (probably related to contraction of the respiratory muscles), various kinds of abnormal eye movements, flushing, sweating, and mild cyanosis are the most common [12, 29, 33, 34, 36]. Other autonomic manifestations have been stressed [31] but in our experience are not common. Laughter has been mentioned [12, 30], but is even less common in our experience, although the cry may simulate a gelastic component. Smiling, also mentioned by several authors, may represent a bilateral facial nerve involvement.

POSTICTAL PHENOMENA

Following a flurry of spasms the infant may exhibit postictal exhaustion and lethargy. Not uncommonly, the opposite occurs. There is a brief period of heightened alertness and responsiveness, which is of interest since it appears to correlate with a brief period of improved background activities in the hypsarrhythmic EEG.

PRECIPITATING FACTORS

The greatest incidence of spasms tends to occur with drowsiness or upon awakening. Handling, feedings, and startles are other triggers for spasms.

CLINICAL COURSE

Infantile spasms may begin without warning, but more often they emerge as a new development in a series of neurologic irregularities. Of 200 patients studied by Matsumoto et al. [45], 68 percent had "delayed development" prior to their spasms; 56 percent had "neurologic abnormality"; 76 percent had abnormal pneumoencephalograms; and 43 percent had "convulsions before onset." Motor deficits of all kinds are the most common pre-existing neurologic abnormalities; spastic or hypotonic forms appear most frequently. Microcephaly and a variety of other CNS deficits are also often present, including many with cortical blindness or deafness, or both.

The onset of IS usually occurs between the ages of 2 and 8 months, although it has ranged from day-old infants to 4½ year olds [33]. The peak incidence of onset occurs between 4 and 6 months of age. In 85 percent of cases reviewed by Jeavons and Bower [29], onset occurred before the age of 1 year. It appeared after the age of 2 years in only 7 percent of cases. One point ignored by most reports dealing with age of onset is that the gestational age of the infant should be considered. If a baby was born at a gestational age of 28 weeks and developed IS 6 months after birth, the actual onset in terms of conceptional age would be 3 months [39, 40].

Although they may appear as full-blown extensor, flexor, or mixed extensor-flexor spasms, the spasms begin most often as isolated events of low intensity. Particularly in the youngest babies, IS may appear in such atypical and fragmentary forms as fleeting myoclonic jerks or unilateral spasms. These eventually develop into classic spasms. As the disease progresses, the spasms tend to increase in intensity and frequency, gathering themselves into clusters. Accompanied by developmental deterioration and an abnormal EEG that usually exhibits hypsarrhythmia or modified hypsarrhythmia, the disease intensifies to a peak stage of many clusters a day. After a period of months or, in some cases, years, the spasms subside, as does the hypsarrhythmia, and the child's development may begin to show some improvement. The course of the disease runs 1 year in approximately 25 percent of cases [33]. Approximately 25 percent more persist up to 2 years [33]. The disease may, rarely, last 5 years or more.

Prior, concomitant, and ensuing seizures and non-hypsarrhythmic EEG abnormalities are common occurrences in patients with IS. Preceding seizures tend to be generalized or focal and, less frequently, tonic, atonic, clonic, or mixed. Concurrent seizures are usually generalized, although focal and mixed patterns are also seen [33]. In addition to short-term relapses of infantile spasms, many seizure types emerge as the spasms subside. In our prospective study [39, 40], tonic or tonic-clonic seizures, often with some focal signature, were found most frequently. The next most common were mixed patterns consisting of myoclonic, atonic, tonic, and modified absences (Lennox-Gastaut syndrome, see Chap. 8). Some of our patients continued to have mainly mixed tonic and myoclonic components that were difficult to classify.

EEG Phenomena

INTERICTAL EEG

Traditionally, infantile spasms are thought to be accompanied by the EEG features of hypsarrhythmia. This term, coined by Gibbs and Gibbs [21], describes

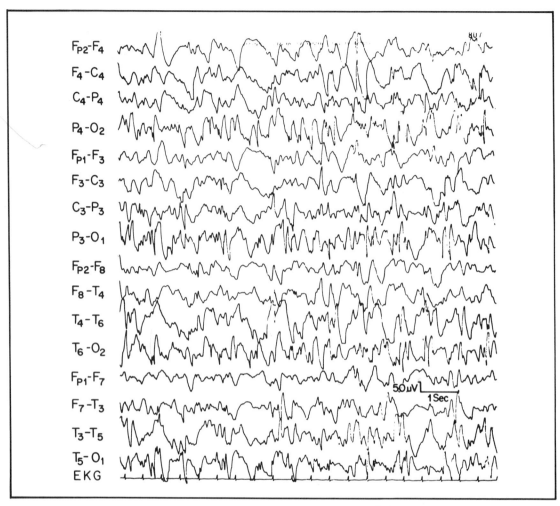

Figure 9-1. Hypsarrhythmic EEG pattern in waking recording of a 6-month-old boy with IS.

the high voltage (*hypso* means high in Greek), arrhythmic, slow EEG patterns prevailing interictally in most babies with IS (see Fig. 9-1). Spikes and sharp waves of various morphologies and with multifocal origin occur almost continuously. Poor synchrony, within and between hemispheres, prevails, although some bilateral synchrony occurs at times, especially in older or treated infants. Curiously, the Gibbs' early descriptions fail to mention another typical EEG feature associated with most cases of IS, namely, "burst-suppression" appearing with slow-wave stages of sleep (see Fig. 9-2). This "periodicity" in the EEG during some sleep stages has caused confusion. The fact that some babies' EEGs at onset of IS may show no hypsarrhythmia while awake but typical burst suppression while asleep has led some authors to label this pattern *modified hypsarrhythmia* [38]. Some cases may fail

to show hypsarrhythmia during the waking state or at the first recording. However, hypsarrhythmia will develop in most cases or is already apparent from the onset in the burst-suppression features during sleep.

In some babies, especially those in the symptomatic group, other types of EEG abnormalities may precede the pattern of hypsarrhythmia. Rarely, the clinical phenomena may precede by a few weeks the EEG appearance of the hypsarrhythmic pattern, although the converse is more common. If the EEG continues to be normal throughout, the diagnosis of true IS may generally be excluded [41].

The EEG pattern of hypsarrhythmia should not be considered pathognomonic for IS because it can be seen in approximately 5 percent of infants who exhibit

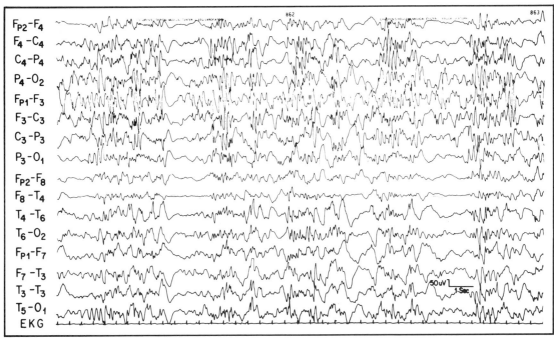

Figure 9-2. Burst-suppression EEG pattern during sleep recording of a 9-month-old girl with IS.

either other ictal phenomena or none at all. Hence, the use of the EEG term for describing clinical syndromes is to be discouraged.

ICTAL EEG

The ictal EEG accompaniments of IS vary. The most common pattern is one in which, following a more or less synchronous burst of high-voltage, atypical spike-and slow-wave activity, there is a profound alteration of the previous ongoing background and the appearance of low-voltage fast rhythms (see Fig. 9-3). These are usually in the beta range, bilateral and diffuse, and coincide with the clinical spasm. Less often, the fast rhythms are in the alpha band. The voltage may be very low, and thus the scalp-derived EEG appears almost isoelectric. These low-voltage discharges have been called "decremental discharges," a term that might cause some misunderstanding because this apparent alteration of EEG activities may well be an epiphenomenon of a "hypersynchronized" discharge. The decremental pattern is also observed in cases of acute brain anoxia, for example, in pallid infantile syncope [42]. The initial burst may be absent, and one sees only the sudden diffuse attenuation. There are instances when the ictal event is accompanied by generalized slow wave and sharp components. Rarely,

only a run of generalized slow waves occurs. All these ictal patterns may be combined or vary from ictus to ictus.

Differential Diagnosis

The differential diagnosis of typical IS is usually an easy one, especially if one can observe the spasms directly. Colic, startle, or exaggerated Moro reflex can be the initial impressions. Less common, and occasionally more difficult in the differential diagnosis, are the abnormal movements that may occur in infants with gastroesophageal reflux ("stomach fits"). Infants who exhibit myoclonic movements for periods of a few weeks to several months but show none of the neurologic or EEG stigmata usually seen in IS, who have no radiologic evidence of gastroesophageal reflux, and who outgrow the abnormal movements with no apparent sequelae, are particularly difficult to diagnose [41]. Differential diagnosis with tonic seizures, mainly encountered within the Lennox-Gastaut syndrome, may be difficult when the spasms last longer than usual and are extensor in pattern. Tonic seizures usually last longer than infantile spasms, occur more often in isolation (instead of in flurries), occur in deeper stages of sleep, and occur in older children. The clinical differentiation from atonic or complex absences is less difficult.

The similarity of some clinical and EEG aspects in

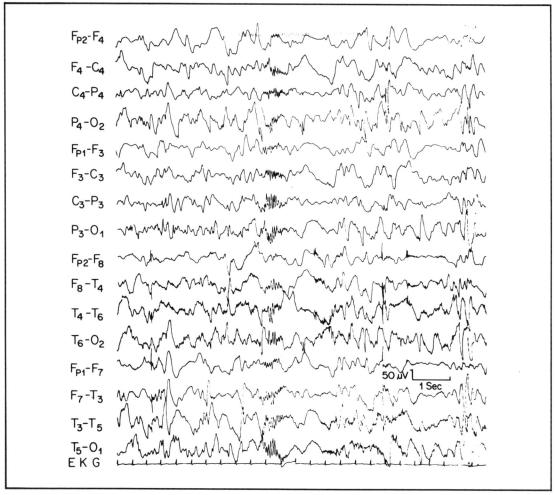

Figure 9-3. Ictal EEG of a 9-month-old girl having a brief infantile spasm. Synchronous high-voltage slow waves are followed by low-voltage fast discharge and disruption of background activity.

IS and in Lennox-Gastaut syndrome have motivated some authors to consider them closely related syndromes, the former evolving into the latter [1, 20, 47, 48] (see Chap. 8). Although it is true that such evolution occurs in a still indefinite number of infants with IS, it should be remembered that a considerable number of infantile spasms evolve into different seizure syndromes. Furthermore, a large number of patients with Lennox-Gastaut syndrome develop it de novo, at a later age, with no preceding history of IS, and even with no history suggestive of a neurologic disorder [40].

Management

ADRENOCORTICOTROPIC HORMONE (ACTH)

Evidence for Efficacy
Comparative studies indicate that nonsynthetic ACTH is the most effective of the available therapies for IS

[40]. However, the evidence regarding the absolute and relative efficacy of all therapies for IS is controversial, and no therapy produces uniformly satisfactory results.

Table 9-3 summarizes some of the reported data on the initial effects of ACTH and oral steroid therapies in IS. Table 9-4 indicates some of the further conflicting observations on long-term outcomes of IS in babies treated with or without steroids. Most studies agree that steroid treatment, whether ACTH or oral steroids, induces early cessation of the spasms and amelioration of EEG abnormalities. The studies differ substantially in their findings on long-term effects (i.e., continuation or resurgence of seizures and intellectual development).

Table 9-3. Initial Effects of Corticotropin and Corticosteroids on Seizure Frequency in IS

Study	No. of Patients	Excellent Response (%)	Good Response (%)	Minimal or No Response (%)	Relapsed (%)
Sorel, 1959	11[a]	36	46	18	—
Low, 1958	10[b]	50	20	30	—
Stamps et al., 1959	60[a]	30	22	48	—
Trojaborg and Plum, 1960	22[b]	32[c]	—	68	—
Dobbs and Baird, 1960	15[a]	20	20	60	—
Pauli et al., 1960	14[b]	21	7	72	75
Millichap and Bickford, 1962	21[b]	24	29	47	—
Ladwig et al., 1962	13[b]	46	31	23	—
Rail, 1963	34[a]	18	47	35	—
Harris, 1964	75[a]	60	—	40	33
Crowther, 1964	20[d]	65[c]	—	35	—
Jeavons and Bower, 1964	56[b]	70	19	11	63
Willoughby et al., 1966	24[a]	25	42	33	—
Wiszczoradamczyk and Koslaczfolga, 1969	29[a]	59	27	14	—

[a]Treated with ACTH alone.
[b]Treated with ACTH and/or corticosteroids.
[c]Good or excellent response.
[d]Treated with oral hydrocortisone alone.
Source: Modified from J. R. Lacy and J. K. Penry [33].

Table 9-4. Intelligence and Mortality in Steroid-Treated and Untreated Patients With IS

Study	Steroid	No. of Patients	Duration of Follow-up (years)	Normal Intelligence (%)	Mild Retardation (%)	Moderate Retardation (%)	Severe Retardation (%)	Deceased (%)
Snyder, 1967	Treated	28	2–7	29	—	—	—	—
	Untreated	20	2–12	10	—	—	—	—
Jeavons et al., 1970	Treated	57	4–12	14[a]	—	7	63	16
	Untreated	41	4–12	15[a]	—	15	49	22
Friedman and Pampiglione, 1971	Treated[b]	49	8–14	24[a]	—	23	33	20
	Untreated[b]	29	8–14	14[a]	—	17	48	21
Jeavons et al., 1973	Treated	105	4–14	26[c]	—	—	52	22
	Untreated	45	4–14	27[c]	—	—	51	22

[a]Includes patients with normal intelligence and mild retardation.
[b]Differences between treated and untreated groups not statistically significant.
[c]Includes patients with normal intelligence and mild and moderate retardation.
Source: Modified from J. R. Lacy and J. K. Penry [33].

Relapses occur often, even in children who have responded promptly to therapy. Long-term studies show relapses in approximately 40 to 50 percent of patients who responded to treatment [33, 49]. Relapses may occur within weeks of ending therapy or up to the age of 4½ years [49].

Pollack et al. [49] and Singer et al. [52, 53] have recently studied the effects of ACTH treatment on intellectual impairment in babies with IS. They found that most IS patients at the end of long-term study were at least as impaired as when they began.

Factors Affecting Response

Hrachovy et al. [25, 26] studied etiologic association, treatment lag, and developmental status at onset in IS. They found that developmental status at onset was an important factor in the patient's response to treatment, but that etiology and treatment lag were not. On the other hand, Singer et al. [52, 53] found that treatment that is begun within 1 month of onset increases the success rate of quick cessation of spasms and of prevention of relapses. Their comparisons with other studies showed that ACTH treatment begun within 1 week of onset produced complete control of spasms in 87 percent (versus 50 percent for other studies) and a 36 percent relapse rate (versus 48 percent for other studies). The lack of correlation between etiology and outcome following steroid treatment found by Hrachovy et al. [25, 26] may be explained by very short-term responses, by the small number of cases, or by mixing symptomatic and idiopathic cases together.

Dosage

We currently employ the following regimen of non-synthetic ACTH for IS: 110 units/sq. m./day for 3 weeks, followed by 70 units/sq. m./day for 2 weeks, followed by 50 units/sq. m./day on alternate days for 3 weeks [39, 40].

Side Effects

Steroid therapy has numerous side effects, including hypertension, electrolyte disturbances, and increased risk of infection. Viral and bacterial infections are enhanced by steroid therapy, especially at large doses. Pneumonia, urinary tract infections, gastroenteritis, and *Candida* infections of the oral mucosa are the most common infectious side effects of steroid therapy [40, 50]. The role of ACTH in such minor infections as skin abscesses, fevers of unknown origin, and otitis is unclear. ACTH may cause latent infections to flare up dangerously in unexpected ways [50].

Some patients experience difficulties upon withdrawal of ACTH therapy [50]. Because of significant disturbances in fluid regulation, patients may have a negative water balance, requiring more fluids, or a positive water balance, requiring diuretics and water restriction. Renal failure may result.

ORAL STEROIDS

Hrachovy et al. [25] question the effectiveness of prednisone as the primary therapy for IS. They found improvement (a 50 percent decrease in IS frequency) in 25 percent of their patients on prednisone. The EEGs of these patients were improved, but all continued to show focal abnormalities. More recently, Hrachovy et al. [26] studied 5 IS patients who were treated for 6 weeks on ACTH at 20 to 30 units/day. Four became seizure-free promptly, and treatment in a fifth was changed to clonazepam owing to hypertension. This patient also became seizure-free. These authors found an immediate rise in serum cortisol levels at that dosage; higher doses did not produce higher serum cortisol levels. They concluded that ACTH is superior to prednisone in treating infantile spasms. Our recently concluded study [40] comparing therapies for IS produced a similar conclusion.

BENZODIAZEPINES AND VALPROIC ACID

The problem of determining the best therapy for IS has been further complicated by recent favorable reports on the use of the benzodiazepines [16, 22, 23, 35, 44, 54, 55] and valproic acid (see Chaps. 20 and 21) [4]. Clonazepam, diazepam, and nitrazepam are the three benzodiazepines used thus far. Nitrazepam has had the highest success rate [33]. These drugs have been used in IS only since the mid-1960s, and because of the predominance of steroid therapy during this period, benzodiazepines have received scant attention. Lacy and Penry [33] report that 63 percent of children in the studies they reviewed benefitted from nitrazepam. Clonazepam seemed to produce less encouraging results, and diazepam had not been studied enough to draw reliable conclusions. Again, the validity of several reports on the effectiveness of the benzodiazepines is marred by the lack of controlled studies and failure to obtain long-term follow-up.

KETOGENIC DIET

The ketogenic diet is sometimes helpful in controlling IS [36] but is seldom used now for reasons reviewed in Chapter 8.

COMPARISON OF THERAPIES

In a study [40] aimed at clarifying some of the controversies still surrounding IS therapy, we sought to determine the following: (1) whether benzodiaze-

Table 9-5. Correlations According to Therapies in Infants with IS After 10 Months From Onset of Treatment

	Symptomatic Group (N = 158)			Cryptogenic Group (N = 119)		
	A Variable Treatment (%)	B Oral Steroids (%)	C ACTH (%)	D Variable Treatment (%)	E Oral Steroids (%)	F ACTH (%)
I. Infantile Spasms						
Abolished/improved > 50%	50	56	65	64	68	86
No significant change	50	44	35	36	32	14
II. EEGs						
Normalized/improved > 50%	55	61	69	68	64	90
No significant change	45	39	31	32	36	10
III. Neurologic Deficits						
None	11	12	18	23	32	34
Present	89	88	82	77	68	66

Statistical significance by χ^2 test: $p < 0.05$ for infantile spasms: D vs. F; E vs. F; and EEGs: D vs. F; E vs. F.
Source: Modified from C. T. Lombroso [40].

pines, valproic acid, or other antiepileptic drugs were as effective as steroid treatment; (2) whether ACTH was superior to oral corticosteroids when steroid therapy alone was used; and (3) whether early institution of therapy makes any difference in outcome.

The short-term effects (10 months after initiation of therapies) were investigated separately from the long-term outcomes (up to 6 years). For the short-term evaluation, we compared three types of therapy for both the symptomatic and cryptogenic groups. The therapies included: (1) only benzodiazepines, valproic acid, and/or other antiepileptic drugs; (2) oral corticosteroids alone (prednisone at 2 mg/kg/day for 8 weeks, tapered to 1 mg/kg/day for 12 to 24 weeks); and (3) nonsynthetic ACTH, using our standard regimen described above.

There seemed to be little difference in short-term effects among the therapies employed (see Table 9-5). A trend favoring ACTH treatment was found but reached statistical significance only for the cryptogenic group.

Long-term outcomes are summarized in Table 9-6. We considered that valid conclusions were more likely to be reached by limiting the prospective follow-up to the cryptogenic group. As mentioned earlier, much of the confusion about various therapies and long-term outcomes may be due to lumping together the symptomatic group of babies, who have very different etiologic and neurologic backgrounds, with the somewhat more homogeneous cryptogenic

group. Therapy with ACTH produced statistically significant better outcomes in terms of later epilepsies and developmental status. Although not completely satisfactory, these prospective observations indicate the superiority of nonsynthetic ACTH over oral steroids or other drugs in long-term outcomes. The mounting evidence that ACTH might directly influence various neuroregulators within the CNS rather than by just cortisol release may explain these differences in part, although the nature of these central effects require elucidation.

Prognosis

COURSE OF SEIZURES
See above.

DEVELOPMENTAL RETARDATION
Most authors report evidence of developmental retardation prior to onset of IS in 55 to 85 percent of patients [33, 45]. Children who develop normally before the onset of IS often show a definite developmental deterioration just before or after onset [33]. The deterioration tends to be more pronounced in psychosocial than in motor function. Lacy and Penry [33] summarized the results of nine studies on the frequency of developmental retardation at initial diagnosis of IS as follows: normal intelligence, 3 to 16 percent (median 9%); mild retardation, 9 to 95 percent (median 19%); moderate retardation, 21 to 84

Table 9-6. Correlations in 102 Cryptogenic Cases of IS Followed up to 6 Years

	A	B	C	D	
	Variable Treatment (%)	Oral Steroids Alone (%)	ACTH (8 wk) (%)	ACTH (8 wk)+Oral Steroids (14 wk)	Statistical Significance by χ^2 test ($p<0.05$)
I. Seizures					
None	25	29	62	65	A vs. D
Present	75	71	38	35	B vs. D
					B vs. C and D
II. EEG					
Normal	33	41	39	41	N.S.
Abnormal	67	59	61	59	N.S.
III. Motor-Sensory Deficits					
None	33	35	47	38	N.S.
Present	67	65	53	62	N.S.
IV. Psychometric Status					
IQ $= 100 \pm 20$	17	12	51	59	B vs. C
IQ ≤ 80	83	88	49	41	B vs. D
					B vs. C and D

Source: Modified from C. T. Lombroso [39, 40].

percent (median 30%); severe retardation, 16 to 79 percent (median 51%).

Once developmental retardation begins, it rarely abates significantly [30, 33, 49, 52, 53]. Long-term follow-up studies report normal intelligence in only 10 to 27 percent of untreated patients and in 14 to 29 percent of patients treated with steroids (see Table 9-4).

DEATH
Death occurs in approximately 20 percent of children with IS (see Table 9-4). Steroid therapy does not appear to reduce this mortality significantly (see Table 9-4).

PROGNOSTIC FACTORS
The presence or absence of certain risk factors can significantly alter the prognosis of a patient with IS. This was documented in our recent follow-up study of 286 patients [40]. A normal outcome was found in 31 percent of IS patients with no history of preceding seizures versus a normal outcome in only 15 percent of IS patients with a history of preceding seizures ($p<.02$). Onset of IS before the age of 3 months was associated with a normal outcome in 1 percent of cases, whereas onset after 3 months of age was associated with a normal outcome in 15 percent of cases

($p<.001$). IS accompanied by hypsarrhythmia EEG pattern was associated with a normal outcome in 36.5 percent of cases, whereas IS accompanied by other abnormal EEG patterns was associated with a normal outcome in 19.5 percent of cases ($p<.01$).

The total duration of IS is considered to be of prognostic importance [33], the outlook worsening as the duration lengthens. This factor has not been as thoroughly explored as some of the others because treatment has interfered with the natural course of the spasms in most series.

References
1. Aicardi, J. The problem of the Lennox syndrome. *Dev. Med. Child. Neurol.* 15:77, 1973.
2. Aicardi, J., Chevrie, J. J., and Rousselie, F. Le syndrome spasmes en flexion, agénésie calleuse, anomalies chorio-rétiniennes. *Arch. Fr. Pediatr.* 26:1103, 1969.
3. Airaksinen, E. M. Tryptophan treatment of infants with Down's syndrome. *Ann. Clin. Res.* 6:33, 1974.
4. Bachman, D. S. Use of valproic acid in treatment of infantile spasms. *Arch. Neurol.* 39:49, 1982.
5. Baird, H. W., and Borofsky, L. G. Infantile myoclonic seizures. *J. Pediatr.* 50:332, 1957.
6. Bray, P. F. The influence of adrenal steroids and

corticotropin on massive myoclonic seizures in infancy. *Pediatrics* 3:169, 1963.

7. Chao, D. H., Taylor, E. M., and Druckman, R. Massive spasms. *J. Pediatr.* 50:670, 1957.

8. Charlton, M. H., and Mellinger, J. F. Infantile spasms and hypsarrhythmia. *Electroencephalogr. Clin. Neurophysiol.* 29:413, 1970.

9. Charlton, M. H. *Myoclonic Seizures.* Amsterdam: Excerpta Medica, 1975.

10. Coleman, M. Infantile spasms associated with 5-hydroxytryptophan administration in patients with Down's syndrome. *Neurology* (Minneap.) 21:911, 1971.

11. Dreifuss, F. E. Proposal for revised clinical and electroencephalographic classification of epileptic seizures. *Epilepsia* 22:489, 1981.

12. Druckman, R., and Chao, D. Massive spasms in infancy and childhood. *Epilepsia* 4:61, 1955.

13. Duffner, P. K., and Cohen, M. E. Infantile spasms associated with histidinemia. *Neurology* (Minneap.) 25:195, 1975.

14. Feré, C. Le tic de salaam. Les salutations neuropathiques. *Proc. Med.* 11:99, 1883.

15. Fleizar, K. A., Daniel, W. L., and Imrey, P. B. Genetic study of infantile spasms with hypsarrhythmia. *Epilepsia* 12:13, 1977.

16. Fukushima, Y. et al. The treatment of infantile spasms with nitrazepam. *Brain Nerve* 20:1297, 1968.

17. Fukuyama, Y. Studies on the etiology and pathogenesis of flexor spasms in infancy. *Adv. Neurol. Sci.* (Tokyo) 4:861, 1960.

18. Fukuyama, Y., Shionaga, A., and Icola, Y. Polygraphic study during whole night sleep in infantile spasms. *Europ. Neurol.* 18:302, 1979.

19. Gastaut, H. Clinical and electroencephalographical classification of epileptic seizures. *Epilepsia* 11:102, 1970.

20. Gastaut, H. et al. Childhood epileptic encephalopathy with diffuse slow spike-waves (otherwise known as the "petit mal variant") or Lennox syndrome. *Epilepsia* 7:139, 1966.

21. Gibbs, F. A., and Gibbs, E. L. Following of ACTH treated and untreated cases of hypsarrhythmia. *Clin. Electroencephalogr.* 7:149, 1976.

22. Hagberg, B. The chlordiazepoxide HCl (Librium) analogue, nitrazepam (Mogadon) in the treatment of epilepsy in children. *Dev. Med. Child. Neurol.* 10:302, 1968.

23. Hanson, R. A., and Menkes, J. H. A new anticonvulsant in the management of minor motor seizures. *Dev. Med. Child. Neurol.* 14:3, 1972.

24. Hellström, B., and Vassella, F. Tryptophan metabolism in infantile spasm. *Acta Paediatr. Scand.* 5:665, 1962.

25. Hrachovy, R. A. et al. A controlled study of prednisone therapy in infantile spasms. *Epilepsia* 20:403, 1979.

26. Hrachovy, R. A. et al. A controlled study of ACTH therapy in infantile spasms. *Epilepsia* 21:631, 1980.

27. Hrachovy, R. A., Frost, J. D., and Kellaway, P. Sleep characteristics in infantile spasms. *Neurology* 31:688, 1981.

28. Huttenlocher, P. R. Dendritic development of neocortex of children with mental defect and infantile spasms. *Neurology* (Minneap.) 24:203, 1974.

29. Jeavons, P. M., and Bower, B. D. Infantile Spasms: A Review of the Literature and a Study of 112 Cases. (Clinics in Developmental Medicine, No. 15.) London: Spastics Society and Heinemann, 1964.

30. Jeavons, P. M., and Bower, B. D. Infantile Spasms. In P. J. Vinken, and G. W. Bruyn (Eds.), *Handbook of Clinical Neurology,* Vol. 15, *The Epilepsies.* Amsterdam: Elsevier, 1974.

31. Kellaway, P. Neurologic Status of Patients with Hypsarrhythmia. In F. A. Gibbs (Ed.), *Molecules and Mental Health.* Philadelphia: Lippincott, 1959.

32. Klawans, H. L., Goetz, C., and Weiner, W. J. 5-Hydroxytryptophan–induced myoclonus in guinea pigs and the possible role of serotonin in infantile myoclonus. *Neurology* (Minneap.) 23:1234, 1973.

32a. Kulenkampff, M., Schwartzman, J. S., and Wilson, J. Neurological complications of pertussis inoculation. *Arch. Dis. Child.* 49:46, 1974.

33. Lacy, J. R., and Penry, J. K. (Eds.). *Infantile Spasms.* New York: Raven Press, 1976.

34. Lennox, W. G., and Davis, J. P. Clinical correlates of the fast and the slow spike-wave electroencephalogram. *Pediatrics* 5:626, 1950.

35. Liske, E., and Forster, F. M. Clinical study of a new benzodiazepine as an anticonvulsant agent. *J. New Drugs* 3:241, 1963.

36. Livingston, S. Diagnosis and treatment of childhood myoclonic seizures. *Pediatrics* 53:542, 1974.

37. Livingston, S., Eisner, V., and Pauli, L. Minor motor epilepsy: Diagnosis, treatment and prognosis. *Pediatrics* 21:916, 1958.

38. Lombroso, C. T. Convulsive Disorders in Newborns. In R. A. Thompson and T. R. Green (Eds.), *Pediatric Neurology and Neurosurgery.* New York: Spectrum, 1978.

39. Lombroso, C. T. Differentiation of Seizures in Newborns and Early Infancy. In P. L. Morselli, J. K.

Penry, and C. E. Pippenger (Eds.), *Antiepileptic Drug Therapy in Pediatrics*. New York: Raven Press, 1982.

40. Lombroso, C. T. A prospective study of infantile spasms: Clinical and therapeutic correlations. *Epilepsia,* in press, 1983.

41. Lombroso, C. T., and Fejerman, M. Benign myoclonus of early infancy. *Ann. Neurol.* 1:138, 1977.

42. Lombroso, C. T., and Lerman, P. Breathholding spells (cyanotic and pallid infantile syncope). *Pediatrics* 39:563, 1967.

43. Majewska, Z. Infantile spasms. Paper presented at the Epilepsy International Workshop on Infantile Spasms, Warsaw, June 9, 1976.

44. Markham, C. H. The treatment of myoclonic seizures of infancy and childhood with LA-1. *Pediatrics* 34:511, 1964.

45. Matsumoto, A. et al. Long-term prognosis after infantile spasms: A statistical study of prognostic factors in 200 cases. *Dev. Med. Child. Neurol.* 23:51, 1981.

46. Millichap, J. G., and Bickford, R. G. Infantile spasms, hypsarrhythmia, and mental retardation: Response to corticotropin and its relation to age and etiology in 21 patients. *J.A.M.A.* 182:523, 1962.

47. Niedermeyer, E. The Lennox-Gastaut syndrome, a severe type of childhood epilepsy. *Dtsch. Z. Nervenheilk.* 195:263, 1969.

48. Otahara, S. et al. Prognosis of West Syndrome with Special Reference to Lennox Syndrome: A Developmental Study. In J. A. Wada, and J. K. Penry (Eds.), *Advances in Neurology: The Tenth Epilepsy International Symposium*. New York: Raven Press, 1980.

49. Pollack, M. A., Thomas, T. E., and Kellaway, P. Long-term prognosis of patients with infantile spasms following ACTH therapy. *Epilepsia* 20:255, 1979.

50. Riikonen, R., and Donner, M. ACTH therapy for infantile spasms: Side effects. *Arch. Dis. Child.* 55:664, 1980.

51. Shih, V. E., Efron, M. L., and Moser, H. W. Hyperornithinemia, hyperammonemia and homocitrullinuria: A new disorder of amino acid metabolism associated with myoclonic seizures and mental retardation. *Am. J. Dis. Child.* 117:83, 1969.

52. Singer, W. O., Rabe, E. F., and Haller, J. S. The effect of ACTH therapy upon infantile spasms. *J. Pediatr.* 96:485, 1980.

53. Singer, W. D., Rabe, E. F., and Haller, J. S. Infantile spasms—substantiation of ACTH therapy and predictors of outcome. *J. Pediatr.* 96:458, 1980.

53a. Swisher, C. N. Neurological sequelae to pertussis infection and immunization. In H. L. Klawans (Ed.), *Handbook of Clinical Neurology,* Vol. 33. Amsterdam: Elsevier, 1978. Pp. 275–303.

54. Vassella, F. et al. Treatment of infantile spasms and Lennox-Gastaut syndrome with clonazepam (Rivotril). *Epilepsia* 14:165, 1973.

55. Weinberg, W. A., and Harwell, J. L. Diazepam (Valium) in myoclonic seizures: A favorable response during infancy and childhood. *Am. J. Dis. Child.* 109:123, 1965.

56. West, W. J. On a peculiar form of infantile convulsions. *Lancet* 1:724, 1841.

57. Westheimer, R., and Klawans, H. L. The role of serotonin in the pathophysiology of myoclonic seizures associated with acute imipramine toxicity. *Neurology* (Minneap.) 24:1175, 1975.

58. Wilson, J. Neurological complications of DPT inoculation in infancy. *Arch. Dis. Child.* 48:829, 1973.

BORDERLINE AREAS

Robert G. Feldman

Is this epilepsy or not? Often, the diagnosis is uncertain because the clinical manifestations of some forms of epilepsy can be mimicked by other conditions. Episodic disturbances of cerebral function and behavioral disturbances of a nonepileptic origin must be considered. If the electroencephalogram (EEG) is abnormal and if loss of consciousness and tonic-clonic movements occur during an attack, a diagnosis of tonic-clonic epilepsy can be made. When the EEG is normal, hysteria or pseudoseizures may be suspected. However, a complex partial seizure without loss of consciousness and with semipurposeful automatisms may show no changes in the EEG from surface recordings made during the seizure, and interictal EEGs are often normal in persons with epilepsy (see Chap. 11). EEGs must be interpreted in light of the clinical data. Some cardiac and respiratory causes of episodic loss of consciousness can be clarified only after all clinical, EEG, and ECG data are reviewed. Examples of conditions that can be called borderline states [16] are described in this chapter.

Migraine

A higher incidence of epilepsy has been found in migrainous patients than would be expected by chance [28]. There is a slightly higher incidence of migraine in persons with epilepsy than in controls. Approximately one sixth of close relatives of persons with epilepsy have migraine attacks. The prodroma of a migraine attack may be similar to the aura of an epileptic attack. When sensorimotor prodromata occur in a migraine attack, they usually develop more slowly than the symptoms of an epileptic aura. In basilar migraine attacks consciousness may be lost. In most (but not all) cases of migraine, other symptoms of the illness such as pulsatile headache, nausea, or vomiting may be associated with the neurologic symptoms, or they may appear at other times alone. There also is a positive family history of migraine in the majority of patients with migraine attacks.

If the EEG shows a pattern pathognomonic of epilepsy, it can be helpful in distinguishing migraine from epilepsy. However, the EEG sometimes shows abnormal features in patients with migraine. Goldensohn [14] studied 200 consecutive patients with recurrent classifiable headache and negative results on neurologic examination. Twenty-seven percent of patients with migraine headaches had abnormal EEG records. Tension headaches and post-traumatic headaches, in which there were no associated neurologic deficits, had lower incidences of EEG abnormalities (12 and 13 percent, respectively). Focal slowing of the EEG typically accompanies the neurologic aura of a migraine attack owing to focal ischemia caused by cerebral vasoconstriction [33]. This focal slowing may end when the aura ends or persist for hours or days after all neurologic signs and symptoms have ended [33]. A permanent slow wave focus may accompany a permanent infarct caused by migraine-induced cerebral vasoconstriction [33]. There are also controversial reports of a high incidence of certain nonspecific (and nondiagnostic) EEG findings between attacks in patients with migraine including higher than normal voltage of driving response to photic stimulation, excess background slowing (focal or diffuse), "dysrhythmic" EEG changes, and excessive response to hyperventilation [14, 28, 31, 33].

The Syncopal Attack

DEFINITIONS

Syncope
Syncope, or fainting, is the sudden loss of tone, collapse of posture, and loss of consciousness associated with a drop in systemic blood pressure. Syncopal attacks begin with a clouding of consciousness accompanied by vertigo, nausea, and a waxy pallor of the skin. The attack usually lasts approximately 10 seconds.

Convulsive Syncope
Convulsive syncope has an onset similar to that of a typical syncopal attack. However, the onset is followed by a tonic spasm in which the back, head, and lower limbs are bent backward and the fists are clenched. This is often accompanied by mydriasis, nystagmus, drooling of saliva, and incontinence. The patient may bite his tongue, although this is extremely rare.

The patient who falls to the floor quickly recovers from a faint when the blood pressure is reestablished. If the person is unable to reach the supine position, as when fainting occurs in a chair or in a phone booth, cerebral circulation is reestablished more slowly. Under these circumstances, convulsive syncope is more likely to occur.

ETIOLOGY
Syncope and convulsive syncope occur when insufficient oxygen reaches the brain by way of the circulation. Thus, syncope is an example of cerebral ischemia and may occur under one or more of the following conditions: bradycardia of less than 40 per minute or tachycardia of more than 150 per minute; asystole of 4 to 15 seconds; systolic blood pressure of less than

70 mm Hg; a decrease in cerebral blood flow of more than 50 percent; or jugular venous O_2 of less than 20 mm Hg [2].

There are a great number of specific causes of syncope, as outlined in Table 10-1. The causes include circulatory disturbances, alterations in the blood reaching the brain, cerebrovascular disturbances, and bulbar lesions. Reflex syncopes are the most common types, accounting for over 90 percent of syncopal attacks [11].

Table 10-1. Causes of Syncope

I. *Circulatory (Deficient Quantity of Blood to Brain)*
  A. Reflex syncope (afferent sensory input activates cardioinhibitory, vasodepressive, and inspiratory efferents in brainstem)
    1. Emotion
    2. Pain
    3. Carotid sinus stimulation
  B. Inadequate vasoconstrictor mechanisms
    1. Postural hypotension
    2. Primary autonomic insufficiency
    3. Sympathectomy (pharmacologic or surgical)
    4. Diseases of central and peripheral nervous systems
  C. Hypovolemia
  D. Mechanical reduction of venous return
    1. Valsalva maneuver
    2. Cough
    3. Micturition
    4. Atrial myxoma, ball-valve thrombus
    5. Exertion
  E. Reduced cardiac output
    1. Obstruction of left ventricular outflow: aortic stenosis, hypertrophic subaortic stenosis
    2. Obstruction to pulmonary flow: pulmonic stenosis, primary pulmonary hypertension, pulmonary embolism
    3. Myocardial: massive myocardial infarction with pump failure
    4. Pericardial: cardiac tamponade
  F. Arrhythmias
    1. Bradyarrhythmias
      a. Atrioventricular block with Stokes-Adams attack
      b. Ventricular asystole
      c. Sinus bradycardia, sinoatrial block, sinus arrest
      d. Breath-holding spells (combination of bradycardia and decreased venous return)
      e. Glossopharyngeal neuralgia and other painful states
    2. Tachyarrhythmias
      a. Episodic ventricular fibrillation
      b. Ventricular tachycardia
      c. Supraventricular tachycardia without atrioventricular block
      d. Premature ventricular contractions (especially if early diastolic)

II. *Altered State of Blood Reaching Brain*
  A. Hypoxia
  B. Anemia
  C. Hypoglycemia

Table 10-1 (Continued)

III. *Cerebrovascular Disturbances*
   A. Extracranial vascular stenosis or occlusion (vertebral-basilar, carotid)
   B. Diffuse constriction of cerebral arteries
      1. Hyperventilation syncope
      2. Hypertensive encephalopathy

IV. *Bulbar Lesions* (directly or indirectly involving cardiac and vasomotor centers)
   A. Poliomyelitis
   B. Rabies
   C. Landry-Guillain-Barré syndrome
   D. Porphyria
   E. Syringobulbia
   F. Bulbopontine paralysis
   G. Amyotrophic lateral sclerosis
   H. Intraparenchymatous tumors

Source: Modified from R. D. Adams et al. [2]. Copyright © 1980 by McGraw-Hill Book Company. Used with the permission of the McGraw-Hill Book Company.

PATHOPHYSIOLOGY

Gastaut [11] has studied the pathophysiology of syncope in detail. Regardless of etiology, hypoxia generally affects the cerebral cortex and basal ganglia first, then several seconds later the hypothalamus and the mesencephalon. The bulbopontine reticular formation, which is more resistant to hypoxia, is affected several minutes after the cerebral cortex. Slow waves are seen on the EEG during the initial stages of syncope, corresponding to a thalamocortical anoxic disturbance. At this stage there is a loss of consciousness and of muscle tone. Electrical silence is then seen on the EEG, corresponding to a greater degree of oxygen deprivation of the mesencephalon. The syncopal attack may stop at this point or go on to convulsive movements. The tonic spasm of convulsive syncope occurs as a result of the release from physiologic cortical inhibition of the tonus-producing structures of the bulbopontine reticular formation, which have been relatively spared hypoxia. This liberation of the caudal reticular system, which is responsible for the tonic spasms and for most of the accompanying autonomic manifestations of convulsive syncope, is also responsible for the reappearance of the cardiac contractions and vascular tone that reestablish effective circulation and terminate syncope. The mechanism of production of convulsive syncope is probably different from the mechanism that produces the tonic phase of tonic-clonic seizures, which appear to be due to spontaneous hyperactivity of the brain stem reticular formation (see Chap. 6).

DIFFERENTIAL DIAGNOSIS

Extent of Problem
Approximately one third of syncopes are unrecognized or are misdiagnosed as epileptic seizures [11]. In some cases the loss of tonus and/or consciousness is confused with absence or complex partial seizures. Convulsive syncope may be mistaken for a tonic-clonic seizure disorder because loss of consciousness, tonic spasms, and clonic jerks can occur in either disorder. Diagnosis can be made only by analyzing each symptom, studying the conditions under which the attack occurs, and reviewing the polygraphic data.

Clinical Differentiation
The features that are valuable in differentiating seizure from syncope are listed in Table 10-2.

EEG Differentiation
The EEG may show nonspecific slow-wave changes during a syncopal episode, whereas specific paroxysms occur during an epileptic attack, followed by postictal slowing. When the EEG is made during an asymptomatic period, the tracing is normal in a patient with syncope. The interictal EEG in a person with epilepsy usually (but not always) shows some evidence of paroxysmal activity (see Chap. 11). Concomitant monitoring of the electrocardiogram (ECG) during the EEG may reveal arrhythmias that may account for the syncope (Fig. 10-1). Continuous ECG monitoring should be specifically requested when ordering an EEG to differentiate seizure from syncope [5, 7, 9, 21].

Role of the ECG
Patients with arrhythmias and cerebral symptoms resulting from impaired cerebral perfusion are common in the neurologic practice [1, 4, 13, 22, 25, 32]. Sometimes a routine ECG will reveal the problem. In other cases a Holter monitor (or an ECG run during an EEG, see Fig. 10-1) will be needed to determine the diagnosis. Jonas et al. [19] employed Holter monitoring in a study of 358 cases of intermittent dizziness, blackout, or both. They found that cardiac arrhythmias could be correlated with cerebral symptoms in 8.9 percent of patients; short-duration predisposing arrhythmias occurred in 11.2 percent, and high-frequency ectopic beats were found in 24.6 percent. Reed et al. [30] concluded that focal neurologic signs were rare during arrhythmias, but symptoms of general cerebral ischemia were common in a study of 290 patients who required pacemakers for rhythm disturbances.

Table 10-2. Differential Diagnosis of Seizure Versus Syncope

Clinical Feature	Syncope	Seizure
Age of onset	Adult or child	Adult or child
Posture	Depends on initial condition or posture (erect)	Any posture
Muscle tone	Flaccid	Increased in tonic-clonic and some absence and complex partial seizures
Duration	10 seconds	3 min. (tonic-clonic); 1–3 min. (complex partial); 10 sec. (absence)
Sleep	Rarely occurs in sleep (but may if cardiac in origin)	May occur during sleep, upon awakening, or after sleep deprivation
Incontinence	Rarely	Often
Biting or injury	Not likely with hypotonia	May occur during tonic phase
Skin color	Pale	Flushed
Respirations	Slow unless syncope is due to hyper-ventilation	Apnea; stertorous
Perspiration	Cold, clammy	Hot, sweaty
EEG	Nonspecific slow	Specific paroxysms
ECG	May show arrhythmia, PVC, asystole, or other abnormality	Usually normal

Special Polygraphic Studies

Special physiologic recordings made concomitantly with routine EEGs may provide objective evidence of several causes of syncope. Concurrent recording of the ECG with a pneumogram and the EEG will show evidence of reflex syncope. Pressure on the eyeballs during polygraph recording provides highly valuable evidence of reflex syncope in children, adolescents, and young adults [24]; a period of asystole of 3 seconds or longer is considered a positive result in this ocular compression test. Carotid sinus massage provokes cardiac arrest and the clinical manifestations of a syncopal episode in some patients with reflex syncope, although the procedure does involve risks. Performing the Valsalva maneuver during an EEG recording may produce clinical and EEG evidence of syncope in patients with syncope due to reduced venous return to the heart. Bradycardia in patients with Stokes-Adams attacks may simulate seizures [18].

When routine EEG and ECG studies fail to provide definitive evidence of the cause of episodic alterations of consciousness, long-term combined EEG and ECG recordings may yield such information in a significant percentage of cases (see Chap. 11).

Meniere's Disease

The differential diagnosis of complex partial epilepsy and Meniere's disease may be difficult when the symptoms of the seizure include vertigo and tinnitus.

Abnormal EEGs have been found in 25 percent of patients with Meniere's disease [3], complicating the differential diagnosis. The chief EEG abnormality found in patients with Meniere's disease is an episodic appearance of slow waves in one or both temporal or frontotemporal regions. It is not diagnostic of the paroxysmal type of disturbance that would be found in epilepsy. Specifically, there are no sharp waves. In otherwise normal adults with recurrent episodes of vertigo and tinnitus with hearing loss the presence of an "abnormal EEG" should not lead the clinician away from a diagnosis of primary Meniere's disease. Complex partial epilepsy with vertiginous symptomatology should be considered when there are other symptoms of complex partial seizures (such as altered consciousness or automatisms) or abnormal sharp activity in the temporal area on the EEG.

Abdominal Epilepsy

Most persons with episodic abdominal pain do not have abdominal epilepsy, but the diagnosis must be kept in mind if other possible causes for the pain have been excluded. Abdominal epilepsy is a nonconvulsive seizure disorder occurring principally in children [8, 12, 15, 27]. The pain of abdominal epilepsy is often colicky, severe, and periumbilical in location. The pain seldom lasts longer than 15 minutes but recurs at unpredictable intervals and may inter-

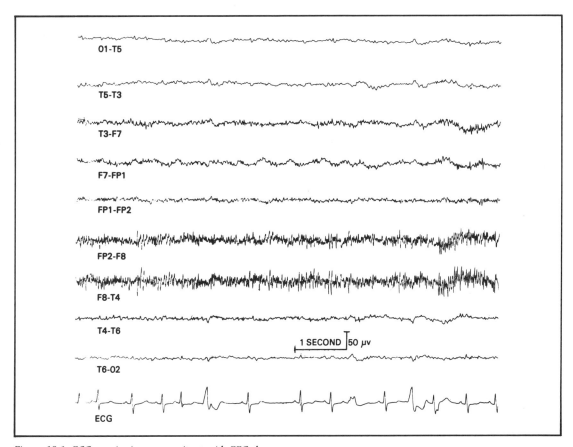

Figure 10-1. ECG monitoring concomitant with EEG shows multifocal ventricular premature contractions during an episode of light-headedness in a patient who had unexplained alterations of consciousness and a normal routine ECG. (From T. R. Browne. Clini-Pearls *3[6]:3, 1980.)*

rupt the child's play. Attacks may be accompanied by other autonomic phenomena (borborygmi, vomiting, emission of gas and feces, paroxysmal sweating, salivation) and by other signs and symptoms typical of seizures (altered consciousness, automatisms, etc.). Cyclic vomiting, singultus, and periodic autonomic dysfunction with or without abdominal pain may also be seizure phenomena. Attacks of abdominal epilepsy, like other forms of seizures, often occur in the morning and may be mistaken for manipulative attempts to avoid school.

EEG changes recorded during abdominal seizures have been bilateral, symmetrical, and synchronous [12]. The specific patterns recorded have included spike and wave, polyspike and wave, simple flattening, low-voltage fast patterns, and 10-Hz fast waves [12].

The diagnosis of abdominal epilepsy is based on the following considerations: (1) ruling out of intra-abdominal causes of recurrent abdominal pain, (2) other symptoms and signs of epilepsy occurring in association with episodes of abdominal pain (altered consciousness, automatisms, etc.), (3) abnormal interictal EEG (usually present), (4) evidence of neurologic abnormality on physical examination or CT scan (sometimes present). Abdominal epilepsy usually responds to antiepileptic medication.

Motivationally Determined Episodic Behavior (Pseudoseizures, Malingering and Hysterical Seizures)

It is sometimes necessary to differentiate motivationally determined episodic behavior (MDEB) or pseudoseizures from seizures (Table 10-3) [26]. The motivation for such behavior may be conscious and purposeful (malingering), or it may be subconscious, the result of failed ego-coping mechanisms (hysteria). Seizures usually occur in an emotionally neutral setting, while MDEB occurs in an emotionally charged setting. However, emotional stress may also exacerbate true seizure disorders (see Chaps. 12 and 24).

Table 10-3. Epilepsy Versus Motivationally Determined Episodic Behavior (MDEB)

Epilepsy	MDEB
Neutral setting	Emotionally charged setting
Stereotyped, with minor variations among attacks	Sometimes rigidly stereotyped; sometimes variable and affected by environment
Abrupt onset and end of attack	Gradual build-up and prolonged resolution
Tongue biting, incontinence, postictal confusion often present	Tongue biting, incontinence, postictal confusion may be present
Self-injury common	Self-injury rare
Family history of more typical epileptic phenomena	May have epilepsy in family
Fragmentary recall or no recall of event	Indifference, apparent amnesia for event; disparity between subjective state of consciousness and objective criteria
Desire to know about attack, to replace lost time (ego-alien)	Denial of details and unwillingness to consider motivational determinants
Secondary gain usually lacking	Secondary gains often identifiable
Abnormal interictal EEG (most)	Normal interictal EEG (63–73%)

Sources: R. J. Cohen and C. Suter [6]; T. A. Gulick et al. [17]; D. W. King et al. [20]; and R. R. Monroe [26].

Seizures are typically stereotyped but with minor variations among attacks. MDEB attacks may be rigidly stereotyped or variable and affected by the environment [6, 17, 26]. The onset and cessation of the attack tend to be more abrupt in seizures than in MDEB [26]. The type of phenomena most often observed during review of videotaped MDEB attacks are motor activity, decreased responsiveness to verbal stimuli, alimentary phenomena, subjective phenomena, semi-purposeful movements resembling seizure automatisms, and nonverbal vocalization [17]. Individual phenomena often simulate epileptic activity, but rarely does the complete episode closely resemble an epileptic seizure [17]. Tongue biting, incontinence, and postictal confusion are more typical of seizures, but may occur during MDEB [6, 26].

With MDEB the patient may not appear to recall the onset of the attack, but he does not seem to mind this. The affect is one of indifference. With complex partial seizures, there is fragmentary or no recall of the event after a seizure, but the patient often desires to know about the attack to replace the lost time. Denial of the details and unwillingness to consider motivational determinants are often good clues to the secondary gains of MDEB. Sometimes the secondary gains are identifiable, but at other times they are not. With epilepsy, however, a secondary gain usually is lacking [26]. Usually there is a cause that excites emotional disturbance during MDEB. This may be obvious or repressed. The type of unresolved emotional conflict may be identifiable on closer investigation [10].

Some additional points are of value in differentiating MDEB from specific seizure types [17, 26]. There is often some degree of warning with complex partial seizures, although an attack in a patient with MDEB may begin with palpitations, malaise, and some difficulties in swallowing. There may be a quasi-volitional vocalization during MDEB, whereas during a complex partial seizure vocalizations are usually stereotyped and repetitive.

Tonic-clonic seizures follow the pattern described in Chapter 6. In MDEB there is a struggling activity involving throwing of the limbs and head, fighting, and kicking, with semipurposeful activity and some degree of interaction with the environment. (This must also be differentiated from the automatic or postictal behavior of complex partial seizures; see Chap. 5). MDEB very rarely occurs during sleep, while tonic-clonic seizures may.

The interictal EEG is abnormal in most patients with epilepsy (see Chap. 11) and is normal in most patients with MDEB. However, 27 percent to 37 percent of patients with MDEB have some abnormality on their interictal EEG, and 12 percent to 37 percent have paroxysmal activity on their interictal EEG [6, 20]. The ictal EEG is invariably normal during MDEB and usually (but not always) abnormal during complex partial seizures (see Chap. 5).

It is not uncommon for patients with MDEB to also have "true" seizures [6, 20]. This phenomenon partially explains the high incidence of paroxysmal EEG abnormalities in patients with MDEB and creates differential diagnostic problems. Persons with both MDEB and seizures often describe two types of events [6]. Cohen and Suter [6] have described a provocative test for MDEB using saline injections and suggestion. While this test is useful, one must be aware that provocation of MDEB by this test does not exclude the possibility of coexisting "true" seizures. When a definitive diagnosis of seizure, MDEB, or both cannot be made on the basis of history and routine EEG, the issue can often be resolved by prolonged EEG recording [20, 29] (see Chap. 11).

Finally, persons thought to have intractable "true" seizures on clinical grounds will sometimes turn out to have MDEB exclusively when subjected to intensive monitoring [20, 29] (see Chap. 31). This possibility must be excluded before submitting a patient to large doses of conventional drugs, experimental drugs, or surgery.

References

1. Abdon, N. J., and Malmcrona, R. High pacemaker implantation rate following "cardiogenic neurology." *Acta Med. Scand.* 198:445, 1975.

2. Adams, R. D., and Brunwald, E. Faintness, Syncope and Episodic Weakness. In K. J. Isselbacher et al. (Eds.), *Harrison's Principles of Internal Medicine* (9th ed.). New York: McGraw-Hill, 1980.

3. Barac, B., Hagbarth, E. E., and Stable, J. EEG in Meniere's disease. A study of EEG and caloric directional preponderance before and after ultrasonic irradiation of the labyrinth. *Acta Otolaryngol.* 62:333, 1966.

4. Braham, J. et al. Reflex cardiac arrest presenting as epilepsy. *Ann. Neurol.* 10:277, 1981.

5. Browne, T. R. Seizure vs. syncope. *Clini-Pearls* 3(6):3, 1980.

6. Cohen, R. J., and Suter, C. Hysterical seizures: Suggestion as a provocative EEG test. *Ann. Neurol.* 11:391, 1982.

7. Daly, D. D. Use of the EEG for Diagnosis and Evaluation of Nonepileptic Episodic Disorders. In D. W. Klass, and D. D. Daly (Eds.), *Current Practice of Clinical Electroencephalography.* New York: Raven Press, 1979.

8. Douglas, E. F., and White, P. T. Abdominal epilepsy: A reappraisal. *J. Pediatr.* 78:59, 1971.

9. Espinosa, R. E., Klass, D. W., and Maloney, J. D. Contribution of the electroencephalogram in monitoring cardiac dysrhythmias. *Mayo Clin. Proc.* 53:119, 1978.

10. Feldman, R. G., and Paul, N. L. Identity of emo-

tional triggers in epilepsy. *J. Nerv. Ment. Dis.* 162:345, 1976.

11. Gastaut, H. Syncopes: Generalized Anoxic Cerebral Seizures. In P. J. Vinken, and G. W. Bruyn (Eds.), *Handbook of Clinical Neurology,* Vol. 15, *The Epilepsies.* Amsterdam: Elsevier, 1974.

12. Gastaut, H. et al. Generalized Nonconvulsive Seizures without Local Onset. In P. J. Vinken, and G. W. Bruyn (Eds.). *Handbook of Clinical Neurology,* Vol. 15, *The Epilepsies.* Amsterdam: Elsevier, 1974.

13. Goldberg, A. D., Raftery, E. B., and Cashman, P. M. Ambulatory electrocardiographic records in patients with transient cerebral attacks or palpitations. *Br. Med. J.* 4:569, 1975.

14. Goldensohn, E. S. Paroxysmal and other features of the electroencephalogram in migraine. *Res. Clin. Stud. Headache* 4:118, 1976.

15. Gowers, W. R. *Epilepsy and Other Chronic Convulsive Diseases.* New York: Wm. Wood, 1881.

16. Gowers, W. R. *The Borderland of Epilepsy.* Philadelphia: P. Blakiston, 1907.

17. Gulick, T. A., Spinks, I. P., and King, D. W. Pseudoseizures: Ictal phenomena. *Neurology* (N.Y.) 32:24, 1982.

18. Haslam, R. H., and Jameson, J. D. Cardiac standstill simulating repeated epileptic attacks. *J.A.M.A.* 224:887, 1973.

19. Jonas, S., Klein, I., and Dimant, J. Importance of Holter monitoring in patients with periodic cerebral symptoms. *Ann. Neurol.* 1:470, 1977.

20. King, D. W., Gallagher, B. B., Murvin, A. J. et al. Pseudoseizures: Diagnostic evaluation. *Neurology* (N.Y.) 32:18, 1982.

21. Klass, D. W., and Reiher, J. Extracerebral uses for electroencephalography. *Med. Clin. North Am.* 52:941, 1968.

22. Laxon, L. M. et al. Controlled study of 24 hour ambulatory electrocardiographic monitoring in patients with transient neurological symptoms. *Neurol. Neurosurg. Psychiatr.* 43:37, 1980.

23. Lennox, W. G., and Lennox, M. *Epilepsy and Related Disorders.* Boston: Little, Brown, 1960.

24. Lombroso, C. T., and Lerman, P. Breathholding spells (cyanotic and pallid infantile syncope). *Pediatrics* 39:563, 1967.

25. McAllen, P. M., and Marshall, J. Cardiac dysrhythmia and transient cerebral ischemic attacks. *Lancet* 1:1212, 1973.

26. Monroe, R. R. *Episodic Behavioral Disorders.* Cambridge, Mass.: Harvard University Press, 1970.

27. Papatheophilou, R., Jeavons, P. M., and Disney, M. E. Recurrent abdominal pain: A clinical and electroencephalographic study. *Develop. Child Med.* 14:31, 1972.

28. Pearce, J. *Migraine: Clinical Features, Mechanisms and Management.* Springfield, Ill.: Thomas, 1969.

29. Porter, R. J., Penry, J. K., and Lacy, J. R. Diagnostic and therapeutic reevaluation of patients with intractible epilepsy. *Neurology* (N.Y.) 27:1006, 1977.

30. Reed, R. L., Siekert, R. V., and Meridith, J. Rarity of transient focal cerebral ischemia in cardiac dysrhythmia. *J.A.M.A.* 223:893, 1973.

31. Townsend, H. R. A. *Background to Migraine.* New York: Springer, 1967.

32. Walter, R. F., Reid, S. D., and Wenger, N. K. Transient cerebral ischemia due to arrhythmia. *Ann. Intern. Med.* 72:471, 1970.

33. Westmoreland, B. F. EEG in Evaluation of Headache. In D. W. Klass, and D. D. Daly (Eds.), *Current Practice of Clinical Electroencephalography.* New York: Raven Press, 1979.

ELECTROENCEPHALOGRAPHY IN THE MANAGEMENT OF EPILEPSY

11

Terrence L. Riley

After early descriptions in the 1930s of characteristic EEG patterns in epilepsy, the EEG quickly became a pivotal tool in the diagnosis and research of the disorder. Because the clinician rarely has the opportunity to observe the patient during a seizure, the EEG can dramatically improve the clinician's diagnostic capability by revealing epileptiform discharges in the interictal period. Electroencephalography alone cannot *establish* a diagnosis of epilepsy, but it may clarify the diagnosis and provide critical information about the anatomic localization or associated metabolic disturbances. With the burgeoning development of neurodiagnostic technology, other instruments such as computerized tomographic (CT) scanners have surpassed the EEG for the evaluation of *structural* disease. However, electroencephalography has continued to grow as a discipline, primarily because of its value in the study of disorders of cerebral *function,* especially epilepsy.

The incidence of truly epileptiform patterns among nonepileptic persons is very low, although many normal EEG patterns often appear epileptiform to inexperienced electroencephalographers or to those who disregard controlled studies. Failing to recognize a benign but "epileptiform appearing" normal variant is a particularly costly error when coupled with an error in clinical interpretation of a nonepileptic spell.

There are currently no enforceable standards of training or practice in electroencephalography, so that techniques and proficiency vary widely among laboratories. The merit of electroencephalography in diagnosis depends on well-trained technologists and interpreters, as well as on the ability of referring physicians to weigh results wisely with clinical observation.

Sensitivity and Specificity of EEG in Patients With Epilepsy

TRUE POSITIVE EEGs

More than 90 percent of patients with epilepsy eventually have abnormal EEG recordings when multiple recordings, noninvasive activation techniques, and sleep recordings are used [2]. The yield of diagnostic abnormalities depends in part on the frequency of the patient's seizures. The child with frequent absence seizures is likely to have spike-wave paroxysms in a routine 30-minute recording, but the person whose tonic-clonic seizures occur only at yearly intervals is less likely to produce an epileptiform discharge. Although the sensitivity of EEG is usually considered higher in the primarily generalized epilepsies, it is also good in many focal epilepsies. More than 90 percent of patients with complex partial seizures have abnormal EEGs when activation procedures and basilar electrodes are used [19, 36].

TRUE NEGATIVE AND FALSE NEGATIVE EEGS

Although 90 percent of patients with epilepsy will have abnormal EEGs if activation procedures are employed, 10 percent of patients with epilepsy will have normal EEGs. These "false negative" EEGs are presumably due to the intermittency of ictal and interictal paroxymal activity in some patients with epilepsy. The frequency of false negative EEGs can be further reduced by prolonged recording techniques (see below). However, the diagnosis of epilepsy can never be excluded on the basis of multiple normal EEGs. The decision must ultimately be made on clinical grounds.

FALSE POSITIVE EEGS

Gastaut and Tassinari [17] reported that only 0.4 percent of the nonepileptic normal population have truly epileptiform bursts in EEG recordings. In another study of 6,497 unselected nonepileptic patients (many with other neurologic diseases), 1.7 percent had epileptiform patterns, including several patients who later had seizures [82].

Lerman and Kivity-Ephraim [41] have stressed that spiking in the central, midtemporal, or (less commonly) occipital area is not uncommon in normal children without epilepsy. Such spikes are usually benign and disappear in the teenage years. Epilepsy should not be diagnosed in patients with such spikes unless there is unequivocal clinical evidence of a seizure disorder.

In early EEG studies and in some clinical practices two types of errors are responsible for most false positive EEGs: (1) misinterpretation of normal EEG patterns as epileptiform discharges, and (2) incidental or irrelevant EEG abnormalities erroneously considered epileptiform. Neither of these types of error should appropriately be called false positive.

EEG IN THE PATIENT WITH A SINGLE SEIZURE
(FIRST SEIZURE)

When presented with a patient who has had a recent single (or "first") seizure, the physician must first exclude a treatable underlying disease. He must then decide whether the patient needs treatment to prevent further seizures. An EEG may be helpful both in diagnosing associated neurologic disease and in deciding about treatment. Approximately one half of adult patients who have had a suspected single seizure but have no other diseases may be susceptible to more seizures if not treated [26, 32]. Johnson et al. [32] followed a group of adults with first seizures who were not given medication. There was a 96 percent recurrence rate when (1) paroxysmal abnormalities appeared on EEG, (2) a physician was convinced that the spell was a seizure, and (3) postictal confusion was present. Recurrences usually occurred within 6 months. In this series, the two best predicters of recurrent seizures were the EEG and a physician's independent conclusion that the initial spell was truly epileptic. Hauser et al. [26] reported the following recurrence rates at 24 months after a first unprovoked seizure and the following EEG findings at initial examination: normal, 14 percent; focal abnormality, 19 percent; generalized spike and wave, 50 percent.

Epileptiform EEG Patterns

Because there are many high-voltage or sharp-contour wave forms in EEG recordings, it has been a continuing challenge to clinicians and physiologists to decide which wave forms constitute reliable evidence of epileptic neuronal activity. Purists justifiably insist that clinical phenomena such as seizures and diagnostic labels such as epilepsy must not be confused with electrophysiologic properties on EEG paper. Daly [9] and others reluctantly accept the use of the term *epileptiform* if it is limited to wave-form patterns that occur only among persons susceptible to recurrent seizures. He disapproves of the term *seizure discharge*, however, because "no electrical event is pathognomonic of epilepsy." Since a seizure is a clinical event it is inaccurate and misleading to apply a clinical term to an EEG pattern.

SPIKES AND SHARP WAVES

Spikes are isolated waves less than 70 msec in duration, and unofficial concensus requires that they have a "paroxysmal" appearance—i.e., abrupt eruption from the background and high voltage (usually more than 100 microvolts [μv]). Sharp waves are isolated waves with a triangular form and a duration of more than 70 msec and less than 200 msec. True epileptic spikes or sharp waves often have a rapidly rising phase followed by a less rapidly declining phase after the potential has reached its peak. A vertical line drawn through the peak would show that the spike or sharp wave is asymmetrical. A rate of voltage increase of at least 2 μv/msec is an important distinguishing feature of reliably pathologic cerebral spikes [38]. Epileptiform spikes or sharp waves are very often polyphasic but usually have a peak (or average) negative polarity at cortical and scalp surfaces. The duration of these waves is at least as brief, but usually briefer, than the background activity from which they arise. Nonepileptic "sharp-looking" waves are distinguished by the following characteristics: (1) duration of single waves is the same as that of the background activity; (2) they are evident only because of their voltage; and (3) symmetry about a vertical line drawn through the peak.

3-Hz Spike-Wave (Typical Spike-Wave) Paroxysms
Typical spike-wave paroxysms consist of bilateral, symmetrical, rhythmic, high-voltage complexes of single spikes followed by single slow waves of similar amplitude. These complexes recur with a frequency of 2 to 4 Hz and are either fully generalized or maximum in voltage in the frontocentral area. The interictal EEG is usually normal, but typical spike-wave paroxysms can usually be precipitated by hyperventilation in untreated patients. Most fully generalized, typical spike-wave paroxysms produce a measurable impairment of performance ("absence"), and most absence seizures are accompanied by typical spike-wave paroxysms on the EEG. See Chap. 7 for details and references.

Slow Spike-Wave (Atypical Spike-Wave) Paroxysms
Atypical spike-wave paroxysms consist of irregular, often asymmetrical, high-voltage complexes of a varying number of spikes (none to three), followed by irregular slow waves that are often higher in voltage than the spikes. These complexes recur with a frequency of 1 to 2½ Hz. The interictal EEG is often abnormal (slow). Slow spike-wave complexes are seldom precipitated by hyperventilation. The relationship between atypical spike-wave paroxysms and clinical seizures is less clear-cut than that between typical spike-wave paroxysms and seizures. See Chap. 8 for details and references.

Other Patterns Indicative of Seizure Disorders
Only definite spikes, sharp waves, or spike-wave complexes are accepted as unequivocal evidence of epileptiform abnormalities by many authorities [22], but other patterns may also indicate seizure disorders. The slow-wave component of a spike-wave discharge is usually more widely distributed and less attenuated by the skull than the spike component. Because deep spike-and-wave discharges may emerge on the skull surface only as rhythmic slow waves [1], paroxysmal rhythmic slow waves may be important signs of an epileptic discharge, particularly when they are focal [5].

During an EEG recording brief seizures may occur that are not clinically recognized but produce ictal EEG patterns during an apparent interictal period. Such patterns include: (1) spike-wave discharges, (2) low-voltage rhythmic fast activity, (3) slow DC potential shifts, and (4) generalized flattening of the EEG pattern.

Following seizures, there is a period of slowing or disruption of normal rhythms ("postictal slowing") that may outlast clinical postictal symptoms. Focal postictal delta waves that resolve in 2 to 4 days may be accepted as strong evidence of epilepsy [35, 39]. Furthermore, asymmetry of the delta waves in the postictal state may be the only localizing abnormality in an EEG suggestive of a mass lesion. Although the value of postictal EEG is generally attributed to diffuse or focal delta waves, at least one study [4] demonstrated spike or sharp waves in postictal records of persons with previously normal records and increased numbers of sharp waves in persons with previously abnormal records.

Specific Interictal and Ictal EEG Patterns Seen in Specific Seizure Types
See Chapters 3–10.

Normal Variant Patterns
A number of normal variant patterns with an "epileptiform" appearance are often found in the EEGs of normal persons and have no value in diagnosing epilepsy. The physician must be aware of these patterns to avoid overinterpreting EEGs and EEG reports.

14- and 6-Hz Positive Spikes
Brief runs of rhythmic spikes may occur at 14 or 6 Hz. Unlike most pathologic spikes, which have a negative polarity, these spikes have a positive polarity when recorded from the scalp. Often a surface negative slow wave is interposed between the spikes, imparting a wicket pattern. Lombroso et al. [44] demonstrated that 58 percent of 212 normal adolescents had 14- and 6-Hz positive spikes during sleep. Noting that occurrence was directly dependent on the duration of sleep during the recording, they concluded that virtually all adolescents would show one or more clusters of the 14- and 6-Hz positive spikes if sleep recording were performed long enough.

6-Hz Spike-Wave ("Phantom Spike-Wave")
This pattern consists of rhythmic repetition of a small spike (seldom exceeding 60 μv) and a larger aftercoming slow wave, both with surface-negative polarity. Bilaterally synchronous and symmetrical with maxi-

mum voltage in the central and frontal regions, the spike is very brief (less than 30 msec), and bursts are characteristically brief, between 0.5 and 1 second. The pattern occurs predominantly during drowsiness and wakefulness [39, 46, 77]. Neither Zivin and Ajmone-Marsan [82] nor Tharp [76] noted the occurrence of seizures in any patient with this pattern. In a survey at the Mayo Clinic the incidence of seizures among persons with 6-Hz spike-wave was no different from that of the general population [77].

Small Sharp Spikes (SSS) or Benign Epileptiform Transients of Sleep (BETS)
The SSS pattern consists of shifting spikes recorded during drowsiness and sleep, especially during the first nocturnal epoch of light sleep. The pattern occurs in up to 20 percent of normal persons in the first light sleep phase of the night [64, 80]. Since the voltage may exceed 100 μv and the duration of the spikes may be up to 90 msec, White et al. [80] argue that these spikes may be neither small nor sharp, and they prefer the term *benign epileptiform transients of sleep* (BETS). This term, however, is misleading in that "epileptiform" is used to describe an EEG pattern that is not reliably associated with epilepsy. Certain features characterize normal and sporadic SSS and serve to distinguish them from pathologic spikes. These features are (1) a remarkably consistent wave form throughout the recording, (2) an occurrence that is always sporadic (rather than the clusters or runs characterizing most epileptiform sharp transients), (3) a low amplitude of 5 to 135 μv (most commonly 25 to 90 μv), (4) a spike duration of 35 to 90 msec (mean, 65 msec), (5) frequently, an aftergoing slow wave 200 to 400 msec in duration, (6) a shifting focus, and (7) a very wide field of distribution and origin (invariably distributed over more than one area of the scalp and eventually bilateral, although seldom bilaterally synchronous). These features contrast with those of sleep-induced epileptic discharges that (1) are often interspersed with other sharp transients (such as theta waves), (2) often occur in clusters or runs, and (3) have varying voltages at different times in the record. SSS and interictal spikes in patients with complex partial seizures tend to occur in the anterior temporal and medial temporal areas; the EEG interpreter must look at spikes in these regions with great care.

Psychomotor Variant
This pattern consists of rhythmic, notched 4- to 7-Hz theta waves with broad temporal lobe distribution. Because of its resemblance to higher voltage patterns often associated with complex partial seizures, the pattern was termed *psychomotor variant*. In several large series the incidence of this pattern in normal subjects (1 to 2%) was at least as high as that among patients with epilepsy [48].

Hypnagogic Slowing in Children
A source of frequent errors is the rhythmic, very high voltage, 2- to 4-Hz generalized slowing that normally occurs in drowsiness and immediately after awakening in children under 6 years. The clusters of "hypersynchronous" slow waves may arise abruptly and continue for several minutes.

Activation Procedures
Because the routine EEG is limited by a relatively short sampling interval for the detection of sporadic, paroxysmal events, several easily performed procedures are helpful in provoking abnormalities in patients whose EEGs at rest fail to disclose abnormalities. Hyperventilation (HV) and photic stimulation are so harmless, easily performed, and effective that they are essential parts of any routine EEG. Sleep, sleep deprivation, and medications are useful activating procedures in certain situations.

HYPERVENTILATION (HV)

Pathophysiology of Hyperventilation
HV produces lowered arterial CO_2, leading to cerebral vasoconstriction, which in turn leads to diminished cerebral oxygenation (see Chap. 12). Decreased cerebral oxygenation appears to be the key factor in producing the EEG changes seen with HV. Breathing oxygen-poor air or pure nitrogen will produce EEG patterns that are identical to those produced by HV [16].

Normal Response to Hyperventilation
There is great variability in the frequency, scalp topography, and wave-form "morphology" induced by HV. The response usually takes the form of rhythmic slow waves that may continue in sequence for 2 to 3 minutes after HV ceases. In adults the slow waves usually have maximum voltage in the frontocentral regions, but they may be found predominantly in the occipital region in young children. In some individuals the background activity may be unaltered except for intermittent or even paroxysmal clusters of generalized slow waves, which are frequently misinterpreted as seizure discharges. Voltages exceeding 200 μv are not uncommon. When normal high-

voltage waves have a duration shorter than 200 msec, they produce a sharpened contour and hence resemble sharp waves. Frequently, a partially biphasic or notched shape in rhythmic slow waves induced by HV may suggest a spike-wave pattern, particularly when such a pattern recurs at 3-Hz intervals. The notched slow waves of HV, however, are seen so commonly among normal individuals that they are without diagnostic significance. Autonomic symptoms such as palpitations, sweating, and syncope in addition to subjective feelings of confusion and unreality often result from vigorous HV. When these symptoms and an exuberant EEG response of generalized slow and sharp waves occur simultaneously, the unwary interpreter may mistake them for a seizure.

In light of the striking range and variability of responses to HV, a response should be considered abnormal only if it is (1) clearly focal or lateralized, (2) accompanied by one of the patient's typical spells, or (3) accompanied by a classic spike-wave or spike paroxysm.

Activating Effect of Hyperventilation

Pupo and Zuckerman [61] reported that the incidence of all types of paroxysmal abnormalities in one group of 665 patients was increased from 29 percent in the resting records to 77 percent with HV. In another series of 313 patients with epilepsy a 34 percent increased yield of paroxysmal abnormalities was reported with HV, including 15 patients with normal resting records and 13 others who had paroxysmal abnormalities at rest but only focal discharges during HV [49].

In patients with untreated absence seizures, 3-Hz spike-wave discharges can almost always be precipitated by HV (see Chap. 7). Once antiabsence medication has begun, it may not be possible to precipitate 3-Hz spike-wave discharges with HV. In one series of EEG recordings made during complex partial seizures, HV was the activation procedure most frequently capable of inducing seizures as well as focal EEG paroxysms [37].

SENSORY STIMULATION

Certain forms of sensory stimulation may evoke paroxysmal activity on the EEG characteristic of primary generalized epilepsy. Sensory stimulation less commonly evokes focal discharges in patients with simple partial seizures and rarely evokes discharges in patients with complex partial seizures. The most common and most effective form of sensory stimulation is stroboscopic photic stimulation, a standard EEG recording procedure.

Photic Stimulation

The normal response to intermittent photic stimulation is an augmented or *driving response* in the occipital region, time-locked to the stimulus. At frequencies of between 1 and 12 Hz, there is most commonly a monophasic or biphasic single response of two or three occipital wave cycles per flash. At more rapid frequencies, occipital driving may continue or disappear, or there may even be a subharmonic response of one occipital wave for every two or three flickers. In some individuals, this time-locked driving response may spread to the central scalp region and attain voltages of nearly 100 μv. Particularly at flicker rates slower than 10 Hz, the time-locked response may evoke a spike-wave pattern. This pattern is completely normal, the spike component apparently representing an excitatory phase and the after-coming slower component a subsequent inhibitory phase of cortical response to repetitive thalamic volley [24]. When such a benign spike wave–like pattern spreads to the central scalp region, it can be distinguished from an abnormal pattern because it is time-locked with the stimulus and because it arises primarily from the occipital region.

Intermittent photic stimulation evokes involuntary myoclonic jerking in as many as 20 percent of normal individuals, affecting predominantly the facial and periorbital muscles and at times even the neck and shoulder muscles [9]. This *photomyoclonic response* is accompanied by spikelike myogenic potentials from frontopolar electrode positions, which are time-locked to the stimulus. Although they may resemble cerebral potentials, these characteristic motor units can be distinguished from brain activity by virtue of their brevity (usually less than 20 msec) and their frontal predominance.

The so-called *photoparoxysmal* or *photoconvulsive response* is characterized by a posteriorly predominant or generalized onset and by a pattern of interspersed spikes (or multiple spikes) and sharp or slow waves; most significantly, the repetition rate is *not* time-locked with the stimulus (it is usually slower). Reilly and Peters [65] compared the duration of photoparoxysmal responses to that of flicker stimulus. In patients in whom the generalized discharge ceased spontaneously as flicker continued or ceased immediately when flicker stopped, only 70 percent had a diagnosis of "convulsive disorder," whereas in those in whom the discharge outlasted flicker ("prolonged" response) 93 percent had convulsive disorders, and most showed generalized epileptiform disturbances at other points in their EEG record. Confining the analysis to patients under 30 years old, they found no higher incidence of epilepsy in patients with the self-limited pattern than among controls. In view of these observations, it seems important to note not only the occurrence of the generalized photoparoxysmal response but also its duration compared to the flicker pattern. In some laboratories the stroboscope is stopped immediately when a generalized spike-wave pattern is recognized to "avoid a seizure." This practice does not allow a distinction to be made between the prolonged and self-limited forms of photoparoxysmal responses.

Photic stimulation can provoke a generalized spike-wave discharge even during sleep in susceptible individuals [71]. For some patients, filtering the light source through red or green lenses may eliminate the photoconvulsive response, and clinical seizures in these patients may be averted by wearing appropriately colored sunglasses.

Photic stimulation is particularly helpful in patients with clonic or myoclonic seizures as well as for absence seizures characterized by a 3-Hz spike-wave pattern [51, 52]. Only 3 percent of patients with complex partial seizures have activation of focal epileptiform patterns by intermittent photic stimulation [22].

Other Sensory Stimuli
Visual, auditory, tactile, or somatosensory stimuli or reading may induce paroxysmal EEG abnormalities or clinical seizures in some patients (see Chaps. 12 and 24).

SLEEP AND SLEEP DEPRIVATION
In one review of 1,620 abnormal EEGs, 11.7 percent of the abnormalities were confined solely to the sleep portions of the record [74]. Sleep recording is particularly important in the diagnosis of temporal lobe abnormalities. In the Gibbs' [19] series, sleep was necessary for identification or accentuation of abnormalities in 73 percent of patients with complex partial seizures and anterior temporal spikes compared with only 0.8 percent of patients with abnormalities in the frontal region. Even fewer patients required sleep for demonstration of paroxysmal abnormalities originating from the parietal or occipital regions. In a series of patients from the Mayo Clinic with complex partial seizures, activation of unilateral temporal lobe abnormalities occurred during sleep in 68 percent and sleep-induced bilateral temporal lobe abnormalities were found in 17 percent [36].

The various stages of sleep affect different types of paroxysmal activity in different ways (see Chap. 12).

Although natural sleep is probably most informative, sleep induced by medications is almost as effective. Because short-acting barbiturates and benzo-diazepines induce prominent beta rhythm activity in the EEG that complicates interpretation, chloral hydrate in oral doses of 500 to 1000 mg is preferable.

Sleep deprivation as an activating technique is useful in more ways than the obvious effect of inducing sleep. In one retrospective study, 26 to 28 hours of sleep deprivation induced generalized epileptiform discharges or focal abnormalities in 34 percent of epileptic patients who had previously normal records and enhanced the abnormalities in 56 percent with known abnormal records [47]. A prospective study later demonstrated activation of EEGs in 41 percent of epileptic patients after 24 to 26 hours of sleep deprivation [60].

DRUGS
Drug activation is most useful for correlating the clinical features of the disease with focal discharges in candidates for surgery. Other techniques, such as telemetry and combined closed circuit television (CCTV) and EEG monitoring, have largely replaced drug activation for diagnosis of epilepsy in patients with normal routine EEGs. Pentylenetetrazol (Metrazol), methohexital (Brevital, Brietal), and thiopental (Pentothal) are the most widely used drugs in the United States. Bemegride (Megimide) is no longer available in the United States, and the phenothiazines are not reliable activating drugs [27].

Methohexital
Methohexital is a barbiturate that is capable of activating both spike-wave discharges in patients with known primarily generalized seizure disorders [81] and temporal lobe discharges in patients with known complex partial seizures [18, 50]. However, methohexital is probably no more effective than natural sleep when used to activate paroxysmal activity in patients with possible epilepsy and normal routine EEGs [8, 73]. Furthermore, there is wide variation among individuals in response to methohexital, and some individuals experience respiratory depression with the "low" dose used for EEG activation studies. Methohexital is not suitable for use as a routine activation procedure for patients with possible epilepsy because it is probably no more effective as an activating procedure than normal sleep and is more dangerous, time-consuming, and expensive.

Pentylenetetrazol
With its potential for lowering the seizure threshold in all humans, pentylenetetrazol has the ability to trigger a patient's characteristic focal seizure so that clinical and physiologic ictal phenomena can be correlated. A disadvantage of this drug is its production of marked

anxiety and general discomfort. More seriously, the drug may cause generalized seizures, apnea, and even death in nonepileptic individuals, and can induce a seizure in an epileptic patient by a different mechanism or focus than that responsible for the patient's usual seizures [22]. For these and other reasons, pentylenetetrazol is now seldom used as an activating drug.

Thiopental Test for Determining Primary Versus Secondary Bilateral Synchrony

Not all patients with bilaterally synchronous spike-wave abnormalities have primary generalized epilepsy. The patient with consistently asymmetrical or irregular spike-wave discharges or distinct focal features may have a focal epileptogenic lesion causing a secondarily generalized bilateral synchronous discharge [22, 23, 43]. This distinction has more than academic importance, because a focal lesion may respond to drugs such as carbamazepine or phenobarbital (or to surgical treatment), whereas a primarily generalized spike-wave discharge may be more appropriately treated with drugs such as ethosuximide or valproic acid. There are three different drug-activated EEG techniques for uncovering or clarifying the process of secondary bilateral synchrony—intravenous thiopental, intracarotid amobarbital, and intracarotid pentylenetetrazol. The intracarotid amobarbital and pentylenetetrazol tests are difficult technical procedures that are limited to a few highly specialized centers [21, 62].

The intravenous thiopental test is the easiest and safest of the three procedures for distinguishing primary versus secondary bilateral synchrony [43]. The test is only useful if there are frequent seizure discharges in the EEG. Small amounts (0.5 mg/kg body weight) of thiopental are injected intravenously while background EEG activity and paroxysmal discharges are observed. There are three classes of response. Type I, indicative of primarily generalized epilepsy, is characterized by prompt suppression of spike-wave discharges bilaterally without the appearance of focal discharges and by prompt appearance of bilateral symmetrical beta activity. Type II, indicative of secondarily generalized epilepsy, is characterized by transient disappearance of spike-wave discharges bilaterally with initial emergence of only focal discharges, or by suppression of beta activity in the area of the presumed primary focus. Type III, indicative of diffuse organic encephalopathy, consists of poor beta activation bilaterally and increased spike-wave activity with or without focal features.

Recent work indicates that primarily generalized spike-wave activity can be distinguished from secon-

darily generalized spike-wave activity without pharmacologic intervention by means of special recording techniques that measure the temporal relationships between arrival of spike-wave activity at homologous EEG channels over the two hemispheres [25]. Primarily generalized spike-wave activity has no significant interhemispheric time differences. Secondarily generalized spike-wave activity is frequently recorded earlier (average, 15 msec) from the side on which it originates.

MEASUREMENTS OF BETA ASYMMETRIES

Barbiturate and benzodiazepine compounds normally induce prominent fast (beta) activity in the fronto-temporal region, particularly in the area recorded by basilar (nasopharyngeal and sphenoidal) electrodes. Asymmetry of normally induced activity may signify a lesion on the side with diminished beta response [54]. Demonstration of such an asymmetry may be useful information for lateralizing the lesion in evaluating patients with seizures for temporal lobectomy.

Special Recording Techniques

NASOPHARYNGEAL AND SPHENOIDAL ELECTRODES

Medial and basal structures in the temporal lobe are often the sites of epileptic foci responsible for complex partial seizures. These sites are not accessible to scalp electrodes but may be recorded by electrodes fixed under the skull of the middle fossa. Nasopharyngeal (NP) electrodes with a silver or platinum electrode surface at the tip of an insulated semiflexible wire are inserted through the nose and positioned against the superior lateral pharyngeal wall, where they lie near the foramen ovale. NP electrodes are difficult to anchor and are vulnerable to many mechanical artifacts, including swallowing, respiration, eye movement, and carotid artery pulsation. Sphenoidal electrodes, consisting of either small-gauge needles or insulated wires, are inserted in a position under the foramen ovale in the sphenopalatine fossa, using either an anterior approach under the maxilla or a lateral approach above the mandible. Sphenoidal electrodes of silver-silver chloride wire inserted from the lateral approach are superior electrically to NP electrodes [2, 7, 29, 67, 68] and have the advantage of being less susceptible to movement artifacts. A patient's fear of needles, pain on insertion, the requirement for a physician for insertion, and occasional breakage of an electrode wire (leaving an irretrievable fragment) are the major drawbacks of sphenoidal electrodes [28]. NP electrodes are located approximately 2 to 2.5 cm more medially and anteriorly than sphenoidal electrodes, but standard placement of both types puts them near the foramen ovale, which affords exposure to the immediate vicinity of the uncinate area of the temporal lobe [22, 53, 67]. Placement of either type of basilar electrode can be guided by roentgenography, and sphenoidal electrodes can be directed at different angles to record from different positions along the inferior and medial portions of the temporal lobe. To record from the orbital surface of the frontal lobe, the same type of electrode used for nasopharyngeal recording may be bent so that the recording surface contacts the roof of the nasal cavity, that is, the floor of the frontal fossa.

Many reports suggest that basilar electrodes may detect critical paroxysmal abnormalities not detectable by scalp electrodes [10, 11, 12, 28, 66, 70], thus increasing the diagnostic yield of EEG, especially in patients with complex partial seizures. Another value of these electrodes is precise localization. In many patients with generalized or bitemporal epileptiform discharges, basilar electrodes can demonstrate a unilateral voltage maximum or origin, or, in the case of a discharge widely distributed over one temporal lobe, a medial or inferior origin. NP electrodes may clarify different phases of physiologic and ictal behavior in complex partial seizures, often yielding as much information as more invasive intracerebral electrodes [11, 12].

NASOETHMOIDAL ELECTRODES
Nasoethmoidal electrodes are inserted through the nose and record from the inferior-mesial surface of the frontal lobe. These special electrodes can detect both frontal lobe paroxysmal activity in patients with normal surface EEGs and independent frontal foci in patients with temporal lobe paroxysmal activity on surface EEGs [62]. This information can be especially helpful in localizing epileptic foci prior to cortical resection procedures.

TELEMETRY AND LONG-TERM RECORDING

Technique
The simplest and theoretically the most desirable manner of increasing the yield from EEG is by prolonging the recording time. Standard EEG equipment can be used for prolonged recording in properly set up recording rooms, although this is rather confining for the patient and expensive in terms of time needed by technicians and equipment. Two widely used methods of prolonged recording employ small EEG amplifiers worn by the patient [56, 58, 71, 72]. The EEG signal can then be recorded directly on electromagnetic tape by a recorder worn by the patient or transmitted by radio signal to a larger recorder (telemetry). Telemetry

is often used in conjunction with prolonged closed circuit television and videotape viewing of the patient.

Miniaturized EEG amplifiers combined with a small recorder utilizing ordinary magnetic tape cassettes can make a continuous EEG record of a mobile subject [42, 56, 63, 71, 72]. This technique allows the patient to perform a normal daily routine while recording cerebral activity, with no geographic restrictions to nearby receivers. It not only allows a long sampling interval but also makes it possible to record brain responses during normal fluctuations in activity, mood, and alertness, all of which may contribute significantly to the numbers of seizures.

The reliability and yield of long-term EEG recording can be increased by recording only those portions of the EEG with abnormal discharges [33]. This can be accomplished by combining prolonged telemetered EEG with quantitative EEG measurements utilizing computer-assisted techniques. Computerization may also eventually allow three-dimensional analysis of EEG signals for better localization.

Differential Diagnosis
of Epilepsy, Syncope, and Hysteria
Several groups have presented convincing evidence that long-term EEG recording can definitively differentiate among epilepsy, syncope, and hysteria in many patients with vague histories and normal or nonspecifically abnormal routine EEGs [6, 7, 14, 40, 56, 57, 63] (see also Chap. 10). The objective information provided on the recording can often resolve an otherwise very difficult differential diagnostic problem.

Differential Diagnosis
of Various Types of Epilepsy
The key to proper management of epilepsy is a proper seizure diagnosis (see Chap. 1). Intensive EEG monitoring of referral patients with "intractable epilepsy" will often reveal that the patient has a type of seizure other than the type diagnosed by the referring physician and that changing the patient's antiepileptic drug regimen to a more appropriate one for the patient's actual seizure type can result in long-term seizure control [57, 59, 75]. Referring physicians are often confused in differentiating between absence and complex partial seizures because both may involve alteration of consciousness and automatisms.

Seizure Management
Long-term EEG recording in patients with refractory (but properly diagnosed) seizure disorders can reveal factors that aggravate the disorder. Correction of these factors can greatly improve seizure control. Factors

that can be demonstrated with long-term monitoring include seizure exacerbation at times of lowest antiepileptic drug serum concentration and exacerbation of seizures by stress, drowsiness, or boredom [6, 30, 57, 59, 71, 75] (see Chap. 31). To correlate the EEG with the patient's activity or the occurrence of a clinical seizure, a digital clock that encodes the hour, minute, and second on the tape can be used to mark the time of recorded events and document the continuity of the recording. An event marker can be added to the recording apparatus so that the patient or observers can indicate on the recording the time of significant events.

Localization of Seizure Foci
Prior to Cortical Resection Procedures
Long-term EEG recording has become a major component of the work-up of patients being evaluated for temporal lobectomy and other cortical resection procedures [31] (see Chap. 25). Using scalp electrodes (sometimes in combination with nasopharyngeal, sphenoidal, or nasoethmoidal electrodes), it is often possible to identify the side(s) and location(s) of origin of a patient's seizures by recording the onset of several spontaneous clinical seizures.

Study of the Clinical Neurophysiology of Seizures
Simultaneous videotape recordings of the patient, his EEG, and other physiological parameters have vastly expanded our knowledge of the clinical and EEG manifestations of many types of seizures (see Chaps. 4-9). Indeed, knowledge gained in this way formed the basis for the changes in the International Classification of Epileptic Seizures in 1981 [13].

DEPTH EEG
See Chapter 25.

CORTICOGRAPHY
See Chapter 25.

Use of EEG to Direct Treatment
The value of the EEG in directing management of absence seizures is well established. There is good evidence that most absence seizures are accompanied by spike-wave paroxysms, that most typical spike-wave discharges produce an absence, and that control of spike-wave paroxysms on the EEG can be equated with clinical seizure control (see Chaps. 7 and 19).

The value of the EEG in guiding medication adjustments for other types of seizures is less certain. Rowan et al. [69, 70] demonstrated that suppression of EEG spikes on long recordings correlated with improved seizure control and increased blood con-

centrations of antiepileptic drugs. Medications were responsible for normal EEGs among many patients with epilepsy in the study of "electroclinical nonconcordance" by Tudor [79]; paroxysmal abnormalities emerged after medications were stopped. Ten of 55 patients in another study had epileptiform EEG findings only when medication was discontinued [45]. With some antiepileptic drugs there may be actual deterioration in the EEG as seizures are controlled, but this usually occurs in the form of slowing of the alpha rhythm or other background activity rather than accentuation of paroxysmal discharges.

The EEG can aid in making the decision of whether or not to discontinue antiepileptic medication. Two groups have investigated cohorts of children whose antiepileptic medication was discontinued after 4 years on medication without seizures [15, 78]. Seizures recurred in 30 to 57 percent of the children whose EEGs were abnormal at the time medication was stopped and in 12 to 19 percent of those whose EEGs were normal at the time medication was stopped.

References
1. Abraham, K., and Ajmone-Marsan, C. Patterns of cortical discharges and their relation to routine scalp electroencephalography. *Electroencephalogr. Clin. Neurophysiol.* 10:447, 1958.
2. Aird, R. B., and Woodbury, D. M. *The Management of Epilepsy.* Springfield, Ill.: Thomas, 1974.
3. Bancaud, J. et al. EEG et SEEG dans les tumeurs cerebrales et l'epilepsie. *Paris Edifor.* 1973.
4. Bauer, G. Personal communication, 1982.
5. Bickford, R. G. Activation Procedures and Special Electrodes. In D. W. Klass, and D. D. Daly (Eds.), *Current Practice of Clinical Electroencephalography.* New York: Raven Press, 1979.
6. Binnie, C. D. et al. Telemetric EEG and video monitoring in epilepsy. *Neurology* 31:298, 1981.
7. Callaghan, C. N., and McCarthy, N. Twenty four hour EEG monitoring in patients with normal routine EEG findings. *Acta Neurol. Scand.* [Suppl. 79] 62:49, 1980.
8. Celesia, G. G., and Paulsen, R. E. Electroencephalographic activation with sleep and methohexital. *Arch. Neurol.* 27:361, 1972.
9. Daly, D. D. Use of the EEG for Diagnosis and Evaluation of Epileptic Seizures and Nonepileptic Episodic Disorders. In D. W. Klass, and D. D. Daly (Eds.), *Current Practice of Clinical Electroencephalography.* New York: Raven Press, 1979.
10. DeJesus, P. V., and Masland, W. S. The role of nasopharyngeal electrodes in clinical electro-

encephalography. *Neurology* (Minneap.) 20:869, 1970.

11. Delgado-Escueta, A. V. Epileptogenic paroxysms: Modern approaches and clinical correlations. *Neurology* (Minneap.) 29:1014, 1979.

12. Delgado-Escueta, A. V. et al. Lapse of consciousness and automatisms in temporal lobe epilepsy: A videotape analysis. *Neurology* (Minneap.) 27:144, 1977.

13. Dreifuss, F. E. Proposal for revised clinical and electroencephalographic classification of epileptic seizures. *Epilepsia* 22:489, 1981.

14. Ebersole, J. S., and Spencer, S. S. The efficacy of 24-hour EEG monitoring in epilepsy diagnosis. *Epilepsia* 22:235, 1981.

15. Emerson, R. et al. Stopping medication in childhood epilepsy: Predictors of outcome. *N. Engl. J. Med.* 304:1125, 1981.

16. Gastaut, H. et al. L'activation hypoxique de l'EEG par inhalation d'azote. 1. Premiers resultats obtenus dans les epilepsies generalisies. *Rev. Neurol.* 100:501, 1959.

17. Gastaut, H., and Tassinari, C. A. Epilepsies. In A. Remand (Ed.), *Handbook of EEG and Clinical Neurophysiology*, Vol. 13, Part A. Amsterdam: Elsevier, 1975.

18. Ghazy, A., Lundervold, A., and Veger, T. Combined activation of EEG with Brevital and Metrazol. *Clin. Electroencephalogr.* 9:60, 1978.

19. Gibbs, F. A., and Gibbs, E. L. *Atlas of Electroencephalography*, Vol. 2, *Epilepsy* (2nd ed.). Reading, Mass.: Addison-Wesley, 1952.

20. Glazer, G. H. Limbic epilepsy in childhood. *J. Nerv. Ment. Dis.* 114:391, 1967.

21. Gloor, P. et al. Fractionized intracarotid Metrazol injection: A new diagnostic method in electroencephalography. *Electroencephalogr. Clin. Neurophysiol.* 17:322, 1964.

22. Gloor, P. Contributions of Electroencephalography and Electrocorticography to the Neurosurgical Treatment of Epilepsy. In D. D. Purpura, J. K. Penry, and R. D. Walter (Eds.), *Advances in Neurology*, Vol. 8. New York: Raven Press, 1975.

23. Gloor, P. Generalized epilepsy with spike-and-wave discharge: A reinterpretation of its electrographic and clinical manifestations. *Epilepsia* 20:571, 1979.

24. Goldensohn, E. S. Neurophysiologic Substrates of EEG Activity. In D. W. Klass, and D. D. Daly (Eds.), *Current Practice of Clinical Electroencephalography*. New York: Raven Press, 1979.

25. Gotman, J. Interhemispheric relationships during bilateral spike-and-wave activity. *Epilepsia* 22:453, 1981.

26. Hauser, W. A. et al. Seizure recurrence after a first unprovoked seizure. *N. Engl. J. Med.* 307:522, 1982.

27. Itil, T. M. Convulsive and Anticonvulsive Properties of Neuropsychopharmaca. In E. Niedermayer (Ed.), *Epilepsy*. Basel: Karger, 1970.

28. Ives, J. R., and Gloor, P. New sphenoidal electrode assembly to permit long-term monitoring of the patient's ictal or inter-ictal EEG. *Electroencephalogr. Clin. Neurophysiol.* 42:575, 1977.

29. Ives, J. R., and Gloor, P. Update: Chronic sphenoidal electrodes. *Electroencephalogr. Clin. Neurophysiol.* 44:789, 1978.

30. Ives, J. R., and Woods, J. F. Four-channel 24-hour cassette recorder or longer-term EEG monitoring of ambulatory patients. *Electroencephalogr. Clin. Neurophysiol.* 39:88, 1975.

31. Ives, J. R., and Woods, J. F. The results of 6000 h of continuous EEG recording on 100 patients suspected of having temporal lobe epilepsy. *Electroencephalogr. Clin. Neurophysiol.* 50:159 P, 1980.

32. Johnson, L. C. et al. Diagnostic factors in adult males following initial seizures: A three-year follow-up. *Arch. Neurol.* 27:193, 1972.

33. Kellaway, P., and Carrie, J. R. G. Relationship Between Quantitative EEG Measurements and Clinical State in Epileptic Patients. In J. K. Penry (Ed.), *Epilepsy, The Eighth International Symposium*. New York: Raven Press, 1975.

34. King, D. W., and Ajmone-Marsan, C. Clinical features and ictal patterns in epileptic patients with EEG temporal lobe foci. *Ann. Neurol.* 2:138, 1977.

35. Klass, D. W. The electroencephalogram in the evaluation of seizures: Current clinical applications. *Med. Clin. North Am.* 52:949, 1968.

36. Klass, D. W. Electroencephalographic Manifestations of Complex Partial Seizures. In J. K. Penry, and D. D. Daly (Eds.), *Advances in Neurology*, Vol. 11. New York: Raven Press, 1975.

37. Klass, D. W., Espinosa, R. E., and Fischer-Williams, M. Analysis of concurrent electroencephalography and clinical events occurring sequentially during partial seizures. *Electroencephalogr. Clin. Neurophysiol.* 34:728, 1973.

38. Kooi, K. A. Voltage-time characteristics of spikes and other rapid EEG transients: Semantic and morphological considerations. *Neurology* (Minneap.) 16:59, 1966.

39. Kooi, K. A., Tucker, R. P., and Marshall, R. E. *Fundamentals of Electroencephalography* (2nd ed.). Hagerstown, Md.: Harper & Row, 1978.

40. Lai, C. W., and Ziegler, D. K. Syncope problem solved by continuous ambulatory simultaneous

EEG/ECG recording. *Neurology* (N.Y.) 31:1152, 1981.

41. Lerman, P., and Kivity-Ephraim, S. Focal epileptic EEG discharges in children not suffering from clinical epilepsy: Etiology, clinical significance, and management. *Epilepsia* 22:551, 1981.

42. Leroy, R. F., and Ebersole, J. S. Three-channel montages for ambulatory EEG monitoring: Are they adequate? *Epilepsia* 22:240, 1981.

43. Lombroso, C. T., and Erba, G. Primary and secondary bilateral synchrony in epilepsy: A clinical and electroencephalographic study. *Arch. Neurol.* 22:321, 1970.

44. Lombroso, C. T. et al. Ctenoids in healthy youths: Controlled study of 14- and 6- per second positive spiking. *Neurology* (Minneap.) 16:1152, 1966.

45. Ludwig, B. E., and Ajmone-Marsan, C. EEG changes after withdrawal of medication in epileptic patients. *Electroencephalogr. Clin. Neurophysiol.* 30:173, 1975.

46. Marshall, C. Some clinical correlates of the wave and spike phantom. *Electroencephalogr. Clin. Neurophysiol.* 7:633, 1955.

47. Mattson, R. H., Pratt, K. L., and Calverley, J. R. Electroencephalograms of epileptics following sleep deprivation. *Arch. Neurol.* 13:310, 1965.

48. Maulsby, R. L. Patterns of Uncertain Significance. In D. W. Klass, and D. D. Daly (Eds.), *Current Practice of Clinical Electroencephalography.* New York: Raven Press, 1979.

49. Morgan, M. H., and Scott, D. F. EEG activation in epileptics other than petit mal. *Epilepsia* 11:255, 1970.

50. Musella, L., Wilder, B. J., and Schmidt, R. P. Electroencephalographic activation with intravenous methohexital in psychomotor epilepsy. *Neurology* (Minneap.) 21:594, 1971.

51. Newmark, M. E., and Penry, J. K. *Photosensitivity and Epilepsy: A Review.* New York: Raven Press, 1979.

52. Niedermeyer, E. *The Generalized Epilepsies.* Springfield, Ill.: Thomas, 1972.

53. Niedermeyer, E., and Walker, A. E. Mesiofrontal epilepsy. *Electroencephalogr. Clin. Neurophysiol.* 31:104, 1971.

54. Niedermeyer, E., Yarworth, S., and Zobniw, A. M. Absence of drug-induced beta activity in electroencephalogram; a sign of severe cerebral impairment. *Eur. Neurol.* 15:77, 1977.

55. Penry, J. K., Porter, R. J., and Dreifuss, F. E. Simultaneous recording of absence seizures with videotape and EEG. *Brain* 98:427, 1975.

56. Porter, R. J. Methodology of Continuous Monitoring With Videotape Recording and Electro-

encephalography. In J. A. Wada, and J. K. Penry (Eds.), *Advances in Epileptology: The Tenth Epilepsy International Symposium.* New York: Raven Press, 1980.

57. Porter, R. J., Penry, J. K., and Lacy, J. R. Diagnostic and therapeutic reevaluation of patients with intractable epilepsy. *Neurology* (Minneap.) 27:1006, 1977.

58. Porter, R. J., Penry, J. K., and Wolf, A. A. Simultaneous Documentation of Clinical and Electroencephalographic Manifestation of Epileptic Seizures. In D. Kellaway, and I. Petersen (Eds.), *Quantitative Analytic Studies in Epilepsy.* New York: Raven Press, 1976.

59. Porter, R. J., Theodore, W. H., and Schulman, E. A. Intensive monitoring of intractable epilepsy: A two year follow up. *Acta Neurol. Scand.* [Suppl. 79]: 62:48, 1980.

60. Pratt, K. L. et al. EEG activation of epileptics following sleep deprivation: A prospective study of 114 cases. *Electroencephalogr. Clin. Neurophysiol.* 24:11, 1968.

61. Pupo, P. P., and Zuckerman, E. Some comparative results of activation methods in electroencephalography. *Electroencephalogr. Clin. Neurophysiol.* 8:154, 1956.

62. Quesney, L. F., Gloor, P., and Andersen, F. Role of nasoethmoidal electrodes in the preoperative localization of seizure activity involving the frontotemporal convexity. *Epilepsia* 22:243, 1981.

63. Ramsey, R. E., and Herskowitz, A. Twenty-four hour ambulatory EEG: A clinical appraisal. *Electroencephalogr. Clin. Neurophysiol.* 51:20P, 1981.

64. Reiher, J., and Klass, D. W. Two common EEG patterns of doubtful clinical significance. *Med. Clin. North Am.* 52:934, 1968.

65. Reilly, E. L., and Peters, J. F. Relationship of some varieties of electroencephalographic photosensitivity to clinical convulsive disorders. *Neurology* (Minneap.) 23:1050, 1973.

66. Remick, R. A., and Wada, J. A. Complex partial and pseudoseizure disorders. *Am. J. Psychiatry* 136:320, 1979.

67. Rovit, R. L., and Gloor, P. Temporal lobe epilepsy: A study using multiple basal electrodes: I. Description of method: II. Clinical EEG findings. *Neurochirurgia* 3:5, 1960.

68. Rovit, R. L., Gloor, P., and Rasmussen, T. Sphenoidal electrodes in the electrographic study of patients with temporal lobe epilepsy: An evaluation. *J. Neurosurg.* 18:151, 1961.

69. Rowan, A. J., and Protass, L. M. Transient global amnesia: Clinical and electroencephalographic

findings in 10 cases. *Neurology* (Minneap.) 29: 869, 1979.

70. Rowan, A. J. et al. Sodium valproate: Serial monitoring of EEG and serum levels. *Neurology* (Minneap.) 29:1450, 1979.

71. Sato, S., Dreifuss, F. E., and Penry, J. K. The effect of sleep on spike-wave discharges in absence seizures. *Neurology* (Minneap.) 23:1335, 1973.

72. Sato, S. et al. Valproic acid versus ethosuximide in the treatment of absence seizures. *Neurology* (N.Y.) 32:157, 1982.

73. Sherwin, I., and Hooge, J. P. Comparative effectiveness of natural sleep and methohexital: Provocative tests in electroencephalography. *Neurology* (Minneap.) 23:973, 1973.

74. Silverman, D., and Morisaki, A. Reevaluation of sleep electroencephalography. *Electroencephalogr. Clin. Neurophysiol.* 10:425, 1958.

75. Sutula, T. P. et al. Intensive monitoring in refractory epilepsy. *Neurology* (N.Y.) 31:243, 1981.

76. Tharp, B. R. The 6 per second spike and wave complex. *Electroencephalogr. Clin. Neurophysiol.* 23:291, 1967.

77. Thomas, J. E., and Klass, D. W. Six-per-second spike-and-wave pattern in the electroencephalogram: A reappraisal of its clinical significance. *Neurology* (Minneap.) 18:587, 1968.

78. Thurston, J. H. et al. Prognosis in childhood epilepsy: Additional follow-up of 148 children 15 to 23 years after withdrawal of anticonvulsant therapy. *N. Engl. J. Med.* 306:831, 1982.

79. Tudor, I. The electroclinical nonconcordance in epilepsy. *Neurol. Psychiatr.* (Bucur.) 15:43, 1977.

80. White, J. C., Langston, J. W., and Pedley, T. A. Benign epileptiform transients of sleep: Clarification of the small sharp spikes controversy. *Neurology* (Minneap.) 27:1061, 1977.

81. Wilder, B. J. Electroencephalogram activation in medically intractable epileptic patients: Activation technique including surgical follow-up. *Arch. Neurol.* 25:415, 1971.

82. Zivin, L., and Ajmone-Marsan, C. Incidence and prognostic significance of epileptiform: Activity in the EEG of nonepileptic subjects. *Brain* 81: 751, 1968.

MANAGEMENT OF UNDERLYING CAUSES AND PRECIPITATING FACTORS OF EPILEPSY

12

Robert G. Feldman

Epilepsy results from the recurrent discharging of neurons due to instability of the cell membrane resulting from excessive depolarization and repolarization. Membrane stability and polarization are maintained by ionic balance across the membrane. When this ionic balance is disturbed or when the intrinsic mechanisms of maintaining membrane stability are affected, there is a tendency for a seizure to occur. Individuals may have, by genetic determination or acquired condition, a lower threshold to spontaneous firing of certain neurons. Others may be exposed to the same conditions that upset membrane stability but will not have seizures because they have an intrinsically higher threshold. Understanding the pathophysiology of epilepsy begins with the knowledge that neurons are capable of paroxysmal discharging given adequate circumstances (see Chap. 2).

A seizure disorder for which no evident cause can be found by history, physical examination, or diagnostic testing is referred to as primary or idiopathic. Secondary or symptomatic epilepsies include those seizures that appear to be manifestations of underlying conditions such as trauma, brain tumor, vascular diseases, malformations, inflammations, infections, or metabolic or toxic disturbances. Once the etiology has been defined, the underlying causes of symptomatic seizures can be addressed. In many cases, seizures are still likely to recur after treatment of the underlying condition. Seizure prevention can be achieved only by instituting an adequate amount of the proper medication and identifying the various triggers or seizure precipitants for the individual patient (Fig. 12-1).

Underlying Causes in Symptomatic (Secondary) Epilepsy

STRUCTURAL CAUSES

Damage to neurons and their supportive structures, glia and blood vessels, renders the brain susceptible to instability and the occurrence of epileptic attacks. Head injury and cerebrovascular accidents disturb the normal anatomy by destruction, phagocytosis, and scar formation (gliosis). Selective loss of inhibitory inputs to neuronal dendrites may be the cause of excessive neuronal discharge in some areas of damaged human cortex [60]. Mass lesions, such as tumors and blood clots, distort cellular membranes. Vascular malformations affect neuronal and glial metabolism by changes in blood flow.

130

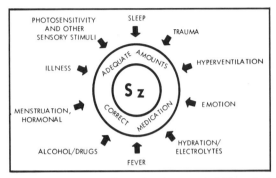

Figure 12-1. Operative factors in seizure control. (From R. G. Feldman. In R. W. Wilkins, and N. G. Levinski [Eds.], Medi-cine: Essentials of Clinical Practice. Boston: Little, Brown, 1978.)

Trauma and Post-Traumatic Epilepsy

The epileptogenic effects of trauma incurred in military injuries have been extensively studied by Caveness et al. [8, 9] and by Walker et al. [59]. Seizures may occur simultaneously with the head trauma or hours, days, weeks, or years later. Seizures occurring minutes to hours after a head injury may be part of the acute injury and do not necessarily predict that seizures will occur later. Seizures occurring days to a few weeks after injury are more likely to result in recurring seizures, and those that begin months to years after an injury are most likely to recur.

The time of onset of recurring seizure disorders after head injury in the military population is as follows: 0 to ½ year, 25 percent; ½ to 1 year, 15 percent; 1 to 2 years, 20 percent; 2 to 5 years, 19 percent; after 5 years, 22 percent. Seizures may develop up to 25 years after a head injury. Post-traumatic seizures develop more slowly in children than in adults.

The incidence of post-traumatic epilepsy in the military population is related to the type of head injury as follows: blow to head without apparent neurologic significance, 7 percent; blow to head with loss of consciousness, 10 percent; blow to head without penetration of dura but with overt evidence of underlying damage to brain, 34 percent; penetration of dura without loss of consciousness or overt neurologic defect, 20 percent; penetration of dura with evident neurologic defect, 51 percent; penetration of dura and brain of profound degree or with significant complications, 57 percent.

In a study performed in a civilian population (Mayo Clinic) the risk of developing post-traumatic epilepsy within 5 years was related to the type of head injury as follows: severe (brain contusion, intracerebral or intracranial hematoma, or 24 hours of either unconscious-

ness or amnesia), 11.5 percent; moderate (skull fracture or 30 minutes to 24 hours of unconsciousness or amnesia), 1.6 percent; mild (briefer periods of unconsciousness or amnesia), 0.6 percent [2].

Prognostic factors associated with a higher incidence of post-traumatic epilepsy include penetration of more than one lobe of the brain, deep injury, injury in the central area, post-traumatic amnesia for more than 24 hours, and depressed skull fracture. Attempts to demonstrate genetic risk factors for developing post-traumatic seizures have been inconclusive.

The seizure types produced by trauma include tonic-clonic only (25%), partial only (25%), and combinations of tonic-clonic and partial seizures (50%). Complex partial seizures seldom occur in the early post-traumatic period but may occur later. Absence seizures are seldom, if ever, produced by head trauma.

Acute head injury involving brain laceration or contusion may be responsible for convulsions that are difficult to control at the time of injury. The presence of persistent seizures under these circumstances must be considered a signal for possible intracerebral hematoma requiring surgical intervention.

Pharmacologic prophylaxis of post-traumatic epilepsy remains controversial. There is considerable data from animal experiments and uncontrolled clinical data indicating that pharmacologic prophylaxis may prevent development of post-traumatic epilepsy [63]. A prospective, double-blind study by the National Institutes of Health compared prophylaxis using phenytoin and phenobarbital with prophylaxis using a placebo and failed to demonstrate a reduction in post-traumatic epilepsy in the treated group [44]. However, the dosages of phenytoin and phenobarbital that were administered produced subtherapeutic blood levels in most patients.

Cerebrovascular Disease

Impairment of cerebral circulation may cause epileptic seizures depending on the severity of the resulting ischemia and the susceptibility of the brain to seizures [48]. Seizures are the most common sign of cerebral anoxia in the newborn, and generally indicate a poor prognosis [15]. Other vascular disorders that may produce seizures in children include: congenital heart disease, Sturge-Weber syndrome, and infantile hemiplegia.

In adults, seizures may occur at the time of an acute cerebral ischemic event (e.g., cerebral embolus), or they may result from long-term ischemia. Occlusive vascular disease occurring in the older age group must be distinguished from postictal hemiplegia, transient ischemic attacks, migraine, and syncope associated with cardiac irregularities (see Chaps. 5 and 10). There is a type of seizure in older patients that is followed by deep coma and often hemiplegia. The patient appears in the postictal period to have had a massive stroke but then hours later is completely recovered. Vascular causes of seizures in adults include cerebral atherosclerosis, cerebral embolism, intracerebral hemorrhage, subarachnoid hemorrhage, arteriovenous malformations, arteritis, cardiac arrhythmias, and disturbed reflex circulatory control [39, 46].

In a study of 107 patients in whom seizures began after the age of 50, cerebrovascular disease was the cause in 32 percent [61]. One or more seizures occur in 12.5 to 14 percent of patients who have had cerebrovascular accidents, and recurrent seizures occur in 5.8 to 8 percent of such patients [22, 46]. Recurring seizures occur in 26 percent of patients with cerebrovascular accidents involving the cerebral cortex, whereas seizures rarely occur after cerebrovascular accidents confined to subcortical structures [46].

In studies of patients with embolic strokes, 21 to 43 percent had seizures (16 to 43% had seizures acutely and 5 to 20% had seizures beginning some time after the stroke) [22, 36, 46]. In studies of patients with thrombotic strokes, 6 to 12 percent had seizures (3 to 4% had seizures acutely and 2% had seizures beginning some time after the stroke) [22, 30, 46]. The incidence of seizures is probably lower after hemorrhagic strokes than after embolic or thrombotic strokes [46].

These data indicate that the clinician must have a high index of suspicion for an embolic cause when a patient presents with an acute onset of a stroke accompanied by a seizure. Cardiac arrhythmias, valvular heart disease, and myocardial infarction (new or old) must be sought in a patient with such a presentation.

Acute cerebral infarction is the most common cause of the PLEDS syndrome in many series [16, 52]. This syndrome consists of periodic, lateralized, epileptiform discharges (PLEDS) on the EEG accompanied clinically by refractory though transient (1 to 14 days) seizures (simple partial, tonic-clonic), altered consciousness, and focal or lateralized neurologic deficits.

Seizures that occur during the first week after a stroke are less likely to recur after recovery. Late-onset seizures, months or years after a stroke, tend to be recurrent and require antiepileptic medication.

The routine EEG done at the time of a cerebrovascular accident can help predict the probability of later development of seizures. Holmes [22] reviewed the outcome after a 2-year follow-up in a group of 250 patients who had had a routine EEG within 1 week of a cerebrovascular accident. The risk of developing chronic epilepsy in relation to the findings on the initial EEG were reported as follows: normal EEG, 0 percent; diffuse slowing, 4 percent; focal slowing, 8 percent; sharp-waves, spikes, or PLEDS, 33 percent.

As many as 50 percent of arteriovenous malformations initially present as a seizure disorder (simple partial, complex partial, or generalized), which may later be followed by intracranial hemorrhage [33, 40]. Onset of epilepsy due to arteriovenous malformations usually occurs during adolescence or the young adult years [33].

Tumors
Epileptic attacks due to an intracerebral mass such as a tumor are caused by changes in the cortex following deprivation of its blood supply, traction on the cortex by the tumor, pressure from edema, or direct deformation of neural tissue by the tumor.

The probability that a tumor is the cause of a first seizure in a given patient varies with age. Only a small percentage of children presenting with a first seizure have a brain tumor. In adults, tumors are found in 1 to 10 percent of newly diagnosed seizure disorders [51]. In adults over the age of 40 years presenting with a first seizure, the probability of finding a brain tumor is 11 to 20 percent [24, 25, 51, 61]. In middle-aged and elderly adults presenting with a first seizure of a *focal* type, the probability of finding a brain tumor is 30 to 60 percent (see Chap. 4).

Overall, 35 percent of patients with cerebral neoplasms will experience one or more seizures [28]. Less malignant tumors of long duration are more likely to cause seizures than more rapidly growing ones [3, 25, 57]. As a group, patients with gliomas who have seizures have a significantly ($p = .0004$) longer survival time than glioma patients who do not have epilepsy [53]. Tumors located deep in the white matter are likely to produce paralysis or other neurologic symptoms before they become manifest as a seizure. Tumors in the infratentorial or pituitary regions rarely cause seizures. Slowly growing gliomas constitute approximately two thirds of brain tumors in patients who present with seizures [28]. A majority of seizures due to slow-growing gliomas begin between the ages of 20 and 50 years.

Meningiomas, which are usually located close to the cortex, are associated with seizures in as many as 67 percent of cases. Small meningiomas or indolent glial tumors are often incidental findings at autopsy or operation in patients considered to have long-standing idiopathic epilepsy [43]. Examination of specimens from patients undergoing surgical procedures (usually temporal lobectomy) for relief of focal epilepsy reveals brain tumors in about 20 percent of specimens (see Chaps. 4 and 5). In about half of these cases, the presence of the tumor was not suspected until it was discovered at operation [28]. The preoperative duration of seizures in these cases of slowly growing gliomas and meningiomas was as much as 15 years in some instances.

Meningitis, Encephalitis, and Brain Abscess

Convulsions may indicate the onset of meningitis or encephalitis [49]. Seizures occur at the onset and during the acute course of inflammation owing to localized cortical venous and arterial occlusion as well as to abnormalities at the membrane level that are caused by changes in glia. Seizures of late onset may be secondary to the meningeal scarring. During purulent encephalitis or brain abscess, neuronal ischemia plays an important role in the epileptogenic process [42]. Seizures are the initial symptom in more than 45 percent of patients with acute abscess. The longer it takes a brain abscess to develop the more likely is the subsequent occurrence of epileptic seizures, which are expressed most often by focal seizures, although generalized convulsions also occur.

Metabolic Causes

Constipation, diarrhea, minor urinary and upper respiratory infections, liver failure, occult neoplasm, anemia, malnutrition, and fluid and electrolyte disturbances (especially of sodium and calcium) are conditions that disrupt the body's homeostasis. Symptomatic epilepsy occurs when such biochemical derangements occur in a susceptible person, thus interfering with normal neuronal functions. In such cases, prompt and proper corrective measures to restore healthy functional metabolism may result in full functional recovery. Metabolic and endocrine imbalances can lead to poor seizure control in epileptic patients and may lower the seizure threshold in nonepileptic patients and in experimental animals under certain conditions.

SODIUM (HYPONATREMIA AND HYPERNATREMIA). Hyponatremic states may cause seizures and slow-wave changes in the EEG [21, 38]. In animals with experimental seizures, a low epileptic threshold is related to a low level of serum sodium and a fall in the ratio of extracellular to intracellular sodium in the brain. Loss of sodium may result from diarrhea, excessive sweating, or increased excretion of sodium in the urine associated with renal disease or diuretics [38]. Hyponatremia may also be associated with central nervous system diseases such as encephalitis or third ventricle tumors affecting hypothalamic structures. Reduced sodium levels may occur after parenteral administration of hyponatremic fluids, acute infections and fever, or acute expansion of the extracellular fluid volume from retention of water. Convulsions due to water intoxication and hyponatremia are resistant to antiepileptic drugs and can be controlled only by correction of the electrolyte imbalance.

Hypernatremic states causing seizures may result from central nervous system lesions that cause diabetes insipidus or from dehydration, sodium retention, or excessive sodium intake [21, 38]. Ironically, too rapid a correction of hypernatremia may lead to seizures owing to rebound hyponatremia. Hypernatremia is corrected by using a 3% solution of sodium chloride with added potassium. Dehydration occurs in infants with diarrhea as well as in patients who have excessive water loss. The seizures may be explained by cerebral cortical damage and alteration in permeability of the nerve cell membrane. Contributory factors in the causation of seizures are hypocalcemia with hypernatremia, a concomitant electrolyte abnormality that results in an alteration in the permeability of the nerve cell membrane, disturbing the normal balance of the intracellular concentration of sodium.

CALCIUM (HYPOCALCEMIA). Normal amounts of ionized calcium in the serum are needed for selective permeability of the cell membranes to sodium and potassium. Hypocalcemia is associated with an instability of cell membranes and neuronal and neuromuscular irritability. Convulsions may be associated with reduction of the diffusable ionized calcium under certain conditions, such as neonatal tetany, hypoparathyroidism, pseudohypoparathyroidism, rickets, steatorrhea, chronic renal disease, treatment of hypernatremia, treatment of acidosis with dehydration, and intravenous administration of fluids low in calcium or blood products containing calcium-chelating agents (e.g., EDTA) [21, 38].

All of these can occur in a nonepileptic patient. However, fluctuations in urinary excretion of electrolytes have been correlated with changes in seizure frequency in adults and children who have centrencephalic epilepsy. There is an exacerbation of seizures coinciding with a marked decrease in urinary sodium in some persons. Calcium excretion parallels that of sodium.

MAGNESIUM. Seizures may occur as a complication of magnesium depletion under the following conditions: malnutrition, alcoholism, diarrhea, vomiting, renal insufficiency, hypoparathyroidism, acute pancreatitis, vitamin B intoxication, hyperthyroidism, or hepatic insufficiency [21, 38]. Other electrolyte disorders that occur with magnesium deficiency may account for some of the symptomatology.

HYPOGLYCEMIA. Hypoglycemia (blood glucose concentration below 40 mg/100 ml) causes seizures by depriving the brain of essential materials for oxidative metabolism [21, 38]. In the absence of sufficient glucose the brain oxidizes other noncarbohydrate substrates such as lipids and amino acids, but none of these is adequate to maintain normal function for any significant length of time. After the stores of cerebral glucose and glycogen are exhausted, the brain's own structural constituents are fed into the glycolytic and Kreb's cycle pathways. Of the many causes of hypoglycemia that may lead to convulsions, overdoses of drugs such as insulin and tolbutamide are the most common. Hypoglycemic seizures may be associated with hyperinsulinism due to tumors of the pancreas, with impaired glycogenolysis and glyconeogenesis resulting from hepatic disease, or with destructive or degenerative lesions of either the anterior lobe of the pituitary or the adrenal cortex. Physiologic (reactive) hypoglycemia occurring after a large meal may precipitate epileptic attacks in some patients.

Renal Failure
Uremia results from the inability to eliminate breakdown products, such as urea, creatine, and uric acid, and the retention of inorganic and organic acids, including sulfate [21]. The accumulated substances are toxic to the brain. Inattention, stupor, coma, and convulsions result. Epilepsy that persists after recovery from uremia suggests neuronal damage. Early in renal failure the EEG shows nonfocal increases in slow-wave activity. Later, spikes and other paroxysmal activity may appear.

Hepatic Failure
Focal, generalized, or myoclonic seizures may occur in hepatic encephalopathy [21]. Stupor and coma are characteristic of the terminal stages of hepatic failure, which is accompanied by an increase in the blood ammonia concentration. Cerebral metabolism, either at the level of glutamine synthesis or in the reductive deamination of alpha-ketoglutarate, may be adversely affected by increased amounts of blood ammonia. The EEG may reflect hepatic failure by slow waves (2 to 3 Hz) or by triphatic waves. The cause of the seizures in hepatic failure may be an interference with pyridoxal function with consequent disruption of glutamic acid–gamma-aminobutyric acid pathways, resulting in

decreased cerebral oxygen consumption. Correction of hepatic dysfunction is the best means of treating these seizures; phenytoin is less effective, and diazepam only masks the problem by adding to the nervous system depression.

Endocrinopathies
A close relationship between the nervous and endocrine systems is well documented because the secretion of hormones is subject to neural control. An antiepileptic action of adrenocorticotropic hormone (ACTH) was first reported in 1950 [26], and ACTH is still used as an antiepileptic drug (see Chap. 9).

The effects of sex hormones, menstruation, and pregnancy on epilepsy are reviewed in Chapter 29.

Precipitating Factors
A seizure is a symptom of instability of the neuronal cell membrane. The initial seizure must be explained, whatever the age of the patient. A cause must be sought, and necessary measures must be taken to prevent recurrence of seizures. Anyone is potentially an epileptic, because seizures are simply a matter of lowering the neuronal discharge threshold far enough. Normally, there are mechanisms that prevent spontaneous neuronal discharging, and seizures are not easily produced. In persons prone to epileptic attacks, the threshold may be lowered by a variety of circumstances. Seizures are controlled by maintaining a balance between factors precipitating them and factors preventing them (Fig. 12-1). Avoidance of seizure threshold-lowering events and medication that raises the threshold combine to make recurrence of seizures less likely.

SLEEP
Many patients have seizures only at night. Clinical seizures and bilateral EEG abnormalities in patients with primarily generalized tonic-clonic seizures are most apt to occur during the slow-wave phase of non-REM sleep and are diminished during REM sleep [20]. Nocturnal partial or focal seizures can arise in all phases of sleep, including REM sleep [50]. Temporal spikes on the EEG are most likely to be seen during stages I and II of non-REM sleep in patients with complex partial seizures and are very rare during REM sleep (see Chaps. 5 and 11). Patients with spike-and-wave discharges on EEGs show maximum discharge rates during stage IV of non-REM sleep, whereas a marked reduction occurs during REM sleep [50]. Recently, techniques that alter sleep patterns have been employed in patients susceptible to nocturnal sei-

134

zures, including medications that enhance deeper stages of sleep or prolong REM sleep.

Sleep deprivation can cause increased seizure frequency and an increased incidence of paroxysmal activity on EEGs, especially in patients with complex partial seizures (see Chaps. 5 and 11). Mattson et al. [31] found that after sleep deprivation of 26 to 28 hours 34 percent of patients whose EEGs had been normal previously showed activation of focal or generalized epileptiform disturbances, and abnormalities that had been present previously increased in 56 percent of patients.

HYPERVENTILATION

Hyperventilation produces a lowering of the CO_2 of the blood, which in turn causes constriction of cerebral arteries and cerebral ischemia [12]. This can cause activation of seizure activity in some patients [7, 12, 27, 38]. It is possible to precipitate absence seizures and 3-Hz spike-wave discharges by hyperventilation in virtually all patients with untreated absence seizures [7], but once antiabsence medication has been started, it may be difficult to precipitate absence seizures in this way [7]. Hyperventilation will occasionally elicit temporal spikes and, less commonly, clinical seizures in patients with complex partial seizures [27].

Involuntary hyperventilation may occur in the course of a patient's daily activities owing to anxiety, sobbing, sexual activity, or other causes and can provoke a seizure in the susceptible patient. Hyperventilation can aggravate a patient's underlying seizure potentialities enough to make control quite difficult. Occasionally, the adjunctive use of sedative drugs (to reduce hyperventilation due to anxiety) or acetazolamide (to reduce the respiratory alkalosis of hyperventilation) is useful in preventing seizures precipitated by hyperventilation [38].

DRUGS

Antiepileptic Drug Withdrawal

Suddenly stopping or rapidly decreasing the dosage of antiepileptic medication may result in increased seizure frequency and/or status epilepticus [54] (see Chaps. 14 and 30).

Sedative Drug Withdrawal

Continued use of relatively high doses of sedative medications for periods of weeks or months followed by abstinence may produce tremors, irritability, and generalized convulsions. Barbiturates, benzodiazepines, opiates, glutethimide, and meprobamate [6, 27,

29] are examples of drugs that may result in seizures on withdrawal.

Tricyclic Antidepressants

Animal work suggests that raising brain monoamine activity raises the seizure threshold and that lowering monoamine activity in the brain lowers the seizure threshold [56]. Tricyclic antidepressants lower the seizure threshold in many animal models of epilepsy, possibly because tricyclics block the reuptake of monoamines into neurons [56].

Seizures are a prominent part of the tricyclic overdosage syndrome in humans [56]. Such seizures have been treated with phenobarbital, paraldehyde, and diazepam [56].

Activation of seizures has been reported in 0.2 to 4 percent of patients receiving the usual therapeutic doses of tricyclics [56]. Many of these patients had a history of either previously diagnosed epilepsy or predisposing risk factors for epilepsy (brain damage, family history of epilepsy, electroconvulsive therapy, drug or alcohol withdrawal) [56]. However, a small number of patients without predisposing risk factors apparently develop seizures while on therapeutic doses of tricyclics [56]. Chlorimipramine, imipramine, and amytriptyline appear to be the tricyclics most likely to exacerbate epilepsy, while maprotiline, flupenthixol, and nomifensine appear to be the least likely [56].

Monoamine Oxidase Inhibitors

Monoamine oxidase inhibitors raise brain monoamine levels and thus might raise the seizure threshold in humans [10, 56]. A clinical trial testing this hypothesis yielded equivocal results [10].

Phenothiazines

Phenothiazines are dopamine-blocking drugs and thus might be expected to lower the seizure threshold [56]. There is clinical, EEG, and animal evidence that this is the case [27, 29, 34, 56].

Other Drugs

Certain drugs appear to lower the seizure threshold directly. These drugs include aminophylline, metrazol, caffeine, and ephedrine [11, 27, 29, 64].

ALCOHOL

Alcohol withdrawal seizures ("rum fits") after heavy alcohol intake characteristically begin in adult life. Ninety percent of alcohol withdrawal seizures occur 7 to 48 hours after decreasing or stopping alcohol intake [58]. The exact mechanism is obscure, but hypomagnesemia and respiratory alkalosis have been suggested as important factors. Associated disturbances in sleep, sleep deprivation, or excessive non-REM sleep have also been considered important factors in alcohol withdrawal seizures.

Mattson et al. [32] studied the effects of single doses of alcohol on nonalcoholic patients with epilepsy. They found a decrease in seizure threshold during the period of falling blood alcohol level. Furthermore, the sedative effect of alcohol can potentiate the sedative effects of antiepileptic drugs, sometimes with disasterous results. For these and other reasons, total abstinence from alcohol should be recommended to patients with epilepsy.

Alcohol-related seizures are discussed in more detail in Chapter 28.

FEVER

Fever may induce febrile convulsions in susceptible children. Fever may precipitate seizures in many patients with epilepsy and is one of the most common causes of status epilepticus. The effects of fever are discussed in more detail in Chapters 27 and 30.

EMOTION

The complicated interactions of emotions with seizures are reviewed in Chapters 5 and 24.

SEX HORMONES, MENSTRUATION, AND PREGNANCY

See Chapter 29.

HOSPITALIZATION

It is a common observation that hospitalization without any change in antiepileptic medication often results in a reduction in seizure frequency, especially in patients with complex partial seizures [47]. Relief from environmental stress and improved compliance with medication schedules may be contributory factors in this phenomenon.

SENSORY OR REFLEX EPILEPSY

The sensory-induced or reflex epilepsies are the most exquisite examples of seizures induced by specific environmental stimuli [4, 14, 18, 23, 41]. Visual, auditory, somatic, olfactory, gustatory, and visceral stimuli can precipitate such seizures. A predisposition to seizures, a facilitation of seizures through moment-to-moment changes in threshold, and the presence of specific stimuli were factors identified by Daube [14] as consistently present in all sensory-precipitated seizures. A propensity for certain EEG features elicited by specific types of stimuli was observed by Bickford and Klass [4]. Visually induced seizures are the largest category.

Photosensitive Epilepsy

Newmark and Penry [41] have exhaustively reviewed the topic of photosensitive epilepsy. An abnormal response occurs most often when photic stimulation of 15 to 20 flashes per second is applied to patients with the eyes open and looking at the flashing light. Several abnormal electrical responses have been described, but generalized spike-wave discharges with an afterdischarge are the most significant response in photosensitive epilepsy.

Extensive clinical correlations with the electrical discharges have been performed. Although exceptions are frequent, most patients are young (under the age of 30), female, and neurologically normal. They usually respond to stroboscopic stimulation with myoclonic, tonic-clonic, or absence seizures. In adults, nonphotic-induced seizures, usually consisting of tonic-clonic or absence attacks, are often present. Patients with partial seizures or seizures secondary to a known cause are not often photosensitive. Among children, the influence of other seizure disorders is not as clear, but febrile convulsions have been correlated with a photoconvulsive response. A prominent family history of photosensitivity and epilepsy has been described in several patients. Nonepileptic patients with abnormal photic responses have also been extensively studied. They often have a positive history of neurologic disease, a family history of epilepsy, and a mixture of neurologic symptoms. Often the photic response is not as significant as the generalized discharges with poststimulus after-discharge. These patients show a sex and age distribution similar to that of patients with photic-induced seizures.

Numerous other visually related seizures have been described, including pattern epilepsy, eye closure epilepsy, epilepsy induced by eye movement, and reading epilepsy.

Television Epilepsy

Watching television may precipitate seizures in some patients. Television epilepsy appears to be a variety of photosensitive epilepsy. The types of clinical seizures (tonic-clonic, absence, myoclonic) that occur are the same for both types, and patients with television epilepsy often have paroxysmal EEG activity in response to the strobe light frequencies (15 to 20 Hz) that typically activate patients with photosensitive epilepsy [23, 41, 62]. The television picture consists of two sets of alternating lines oscillating out of phase at 30 per second (25 per second in Europe) [62]. Viewing at close range (less than 8 feet), where the lines can be seen, is far more likely to elicit a seizure than viewing from a distance [41, 62]. The exact stimulus from the television picture that induces the seizure is controversial and may include photic stimulation, eye movements, patterned stimuli, and flickering light [41, 62].

Self-Induced Seizures
Some patients deliberately induce seizures to produce a pleasurable sensation, to escape from stress, or to satisfy a compulsion [13, 41]. Some patients induce their attacks by hyperventilation, and a few can bring on a seizure by means of no obvious maneuver except concentrating on doing so [13, 41]. However, the overwhelming majority of patients are photosensitive and employ some form of visual stimulus to induce seizures [13, 41]. This may take the form of waving one hand in front of the eyes while looking at the sun or a bright light, blinking, or closing the eyes in unusual ways [13, 41].

Overall, the age and sex characteristics of patients with self-induced seizures are similar to those of patients with photic-induced seizures [41]. However, patients with self-induced seizures have a slightly higher prevalence of mental retardation and a significantly higher prevalence of induced absence attacks [41].

Studies using video analysis suggest that the method of inducing the seizure is actually a part of the seizure in some patients [41]. Self-induced seizures require more study to resolve the issue of how many are brought on voluntarily [41].

Reading Epilepsy
Bickford et al. [5] described two groups of patients with seizures precipitated by reading. Group I had the following features: (1) seizures occur *only* with reading; (2) onset with clicking sensation in the jaw or jaw movement, followed by generalized seizure activity if reading was not stopped; (3) paroxysmal discharges of bilaterally synchronous 3- to 6-Hz activity, which is the maximal posteriorly; (4) normal resting EEG; and (5) no evidence of brain pathology. Group II had the following features: (1) seizures sometimes precipitated with stimuli other than reading (photic stimulation, visual patterns, writing, calculation, recall); (2) jaw clicking does not occur; and (3) sometimes evidence for brain damage. Reading epilepsy is reviewed by Merlis [35].

Eating Epilepsy
There are at least 32 reports of seizures provoked by eating a meal, chewing, holding water in the mouth, or bringing food to the mouth with the upper extremity [1, 45]. Complex partial seizures were the most common type of seizure reported in association with eating

epilepsy, and a temporal lobe focus was seen with EEG recording [1, 45] in 17 of 24 reported cases of eating epilepsy. This suggests that input to temporal lobe structures involved in alimentary functions (especially the amygdala) may have a role in the genesis of eating epilepsy [1, 45].

"Musicogenic" Epilepsy
Seizures induced by some aspect of music are called musicogenic epilepsy [55]. Characteristic features include older age at onset than with idiopathic seizures, sensitivity to different types of music, complex partial or tonic-clonic seizure type, and favorable prognosis. Precipitating factors can be quite specific, such as listening to only one composition or the actual playing of music on an instrument.

References

1. Ahuja, G. K. et al. Eating epilepsy. *Epilepsia* 21:85, 1980.
2. Annegers, J. F. et al. Seizures after head trauma: A population study. *Neurology* (N.Y.) 30:683, 1980.
3. Arseni, C., and Petrovici, I. N. Epilepsy in temporal lobe tumors. *Eur. Neurol.* 5:201, 1971.
4. Bickford, R. G., and Klass, D. W. Sensory Precipitation and Reflex Mechanisms. In H. H. Jasper, A. A. Ward, and A. Pope (Eds.), *Basic Mechanisms of the Epilepsies.* Boston: Little, Brown, 1969.
5. Bickford, R. et al. Reading epilepsy: Clinical and electroencephalographic studies of a new syndrome. *Trans. Am. Neurol. Assoc.* 81:100, 1975.
6. Browne, T. R., and Penry, J. K. Benzodiazepines in the treatment of epilepsy: A review. *Epilepsia* 14:277, 1973.
7. Browne, T. R. et al. Clinical and electroencephalographic estimates of absence seizure frequency. *Arch. Neurol.,* in press, 1983.
8. Caveness, W. F. Etiological and Provocative Factors. Trauma. In P. J. Vinken, and G. W. Bruyn (Eds.), *Handbook of Clinical Neurology,* Vol. 15, *The Epilepsies.* Amsterdam: Elsevier, 1974.
9. Caveness, W. F. et al. The nature of posttraumatic epilepsy. *J. Neurosurg.* 50:545, 1979.
10. Chadwick, D. et al. Manipulation of cerebral monoamines in the treatment of human epilepsy: A pilot study. *Epilepsia* 19:3, 1978.
11. Chu, N. A. Caffeine- and aminophylline-induced seizures. *Epilepsia* 22:85, 1981.
12. Cooper, R. Influence on the EEG of Certain Physiological States and Other Parameters. In A. Redmond (Ed.), *Handbook of Electroencephalography*

and *Clinical Neurophysiology,* Vol. 7. Amsterdam: Elsevier, 1974.

13. Darby, C. E. et al. The self-induction of epileptic seizures by eye closure. *Epilepsia* 22:31, 1980.

14. Daube, J. R. Sensory precipitated seizures: A review. *J. Nerv. Ment. Dis.* 141:524, 1966.

15. Del Mundo-Valarta, J., and Robb, J. P. A follow-up study of newborn infants with perinatal complications. Determination of etiology and predictive value of abnormal histories and neurological signs. *Neurology* (Minneap.) 14:413, 1964.

16. Erkulvrawatr, S. Occurrence, evolution and prognosis of periodic lateralized epileptiform discharges in EEG. *Clin. Electroencephalogr.* 8:89, 1977.

17. Feldman, R. G. Neurological Diseases: A Symptomatic Approach. In R. W. Wilkins, and N. G. Levinski (Eds.), *Medicine: Essentials of Clinical Practice.* Boston: Little, Brown, 1978.

18. Forster, F. *Reflex Epilepsy, Conditional Reflexes and Behavioral Treatment.* Springfield, Ill.: Thomas, 1975.

19. Gastaut, H., and Tassinari, C. A. Triggering mechanisms in epilepsy. *Epilepsia* 7:85, 1966.

20. Gastaut, H. et al. Generalized Convulsive Seizures Without Local Onset. In P. J. Vinken, and G. W. Bruyn (Eds.), *Handbook of Clinical Neurology,* Vol. 15, *The Epilepsies.* Amsterdam: Elsevier, 1974.

21. Glaser, G. H. Metabolic, Endocrine, and Toxic Diseases. In A. Redmond (Ed.), *Handbook of Electroencephalography and Clinical Neurophysiology,* Vol. 7. Amsterdam: Elsevier, 1974.

22. Holmes, G. L. The electroencephalogram as a predictor of seizures following cerebral infarction. *Clin. Electroencephalogr.* 11:83, 1980.

23. Jeavons, P. M., and Harding, G. F. A. *Photosensitive Epilepsy: A Review of the Literature and a Study of 460 Patients.* London: Heinemann, 1975.

24. Jüül-Jensen, P. Epilepsy, A clinical and social analysis of 1,020 adult patients with epileptic seizures. *Acta Neurol. Scand.* 40 [Suppl. 5]:1, 1964.

25. Ketz, E. Brain Tumors and Epilepsy. In P. J. Vinken, and G. W. Bruyn (Eds.), *Handbook of Clinical Neurology,* Vol. 16, *Tumors of the Brain and Skull.* Amsterdam: Elsevier, 1975.

26. Klein, R., and Livingston, S. The effects of adrenocorticotropic hormone in epilepsy. *J. Pediatr.* 37:733, 1950.

27. Kooi, K. E., Tucker, R. P., and Marshall, R. E. *Fundamentals of Electroencephalography.* New York: Harper & Row, 1978.

28. Leblanc, F. E., and Rasmussen, T. Cerebral Seizures and Brain Tumors. In P. J. Vinken, and G. W.

Bruyn (Eds.), *Handbook of Clinical Neurology,* Vol. 15, *The Epilepsies.* Amsterdam: Elsevier, 1974.

29. Longo, V. G. Effects of Drugs on the EEG. In A. Redmond (Ed.), *Handbook of Electroencephalography and Clinical Neurophysiology,* Vol. 7. Amsterdam: Elsevier, 1974.

30. Louis, S., and McDowell, F. Epileptic seizures in nonembolic cerebral infarction. *Arch. Neurol.* 17:414, 1967.

31. Mattson, R. H., Pratt, K. L., and Calverley, J. R. Electroencephalograms of epileptics following sleep deprivation. *Arch. Neurol.* 13:310, 1965.

32. Mattson, R. H. et al. Effect of alcohol intake in nonalcoholic epileptics. *Neurology* (Minneap.) 25:361, 1975.

33. McCormick, N. F., and Schochet, S. *Atlas of Cerebrovascular Disease.* Philadelphia: Saunders, 1976.

34. Meldrum, B. S., Anlezark, G., and Trimble, T. R. Drugs modifying dopaminergic and behavior, the EEG, and epilepsy in *Papio papio. Eur. J. Pharmacol.* 32:203, 1975.

35. Merlis, J. K. Reflex Epilepsy. In P. J. Vinken, and G. W. Bruyn (Eds.), *Handbook of Clinical Neurology,* Vol. 15, *The Epilepsies.* Amsterdam: Elsevier, 1974.

36. Meyer, J. S. et al. Cerebral embolization: Prospective analysis of 42 cases. *Stroke* 2:541, 1971.

37. Millichap, J. G. *Febrile Convulsions.* New York: Macmillan, 1968.

38. Millichap, J. G. Metabolic and Endocrine Factors. In P. J. Vinken, and G. W. Bruyn (Eds.), *Handbook of Clinical Neurology,* Vol. 15, *The Epilepsies.* Amsterdam: Elsevier, 1974.

39. Mohr, J. P. et al. The Harvard Cooperative Stroke Registry: A prospective registry. *Neurology* (Minneap.) 28:754, 1978.

40. Murphy, M. J., and Wilkinson, J. T. Long term follow-up of seizures associated with cerebral arteriovenous malformations: Results of therapy. *Epilepsia.* In press, 1982.

41. Newmark, M. E., and Penry, J. K. *Photosensitivity and Epilepsy: A Review.* New York: Raven Press, 1979.

42. Ounsted, C. Significance of convulsions in children with purulent meningitis. *Lancet* 1:1245, 1951.

43. Penfield, W., Erickson, T. C., and Tarlov, I. M. Relation of intracranial tumors and symptomatic epilepsy. *Arch. Neurol. Psychiatry* 44:300, 1940.

44. Penry, J. K., White, B. G., and Brackett, C. E. A controlled prospective study of the pharmacologic prophylaxis of posttraumatic epilepsy. *Neurology* (N.Y.) 29:600, 1979.

138

45. Reder, A. T., and Wright, F. S. Epilepsy provoked by eating: The role of peripheral input. *Neurology* (N.Y.) 32:1065, 1982.
46. Richardson, E. P., and Dodge, P. R. Epilepsy in cerebral vascular disease. A study of the incidence and nature of seizures in 104 consecutive autopsy-proven cases of cerebral infarction and hemorrhage. *Epilepsia* 3:49, 1954.
47. Riley, T. L. et al. The hospital experience and seizure control. *Neurology* (N.Y.) 31:912, 1981.
48. Robb, R., and McNaughton, F. Vascular Disease. In P. J. Vinken, and G. W. Bruyn (Eds.), *Handbook of Clinical Neurology,* Vol. 15, *The Epilepsies.* Amsterdam: Elsevier, 1974.
49. Robb, R., and McNaughton, R. Infections. In P. J. Vinken, and G. W. Bruyn (Eds.), *Handbook of Clinical Neurology,* Vol. 15, *The Epilepsies.* Amsterdam: Elsevier, 1974.
50. Sato, S., Dreifuss, F. E., and Penry, J. K. The effect of sleep on spike-wave discharges in absence seizures. *Neurology* (Minneap.) 23:1335, 1973.
51. Schmidt, R. P., and Wilder, B. J. *Epilepsy.* Philadelphia: Davis, 1968.
52. Schwartz, M. S., Prior, P. F., and Scott, D. F. The occurrence and evolution of the EEG of a lateralized periodic phenomenon. *Brain* 96:613, 1973.
53. Scott, G. M., and Gibberd, F. B. Epilepsy and other factors in the prognosis of glioma. *Acta Neurol. Scand.* 61:227, 1980.
54. Spencer, S. S. et al. Ictal effects of anticonvulsant medication withdrawal in epileptic patients. *Epilepsia* 22:297, 1981.
55. Sutherling, W. W., Hershman, L. M., and Lee, S. I. Seizures induced by playing music. *Neurology* (N.Y.) 30:1001, 1980.
56. Trimble, M. Non-monoamine oxidase inhibitor antidepressants and epilepsy: A review. *Epilepsia* 19:241, 1978.
57. Van Rensburg, M. J. et al. Temporal lobe epilepsy due to intracerebral Schwannoma: Case report. *J. Neurol. Neurosurg. Psychiatry* 38:703, 1975.
58. Victor, M., and Brausch, C. The role of abstinence in the genesis of alcoholic epilepsy. *Epilepsia* 8:1, 1967.
59. Walker, A. E., Caveness, W. F., and Critchley, M. *The Late Effects of Head Injury.* Springfield, Ill.: Thomas, 1969.
60. Ward, A. A. Basic Mechanisms of the Epilepsies. In M. Critchley, J. J. O'Leary, and B. Jennett (Eds.), *Scientific Foundations of Neurology.* Philadelphia: Davis, 1972.
61. White, P. T., Bailey, A. A., and Bickford, R. G. Epileptic disorders in the aged. *Neurology* (Minneap.) 3:674, 1953.
62. Wilkins, A. J. et al. Television epilepsy: The role of pattern. *Electroencephalogr. Clin. Neurophysiol.* 47:163, 1979.
63. Young, B. et al. Posttraumatic epilepsy prophylaxis. *Epilepsia* 20:671, 1979.
64. Zwillich, C. W. et al. Theophylline-induced seizures in adults. Correlation with serum concentrations. *Ann. Intern. Med.* 82:784, 1975.

RESOURCES AVAILABLE TO THE PATIENT WITH EPILEPSY

13

Edward B. Shaw

Like everyone else, people with epilepsy have many needs, but for many, epilepsy creates additional special needs. These needs vary from counseling to education. The way in which people with epilepsy approach their needs often reveals how well they are coping with their condition. Some patients are hostile and demanding, others are shy and withdrawn. Social and health care facilities often complicate matters by presenting to patients and their families an uncoordinated, tangled web of resources that compounds their confusion and frustration. The purpose of this chapter is to present a resource checklist that can be utilized in the patient's local area.

The Patient as a Resource

Persons with epilepsy are often called upon in the home, school, or work environment to explain or define their epilepsy. Frequently, there is a need to explain specific seizures, their causes and manifestations, and what others should do when a seizure occurs. Patients must be able to understand and explain their disorder in basic layman's terms. This is not always easy, since patients cannot observe their own seizures and may never have seen another person's seizures.

A failure to explain often leads people to conclude that the patient is unable to cope with their epilepsy. This perception can label the person with epilepsy as a social outcast. On the other hand, when the individual is well informed about their condition and is comfortable with it, communication is smooth, and the patient is understood as a person rather than as an "epileptic."

Family and Friends

The family and the patient's personal and social network are valuable resources. To a considerable extent, we all see ourselves as others see us, and positive perceptions by family and friends are important to our self-image.

Persons with newly diagnosed epilepsy are suddenly and unwillingly thrust into a new relationship with the rest of their personal universe. Many people feel that they are no longer in control of their lives. Family and friends can be of great help at this often devastating time by providing emotional support, by helping to make certain that the patient follows the medical regimen, and by assisting in vocational readjustments. To provide such assistance, family and friends must be educated to understand the nature of epilepsy and the role of antiepileptic drugs. They must also be cautioned not to overprotect the patient.

Epilepsy Organizations and Agencies

There are over 135 separate epilepsy organizations in the United States. Some are affiliated with the Epilepsy Foundation of America (EFA), a national organization,* and some are autonomous.

Such organizations generally offer many valuable resources to meet the needs of those with epilepsy. The local group is typically an excellent information and referral source. Here the person with epilepsy can receive up-to-date pamphlets and other suggested reading material as well as referrals for neurologic advice and other professional services. Many agencies also offer programs, seminars, and other contacts that many patients find valuable. They may publish newsletters, hold social events, and welcome volunteers. A recent very popular service is the self-help group, in which people with epilepsy and/or their parents or close family members share experiences, thereby providing mutual support and encouragement. Local epilepsy organizations often have resource directives that are of value both to patients with epilepsy and to social and health care professionals [5].

To find local epilepsy groups, write to the Epilepsy Foundation of America, check the white pages of the local phone book under the heading *epilepsy*, or call the local United Way agency.

Medications

Costs of antiepileptic medications vary widely from state to state and from pharmacy to pharmacy. The patient with epilepsy should be encouraged to comparison-shop. Because epilepsy generally entails a lifelong requirement for medication, a few dollars saved on each prescription will easily amount to a saving of several thousand dollars during a lifetime.

At the Epilepsy Society of Massachusetts, we regularly survey drug costs and publish the results in our newsletter. We have found that once we have contacted a pharmacy chain and expressed our concerns, their prices for antiepileptic drugs often go down dramatically. The consumer should not be afraid to ask the local pharmacy for the discount rate available at other pharmacies in exchange for continued patronage. The use of generic medications can also reduce costs. However, patients should first check with their physicians before changing generic brands of an antiepileptic drug because the pharmacologic proper-

ties of different generic preparations of the same drug may vary considerably (see Chap. 14).

Many medical or health insurance plans (individual, family, or group) will reimburse subscribers for 80 percent of their paid medical expenses, including prescription drugs, after a fixed deductible. For example, medical expenses for the insured person, including medications and doctor's visits, for a given year equal $400. The deductible is $100; 80 percent of the remaining $300 equals $240 that will be reimbursed. Insurance policies vary considerably, so it is important to read the terms and check all the fine print; insurers rarely publicize all reimbursable items. People under age 21 may be eligible for free antiepileptic medications through the federal government's Crippled Children's Services. These programs often include clinical services for children with neurologic problems and are administered by state health departments.

Discount medications in any quantity are available by mail through Pastors Pharmacy, 126 South York Avenue, Hatboro, Pa., 01940 (215-674-1565).

Free Medical Care

Under the federally sponsored Crippled Children's Services,* each state receives funds to operate various clinical programs. A check with the state health department should reveal the locations of neurology clinics that service those under age 21. The quality of service is generally very high, and this resource is especially valuable for a family that has no insurance and is unable to afford the cost of medical care.

Low-income people with severe epilepsy who are over 21 and have no insurance, may qualify for Medicaid, a public (federal-state) medical insurance program. A patient in need should be encouraged to apply at the local office of the state welfare, social service, or human resource agency.

Patients with epilepsy who are veterans can often qualify for free medical care and free medication at a Veterans Administration (VA) Medical Center. Excellent care for patients with epilepsy is available at many such centers.

Education

Until very recently, many children with epilepsy were denied education or were inappropriately relegated to "special" classes. Teachers and school systems frequently believed that a child with epilepsy should not be allowed to associate with "normal" children. Fortunately, such denial or inappropriate segregation is

---

*Located at 4351 Garden City Drive, Landover, Md., 20785 (301-459-3700).

*The program in a particular state may or may not be identified by this name. Some states refer to the program as Handicapped Children's Services.

now against the law. The Education for All Handicapped Children Act is a federal law (P.L. 94-142, signed in 1975) that guarantees the right to a publicly financed and individually determined special education program for each child with a handicapped condition, broadly defined. This includes the child with epilepsy. If a child with any kind of handicap or special educational need is denied an appropriate education, the parent should complain to the Office of Civil Rights of the US Department of Education. The purpose of this law is to ensure that every handicapped child receives an appropriate education; it encourages "mainstreaming" (i.e., integrating) handicapped children into regular educational settings as far as possible.

Many states also have their own special education laws. Massachusetts, for example, has a program for children with special needs. Of course, not all children with epilepsy will have special educational problems or needs. For the post–elementary school student, states and local school districts support numerous programs of vocational and technical education, which are usually available through both special and regular routes. For adults, the Department or Division of Education in each state should be consulted about programs such as high school equivalency, community colleges, adult education, and correspondence courses. Veterans with epilepsy may qualify for VA educational benefits.

Vocational Rehabilitation
Each state has a federally funded vocational rehabilitation program. For the older teenager or disabled adult of any age who needs or wants better employment opportunities, a check with the state vocational rehabilitation (VR) agency is recommended.

Epilepsy constitutes a "physical disability" for the purposes of eligibility requirements. The following rehabilitation services may be provided to an eligible person, although some depend on availability of funds, and all depend on the needs and interests of the disabled person:

1. Medical, psychologic, and vocational evaluation to determine the nature and degree of disability and to assess work capacity.
2. Counseling and guidance to achieve vocational goals or adjustment.
3. Medical, surgical, psychiatric, and hospital care, and related therapies to reduce or remove disability.
4. Vocational training in accordance with abilities, capacities, and limitations.
5. Transitional employment or extended employ-

ment for those who cannot be readily absorbed into the competitive labor market.
6. Placement and follow-up.

Employment
Patients with epilepsy who have employment problems resulting from inadequate training or preparation should be encouraged to seek the assistance of the state vocational rehabilitation agency. The counseling, rehabilitation training, and placement offered by these programs can often enable a person to achieve and maintain gainful employment. Each state has an Employment Security Office that is funded and administered under the Unemployment Insurance Program. This program offers services to handicapped individuals. Some of the services offered by the Employment Security Office include occupational listing, employment counseling, training programs, and placement.

State employment services are free and definitely worth checking out; some have special testing and other services for handicapped people that can be used by the job-seeker with epilepsy. Until recently, people with epilepsy frequently encountered employment discrimination regardless of the degree of seizure control. Recent federal laws that prohibit discrimination based upon a handicapped or health-related condition have encouraged many employers to consider positively an "otherwise qualified" handicapped applicant, including those with epilepsy. Employers may legally consider safety-related factors, however, and people with incomplete seizure control should plan their job prospects accordingly. Unfortunately, discrimination persists despite improved legal protections. Local epilepsy organizations can be consulted about both resources and discrimination problems.

The EFA administers a Training and Placement Service (TAPS) in six cities under a grant from the US Department of Labor. TAPS has developed many satellite programs throughout the country, and its services are unique in that they are designed especially and exclusively for job-seekers with epilepsy. Check with EFA or a local epilepsy organization.

A job-hunter with epilepsy should, of course, be encouraged to seek employment actively through help-wanted advertisements, employment agencies, referrals from friends, and all other normal channels.

People with epilepsy usually wonder whether, ethically or legally, they should tell a prospective employer about their condition. The general rule is that disclosure is not necessary unless the individual's condition would in some way affect job performance or raise potential safety hazards for the person or others. However, it is a personal decision, and some state laws will apply where federal law does not. (Federal employment discrimination laws generally apply only when the federal government or federal funds are involved; the "general rule" cited above is consistent with federal law.)

Insurance

Until recently obtainment of life insurance and health insurance has been difficult and expensive, if not impossible, for people with epilepsy. Whenever possible, a person with epilepsy is well advised to enroll in group insurance plans that are available through their own or their parents' places of employment or a membership association. Often, however, group coverage is not available, and a person desires to apply for an individual policy. According to the Underwriters Service Agency,* an agency that represents companies around the United States that specialize in writing life and health insurance, a variety of plans are now available to people with epilepsy. Several companies will underwrite people whose epilepsy is well controlled at standard rates; some companies will underwrite those with incomplete control. As a general rule, it is easier to get life insurance than full-coverage health insurance. Although many people are still denied coverage, at least decisions are now being made more and more on the basis of a person's insurability rather than on a categorical "epilepsy equals denial" basis.

Health insurance is available in several forms. Membership in Health Maintenance Organizations (HMOs) is increasingly available through either group or individual plans. With HMOs, however, as well as with more conventional medical insurance plans, there often is a waiting period or an exclusion of a preexisting condition such as epilepsy. The person with epilepsy should investigate the various insurance companies that sell life or health insurance and should thoroughly understand the costs and benefits and the extent of coverage before purchasing any plan.

In each state there is a state insurance regulatory agency, which can be located by a call to the governor's office or citizens' information service. The consumer affairs or legal staff of the state insurance agency can be a valuable resource when there are insurance-related problems.

If a person with epilepsy wishes to purchase a life or health insurance policy and cannot obtain satisfaction

locally, we recommend that he or she contact the Underwriters Service Agency at the address below.

Protection and Advocacy Programs

Many times the person with epilepsy and the family are faced with confusing and contradictory information. Such confusion can mean a reduced ability to "trouble-shoot" or advocate effectively to meet needs associated with this condition.

Each state offers a "protection and advocacy" (P and A) program for those who are "developmentally disabled." Epilepsy in its more severe forms is usually considered a developmental disability. Parents of children with epilepsy and adults who may need information about laws, legal rights, and state and federal programs serving the disabled should contact their state's P and A program. Check with the governor's office to locate the department responsible for developmental disabilities; that department will know who runs the P and A program. The P and A may or may not be within the state government, but it will be independent of all service-providers and will be oriented solely toward assisting developmentally disabled people to protect their rights and receive needed services.

Social Security Administration Programs

There are two separate programs with disability provisions for which the person disabled by epilepsy may be eligible; a qualified individual can receive benefits from one or both programs. The requirements for establishing disability, which basically involves both medical severity and chronic unemployability, are the same under both programs, but financial and other eligibility requirements are different.

SUPPLEMENTAL SECURITY INCOME (SSI)

This national program, created in 1974, replaced many preexisting and locally administered welfare programs to aid the disabled. The program is administered by the Social Security Administration, but it is not related to regular social security programs. It is a cash-assistance program; the amount of the monthly check, up to a ceiling amount, depends on the person's other resources. A person of any age who is disabled and has limited financial resources may be eligible for SSI. A disabled person is one who has a physical or mental impairment that prevents that person from doing substantial work and that is expected to last 12 months or result in death, or both; in the case of a child under 18, the label applies to an impairment of comparable severity that greatly interferes with normal growth and development.

*Contact Wilbur Bullen, Vice President, Underwriters Service Agency, Inc., 89 State Street, Boston, Mass. 02109.

In most states, SSI assistance automatically entitles the recipient to Medicaid benefits. This program is well worth looking into if income and personal resources are low and if epilepsy is severe. Information and applications are available from the local Social Security office.

People denied these benefits are advised to appeal such denials, because many mistakes are made in the determination process. Assistance may be available from the P and A program or from a legal aid or legal services office. One may also contact the local Bar Association for referrals to private attorneys who are specialists in social security disability.

SOCIAL SECURITY DISABILITY INSURANCE (SSDI)
The Social Security Disability Insurance program provides benefits for individuals who have worked long enough to be covered by Social Security and for disabled widows, widowers, and children of wage-earners, spouses, or parents who have become disabled, died, or retired. The local Social Security office should be able to assist the applicant with epilepsy.

The disability criteria are the same as those for SSI, but the person need not be low-income, only eligible through an insured person's payments into Social Security funds. SSDI recipients are not eligible for Medicaid but are eligible for Medicare after 24 months. A low-income SSDI recipient may be eligible for SSI as well; the Social Security office should advise and assist in this regard. Again, those who are denied benefits should seek legal assistance to prepare for formal appeal.

MEDICARE
Medicare is a health insurance program administered by the Social Security Administration. It is a program for people 65 years of age and older and some people who are under 65 and disabled. The program provides two types of medical insurance, Part A, hospital insurance, and Part B, supplemental protection against costs of physicians' services and other medical services and supplies. Contact a local or regional Social Security office with any questions concerning Medicare benefits. (Note: Medicaid is not administered by the Social Security Administration. For information about Medicaid, contact the state welfare or health agency.)

Miscellaneous Resources
Many services and resources are available to people with epilepsy and their families that are local or regional in scope, for example, discounts or half-fare rides are often offered by public transportation authorities.

AmTrak offers special fares for handicapped citizens, and there are many publicly funded, nonprofit corporations throughout the country that offer transportation for the elderly and handicapped.

In the private sector, Greyhound Bus Lines provides a Helping Hand Program that allows a handicapped person to have a travelling companion for the price of one ticket. There are many other programs of this nature.

When All Else Fails
Local epilepsy groups and other advocacy groups can often lead the person with epilepsy to the right resource. Groups representing other disabilities (e.g., cerebral palsy or multiple sclerosis) may have information useful to the person with epilepsy. We encourage people to ask forcefully and seek out the resources they need.

When all else fails, try the state attorney general's office. It is responsible for protecting its citizens, for civil rights and consumer rights, and can offer advice about state agency responsibilities, for example, special education or mental health or retardation services.

References
1. Aird, R. B., and Woodbury, D. *The Management of Epilepsy*. Springfield, Ill.: Thomas, 1974.
2. Boshes, L., and Gibbs, F. E. *Epilepsy Handbook* (2nd ed.). Springfield, Ill.: Thomas, 1972.
3. Epilepsy Foundation of America. *A Guide to Epilepsy Services*. Washington, D.C., 1976.
4. Epilepsy Foundation of America. *Legal Rights of Persons with Epilepsy*. Washington, D.C., 1976.
5. Epilepsy Society of Massachusetts, Inc. *Epilepsy in Massachusetts: A Reference Handbook* (revised ed.). Boston: January, 1981.
6. Goldin, G. J. *The Rehabilitation of the Young Epileptic*. Boston: D. C. Heath, 1971.
7. Sands, H., and Minters, F. C. *The Epilepsy Fact Book*. Philadelphia: Davis, 1977.
8. Silverstein, A., and Virginia, B. *Epilepsy*. Philadelphia: Lippincott, 1975.
9. Temkin, O. *The Falling Sickness: A History of Epilepsy from the Greeks to the Beginning of Modern Neurology* (2nd ed.). Baltimore: Johns Hopkins, 1971.
10. Volle, F. E., and Heron, P. A. *Epilepsy and You*. Springfield, Ill.: Thomas, 1977.
11. Wright, G. N., ed. *Epilepsy Rehabilitation*. Boston: Little, Brown, 1975.

Thomas R. Browne

...ug [24]. Free drug concentration is
by the dosing rate and the ability of
..o biotransform or excrete the free
...ate and free drug clearance remain
...ncentration of the drug will fall and
... increase when protein binding de-
...concentration, and therefore clinical
...ain unchanged.

...on of free drug is the same in intra-
...d in serum for most antiepileptic
..., the total concentration of the drug
...gher in cells than in serum if the drug
...mponents (proteins, nucleoproteins,
... of the cell [20, 76]. Most antiepi-
...re lipid-soluble and accumulate in
...Persons with large amounts of adipose
...rly and the obese) have more extensive
...ion of lipid-soluble drugs, but no
...y-state serum concentration [25].

...LUIDS: CSF, SALIVA, AND TEARS
...ved as a plasma ultrafiltrate with a low
...ration (and hence little protein bind-
...entrations of phenytoin, phenobarbi-
...carbamazepine, and ethosuximide in
...ially identical to the concentrations of
...he serum [6]. Similar considerations
...and tears, and the possibility that the
...of antiepileptic drugs in saliva or tears
...nely determined as a means of determin-
...ntration of free drug in the serum is
...ated [32, 36, 42, 43, 44, 46, 51].

...ation and Excretion

...s
...ptic drugs are inactivated and eliminated
...biotransformation by the hepatic micro-
... function oxidase system (cytochrome
..., which transforms antiepileptic drugs
...d metabolites. These metabolites are
...effective antiepileptic drugs than the
...out biotransformation to active metabo-
...urs (see below). The oxidized metabo-
...lly more polar than the parent drug and
...xcreted by the kidney.

...S OF BIOTRANSFORMATION AND EXCRETION
...phenobarbital, and ethosuximide first
...oxidation reaction and are then excreted
...: oxidized metabolite and partly as con-
...lized metabolite (see Chaps. 16, 17, 19).
...xidation step renders these drugs inactive

as antiepileptic drugs. Primidone is oxidized to two
active metabolites, phenobarbital and phenylethylmalonamide (see Chap. 17). Carbamazepine may
undergo oxidation to form carbamazepine-10,11-
epoxide or carbamazepine-10,11-dihydroxide (see
Chap. 18). Carbamazepine may also undergo loss of
the carbamide group to form iminostilbene (see Chap.
18). Carbamazepine-10,11-dihydroxide has antiepileptic activity [6]. Methsuximide is first demethylated
to form N-desmethyl-methsuximide (NDM), an active
metabolite that is the major antiepileptic substance
in the plasma of patients taking methsuximide (see
Chap. 19). Methsuximide and NDM are then inactivated by oxidation and excreted as oxidized and
conjugated oxidized metabolites (see Chap. 19).
Valproic acid is eliminated by direct conjugation of the
parent drug and by oxidation of the parent drug (see
Chap. 20). The major metabolic pathway of clonazepam is reduction of the nitro group to form an inactive
7-amino derivative (see Chap. 21).

Acetazolamide, bromine, and dimethadione are
eliminated almost entirely by direct renal excretion
(see Chap. 22). Phenobarbital, primidone, and ethosuximide are partly eliminated by direct renal excretion but principally as biotransformed metabolites
(see Chaps. 17 and 19).

EFFECTS OF AGE
The rates of biotransformation of drugs may change
with age. Many drugs are slowly metabolized by neonates because of their immature hepatic microsomes.
Hydroxylation of phenytoin and conjugation of phenobarbital proceed more slowly in neonates than in
children or adults [5, 6, 45, 54, 60]. On the other hand,
children metabolize phenytoin and phenobarbital
more rapidly than adults and require higher doses of
phenytoin and phenobarbital (in mg/kg) to achieve a
given serum concentration [6, 45, 54, 60] (see Chaps.
16 and 17). Biotransformation rates may change (decrease) very abruptly at puberty [54].

At the other end of the age spectrum, there is evidence that the elimination half-lives of phenytoin,
phenobarbital, and diazepam are longer in the elderly
than in young adults [3, 61]. These changes appear to
be due chiefly to slower metabolism [25, 61].

Renal excretion also changes with age. Neonates
have a lower renal clearance of drugs than older infants or children [45, 54]. The glomerular filtration
rate and renal excretion of intact drug decline predictably in old age, with a mean 35 percent reduction
in the elderly as compared with young adults [25].

EFFECTS OF HEPATIC FAILURE
In patients with hepatic disease the rate of hepatic
biotransformation of drugs and hepatic blood flow are

The physician who understands the pharmacologic
principles of antiepileptic drug administration can
greatly improve the effectiveness with which he uses
these drugs. This chapter will first review the principles
of absorption, distribution, biotransformation, excretion, pharmacokinetics, and drug interactions that
are of special clinical significance for antiepileptic
drugs. This will be followed by a discussion of how
these principles can be applied to develop guidelines
for optimal administration of antiepileptic drugs.
Finally, the drugs of choice for various types of seizures will be reviewed.

Absorption

ORAL ROUTE

Effect of Generic Preparations
Different oral preparations of the same generic drug
may have different bioavailability [6, 12, 52, 60]. There
may be lowered drug serum concentration with increased seizure frequency or increased drug serum
concentration with increased drug toxicity if the
brand of antiepileptic drug capsule or tablet used by a
patient is changed [19, 57, 60, 69]. It is best to specify
that the patient take only one generic form of an antiepileptic drug.

Oral Suspension Preparations
The oral suspension form of phenytoin has significantly greater bioavailability than many capsule
preparations of the same drug [52]. Patients who do
not absorb phenytoin capsules well may have a significant increase in serum phenytoin concentration when
switched to the oral suspension form. Ethosuximide
has a high bioavailability in both capsule and liquid
forms [10].

Effect of Age and Pregnancy
Absorption of phenytoin in neonates is incomplete
and erratic [5, 49]. There is no evidence that drug
absorption is impaired in old age [25]. The effect of
pregnancy on drug absorption is reviewed in Chapter 29.

INTRAMUSCULAR ROUTE
There are many problems with administration of antiepileptic drugs by the intramuscular route [23].

This work was supported in part by the Veterans Administration.

Phenytoin is a weak acid with a pK$_a$ of approximately 9.0 [76]. To get phenytoin into solution in a small volume of liquid, it must be prepared in a solution of pH 12. When it is injected intramuscularly (i.e., into a medium with a pH of about 7.4), the water solubility of the drug decreases considerably, phenytoin crystals precipitate in the muscle [66, 75], and the drug is absorbed very slowly [35, 71].

Peak serum phenytoin concentrations occur approximately 24 hours after a single intramuscular injection and are significantly less than the peak concentrations produced by the same dose given by rapid intravenous infusion [35]. Peak phenobarbital and diazepam concentrations are reached 1 to 12 hours and 45 to 60 minutes, respectively, after intramuscular injection (see Chap. 30). Peak serum concentrations of diazepam after intramuscular injection are substantially less than the peak concentrations produced by the same dose given as an intravenous bolus (see Chap. 30). Antiepileptic drugs should not be given via the intramuscular route in status epilepticus and other emergencies because of the slowness of absorption and the relatively low peak serum concentrations produced by this route.

Use of the intramuscular route for administration of maintenance doses of antiepileptic drugs remains controversial. Eventually, almost all of an intramuscular injection of phenytoin is absorbed, and regimens for intramuscular administration of maintenance doses of phenytoin have been published [53, 73]. However, the following problems are associated with intramuscular administration: (1) peak phenytoin serum concentrations occur 24 hours after an intramuscular injection; (2) there is variability in the phenytoin serum concentrations produced by these regimens; (3) phenytoin serum concentrations may fall below therapeutic levels shortly after switching to the intramuscular route from the oral or intravenous route; (4) toxic serum concentrations of phenytoin may accumulate after switching back from the intramuscular route to the oral route [13, 35, 66, 73, 75]. Intramuscular phenobarbital and diazepam are slowly absorbed, and the bioavailability of these drugs by this route is not known. In most situations maintenance doses of antiepileptic drugs should not be given by the intramuscular route because of the slowness and variability of absorption and because of the danger of overmedication and undermedication when switching to and from other routes of administration.

Distribution

ROUTE OF ADMINISTRATION

Following administration of an antiepileptic drug by the oral or intramuscular route, there is a rise and then a fall in serum concentration of the drug. The rates of rise and fall of serum concentration of the drug depend on the rates of absorption, distribution, and elimination of the drug [18, 22]. Following intravenous administration of a drug there is a high initial peak drug serum concentration followed by a rapid fall in serum concentration, corresponding to the distribution of the drug into various compartments [18, 22]. Then there is a second phase in which serum concentration declines more slowly, corresponding to the elimination of the drug by the processes of biotransformation and excretion [18, 22]. Phenytoin and diazepam demonstrate this type of "biphasic" fall in serum concentration after intravenous administration [6]. The pharmacokinetics of intravenous phenobarbital have not been extensively studied. The half-life of the fall of serum concentration during the "distribution" phase after intravenous injection is 0.38 to 1.23 hours for phenytoin, and 15 to 60 minutes for diazepam [6] (see Chap. 30). When administering a loading dose of intravenous phenytoin, it is necessary to give a large enough dose so that a therapeutic serum concentration will be present after the rapid fall in serum concentration during the distribution phase (see below). The rapid fall in serum diazepam concentration following an intravenous injection may account for the observation that status epilepticus frequently recurs after a single intravenous injection of diazepam if a long-acting antiepileptic drug is not also given (see Chap. 30).

DISTRIBUTION TO ACTIVE SITE

Antiepileptic drugs presumably act on neurons and/or glial cells of the central nervous system. To enter these cells, the drug molecules must pass the blood-brain barrier and the cell membrane. The rate of penetration of brain cells by an antiepileptic drug depends on lipid solubility and other factors. The concentration of phenytoin and phenobarbital in the brain parenchyma and cerebrospinal fluid (CSF) may not reach peak levels in humans until an hour or more after an intravenous injection [50, 74]. However, animal and human work indicate that the concentration of phenytoin in the brain parenchyma remains greater than the serum concentration of unbound phenytoin once peak brain concentrations have been reached, presumably because of binding by tissue protein and phospholipids [20]. Diazepam enters the brain parenchyma very rapidly and the brain concentration of diazepam closely parallels the serum concentration [6, 50]. Thus the brain concentration of diazepam peaks soon after an intravenous injection but falls rapidly in association with the rapidly falling serum concentration. These observations provide a

Table 14-1. Pharmacologic Data on Antiepileptic Drugs

Drug	Elimination Half-Life in Adults (hr.)	Elimination Half-Life in Children (hr.)	Time to Reach Stead State (days)
Acetazolamide	—	—	—
Carbamazepine	14–27	14–27 (children) 8–28 (neonates)	3–4
Clonazepam	20–40	20–40	—
Ethosuximide	20–60	20–60	7–10
Ethotoin	5	—	—
Mephenytoin	7	—	—
Nirvanol[b]	96	—	21
Methsuximide	1–3	—	—
N-desmethyl-methsuximide[d]	34–80	—	8–17
Paraldehyde	—	3–10	—
Phenobarbital	46–136	37–73 (children) 61–173 (neonates)	14–21
Phenytoin	10–34	5–14 (children) 10–60 (neonates) 10–140 (prematures)	7–28
Primidone[e]	6–18	5–11	4–7
Trimethadione	16	16	—
Dimethadione[f]	240	240	30
Valproic acid	6–15	8–15	1–2

[a]See Appendix I for conversion to other units.
[b]Active metabolite of mephenytoin and major antiepileptic drug in plasma of patients taking m
[c]Sum of nirvanol plus mephenytoin plasma concentrations.
[d]Active metabolite of methsuximide and major antiepileptic drug in plasma of patients taking n
[e]Metabolized to phenobarbital and phenylethylmalonamide. Both these derivatives have antiepi
[f]Active metabolite of trimethadione and major antiepileptic drug in serum of patients taking trim

basis for the therapeutic strategy of treating status epilepticus with a single dose of intravenous diazepam (to stop the seizures quickly) followed immediately by a loading dose of phenytoin to provide long-term antiepileptic activity.

PROTEIN BINDING

Upon entering the bloodstream antiepileptic drugs are bound to differing degrees by plasma proteins, principally albumin. The extent of protein binding by various antiepileptic drugs is listed in Table 14-1. Protein binding has several important clinical implications. First, the serum drug concentration determinations performed by most laboratories measure the total drug serum concentration, not the free (non-protein-bound) serum concentration. Second, only the free drug can enter active sites from the plasma, and there is evidence that the concentration of free antiepileptic drug in the serum correlates better with efficacy and toxicity than does the total drug concen-

tration of free d
determined only
clearing organs
drug. If dosing
constant, total c
free fraction wi
creases, but free
activity, will rem

CELL STORAGE

The concentrat
cellular fluid a
drugs. Howeve
can be much h
is bound by c
phospholipids)
leptic drugs a
adipose tissue.
tissue (the elde
tissue distribu
change in stea

TRANSCELLULAR F
CSF may be vie
protein concer
ing). The con
tal, primidone
CSF are essen
free drug in
apply to saliva
concentration
might be routi
ing the conce
being investig

Biotransfor

BASIC PRINCIPL
Most antiepil
as a result of
somal mixed
P-450 system
into oxidize
usually less
parent drug,
lites also oc
lites are usu
more easily

USUAL ROUT
Phenytoin,
undergo an
partly as th
jugated ox
The initial

tration [4]. Thir
serum is inverse
centration. Patien
trations have a l
concentration) of
probability of dev
for a given total c
patients with a h
[6, 34, 56]. Fourth
antiepileptic drug
from its protein-bi

Plasma protein b
children and young
of the age spectr
creases by 18 perce
decrease correlates
trations and does no
in binding affinity.

Reduced protein b
of a drug does *not*

slowed, resulting in slowing of inactivation and/or conversion to active metabolites of antiepileptic drugs [6, 37, 60]. In addition, the protein binding of antiepileptic drugs may be reduced by any of three mechanisms: (1) hypoalbuminemia, (2) displacement by bilirubin or other substances, and (3) changes in the configuration of albumin [60]. These alterations tend to increase both the total serum drug concentration and the percentage of free drug in the serum.

Unfortunately, there is no formula for predicting the proper dose of an antiepileptic drug in a patient with hepatic dysfunction based on serum albumin concentration and/or liver function tests. One must adjust drug dosage on the basis of frequent determinations of drug serum concentration.

EFFECTS OF RENAL FAILURE
The clearance of drugs eliminated entirely by the kidney (acetazolamide, bromine, dimethadione) may be considerably slowed by renal disease, resulting in a large rise in serum concentration [37]. The serum concentration of drugs partly eliminated by the kidney (phenobarbital, primidone, ethosuximide) may also rise in renal failure [37, 38].

The effects of renal failure on elimination of drugs that are principally eliminated by the liver have been illustrated by clinical studies with phenytoin. Uremic patients receiving phenytoin have lower total serum phenytoin concentrations, higher serum hydroxyphenyl-phenylhydantoin (HPPH, the principal metabolite of phenytoin) concentrations, and shorter phenytoin elimination half-lives than nonuremic patients receiving the same dosage of phenytoin [27, 39, 47]. In renal failure the hepatic biotransformation processes continue and may accelerate, but renal excretion of metabolites is slowed [37]. The high serum concentration of HPPH is presumably due to impaired renal excretion of the metabolite. The short elimination half-life is presumably due to increased accessibility of phenytoin to hepatic biotransformation enzymes due to decreased protein binding caused by low serum albumin concentration, by displacement of phenytoin from protein-binding sites by HPPH and endogenous metabolites, and by structural alterations of plasma proteins [37]. The low serum phenytoin concentration is presumably due to the low serum albumin concentration or to an increased rate of hepatic biotransformation, or both.

EFFECTS OF HEMODIALYSIS AND PLASMAPHERESIS
Hemodialysis has little effect on the serum concentration of lipid-soluble drugs (e.g., phenytoin) [41]. However, hemodialysis can remove significant quantities of water-soluble drugs, which normally are ex-creted in part by the kidney (e.g., primidone) with a resulting fall in serum concentration [38]. Plasmapheresis has been reported to remove significant quantities of phenytoin [41].

Pharmacokinetics of Antiepileptic Drugs

DEFINITIONS

Pharmacokinetics
Pharmacokinetics is the quantitative study of the combined processes of drug absorption, distribution, biotransformation, and excretion to produce mathematical models that will predict the concentration of a drug in various parts of the body as a function of dosage, route of administration, and time after administration [22]. Knowledge of basic pharmacokinetic principles [18, 22, 26] allows the physician to administer antiepileptic drugs in a safer and more effective manner. This section will review the application of pharmacokinetic principles to the administration of antiepileptic drugs and will summarize the pharmacokinetic values that one must know in order to apply these principles to the administration of the most frequently used antiepileptic drugs. Before these topics are reviewed, certain other terms must be defined.

First Order Enzyme Kinetics
In first order enzyme processes (e.g., many biotransformation reactions) the rate of the reaction varies directly with the concentration of the drug. This can be expressed mathematically as:

$$\frac{dc}{dt} = -kc$$

where c = concentration of drug, t = time, and k = a constant. This is the type of reaction seen when an enzyme system is not saturated.

Zero Order Enzyme Kinetics
In zero order processes the rate of the reaction is the same regardless of drug concentration. This can be expressed mathematically as:

$$\frac{dc}{dt} = -k.$$

This is the type of reaction seen when an enzyme system is saturated.

With first order elimination kinetics, the steady state serum concentration of a drug increases proportionally with increasing dosage, while the elimination half-life remains constant. With zero order elimination

150

kinetics, the enzymes responsible for elimination of the drug are saturated, the concentration of the drug increases disproportionally with increases in dosage, and the apparent elimination half-life increases with increasing dosage.

These considerations are particularly important in the case of phenytoin. With doses up to 4 to 12 mg/kg/day there is a proportional increase in phenytoin serum concentration with increasing dosage, and the elimination half-life remains constant at about 24 hours (i.e., first order kinetics) [6, 60]. When the dosage exceeds 4 to 12 mg/kg/day, a small increase in dosage may produce a large increase in phenytoin serum concentration, an increase in apparent elimination half-life, and unexpected drug toxicity [6, 60]. This phenomenon is presumably due to saturation of the enzyme system that eliminates phenytoin and a change from first order to zero order kinetics [6, 33, 60].

Compartments
Compartments are fictitious, nonanatomic volumes into which drugs are assumed to be taken up after administration. The simplest pharmacokinetic model is the one-compartment model, which views the body as a single compartment with only two unit processes, absorption and elimination (i.e., biotransformation plus excretion). Distribution is assumed to be uniform in all body tissues and to occur rapidly in relation to absorption and elimination. This simple model often accurately predicts the clinical pharmacokinetics of antiepileptic drugs during chronic oral administration. A more complex two or more compartment model is usually necessary to predict the pharmacokinetics of single doses of a drug because of the dramatic changes in drug concentration in body tissues that occur during distribution [22].

"Therapeutic Range" of Serum Concentration
The lower limit of the therapeutic range of serum concentration of antiepileptic drugs is usually defined as the serum concentration below which a majority of patients fail to have a significant reduction in seizure frequency. The upper limit of the therapeutic range of serum concentration is usually defined as the serum concentration above which a majority of patients develop disturbing signs or symptoms of intoxication. Published therapeutic ranges of serum concentration of antiepileptic drugs thus represent values indicative of the majority of patients, but not all patients. Some patients may have good therapeutic responses with drug serum concentrations below the lower limit of the therapeutic range [16]. Some patients may exhibit

considerable intoxication with serum concentrations that are within the therapeutic range. Other patients may require serum concentrations above the therapeutic range for seizure control and show no signs or symptoms of intoxication with such concentrations. The therapeutic ranges of serum concentration of antiepileptic drugs are listed in Table 14-1.

CLINICAL APPLICATIONS

Fundamental Principles
Figure 14-1 shows the fundamental pharmacokinetic relationships predicted by the one-compartment model assuming first order elimination kinetics. When administration of a drug is stopped, the concentration of the drug in the serum decreases exponentially. After one elimination half-life the concentration of the drug has decreased by 50 percent, and after five elimination half-lives the concentration of the drug has decreased by more than 95 percent.

Many physicians are not aware of the converse relationship shown in Figure 14-1. When a constant intravenous infusion of a drug is begun, the concentration of the drug in the serum will accumulate at a rate that is the reciprocal of its rate of elimination. After one elimination half-life the concentration of drug in the serum is 50 percent of the steady state concentration. After five elimination half-lives the serum concentration is essentially at its steady state value. At this point the rate of infusion is equal to the rate of elimination of the drug from the body.

Most drugs are not given as constant intravenous in-

Figure 14-1. Fundamental pharmacokinetic relationships predicted by one-compartment model with first order elimination kinetics. Inset table indicates the percentages of completion of elimination or build-up to steady state concentration after multiples of drug's elimination half-life. (From T. R. Browne, Clinical pharmacology of antiepileptic drugs. Drug Ther. Rev. 2:469, 1979.)

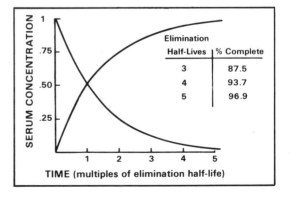

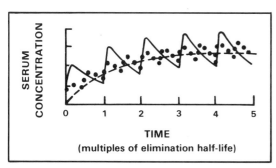

Figure 14-2. Predicted kinetic patterns when the same dose per unit time of a drug is given by constant intravenous infusion (dashed line), at intervals equal to the elimination half-life (solid line), and at intervals equal to one half the elimination half-life (dotted line). (From T. R. Browne, Clinical pharmacology of antiepileptic drugs. Drug. Ther. Rev. 2:469, 1979.)

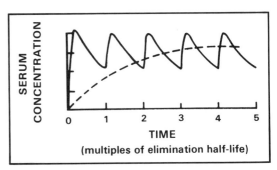

Figure 14-3. Predicted kinetic pattern during repeated administration of unit doses of a drug at intervals equal to its elimination half-life after initial loading dose equal to two unit doses. Dashed line shows predicted kinetic pattern for continuous intravenous infusion of drug at a rate of one unit dose per elimination half-life. (From T. R. Browne, Clinical pharmacology of antiepileptic drugs. Drug Ther. Rev. 2:469, 1979.)

fusions but as fixed doses at fixed intervals. Figure 14-2 shows the rise in serum concentration when the same dose per unit time of a drug is given by constant infusion at intervals equal to the elimination half-life and at intervals equal to one half the elimination half-life. The time required to reach steady state and the mean serum drug concentration are the same for all three schedules; all that varies is the range of fluctuation of serum concentration between doses. The relationships shown in Figure 14-2 apply to intravenously administered drugs and to orally administered drugs that have rapid absorption and distribution relative to elimination.

Table 14-1 lists the elimination half-lives and the time required to reach steady state serum concentration with chronic oral administration for the most commonly prescribed antiepileptic drugs. It will be seen that the time required to reach steady state serum concentration is approximately five times the elimination half-life.

Probably the most important pharmacokinetic relationship to be aware of when administering antiepileptic drugs is that every time a new drug is begun, or the dosage of a drug is raised or lowered, five elimination half-lives must elapse before the new steady state serum concentration is known and the full therapeutic effect of the medication change can be judged. Too often an antiepileptic drug is discarded as ineffective because inadequate time has been allowed for build-up of a steady state concentration. Similarly, the dosage of a drug is sometimes increased too rapidly because not enough time is allowed for the serum concentration to reach a steady state before the dose of the drug is raised again. This may result in the accumulation of toxic concentrations of the drug.

Another frequent error is to make two changes at the same time in the dosage or type of antiepileptic drug being given. This results in a very complex situation because (1) different antiepileptic drugs work by different mechanisms, (2) different antiepileptic drugs often have similar side effects, (3) the concentration of the two drugs is changing at the same time but at different rates, and (4) addition or subtraction of drugs may alter the metabolism of other drugs whose dosage is not changed. If good seizure control, increased seizure frequency, drug toxicity, or a large change in the serum concentration of a drug whose dosage was not altered occurs after two or more changes in drug regimen are made simultaneously, one does not know which change is responsible for the observed effect. In nonemergency situations it is usually best to make only one change at a time in the antiepileptic drug regimen.

Loading Dose

The one-compartment, first order kinetics model predicts that if unit doses of a drug are given intravenously at intervals equal to its elimination half-life, the initial serum concentration after the initial intravenous dose will be one-half the peak value reached during chronic administration (Fig. 14-2). Figure 14-3 shows that under these conditions steady state serum concentration can be achieved immediately if the initial dose is twice the maintenance dose per elimination half-life. This is the principle of the loading dose. It is necessary to give such a loading dose if one wishes to reach a therapeutic serum concentration of an antiepileptic drug immediately. Figure 14-4 shows that the administration of 500 mg of phenytoin intra-

152

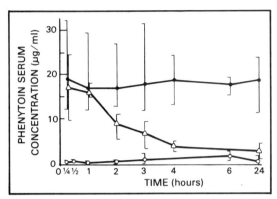

Figure 14-4. Range and mean of phenytoin serum concentrations over 24 hours with parenteral phenytoin. Dark dots: Twenty-six patients treated with 1000 mg IV, 500 mg IM, and 300 to 500 mg IV or orally daily as maintenance doses. Triangles: Five volunteers treated with 500 mg IM, 500 mg IV, and 100 mg IV every 6 hours as maintenance doses. Open circles: Six volunteers treated with 500 mg IM. (From W. Wallis, H. Kutt, and F. McDowell, Intravenous diphenylhydantoin in treatment of acute repetitive seizures. Neurology [Minneap.] 18:513, 1968.)

venously (a little more than the usual maintenance dose of 300 to 400 mg per half-life of about 24 hours) fails to produce consistently a therapeutic serum concentration (10 to 20 μg/ml), whereas 1000 mg of phenytoin administered intravenously does produce this concentration. Figure 14-4 also demonstrates that intramuscular phenytoin is absorbed very slowly. In adults it is necessary to administer an intravenous loading dose of 13 to 14 mg/kg of phenytoin to achieve therapeutic serum concentrations consistently (see Chap. 30). In infants, the proper loading dose of phenytoin is probably the same as it is in adults or slightly greater [49]. The loading dose of intravenous phenobarbital necessary to achieve therapeutic serum concentrations has not been extensively studied but is probably 10 to 20 mg/kg (see Chap. 30).

Choice of Dosage Interval

Pharmacokinetic principles can also assist in choosing a dosage interval for an antiepileptic drug. Ideally, such a drug should be administered using as long an interval between doses as practical. Drug regimens requiring more frequent administration than once per day are not followed as well by outpatients as regimens requiring once daily administration [17, 48, 55]. The one-compartment first order kinetics model predicts that peak serum concentration will increase proportionally with increasing dosage, whereas the duration of the serum drug concentration at or above a given minimal therapeutic concentration increases by

Table 14-2. Phenytoin Serum Concentration Fluctuation in Six Patients Receiving Once-Daily Doses*

	Serum Concentration (μg/ml)	
Dose (mg/kg)	High	Low
8.0	15	8
5.2	37	19
4.8	26	18
7.5	40	27
5.3	16	7
8.2	29	20

*Serum phenytoin concentrations were determined 0, 2, 4, 6, 8, 10, 12, 14, 16, and 24 hours after oral dose.
Source: Modified from B. J. Wilder, R. R. Streiff, and R. H. Hammer. Diphenylhydantoin Absorption, Distribution, and Excretion: Clinical Studies. In D. M. Woodbury, J. K. Penry, and R. P. Schmidt (Eds.), *Antiepileptic Drugs.* New York: Raven Press, 1972. Pp. 137–148.

one elimination half-life with each doubling of dose [26]. Increasing the dosage by twofold will increase the peak serum concentration twofold and will increase the duration of the minimal therapeutic serum concentration by one elimination half-life. Increasing the dosage by fourfold will increase the peak serum concentration fourfold but will increase the duration of the minimal therapeutic serum concentration by only two elimination half-lives. Increasing the dosage by eightfold will increase the peak serum concentration eightfold but will increase the duration of the minimal therapeutic serum concentration by only three elimination half-lives. Because of the toxicity associated with high peak serum concentrations of antiepileptic drugs, the choice of dosage interval must represent a compromise that maximizes the duration of effective serum concentration and minimizes the toxicity associated with peak serum concentrations. In practice, antiepileptic drugs whose elimination half-lives are 24 hours or longer usually need to be given only once daily to maintain a therapeutic serum concentration [8, 9, 21, 28, 56, 72]. Table 14-2 illustrates that there is approximately a twofold range in phenytoin serum concentration when the drug is given once every elimination half-life (i.e., once every 24 hours). The daily dose is usually best given at bedtime to avoid the sedative effect associated with peak levels of antiepileptic drugs.

Limits of Pharmacokinetic Principles

The pharmacokinetic principles discussed in this section are not intended to be a substitute for clinical judgment or a substitute for the measurement of the

PHARMACOLOGIC PRINCIPLES OF ANTIEPILEPTIC DRUG ADMINISTRATION

14

Thomas R. Browne

The physician who understands the pharmacologic principles of antiepileptic drug administration can greatly improve the effectiveness with which he uses these drugs. This chapter will first review the principles of absorption, distribution, biotransformation, excretion, pharmacokinetics, and drug interactions that are of special clinical significance for antiepileptic drugs. This will be followed by a discussion of how these principles can be applied to develop guidelines for optimal administration of antiepileptic drugs. Finally, the drugs of choice for various types of seizures will be reviewed.

Absorption

ORAL ROUTE

Effect of Generic Preparations
Different oral preparations of the same generic drug may have different bioavailability [6, 12, 52, 60]. There may be lowered drug serum concentration with increased seizure frequency or increased drug serum concentration with increased drug toxicity if the brand of antiepileptic drug capsule or tablet used by a patient is changed [19, 57, 60, 69]. It is best to specify that the patient take only one generic form of an antiepileptic drug.

Oral Suspension Preparations
The oral suspension form of phenytoin has significantly greater bioavailability than many capsule preparations of the same drug [52]. Patients who do not absorb phenytoin capsules well may have a significant increase in serum phenytoin concentration when switched to the oral suspension form. Ethosuximide has a high bioavailability in both capsule and liquid forms [10].

Effect of Age and Pregnancy
Absorption of phenytoin in neonates is incomplete and erratic [5, 49]. There is no evidence that drug absorption is impaired in old age [25]. The effect of pregnancy on drug absorption is reviewed in Chapter 29.

INTRAMUSCULAR ROUTE
There are many problems with administration of antiepileptic drugs by the intramuscular route [23].

This work was supported in part by the Veterans Administration.

Phenytoin is a weak acid with a pK_a of approximately 9.0 [76]. To get phenytoin into solution in a small volume of liquid, it must be prepared in a solution of pH 12. When it is injected intramuscularly (i.e., into a medium with a pH of about 7.4), the water solubility of the drug decreases considerably, phenytoin crystals precipitate in the muscle [66, 75], and the drug is absorbed very slowly [35, 71].

Peak serum phenytoin concentrations occur approximately 24 hours after a single intramuscular injection and are significantly less than the peak concentrations produced by the same dose given by rapid intravenous infusion [35]. Peak phenobarbital and diazepam concentrations are reached 1 to 12 hours and 45 to 60 minutes, respectively, after intramuscular injection (see Chap. 30). Peak serum concentrations of diazepam after intramuscular injection are substantially less than the peak concentrations produced by the same dose given as an intravenous bolus (see Chap. 30). Antiepileptic drugs should not be given via the intramuscular route in status epilepticus and other emergencies because of the slowness of absorption and the relatively low peak serum concentrations produced by this route.

Use of the intramuscular route for administration of maintenance doses of antiepileptic drugs remains controversial. Eventually, almost all of an intramuscular injection of phenytoin is absorbed, and regimens for intramuscular administration of maintenance doses of phenytoin have been published [53, 73]. However, the following problems are associated with intramuscular administration: (1) peak phenytoin serum concentrations occur 24 hours after an intramuscular injection; (2) there is variability in the phenytoin serum concentrations produced by these regimens; (3) phenytoin serum concentrations may fall below therapeutic levels shortly after switching to the intramuscular route from the oral or intravenous route; (4) toxic serum concentrations of phenytoin may accumulate after switching back from the intramuscular route to the oral route [13, 35, 66, 73, 75]. Intramuscular phenobarbital and diazepam are slowly absorbed, and the bioavailability of these drugs by this route is not known. In most situations maintenance doses of antiepileptic drugs should not be given by the intramuscular route because of the slowness and variability of absorption and because of the danger of overmedication and undermedication when switching to and from other routes of administration.

Distribution

ROUTE OF ADMINISTRATION
Following administration of an antiepileptic drug by the oral or intramuscular route, there is a rise and then a fall in serum concentration of the drug. The rates of rise and fall of serum concentration of the drug depend on the rates of absorption, distribution, and elimination of the drug [18, 22]. Following intravenous administration of a drug there is a high initial peak drug serum concentration followed by a rapid fall in serum concentration, corresponding to the distribution of the drug into various compartments [18, 22]. Then there is a second phase in which serum concentration declines more slowly, corresponding to the elimination of the drug by the processes of biotransformation and excretion [18, 22]. Phenytoin and diazepam demonstrate this type of "biphasic" fall in serum concentration after intravenous administration [6]. The pharmacokinetics of intravenous phenobarbital have not been extensively studied. The half-life of the fall of serum concentration during the "distribution" phase after intravenous injection is 0.38 to 1.23 hours for phenytoin, and 15 to 60 minutes for diazepam [6] (see Chap. 30). When administering a loading dose of intravenous phenytoin, it is necessary to give a large enough dose so that a therapeutic serum concentration will be present after the rapid fall in serum concentration during the distribution phase (see below). The rapid fall in serum diazepam concentration following an intravenous injection may account for the observation that status epilepticus frequently recurs after a single intravenous injection of diazepam if a long-acting antiepileptic drug is not also given (see Chap. 30).

DISTRIBUTION TO ACTIVE SITE
Antiepileptic drugs presumably act on neurons and/or glial cells of the central nervous system. To enter these cells, the drug molecules must pass the blood-brain barrier and the cell membrane. The rate of penetration of brain cells by an antiepileptic drug depends on lipid solubility and other factors. The concentration of phenytoin and phenobarbital in the brain parenchyma and cerebrospinal fluid (CSF) may not reach peak levels in humans until an hour or more after an intravenous injection [50, 74]. However, animal and human work indicate that the concentration of phenytoin in the brain parenchyma remains greater than the serum concentration of unbound phenytoin once peak brain concentrations have been reached, presumably because of binding by tissue protein and phospholipids [20]. Diazepam enters the brain parenchyma very rapidly and the brain concentration of diazepam closely parallels the serum concentration [6, 50]. Thus the brain concentration of diazepam peaks soon after an intravenous injection but falls rapidly in association with the rapidly falling serum concentration. These observations provide a

Table 14-1. Pharmacologic Data on Antiepileptic Drugs

Drug	Elimination Half-Life in Adults (hr.)	Elimination Half-Life in Children (hr.)	Time to Reach Steady State (days)	Therapeutic Range of Serum Concentration (μg/ml)[a]	Protein Binding (%)
Acetazolamide	—	—	—	10–14	83–95
Carbamazepine	14–27	14–27 (children) 8–28 (neonates)	3–4	4–12	66–89
Clonazepam	20–40	20–40	—	0.005–0.070	47
Ethosuximide	20–60	20–60	7–10	40–100	0
Ethotoin	5	—	—	15–50	46
Mephenytoin	7	—	—	—[c]	39
Nirvanol[b]	96	—	21	10–35[c]	27
Methsuximide	1–3	—	—	—	—
N-desmethyl-methsuximide[d]	34–80	—	8–17	10–40	—
Paraldehyde	—	3–10	—	—	—
Phenobarbital	46–136	37–73 (children) 61–173 (neonates)	14–21	15–40	40–60
Phenytoin	10–34	5–14 (children) 10–60 (neonates) 10–140 (prematures)	7–28	10–20	69–96
Primidone[e]	6–18	5–11	4–7	5–12	0
Trimethadione	16	16	—	—	0
Dimethadione[f]	240	240	30	over 700	0
Valproic acid	6–15	8–15	1–2	40–150	80–95

[a]See Appendix I for conversion to other units.
[b]Active metabolite of mephenytoin and major antiepileptic drug in plasma of patients taking mephenytoin.
[c]Sum of nirvanol plus mephenytoin plasma concentrations.
[d]Active metabolite of methsuximide and major antiepileptic drug in plasma of patients taking methsuximide.
[e]Metabolized to phenobarbital and phenylethylmalonamide. Both these derivatives have antiepileptic activity.
[f]Active metabolite of trimethadione and major antiepileptic drug in serum of patients taking trimethadione.

basis for the therapeutic strategy of treating status epilepticus with a single dose of intravenous diazepam (to stop the seizures quickly) followed immediately by a loading dose of phenytoin to provide long-term antiepileptic activity.

PROTEIN BINDING

Upon entering the bloodstream antiepileptic drugs are bound to differing degrees by plasma proteins, principally albumin. The extent of protein binding by various antiepileptic drugs is listed in Table 14-1. Protein binding has several important clinical implications. First, the serum drug concentration determinations performed by most laboratories measure the total drug serum concentration, not the free (non-protein-bound) serum concentration. Second, only the free drug can enter active sites from the plasma, and there is evidence that the concentration of free antiepileptic drug in the serum correlates better with efficacy and toxicity than does the total drug concen-

tration [4]. Third, the percentage of free drug in the serum is inversely proportional to the albumin concentration. Patients with low plasma albumin concentrations have a higher percentage (but not higher concentration) of free antiepileptic drug and a greater probability of developing antiepileptic drug toxicity for a given total drug serum concentration than do patients with a high plasma albumin concentration [6, 34, 56]. Fourth, other drugs given in addition to an antiepileptic drug may displace the antiepileptic drug from its protein-binding sites (see below).

Plasma protein binding is less in neonates than in children and young adults [45, 54]. At the other end of the age spectrum, plasma protein binding decreases by 18 percent in the elderly [25, 31, 61]. This decrease correlates well with plasma albumin concentrations and does not appear to be caused by changes in binding affinity.

Reduced protein binding (increased *free fraction*) of a drug does *not* result in a change in the *concen-*

tration of free drug [24]. Free drug concentration is determined only by the dosing rate and the ability of clearing organs to biotransform or excrete the free drug. If dosing rate and free drug clearance remain constant, total concentration of the drug will fall and free fraction will increase when protein binding decreases, but free concentration, and therefore clinical activity, will remain unchanged.

CELL STORAGE

The concentration of free drug is the same in intracellular fluid and in serum for most antiepileptic drugs. However, the total concentration of the drug can be much higher in cells than in serum if the drug is bound by components (proteins, nucleoproteins, phospholipids) of the cell [20, 76]. Most antiepileptic drugs are lipid-soluble and accumulate in adipose tissue. Persons with large amounts of adipose tissue (the elderly and the obese) have more extensive tissue distribution of lipid-soluble drugs, but no change in steady-state serum concentration [25].

TRANSCELLULAR FLUIDS: CSF, SALIVA, AND TEARS

CSF may be viewed as a plasma ultrafiltrate with a low protein concentration (and hence little protein binding). The concentrations of phenytoin, phenobarbital, primidone, carbamazepine, and ethosuximide in CSF are essentially identical to the concentrations of free drug in the serum [6]. Similar considerations apply to saliva and tears, and the possibility that the concentration of antiepileptic drugs in saliva or tears might be routinely determined as a means of determining the concentration of free drug in the serum is being investigated [32, 36, 42, 43, 44, 46, 51].

Biotransformation and Excretion

BASIC PRINCIPLES

Most antiepileptic drugs are inactivated and eliminated as a result of biotransformation by the hepatic microsomal mixed function oxidase system (cytochrome P-450 system), which transforms antiepileptic drugs into oxidized metabolites. These metabolites are usually less effective antiepileptic drugs than the parent drug, but biotransformation to active metabolites also occurs (see below). The oxidized metabolites are usually more polar than the parent drug and more easily excreted by the kidney.

USUAL ROUTES OF BIOTRANSFORMATION AND EXCRETION

Phenytoin, phenobarbital, and ethosuximide first undergo an oxidation reaction and are then excreted partly as the oxidized metabolite and partly as conjugated oxidized metabolite (see Chaps. 16, 17, 19). The initial oxidation step renders these drugs inactive

as antiepileptic drugs. Primidone is oxidized to two active metabolites, phenobarbital and phenylethylmalonamide (see Chap. 17). Carbamazepine may undergo oxidation to form carbamazepine-10,11-epoxide or carbamazepine-10,11-dihydroxide (see Chap. 18). Carbamazepine may also undergo loss of the carbamide group to form iminostilbene (see Chap. 18). Carbamazepine-10,11-dihydroxide has antiepileptic activity [6]. Methsuximide is first demethylated to form N-desmethyl-methsuximide (NDM), an active metabolite that is the major antiepileptic substance in the plasma of patients taking methsuximide (see Chap. 19). Methsuximide and NDM are then inactivated by oxidation and excreted as oxidized and conjugated oxidized metabolites (see Chap. 19). Valproic acid is eliminated by direct conjugation of the parent drug and by oxidation of the parent drug (see Chap. 20). The major metabolic pathway of clonazepam is reduction of the nitro group to form an inactive 7-amino derivative (see Chap. 21).

Acetazolamide, bromine, and dimethadione are eliminated almost entirely by direct renal excretion (see Chap. 22). Phenobarbital, primidone, and ethosuximide are partly eliminated by direct renal excretion but principally as biotransformed metabolites (see Chaps. 17 and 19).

EFFECTS OF AGE

The rates of biotransformation of drugs may change with age. Many drugs are slowly metabolized by neonates because of their immature hepatic microsomes. Hydroxylation of phenytoin and conjugation of phenobarbital proceed more slowly in neonates than in children or adults [5, 6, 45, 54, 60]. On the other hand, children metabolize phenytoin and phenobarbital more rapidly than adults and require higher doses of phenytoin and phenobarbital (in mg/kg) to achieve a given serum concentration [6, 45, 54, 60] (see Chaps. 16 and 17). Biotransformation rates may change (decrease) very abruptly at puberty [54].

At the other end of the age spectrum, there is evidence that the elimination half-lives of phenytoin, phenobarbital, and diazepam are longer in the elderly than in young adults [3, 61]. These changes appear to be due chiefly to slower metabolism [25, 61].

Renal excretion also changes with age. Neonates have a lower renal clearance of drugs than older infants or children [45, 54]. The glomerular filtration rate and renal excretion of intact drug decline predictably in old age, with a mean 35 percent reduction in the elderly as compared with young adults [25].

EFFECTS OF HEPATIC FAILURE

In patients with hepatic disease the rate of hepatic biotransformation of drugs and hepatic blood flow are serum concentration of antiepileptic drugs. These principles are intended to help the physician decide when to change the dosage or type of drug being administered and to help in the interpretation of measured serum concentrations of antiepileptic drugs. The pharmacokinetic principles described here are based on simple models that make many assumptions and have several limitations [18, 22, 26, 62].

Drug Interactions

Antiepileptic drugs are frequently administered in combination, creating the possibility of pharmacodynamic and pharmacokinetic drug interactions.

PHARMACODYNAMIC DRUG INTERACTIONS

Pharmacodynamic drug interactions are those involving the effects of two or more drugs at a common receptor site [40]. Such effects may be agonistic or antagonistic and may be more or less than the mathematical sum of the effects of the drugs given singly.

PHARMACOKINETIC DRUG INTERACTIONS

Definition

Pharmacokinetic drug interactions are those resulting from alterations in absorption, distribution, biotransformation, or excretion of a drug as a consequence of coadministration of one or more additional drugs [40]. In addition, some drugs alter their own biotransformation · as a consequence of chronic administration. Five forms of clinically important pharmacokinetic drug interactions have been found for antiepileptic drugs: (1) self-induction of biotransformation, (2) self-inhibition of biotransformation, (3) induction of biotransformation of coadministered drug, (4) inhibition of biotransformation of coadministered drug, and (5) displacement from protein-binding sites by coadministered drug [40]. Pharmacokinetic drug interactions may be bidirectional (i.e., the pharmacokinetics of both drugs are affected by the presence of the other drug), and one drug may have more than one type of pharmacokinetic drug interaction with the other drug [40].

Methods of Study

Most studies of drug interactions merely report how the addition of a second drug affects the serum concentration of the first drug. Such studies fail to determine the cause of the change in serum drug concentration (change in biotransformation rate, protein binding, etc.).

Proper study of pharmacokinetic drug interactions requires the performance of serial studies to measure the changes in pharmacokinetic values brought about by prolonged administration of one drug or the addition of a second drug to a patient's regimen. The conventional methods of performing serial pharmacokinetic studies involve either temporarily discontinuing the drug at specified times to measure its elimination or serial administration of radioactive tracer doses of the drug. The former technique exposes the patient to the risk of increased seizure frequency, and the latter technique exposes the patient to radiation. Serial pharmacokinetic studies using newly developed stable isotope-labeled tracer doses of drug eliminate these hazards [7]. Stable isotopes (e.g., deuterium, ^{13}C, ^{15}N) are naturally occurring *nonradioactive* isotopes that contain one additional neutron. Drugs can be labeled with such isotopes, and the concentration of both the labeled drug and the nonlabeled drug in body fluids can be determined by gas chromatography-mass spectrometry (see Chap. 15). Stable isotope-labeled tracer doses of an antiepileptic drug can be used to measure steady state pharmacokinetic values and metabolite formation without interrupting a patient's drug regimen [7].

Self-Induction of Biotransformation

Several antiepileptic drugs are known to be inducers of the hepatic microsomal mixed function oxidase-system enzymes. Carbamazepine and valproic acid have been shown to stimulate their own metabolism during chronic administration [7] (see Chaps. 18 and 20).

Self-Inhibition of Biotransformation

Certain drugs bind tightly to the hepatic, mixed function oxidase-system enzymes and inhibit their own biotransformation at therapeutic drug serum concentrations. This phenomenon has been documented for phenytoin [7].

Induction and Inhibition of Biotransformation
of Coadministered Drugs

The hepatic mixed function oxidase system has a low substrate specificity and metabolizes many drugs. Because antiepileptic drugs are often given in combination, their common metabolism by the mixed function oxidase system may result in clinically important drug interactions. Certain antiepileptic drugs have a relatively high affinity for the mixed function oxidase system and may competitively inhibit the metabolism of other drugs given simultaneously. Other antiepileptic drugs may stimulate the mixed function oxidase system (hepatic microsomal enzyme induction) and increase the rate of metabolism of other drugs given simultaneously.

154

Table 14-3 summarizes the published data on observed interactions of antiepileptic drugs. Enzyme induction is the proven or presumed mechanism for decreases in serum concentration of the original drug in most cases, although a few of the decreases may be due to reduced protein binding. Inhibition of hepatic metabolism is the proven or presumed mechanism for increases in serum concentration of the original drug. It should be noted that the data in Table 14-3 are from small and sometimes conflicting studies. This list of interactions will be modified and expanded as more data are collected.

Antiepileptic drugs may also influence the metabolism of other drugs and vice versa. These types of drug interactions have been reviewed elsewhere [30].

Displacement from Protein-Binding
Sites by Coadministered Drugs
Coadministration of two or more drugs may result in displacement of a drug from its protein-binding sites. This will result in a lower total drug level but a higher percentage of unbound drug [6, 30, 40, 56, 76]. Valproic acid significantly displaces phenytoin from protein-binding sites (see Chap. 20). Evidence thus far indicates that coadministration of other antiepileptic drugs probably does not significantly alter the protein binding of phenytoin or carbamazepine [6]. The effect of drugs other than antiepileptic drugs on the protein binding of antiepileptic drugs is reviewed elsewhere [6, 30, 56, 76].

Guidelines for Antiepileptic Drug Therapy

BEGIN WITH MONOTHERAPY
WITH LEAST TOXIC DRUG
Once the exact type of seizure(s) a patient has is determined, the physician should initiate monotherapy with the least toxic drug that is likely to produce good long-term seizure control. If a patient has more than one type of seizure, therapy should begin with the least toxic drug for the most bothersome type of seizure. The choice of drug must be made on an individual basis, and there is no one "best" drug for all patients with a given type of seizure disorder (see below).

The monotherapy approach for initial treatment is based on a growing body of scientific evidence indicating that monotherapy with an appropriately selected drug "pushed" to adequate serum concentration will control seizures in a majority of patients and that polytherapy exposes the patient to several unnecessary risks. Monotherapy of simple partial, complex partial, and tonic-clonic seizures with pheny-

toin, phenobarbital, primidone, or carbamazepine using the guidelines outlined here will result in satisfactory long-term seizure control in 56 to 88 percent of patients and complete seizure control in 31 to 80 percent of patients [29, 58, 59, 70]. Monotherapy of absence seizures with ethosuximide, valproic acid, or clonazepam will result in satisfactory long term seizure control in 50 to 90 percent of patients and complete seizure control in 50 percent of patients (see Chaps. 19, 20, 21). The principal reason for the high rate of success of modern monotherapy trials when compared with older monotherapy trials is the availability of drug level monitoring which detects low drug serum concentration, the major reason for failure of monotherapy in the past. Factors that appear to be associated with failure of modern monotherapy include persistent noncompliance, drug allergy, large or progressive brain lesions, partial seizures, more than one type of seizure, neuropsychiatric handicaps, and high pretreatment seizure frequency [1, 58, 59, 70].

The risks of unnecessary polytherapy are many. Chronic toxicity is associated with the use of any antiepileptic drug, and minimizing the number of drugs taken minimizes the risks of toxicity [58]. Unnecessary polytherapy is particularly likely to include barbiturates with their high risk for cognitive and behavioral toxicity [1, 58]. Other risks of unnecessary polytherapy include drug interactions, exacerbation of seizures, and inability to evaluate the effectiveness of individual antiepileptic drugs [58, 59, 65].

"PUSH" THE FIRST DRUG TRIED
The first drug tried for a seizure disorder is usually the least toxic drug available, and the physician must be certain he has obtained the maximum possible therapeutic effect from the first drug before adding other drugs. Therapy usually begins with an "average" dose of antiepileptic drug. If the seizures are controlled with this average dose and there are no serious side effects, no further changes are necessary. If the seizures are not controlled with this dose and there is no serious drug toxicity, the dosage of the drug should be systematically increased until the seizures are controlled or side effects preclude further dosage increase [59].

The drug serum concentration should be determined if a patient's seizures are not controlled by an average or high drug dosage. There are many causes of a lower-than-expected drug serum concentration, especially noncompliance (see Chap. 15). It would be a serious error to substitute or to add a more toxic drug because the patient has a low serum concentration of the first drug. Causes of low drug serum con-

Table 14-3. *Effect of Adding a Second Antiepileptic Drug on Serum Concentration of First Antiepileptic Drug*

Original Drug	Added Drug	Effect of Added Drug on Serum Concentration of Original Drug
Carbamazepine	Clonazepam	No change
	Mephenytoin	Decrease
	Phenobarbital*	Decrease*
	Phenytoin*	Decrease*
	Primidone*	Decrease*
Clonazepam	Phenobarbital	Decrease
	Phenytoin	Decrease
	Valproic acid	No change
Ethosuximide	Carbamazepine	Decrease
	Methylphenobarbital	Increase
	Phenobarbital	No change
	Phenytoin	No change
	Primidone	No change
	Valproic acid	Increase or no change
Mephenytoin	Carbamazepine	Decrease
	Phenobarbital	Decrease
	Phenytoin	Decrease or increase
Phenobarbital	Carbamazepine	No change
	Clonazepam	Data conflicting
	Mephenytoin	Decrease
	Methsuximide*	Increase*
	Phenytoin	Increase
	Valproic acid*	Increase*
Phenytoin	Carbamazepine	Increase*
	Clonazepam	Data conflicting
	Ethosuximide	No change
	Mephenytoin	Decrease
	Methsuximide*	Increase*
	Phenobarbital	Decrease, increase, or no change
	Primidone	No change
	Valproic acid*	Decrease*
Primidone	Carbamazepine	Increased concentration of derived phenobarbital
	Clonazepam	No change
	Ethosuximide	No change
	Phenytoin	Increased concentration of derived phenobarbital
	Valproic acid	Increase
Valproic acid	Carbamazepine*	Decrease*
	Clonazepam	No change
	Ethosuximide	No change
	Phenobarbital*	Decrease*
	Phenytoin*	Decrease*
	Primidone*	Decrease*

*Interactions particularly likely to be encountered in clinical practice.

centration can usually be identified and dealt with (see Chap. 15). A drug cannot be said to be ineffective until it is documented that the seizures are not controlled with a high therapeutic serum concentration of the drug unless drug toxicity precludes reaching such concentrations.

The "therapeutic range" of drug serum concentrations represents values applicable to "average" patients (see Chap. 15). Some patients require higher drug serum concentrations than the therapeutic range for good seizure control. If a patient has a high therapeutic serum concentration of a nontoxic drug, poor seizure control, and no drug side effects, the best approach usually is to increase the dosage of the first drug rather than add a more toxic second drug.

ADD ADDITIONAL DRUGS
If the first drug tried is pushed to its maximum tolerated dosage and/or high therapeutic serum concentration and seizures are still not controlled, a second antiepileptic drug should be added. In general, it is best to add the second drug and continue administration of the first drug (at least temporarily) because (1) the first drug will provide protection while the serum concentration of the second drug is being built up, (2) discontinuing the first drug may result in withdrawal activation of the seizure disorder, and (3) there is evidence that two antiepileptic drugs in combination may control seizures in some patients when either drug alone will not [11, 14, 29]. Unfortunately, only a minority of patients with partial or tonic-clonic seizures whose seizures were not controlled with a proper trial of monotherapy will obtain good seizure control with two drugs [29, 58, 65, 70].

If complete seizure control is obtained after adding a second drug, the physician should consider tapering the patient off the first drug because of the many hazards of chronic polytherapy. The decision to taper the patient off the first drug must be individualized and take into consideration the antiepileptic effect of the first drug when given alone, the side effects of the first drug, and the psychosocial consequences to the patient of having a seizure if withdrawal of the first drug results in loss of complete seizure control. The many adverse effects of antiepileptic drugs on behavior and cognition argue strongly for strenuously attempting to minimize the number of such drugs given to children. In adults, the hazards of polytherapy must be weighed against the risk of loss of job and/or driver's license if withdrawal of the first drug results in a recurrence of seizures. If it is elected to withdraw the first drug, the withdrawal should be done very slowly (e.g., withdrawal of one tablet or capsule every five

elimination half-lives or longer). This will minimize the chance of withdrawal activation of seizures [64, 67] and, if seizures should return, will establish the steady state serum concentration at which seizures return.

A third drug should not be added until it is documented that seizures cannot be controlled with maximum tolerated doses and/or high therapeutic serum concentrations of the first two drugs tried. It is usually better to add a third drug (at least temporarily) than to substitute the third drug for the first and/or second drug for reasons similar to those cited above for adding rather than substituting the second drug [11, 63]. If complete seizure control is obtained after addition of a third drug, the physician may elect to withdraw one of the first two drugs using the guidelines outlined above.

DURATION OF THERAPY
Uncontrolled seizures and seizures due to a progressive neurologic illness (e.g., astrocytoma) are indications for continuing antiepileptic drug therapy indefinitely. Antiepileptic drug therapy should usually be maintained for a minimum of 2 to 5 years after diagnosis of epilepsy, even if the patient has no further seizures [64]. When a patient has been free of seizures for 2 to 5 years on antiepileptic drug therapy, the need for continued therapy can be reevaluated. Risk factors have been identified that help the physician evaluate the likelihood of seizures recurring after medication has been discontinued. Patients who continue to have an abnormal electroencephalogram (EEG) (spikes, sharp waves, paroxysmal activity, or nonparoxysmal abnormalities) have a 30 to 57 percent chance of seizures recurring if antiepileptic medication is discontinued [15, 68]. Other risk factors include (1) occurrence of many generalized seizures before control with medication, (2) long duration between onset of therapy and seizure control, (3) presence of a known structural lesion and/or neurologic deficit, (4) mental retardation, (5) onset of seizures before 2 years of age, (6) adult onset of complex partial seizures, and (7) more than one seizure type [2, 15, 68].

Each decision must be made on an individual basis. A history of seizure frequency and risk factors must be obtained. A routine EEG is mandatory, and a long-term EEG recording is sometimes desirable. The probability of recurrent seizures, the consequences of having another seizure (loss of driver's license or job, physical injury), and the benefits of living without medication (reduction in side effects and cost of management) must be discussed with the patient, and a judgment must be made weighted by the patient's needs.

If it is decided to discontinue antiepileptic therapy, medication should be withdrawn slowly. Eliminating one pill per day every five elimination half-lives is probably the optimal regimen. More rapid tapering of therapy may precipitate seizures [67], and more prolonged withdrawal probably does not reduce the risk of seizure recurrence [64].

Antiepileptic Drugs of Choice for Tonic-Clonic, Complex Partial, and Simple Partial Seizures

These are the most common types of seizure disorder, and phenytoin, phenobarbital, primidone, and carbamazepine are the drugs usually employed to treat them. Phenytoin, phenobarbital, and primidone are approved by the Food and Drug Administration (FDA) for use as primary antiepileptic drugs. Carbamazepine is currently approved for use only in patients refractory to phenytoin and phenobarbital and/or primidone. However, carbamazepine is being tested as a primary antiepileptic drug for tonic-clonic and partial seizures, and some authorities already believe that it is more desirable than the other three drugs (see Chap. 18).

There is overwhelming evidence that phenytoin, phenobarbital, primidone, and carbamazepine are all effective for tonic-clonic and partial seizures. However, there is no definitive evidence establishing which of these four drugs is most effective and/or least toxic in the treatment of any given type of seizure. Cereghino et al. [11] found similar efficacy in a cross-over study of phenytoin, phenobarbital, and carbamazepine in a small group of institutionalized patients with a variety of seizure disorders. Several studies have compared two of the four drugs in question, but the results of these studies are inconclusive and contradictory. The Veterans Administration is currently conducting a large, prospective, randomized, double-blind study to determine which of the four drugs in question is the drug of choice for tonic-clonic, complex partial, and simple partial seizures [70]. At the present time the choice of antiepileptic drug varies in different centers depending upon how local experts weigh the advantages and disadvantages of the four available drugs and upon how the known side effects of the drugs might affect a given patient's life cycle.

PHENYTOIN

Advantages
Phenytoin (see Chap. 16) (1) is relatively nonsedating, (2) rarely causes serious toxicity, (3) can be administered parenterally, (4) may be given in a loading dose by the oral or intravenous route, (5) need be taken only once a day by many adults.

Disadvantages
The drug (1) may cause some sedation or impairment of higher intellectual function, (2) has a relatively high incidence of annoying side effects with chronic administration, including gingival hyperplasia, hirsutism, acne, coarsening of facial features, and cholasmalike pigmentation.

PHENOBARBITAL

Advantages
Phenobarbital (see Chap. 17) (1) rarely causes serious toxicity, (2) can be administered parenterally, (3) may be given in a loading dose by the oral or intravenous route, (4) is inexpensive, (5) need be taken only once a day by many adults.

Disadvantages
The drug causes sedation, irritability, or impairment of higher intellectual functions in a high percentage of patients.

PRIMIDONE

Advantages
Primidone (see Chap. 17) rarely causes serious toxicity.

Disadvantages
The drug (1) causes sedation, irritability, or impairment of higher intellectual functions in a high percentage of patients, (2) has an incidence of sedation and drowsiness that is probably higher than that with phenobarbital during period of initiation of therapy, (3) cannot be administered parenterally, (4) cannot be administered in a loading dose by the oral or intravenous route, (5) is considerably more expensive than phenobarbital, (6) requires determination of two blood levels (primidone and phenobarbital) each time the blood level is checked, (7) must be given in divided doses.

CARBAMAZEPINE

Advantages
Carbamazepine (see Chap. 18) (1) definitely causes less sedation and impairment of intellectual functions than phenobarbital or primidone, (2) probably causes less sedation and impairment of intellectual functions than phenytoin, (3) does not have the annoying cosmetic side effects of phenytoin.

Disadvantages
This drug (1) has been reported to cause serious bone marrow depression and other idiosyncratic reactions

158

in a very small percentage of patients, (2) requires routine obtaining of the laboratory tests recommended by the FDA (complete blood count, liver function tests, BUN, urinalysis, slit lamp examination, funduscopy, and tonometry) and is therefore extremely expensive and time consuming for the patient, (3) may cause diplopia, dizziness, drowsiness, ataxia, or nausea, especially at onset of therapy, (4) cannot be administered parenterally, (5) cannot be administered in a loading dose by the oral or intravenous route, (6) must be given in divided doses, (7) is more expensive than alternative drugs.

Other Drugs for Tonic-Clonic and Partial Seizures
Clorazepate dipotassium, phenacemide, mephenytoin, and ethotoin are less consistently effective and/or more toxic than phenytoin, phenobarbital, primidone, and carbamazepine in the treatment of tonic-clonic and partial seizures (see Chaps. 16, 21, and 22). However, an occasional patient whose seizures cannot be controlled with the four first line drugs may respond to these alternative medications.

Antiepileptic Drugs of Choice for Other Seizure Types
Drugs of choice for other seizure types are discussed in the chapters on specific seizure types (see Chaps. 7, 8, 9, 26, 27, 28, and 30).

References

1. Albright, P. S., and Bruni, J. Monotherapy versus polypharmacy in the treatment of epilepsy. *Epilepsia.* In press, 1983.
2. Annegers, J. F., Hauser, W. A., and Elveback, L. R. Remission of seizures and relapse in patients with epilepsy. *Epilepsia* 20:729, 1979.
3. Bauer, L. A., and Blouin, R. A. Age and phenytoin kinetics in adult epileptics. *Clin. Pharmacol. Ther.* 31:301, 1982.
4. Booker, H. E., and Darcy, B. Serum concentrations of free diphenylhydantoin and their relationship to clinical intoxication. *Epilepsia* 14:177, 1973.
5. Bourgeois, B. F. D., and Dodson, W. E. Phenytoin bioavailability and kinetics in newborns. *Epilepsia* 23:436, 1982.
6. Browne, T. R. Clinical pharmacology of antiepileptic drugs. *Drug Ther. Rev.* 2:469, 1979.
7. Browne, T. R. et al. Applications of stable isotope methods to studying the clinical pharmacology of antiepileptic drugs in newborns, infants, children, and adolescents. *Ther. Drug Monit.* In press, 1983.
8. Buchanan, R. A. et al. The metabolism of diphenylhydantoin (Dilantin®) following once daily administration. *Neurology* (Minneap.) 22:126, 1972.
9. Buchanan, R. A. et al. Single daily dose of diphenylhydantoin in children. *J. Pediatr.* 83:479, 1973.
10. Buchanan, R. A. Personal communication, 1977.
11. Cereghino, J. J. et al. The efficacy of carbamazepine combinations in epilepsy. *Clin. Pharmacol. Ther.* 18:733, 1975.
12. Chen, S. S. et al. Comparative bioavailability of phenytoin from generic formulations in the United Kingdom. *Epilepsia* 23:149, 1982.
13. Dam, M., and Olesen, V. Intramuscular administration of phenytoin. *Neurology* (Minneap.) 16:288, 1966.
14. Diamond, W. D., and Buchanan, R. A. Clinical studies of the effect of phenobarbital on diphenylhydantoin plasma levels. *J. Clin. Pharmacol.* 10:306, 1970.
15. Emerson, R. et al. Stopping medication in children with epilepsy: Predictors of outcome. *N. Engl. J. Med.* 304:1125, 1981.
16. Feldman, R. G., and Pippenger, C. E. The relation of anticonvulsant drug levels to complete seizure control. *J. Clin. Pharmacol.* 16:51, 1976.
17. Gatley, M. S. To be taken as directed. *J. R. Coll. Gen. Pract.* 16:39, 1968.
18. Gibaldi, M., and Levy, G. Pharmacokinetics in clinical practice. *J.A.M.A.* 235:1864, 1976.
19. Glazko, A. J., and Chang, T. Diphenylhydantoin: Absorption, Distribution, Biotransformation, and Excretion. In D. M. Woodbury, J. K. Penry, and R. P. Schmidt (Eds.), *Antiepileptic Drugs.* New York: Raven Press, 1972. Pp. 127–136.
20. Goldberg, M. A., and Crandall, P. H. Human brain binding of phenytoin. *Neurology* (Minneap.) 28:881, 1978.
21. Goulet, J. R., Kinkel, A. W., and Smith, T. C. Metabolism of ethosuximide. *Clin. Pharmacol. Ther.* 20:213, 1976.
22. Greenblatt, D. J., and Koch-Weser, J. Clinical pharmacokinetics. *N. Engl. J. Med.* 293:702, 964, 1975.
23. Greenblatt, D. J., and Koch-Weser, J. Intramuscular injection of drugs. *N. Engl. J. Med.* 295:542, 1976.
24. Greenblatt, D. J., Sellers, E. M., and Koch-Weser, J. Importance of protein binding for the interpretation of serum or plasma drug concentrations. *J. Clin. Pharmacol.* 22:259, 1982.
25. Greenblatt, D. J., Sellers, E. M., and Shader, R. I. Drug therapy: Drug disposition in old age. *N. Engl. J. Med.* 306:1081, 1982.
26. Guelen, P. J. M., and Van Derkleijn, E. Practical Pharmacokinetics. In D. M. Woodbury, J. K. Penry,

and C. E. Pippenger (Eds.), *Antiepileptic Drugs.* New York: Raven Press, 1982.

27. Gugler, R. et al. Pharmacokinetics of drugs in patients with nephrotic syndrome. *J. Clin. Invest.* 55:1132, 1975.

28. Haerer, A. F., and Buchanan, R. A. Effectiveness of single daily doses of diphenylhydantoin. *Neurology* (Minneap.) 22:1021, 1972.

29. Hakkarainen, H. Carbamazepine vs. diphenylhydantoin vs. their combination in adult epilepsy. *Neurology* 30:354, 1980.

30. Hansten, P. D. *Drug Interactions.* Philadelphia: Lea & Febiger, 1979.

31. Hayes, M. J., Langman, M. J. S., and Short, D. H. Changes in drug metabolism with increasing age: II. Phenytoin clearance and protein binding. *Br. J. Clin. Pharmacol.* 2:73, 1975.

32. Horning, M. G. et al. Use of saliva in therapeutic drug monitoring. *Clin. Chem.* 23:157, 1977.

33. Houghton, G. W., and Richens, A. Rate of elimination of tracer doses of phenytoin at different steady-state serum phenytoin concentrations in epileptic patients. *Br. J. Clin. Pharmacol.* 1:155, 1974.

34. Jusko, W. J., and Gretch, M. Plasma and tissue protein binding of drugs in pharmacokinetics. *Drug Metab. Rev.* 5:43, 1976.

35. Kostenbauder, H. B. et al. Bioavailability and single-dose pharmacokinetics of intramuscular phenytoin. *Clin. Pharmacol. Ther.* 18:449, 1975.

36. Kristensen, O., and Larsen, H. F. Value of saliva samples in monitoring carbamazepine concentrations in epileptic patients. *Acta Neurol. Scand.* 61:344, 1980.

37. Kutt, H. Effect of Acute and Chronic Illness on the Disposition of Antiepileptic Drugs. In P. L. Morselli, J. K. Penry, and C. E. Pippenger (Eds.), *Antiepileptic Drug Therapy in Pediatrics.* New York: Raven Press, 1982.

38. Lee, C. S. et al. Pharmacokinetics of primidone elimination by uremic patients. *J. Clin. Pharmacol.* 22:301, 1982.

39. Letteri, J. M. et al. Diphenylhydantoin metabolism in uremia. *N. Engl. J. Med.* 285:648, 1971.

40. Levy, R. Drug Interactions. In P. L. Morselli, J. K. Penry, and C. E. Pippenger (Eds.), *Antiepileptic Drug Therapy in Pediatrics.* New York: Raven Press, 1982.

41. Liu, E., and Rubenstein, M. Phenytoin removal by plasmapheresis in thrombotic thrombocytopenic purpura. *Clin. Pharmacol. Ther.* 31:762, 1982.

42. Monaco, F. et al. Tears as the best practical indicator of the unbound fraction of an anticonvulsant drug. *Epilepsia* 20:705, 1979.

43. Monaco, F. et al. Diphenylhydantoin and primidone in tears. *Epilepsia* 22:185, 1981.

44. Monaco, F. et al. The free fraction of valproic acid in tears, saliva, and cerebrospinal fluid. *Epilepsia* 22:23, 1982.

45. Morselli, P. L. Maturation of Physiological Variables Regulating Drug Kinetics. In P. L. Morselli, J. K. Penry, and C. E. Pippenger (Eds.), *Antiepileptic Drug Therapy in Pediatrics.* New York: Raven Press, 1982.

46. Nishihara, K. et al. Estimation of plasma unbound phenobarbital concentration by mixed saliva. *Epilepsia* 20:37, 1979.

47. Odar-Cederlof, I., and Borga, O. Kinetics of diphenylhydantoin in uremic patients: Consequences of decreased plasma protein binding. *Eur. J. Clin. Pharmacol.* 7:31, 1974.

48. Nugent, C. A. et al. Glucocorticoid toxicity: Single contrasted with divided daily doses of prednisolone. *J. Chronic Dis.* 18:323, 1965.

49. Painter, M. J. et al. Phenobarbital and phenytoin in neonatal seizures: Metabolism and tissue distribution. *Neurology* (N.Y.) 31:1107, 1981.

50. Paulson, O. B., Gyory, A., and Hertz, M. M. Blood brain transfer and cerebral uptake of antiepileptic drugs. *Clin. Pharmacol. Ther.* 32:466, 1982.

51. Paxton, J. W., and Donald, R. A. Concentrations and kinetics of carbamazepine in whole saliva, parotid saliva, serum ultrafiltrate, and serum. *Clin. Pharmacol. Ther.* 28:695, 1980.

52. Pentikainen, P. J., Neuvonen, P. J., and Elfving, S. M. Bioavailability of four brands of phenytoin tablets. *Eur. J. Clin. Pharmacol.* 9:213, 1975.

53. Perrier, D. et al. Maintenance of therapeutic phenytoin plasma levels via intramuscular administration. *Ann. Intern. Med.* 85:318, 1976.

54. Pippenger, C. E. Absorption, Distribution, Protein Binding, Biotransformation, and Excretion of Antiepileptic Drugs. In P. L. Morselli, J. K. Penry, and C. E. Pippenger (Eds.), *Antiepileptic Drug Therapy in Pediatrics.* New York: Raven Press, 1982.

55. Porter, A. M. W. Drug defaulting in general practice. *Br. Med. J.* 1:218, 1969.

56. Porter, R. J., and Layzer, R. B. Plasma albumin concentration and diphenylhydantoin binding in man. *Arch. Neurol.* 32:298, 1975.

57. Rail, L. Dilantin overdosage. *Med. J. Aust.* 2:339, 1968.

58. Reynolds, E. H., and Shorvon, S. D. Monotherapy or polytherapy for epilepsy? *Epilepsia* 22:1, 1981.

59. Reynolds, E. et al. Phenytoin monotherapy for epilepsy: A long-term prospective study, assisted

by serum level monitoring, in previously untreated patients. *Epilepsia* 22:475, 1981.

60. Richens, A. Clinical pharmacokinetics of phenytoin. *Clin. Pharmacokinet.* 4:153, 1979.

61. Richey, D. P., and Bender, D. Pharmacokinetic consequences of aging. *Annu. Rev. Pharmacol. Tox.* 17:49, 1977.

62. Riegelman, S., Loo, J. C. K., and Rowland, M. Shortcomings in pharmacokinetic analysis by conceiving the body to exhibit properties of a single compartment. *J. Pharm. Sci.* 57:117, 1968.

63. Rodin, E. A., Rim, C. S., and Rennick, P. M. The effects of carbamazepine on patients with psychomotor epilepsy: Results of a double-blind study. *Epilepsia* 15:547, 1974.

64. Rothman, S. J. et al. Discontinuation of antiepileptic drugs: Preliminary report of a prospective randomized study of two-years versus four-years seizure-free interval, and nine-months versus six-weeks taper schedules. *Epilepsia* 23:437, 1982.

65. Schmidt, D. Two antiepileptic drugs for intractable epilepsy. *Epilepsia.* In press, 1983.

66. Serrano, E. E., and Wilder, B. J. Intramuscular administration of diphenylhydantoin. *Arch. Neurol.* 31:276, 1974.

67. Spencer, S. S. et al. Ictal effects of anticonvulsant medication withdrawal in epileptic patients. *Epilepsia* 22:297, 1981.

68. Thurston, J. H. et al. Prognosis in childhood epilepsy: Additional follow-up of 148 children 15 to 23 years of age after withdrawal of anticonvulsant therapy. *N. Engl. J. Med.* 306:831, 1982.

69. Tyrer, J. H. et al. Outbreak of anticonvulsant intoxication in an Australian city. *Br. Med. J.* 4:271, 1970.

70. Veterans Administration Cooperative Study #118: A Prospective Study of Relative Efficacy and Toxicity of Antiepileptic Drugs on Well-Defined Types of Seizures. Unpublished data, 1982.

71. Wallis, W., Kutt, H., and McDowell, F. Intravenous diphenylhydantoin in treatment of acute repetitive seizures. *Neurology* (Minneap.) 18:513, 1968.

72. Wilder, B. J., Streiff, R. R., and Hammer, R. H. Diphenylhydantoin Absorption, Distribution, and Excretion: Clinical Studies. In D. M. Woodbury, J. K. Penry, and R. P. Schmidt (Eds.), *Antiepileptic Drugs.* New York: Raven Press, 1972.

73. Wilder, B. J. et al. A method for shifting from oral to intramuscular diphenylhydantoin administration. *Clin. Pharmacol. Ther.* 16:507, 1974.

74. Wilder, B. J. et al. Efficacy of intravenous phenytoin in the treatment of status epilepticus: Kinetics of central nervous system penetration. *Ann. Neurol.* 1:511, 1977.

75. Wilensky, A. J., and Lowden, J. A. Inadequate serum levels after intramuscular administration of diphenylhydantoin. *Neurology* (Minneap.) 23:318, 1973.

76. Woodbury, D. M. Phenytoin: Absorption, Distribution, and Excretion. In D. M. Woodbury, J. K. Penry, and C. E. Pippenger (Eds.), *Antiepileptic Drugs.* New York: Raven Press, 1982.

ANTIEPILEPTIC DRUG SERUM CONCENTRATION DETERMINATIONS ("BLOOD LEVELS")

15

Thomas R. Browne
Joyce A. Cramer

Definitions

Serum concentration of a drug refers to the amount of drug (by weight) dissolved in a unit volume of serum. "Blood level" is a term often used as a synonym for serum concentration. Strictly speaking, "blood level" is not a proper synonym for serum concentration because measurements are made using serum (or plasma), not blood, and because there are no units for a "level." However, the term "blood level" is so entrenched in the medical literature that it would be impractical to suggest it be abolished.

UNITS

The units for antiepileptic drug serum concentration determinations most widely used in the United States are weight-per-volume units. Micrograms per milliliter (μg/ml) is the unit most commonly used by laboratories in the United States and therefore is the unit used in this book. Other weight-per-volume units in use include milligrams per liter (mg/L), milligrams per 100 milliliters (mg/100 ml), and milligrams per deciliter (mg/dl).

In Europe and in many other areas of the world molar units are used. The most widely used molar unit is micromoles (μM). Although molar units are more physiologic and have many theoretical advantages over weight-per-volume units, they have not yet gained widespread acceptance in the United States.

The physician must be familiar with the conversion factors among these units (see Appendix I) because different laboratories may use different units, and one laboratory may use different units for different drugs.

Indications for Determining Antiepileptic Drug Serum Concentration

POOR SEIZURE CONTROL

Poor seizure control is the most frequent indication for obtaining antiepileptic drug serum concentration determinations. Use of such determinations may decrease by as much as 50 percent the number of patients whose seizures are poorly controlled when compared with patients whose therapy is empirically determined

Our appreciation to Peter Jatlow, M.D., Richard H. Mattson, M.D., and George K. Szabo for reviewing this chapter. This work was supported in part by the Veterans Administration.

without the assistance of antiepileptic drug serum concentration determinations [6, 10, 21, 38].

When a patient's seizures are not controlled with an average dose of an antiepileptic drug appropriate for the type of seizure being treated, the serum concentration of the drug should be determined. The first drug used in treating a given patient's seizure disorder is usually chosen because the drug should have the best efficacy-to-toxicity ratio for the patient. There are many causes for a lower than expected drug serum concentration, and these causes can often be identified and corrected. Patients with subtherapeutic drug serum concentrations often obtain good seizure control when a therapeutic drug serum concentration is attained (see Chap. 14). Some patients whose seizures are not controlled with drug serum concentrations in the lower part of the therapeutic range will obtain good seizure control with drug serum concentrations in the upper part of the therapeutic range [23, 38]. It would be an error to add a second, more toxic, drug to a patient's antiepileptic drug regimen until it has been documented that the patient's seizure disorder cannot be controlled with a high therapeutic serum concentration of the first (least toxic) drug tried. Similarly, a third drug should not be added to an antiepileptic drug regimen until it has been documented that the patient's seizure disorder cannot be controlled with high therapeutic serum concentrations of the first two drugs tried.

EVALUATION OF ANTIEPILEPTIC DRUG INTOXICATION

Antiepileptic drug serum concentration determinations can assist in evaluating antiepileptic drug intoxication in at least two ways. First, many antiepileptic drugs produce similar toxic symptoms (e.g., drowsiness, ataxia, diplopia). If a patient is taking more than one drug, antiepileptic drug serum concentration determinations can determine which drug in the serum is present in supratherapeutic concentration and is therefore presumably responsible for the patient's toxic symptoms. Second, knowledge of a drug's serum concentration and elimination half-life can enable the physician to make an educated guess as to how long the drug causing intoxication must be withheld before therapy is resumed at a lower dose (see Chap. 14). However, this "educated guess" should not be the sole factor determining when drug therapy should be resumed because drug elimination half-lives vary considerably among patients; also, the elimination half-life of a drug, especially phenytoin, may be greater when the drug serum concentration is high than when it is low (see Chap. 14). Therapy should be resumed when the patient's symptoms of intoxication have disappeared or are minimal, and

when the patient's serum concentration of the drug causing intoxication is back in the therapeutic range. The drug serum concentration should not be allowed to fall to a subtherapeutic concentration.

DOCUMENTATION OF DRUG SERUM CONCENTRATION UNDER SUPERVISED ADMINISTRATION

Some patients continue to have subtherapeutic serum concentrations of an antiepileptic drug despite a large prescribed dose. It is sometimes necessary to hospitalize a patient, administer drugs under strict supervision, and measure drug serum concentration sequentially to determine if noncompliance was the cause of the apparently low drug serum concentration.

DOCUMENTATION OF CONTINUED COMPLIANCE

There is a great tendency for patients whose seizures are controlled to begin omitting some of their medication. One estimate is that patients who are seizure free omit one pill per day for every 6 months they are seizure free. Antiepileptic drug serum concentrations should be determined every 6 to 12 months in patients whose seizures are controlled to detect noncompliance and prevent recurrence of seizures. Sometimes it will be found that the patient has discontinued his medication entirely. In this case the physician must confront the patient, and they must decide either to discontinue the medication or to resume it at full dosage.

Expected Serum Concentrations

Expected serum concentrations of antiepileptic drugs are determined by measuring the drug serum concentration in a large group of patients at carefully specified times during closely supervised drug administration. The expected serum concentrations of the most commonly prescribed antiepileptic drugs are summarized in Table 15-1. Even under such carefully controlled conditions the range of drug serum concentrations produced by a given dose (in mg/kg) of a given antiepileptic drug varies two- to threefold among patients. This variability is caused by interindividual differences in drug absorption, protein binding, biotransformation, and excretion. For a given patient it is impossible to predict what antiepileptic drug serum concentration will be produced by a given dose of drug. This can be determined only by actual measurement.

Causes of Lower Than Expected Drug Serum Concentrations

NONCOMPLIANCE

Noncompliance is the most frequent cause of lower than expected antiepileptic drug serum concentrations. A review of over 50 studies found that complete

Table 15-1. Expected Serum Concentrations of Antiepileptic Drugs

Drug	Dosage		Expected Serum Concentration (μg/ml[a])	
	mg/kg	mg/day	Range	Average
Phenytoin	5	300–400	8–20	15
Phenobarbital	2	120–180	15–40	20
Primidone	10	750–1,000	5–15	6
Phenobarbital derived from primidone	—	—	5–32	20
Carbamazepine	15	1,000–1,200	4–12	6
Ethosuximide	15	1,000–1,250	40–100	60
Methsuximide	13	600–1,200	—	20[b]
Valproic acid	45	1,500–2,500	50–100	80
Clonazepam	0.03–0.10	2–7	Highly variable	Highly variable

[a]See Appendix I for conversion to other units.
[b]N-desmethyl-methsuximide derived from methsuximide.
Note: See Kutt and Penry [21] and Chapters 16 to 21 for references.

failure to take medication occurred in 25 to more than 50 percent of outpatients taking medications prescribed for a variety of conditions [3]. Similar figures probably apply to patients taking antiepileptic drugs [14, 38, 39]. Incomplete compliance is probably even more common than total noncompliance. Noncompliance may be due to active, volitional, conscious efforts or to passive, unconscious processes [11]. The factors involved in inducing noncompliance in a given patient are multiple and complex [11, 39]. They include the patient's psychological make-up, the illness, the physician, the medication regimen (see Chap. 14), and the treatment milieu. A family physician who studied this problem in detail [33] concluded that "It has not proved possible to identify an uncooperative type. Every patient is a potential defaulter; compliance can never be assumed." The topic of noncompliance is reviewed in more detail elsewhere [4, 35, 40].

STEADY STATE NOT REACHED
If the serum concentration of a drug is determined before sufficient time has elapsed for the serum concentration to rise to steady state (see Chap. 14), the serum concentration will be less than expected.This fact must be remembered especially when administering phenobarbital, which requires 14 to 21 days to reach steady state serum concentration.

POOR ABSORPTION
Certain antiepileptic drugs are marginally soluble in water and are not well absorbed by the oral route in some persons. This is particularly true of phenytoin (see Chap. 14). Low serum phenytoin concentration on the basis of poor absorption of phenytoin capsules

is not an uncommon problem. The oral suspension form of phenytoin is more completely absorbed than the capsule form by normal people [27], and changing to the oral suspension in a patient who absorbs phenytoin capsules poorly may result in a dramatic increase in phenytoin serum concentration. There is also evidence that neonates do not absorb oral phenytoin well, although they do absorb oral phenobarbital [26].

CHANGE IN DRUG FORMULATION
Different generic preparations of the same antiepileptic drug may have different bioavailabilities [25, 27] (see Chap. 14). A fall in antiepileptic drug serum concentration (and an increase in seizure frequency) may result if a patient switches from one generic brand of a drug to another [15].

RAPID METABOLISM
There are differences among patients in the rate of metabolism of antiepileptic drugs [29]. These differences are caused by genetic differences in the rate at which biotransformation reactions are carried out and by differences in the extent to which the individual has been exposed to enzyme-inducing agents [29]. Thus, some people will metabolize antiepileptic drugs more rapidly than others. However, in the authors' experience, much lower than expected antiepileptic drug serum concentrations are seldom due to rapid metabolism but are usually the result of noncompliance or poor absorption.

DRUG INTERACTIONS
Drug interactions can lower the serum concentration of an antiepileptic drug in at least two ways. First, the

interacting drug can cause microsomal enzyme induction, thereby increasing the rate of metabolism of the antiepileptic drug. Second, the interacting drug may displace the antiepileptic drug from protein-binding sites. This will lower the total serum concentration of antiepileptic drug, but will not alter the concentration of free drug (see Chap. 14). Drug interactions are discussed in more detail in Chapter 14.

LOW PLASMA PROTEIN-BINDING CAPACITY
Antiepileptic drug serum concentration determinations reported by most laboratories measure total drug serum concentration, including both free and protein-bound drug. Patients with a low plasma albumin (the principal binding protein) concentration have a lowered capacity to carry protein-bound antiepileptic drug and relatively low total serum concentrations of drug. However, the serum concentration of free drug remains unchanged (see Chap. 14).

RENAL DYSFUNCTION
This topic is discussed in Chapter 14.

PREGNANCY
This topic is discussed in Chapter 29.

PATIENT TAKING WRONG DOSE
Errors in instructing the patient by the physician, errors in filling or labeling prescriptions by the pharmacist, or errors in comprehension of instructions by the patient may result in the patient's taking less or more medication than the physician intended. In patients with lower or higher than expected antiepileptic drug serum concentrations, the physician should be certain that the patient is taking the proper number of the proper size of tablets or capsules each day. Also, patients taking the oral suspension form of medication may at first receive less than the prescribed amount of drug if the bottle is not shaken properly before each dose. As the bottle is used up, the suspended drug becomes concentrated at the bottom of the bottle, and the patient will then receive more than the prescribed dosage. Errors can also result when oral suspension is given using a tablespoon instead of a teaspoon or vice versa.

LABORATORY ERROR
See discussion of this topic below.

Causes of Higher Than Expected Drug Serum Concentrations

PATIENT WILLFULLY TAKING ADDITIONAL MEDICATION
Patients who are apprehensive of having seizures will sometimes take more antiepileptic drug than pre-scribed, especially if they are about to participate in some important event (e.g., high school dance or job interview). Also, patients who know that drug serum concentration determinations are being used as a measure of compliance will sometimes take additional medication just before visiting the physician.

PATIENT TAKING WRONG DOSE
See discussion of this topic above.

INDIVIDUAL VARIABILITY IN RATE OF DRUG METABOLISM
There is a considerable range of variability among individuals in the rate at which they metabolize antiepileptic drugs. Patients with slower than average rates of metabolism may have higher than expected drug serum concentrations. Also, some people have an extremely limited capacity to metabolize specific antiepileptic drugs, presumably because of a genetically determined biochemical abnormality [22, 45].

CHANGE IN DRUG FORMULATION
A rise in antiepileptic drug serum concentration and unexpected drug toxicity may result if a patient switches from one generic brand of drug to another [34, 44] (see Chap. 14).

DRUG INTERACTIONS
Other antiepileptic drugs and drugs of other types may elevate the serum concentration of an antiepileptic drug by interfering with its metabolism. Such interactions are reviewed in Chapter 14 and elsewhere [16, 21].

HEPATIC DISEASE
This topic is discussed in Chapter 14.

IMMATURITY OF ENZYME SYSTEMS IN INFANTS
The enzyme systems for biotransformation are sometimes not fully functional at birth. Thus, serum concentration of a drug may be greater for a given dose (in mg/kg) in infants than in children and adults [26] (see Chap. 14).

LABORATORY ERROR
Antiepileptic drug serum concentration determinations are usually reported with an implied accuracy of 1.0 to 0.1 μg/ml (e.g., 14.3 μg/ml). Clinicians who lack a sophisticated knowledge of clinical chemistry often assume that techniques with such imposing names as *high performance liquid chromatography* and *enzyme multiplied immunoassay technique* must unquestionably be very accurate all of the time. Un-

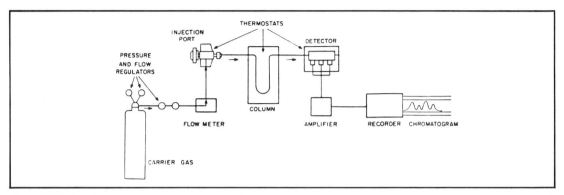

Figure 15-1. Gas chromatographic system. The gas chroma-tographic system starts with an inert gas flowing through the column under pressure. The sample enters the column via the injector port, where it is volatilized and enters the gas-mobile phase. As the separated compounds leave the column, electronic components detect the compounds and amplify and relay the signal to a recorder. The chromatogram appears as a series of peaks representing the quantity of drug. (Reprinted with permission from G. Zweig and J. Sherma, Handbook of Chromatography, Vol. 2. Cleveland: CRC Press, 1972. Copyright 1972, The Chemical Rubber Co., CRC Press, Inc.)

fortunately, this faith is not always justified. A blind survey of 112 laboratories sponsored by the Epilepsy Foundation of America found that antiepileptic drug serum concentrations reported by half of the labora-tories were outside ±1 standard deviation of the mean of five reference laboratories [31]. The physician using antiepileptic drug serum concentrations to guide therapy should do all of the following: (1) be aware that there are many sources of error in any method of determining the serum concentration of an antiepi-leptic drug; (2) learn the basic principles and sources of error in the method(s) employed by the clinical laboratory he uses to determine antiepileptic drug serum concentrations; (3) check to be certain that the quality control measures suggested below are fol-lowed by the clinical laboratory; (4) ask for a repeat drug serum concentration determination (at no charge to the patient) when the serum concentration re-ported by the laboratory seems inconsistent with the patient's clinical condition.

The optimum procedure for determining antiepi-leptic drug serum concentrations would be a reliable, simple, inexpensive, rapid, qualitative, and quantita-tive analysis of all major antiepileptic drugs and their metabolites simultaneously. No single method fulfills all these criteria. The most popular methods for quan-tification of antiepileptic drugs are gas chromatog-raphy, liquid chromatography, and enzyme multiplied immunoassay technique.

Gas Chromatography

BASIC PRINCIPLES

All modes of chromatography have two compartments: the mobile phase and the stationary phase [47]. The mobile phase contains a mixture of drugs or other molecules in a gas or liquid form. The stationary phase is usually a liquid or solid bound to an inert support, such as particles of silicone or alumina, which is packed into a column. Separation of drugs is accom-plished by partition of the drugs between the mobile phase and the stationary phase as the mobile phase passes through the column. Compounds that are least retained by the stationary phase will pass through the column (elute) rapidly, whereas compounds that are most attracted to the stationary phase will elute slowly. The length of time required to reach the end of the column is called the retention time.

In gas chromatography (GC) the mobile phase is a gas. Therefore, compounds must be volatile in order to be analyzed by this technique. The gas chromato-graph is an intricate instrument with several com-ponents (Fig. 15-1). The drug sample is injected by syringe into the system through a rubber septum, made volatile by heating, and carried by an inert gas under pressure. The mobile phase carrier gas (usually nitro-gen) flows through a 3- to 6-foot-long glass column placed in a temperature controlled oven. The column contains a liquid stationary phase bonded to an inert support. As the gaseous forms of the drugs flow over the liquid, the drugs are separated from each other according to differences in attraction to the liquid phase. This is gas-liquid chromatography. When separated compounds reach the end of the column, electronic components detect the molecules leaving the system by means of a detector head that registers on a chart recorder. The pens of the recorder respond to the detector by moving away from the baseline to inscribe a peak the instant the drug passes through the detector. The quantity of each separate drug determines the size of the peak. Finally, the concentration of drug is calculated from the height and width of the peak.

DETECTORS
The flame ionization detector is widely used for routine GC procedures because it is sensitive to all organic compounds. This detector measures the charged molecules generated when a combustible material in the carrier gas enters a hydrogen-air flame. A DC potential is applied across this flame by means of electrodes that also collect the charged molecules. An electrometer then amplifies the current resulting from the flow of charged molecules, and the amplified current causes deflection of the pen of the chart recorder.

The electron capture detector is a special detector used to detect compounds containing strong electronegative functional groups such as halogen-containing compounds (e.g., benzodiazepines). The electron capture detector has a standing electron flux (supplied by a radioactive source) that results in a standing electrical current. When a chemical passing through the electron flux is capable of capturing electrons, a reduction in the amount of standing current is produced. The decreased standing current is amplified to appear as a peak on the recorder.

EXTRACTION AND DERIVITIZATION
Whereas determination of the concentration of drugs as solutions of pure chemicals is relatively easy once the optimum chromatographic conditions are known, their determination in blood requires careful sample preparation steps including extraction, purification, concentration, and derivitization.

Blood samples are centrifuged to give serum or plasma ready for extraction. A solvent is selected that must efficiently extract only the desired compounds from aqueous serum into organic solvent [30], leaving behind all the undesirable components present in blood. After extraction, the large volume of solvent (usually chloroform or ether) is evaporated to concentrate and dry the drug mixture. The purified residue, containing only the desired drugs, is redissolved in a few drops of suitable solvent. The highly concentrated sample is then ready for chromatographic analysis or for conversion into derivatives.

For some drugs or their metabolites, direct GC separation is difficult or impossible [30]. Compounds that are nonvolatile, or unstable at high temperatures, or have certain functional groups that absorb onto column material will give erratic results. Many of these difficulties can be overcome by converting the extracted drugs to stable, volatile derivatives.

Methylation is the most commonly employed technique for derivitization of antiepileptic drugs [13, 20]. Tetramethyl ammonium hydroxide (TMAH) [41] or trimethylphenyl ammonium hydroxide (TMPAH) [13] solutions are used to redissolve the dried drug after extraction. No further preparation is necessary before the concentrated sample is injected into the gas chromatograph. The methyl derivatives of the drug are formed spontaneously in the hot injector block of the instrument ("flash methylation"), and the concentration of the methyl derivative is then measured by GC.

INTERNAL STANDARD
The principle of an internal standard (IS) is the addition of a known concentration of a drug ("internal standard") similar to the one being assayed to the serum (or other fluid) being tested. The ratio of the chromatographic peaks of the IS and the drug being assayed is then compared in order to calculate the concentration of the drug being assayed. An IS is a molecule that is structurally similar to the drug being assayed and has analogous chemical properties during the extraction process. In the chromatographic process, the IS should elute near the drug being assayed (Fig. 15-2). The ratio of the assayed drug peak area to the IS peak area is obtained from the chromatogram. The serum concentration of the assayed drug is determined from this ratio using standard curves prepared in advance.

Exact amounts of IS must be added to the serum as the first step in sample handling. In this way, any losses during manipulation of the sample during extraction, concentration, or derivitization or any degradation on injection during passage through the column will be reflected in the IS peak.

Because several antiepileptic drugs are structurally related, many investigators [20, 41] have used only one IS, usually 5(p-methylphenyl)-5-phenylhydantoin (MPPH), to represent the basic molecule. However, correlation of nonhydantoin drugs with MPPH is often poor because other drugs have specific properties not shared with hydantoins during extraction or chromatography. A separate IS for each drug allows for the different disposition of each drug during derivitization and GC analysis.

APPLICATIONS
GC is a reliable method that uses inexpensive reagents and can be applied to assaying the concentration of drugs that are volatile and heat stable, such as phenytoin [9, 20, 41], phenobarbital [9, 20, 41], ethosuximide [13], valproic acid [24], and benzodiazepines [12]. The variety of chemical properties of antiepileptic drugs makes it difficult to use a single procedure to analyze all major drugs. Several different tech-

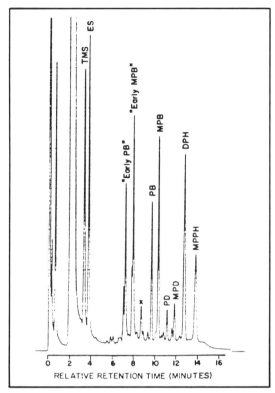

Figure 15-2. A typical gas chromatogram of plasma containing antiepileptic drugs and their internal standards, as permethylated derivatives. The plasma contained ethosuximide (ES) and α,α,β-trimethylsuccinimide (TMS); phenobarbital (PB) and 5-ethyl-5-(p-tolyl)barbituric acid (MPB); primidone (PD) and 5-ethyl-5-(p-tolyl)hexahydropyrimi'ine-4,6-dione (MPD); phenytoin (DPH) and 5-(p-tolyl)-5-phenylhydantoin (MPPH). Early PB and early MPB are the methylated degradation products of PB and MPB. (From K. H. Dudley et al. Gas chromatographic on-column methylation technique for simultaneous determination of antiepileptic drugs in blood. Epilepsia 18:259, 1977. Reprinted with permission of Raven Press, New York.)

niques are used in most laboratories, each specific for one class of drugs. Compounds that are nonvolatile (e.g., conjugated metabolites of antiepileptic drugs) or that are not heat stable (e.g., carbamazepine) are usually best assayed by another technique. Primidone is not extracted efficiently in methods designed for multiple drug analyses but can be assayed by GC using an appropriate IS [13].

SOURCES OF ERROR
There are many potential sources of error in all methods used to determine the serum concentration of drugs. Some of the main sources of error for each method will be outlined in this chapter. These outlines illustrate that no method is perfect and that labora-

tories must constantly strive to maintain quality control. More comprehensive reviews of the sources of error for each method can be found elsewhere [30, 47].

Improper requisitions, improper specimens, and reporting errors are potential sources of error with any method. The other sources of error listed below are specific for chromatography.

Improper Requisitions
All drugs taken by the patient should be indicated on the requisition for an antiepileptic drug serum concentration determination because other drugs may interfere with the quantification of a given antiepileptic drug. The laboratory must know all the drugs the patient takes to select a method of determination and interpret the results properly. The requisition should also indicate the total daily dosage and the time of last dose for each drug as well as the time the blood sample was drawn. There can be considerable hour-to-hour fluctuation in the serum concentration of antiepileptic drugs as the processes of absorption and elimination take place (see Chap. 14). An apparent rise or fall in the serum concentration of an antiepileptic drug may be due entirely to the fact that specimens were obtained at different times after the previous dose.

Improper Specimens
Because red blood cells contain antiepileptic drugs in concentrations different from those in serum, the use of hemolyzed serum will yield spurious results. Frozen specimens must be allowed to come to room temperature and must be mixed thoroughly because crystallized drug may collect at the bottom of the sample.

Improper Reports
Errors in transcription and decimal errors can result in improper reports. Also, errors can result if the laboratory reports the proper number with the wrong units, or if the physician confuses the different units used by different laboratories to report antiepileptic drug serum concentrations (see Appendix I).

Extraction
Sources of error include (1) extraction of unexpected drugs or serum constituents that cause interference with chromatography and detection procedures, and (2) contaminants and stabilizers in reagents and glassware that cause interference.

Injection
Sources of error include (1) incomplete injection from syringe, (2) degradation of extracted drug while

waiting for injection, (3) decomposition of drug in hot injector block, (4) faulty septum, and (5) contamination of specimens by septum compounds ("septum bleed").

Derivitization
Sources of error include (1) incomplete derivitization, (2) remethylation of drugs that are demethylated as part of their usual metabolism (e.g., methsuximide, mephobarbital).

Chromatographic Column
Sources of error include (1) variability of column temperature, (2) variability of carrier gas flow rate, and (3) decomposition of drug and/or reagent at high temperature.

Detection
Sources of error include (1) contamination of drug peaks by drug metabolites, other drugs, serum components, reagents, or septum material, and (2) improper choice of IS.

Quantitation
Sources of error include (1) failure to determine the standard curve each day (see below under Quality Control), (2) decomposition or evaporation of calibration standards (see below under Quality Control), and (3) failure to use an IS.

GAS CHROMATOGRAPHIC MASS SPECTROMETRY
In gas chromatographic mass spectrometry (GCMS) a conventional gas chromatograph is combined with a mass spectrometer to identify and quantify compounds as they elute from the GC column [17]. This technique is extremely accurate but also very expensive and at present is suited only to research applications. Such applications include (1) quantitation of stable isotope-labeled tracer doses of drug in human pharmacokinetic and bioavailability studies (see Chap. 14), (2) identification of drug metabolites, (3) quantitation of drugs and drug metabolites in very small volumes of biologic fluids [7, 17].

Liquid Chromatography

BASIC PRINCIPLES
Liquid chromatography (LC) shares some characteristics with all chromatographic methods [47]. The sample is injected into the LC system dissolved in a liquid mixture (mobile phase) and is pushed through a column under pressure from a pump (Fig. 15-3). As in GC, the stationary phase is a liquid that is bonded to the solid support in the column. While in the column,

the compounds in the sample mixture are separated according to differences in solubility between the mobile phase liquid and the stationary phase liquid, which must be immiscible. Therefore, LC is liquid: liquid chromatography. Some columns contain a polar stationary phase and utilize a nonpolar solvent to elute compounds in the sample in order of increasing polarity. An alternative system contains a nonpolar stationary phase and a polar mobile phase; elution in this system takes place in order of decreasing polarity. When the separated compounds reach the end of the column, they pass through an ultraviolet detector that monitors the change in light absorbance to measure the separate substances in the solvent flow. A chart recorder is attached to the spectrophotometer to record the presence of compounds as peaks. The size of the peak represents the quantity of drug in the original sample.

The extraction procedures for LC are simpler than those for GC, but they must still remove background material from the serum or plasma sample that might otherwise interfere with the analysis. After the IS is added, the sample is extracted into an organic solvent. The sample is evaporated to dryness before being redissolved in an appropriate solvent for injection directly onto the column. No derivitization is used.

The chromatogram obtained for LC is similar to that for GC (as in Fig. 15-2) except that individual ISs are not used for each drug [1, 43]. Only a single IS such as toly-barbital or phenacetin is used.

APPLICATIONS
Unlike GC, LC does not involve volatilization, derivitization, or destruction of drug molecules. LC separates polar molecules more easily than GC. LC can be useful in analyzing thermally labile compounds (e.g., carbamazepine) [2, 43] and polar or nonvolatile compounds such as drug metabolites [18, 28]. It is possible to separate a mixture of antiepileptic drugs and their metabolites by LC. Methods are available for LC analysis of carbamazepine, clonazepam, diazepam, ethusuximide, methsuximide, N-desmethyl-methsuximide, phenobarbital, phenytoin, primidone, and valproic acid [1, 19, 28, 30, 36, 43].

Many laboratories have established GC methods (the first method to be widely utilized) and prefer not to change instrumentation. However, because of the versatility and simplicity of LC it is becoming the preferred chromatographic system.

SOURCES OF ERROR
Many of the sources of error listed in the section on GC also apply to LC. These sources will not be repeated.

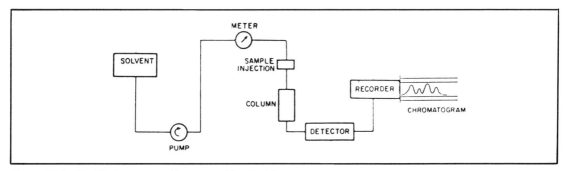

Figure 15-3. Liquid chromatographic system. The liquid chromatographic system starts with a solvent which is pumped under pressure through the column. The sample is injected into the column and enters the moving solvent. The separated compounds leaving the column pass through the UV detector which is attached to a recorder. The chromatogram appears as a series of peaks representing quantity of drug. (Reprinted with permission from G. Zweig and J. Sherma, Handbook of Chromatography, Vol. 2. Cleveland: CRC Press, 1972. Copyright 1972, The Chemical Rubber Co., CRC Press, Inc.)

Because the LC detector is sensitive to any compound absorbed at the preset wavelength, many metabolites of antiepileptic drugs or other drugs present will produce peaks. To verify the identity of the unusual peaks, the suspected pure chemical must undergo chromatography to determine its retention time. Other sources of error are dissolved gases, impurities, and additives to prevent decomposition in organic solvents.

Enzyme Multiplied Immunoassay Technique (EMIT)

BASIC PRINCIPLES

A method of analysis of drugs that is entirely different from chromatography is based on the immunoassay principle of competition for binding sites on an antibody. Antibodies specific for each antigen (drug) are produced by injecting animals with a modified form of the drug. The Enzyme Multiplied Immunoassay Technique (EMIT) uses, as one of its two reagents, antidrug antibody preparations of gamma globulin from sheep immunized to form antibodies against a specific antiepileptic drug.

The second reagent in the EMIT method is an enzyme that has a molecule of the drug to be quantified attached to it (enzyme-labeled drug) (Fig. 15-4). The enzyme is a bacterial glucose 6-phosphate dehydrogenase. This enzyme converts nicotinamide-adenine dinucleotide (NAD^+) to NADH.

In the drug assay [37], patient serum, antidrug antibody, enzyme-labeled drug, and NAD^+ are mixed (Fig. 15-4). When antibody attaches to the enzyme-labeled drug, the active site of the enzyme is blocked by the attachment of the antibody, preventing the enzyme from acting upon the NAD^+ substrate (Fig. 15-4). The enzyme-labeled drug is competitively displaced from its complex with the antibody by the endogenous unlabeled drug from the patient serum sample. When a high concentration of the drug in the serum sample binds to most of the antibody, very little of the enzyme is deactivated. The enzyme substrate reaction will convert a large quantity of NAD^+ to NADH. Conversely, when the serum contains a small amount of drug, most of the antibody is free to bind with the enzyme-labeled drug. Therefore, only a small amount of enzyme is free to react with the substrate. The activity of the unbound enzyme is directly related to the concentration of drug in serum. The rate of change in concentration of substrate (NAD^+) is measured using a spectrophotometer. The drug serum concentration is determined by comparing the observed change in substrate concentration during a period of time with the changes produced by known drug serum concentrations in "calibrator" serum specimens used to produce a standard curve (see section on Quality Control below).

METHOD

A small quantity (50 μl) of plasma or serum is serially diluted twice in buffer (step 1) and added to the reaction vessel (Fig. 15-5). As antidrug antibody and NAD^+ substrate (reagent A) are added (step 2), the molecules of the drug in serum bind to the antibody. Those antibody sites not filled by free drug in serum are available to bind to the enzyme-labeled drug, which is added last (step 3). Some enzyme-labeled drug is left over, unbound to the antibody, and is capable of accepting the substrate (NAD^+) present in the reaction vessel. The enzyme substrate reaction is initiated while the solution is transferred into a temperature-regulated cuvette in the spectrophotome-

170

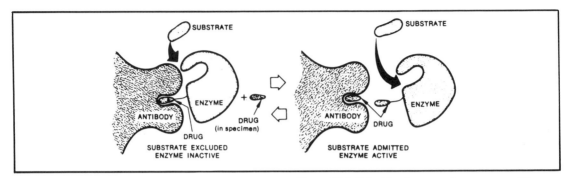

Figure 15-4. Principle of enzyme immunoassay. When enzyme-labeled drug is bound to antibody, the substrate is excluded and cannot react with enzyme (left). When antibody binds to drug in serum, the enzyme-labeled drug is excluded and can accept substrate (right). (From R. S. Schneider et al. Homogeneous enzyme immunoassay for opiates in urine. Clin. Chem. 19:821, 1973. Copyright 1973, Clinical Chemistry.)

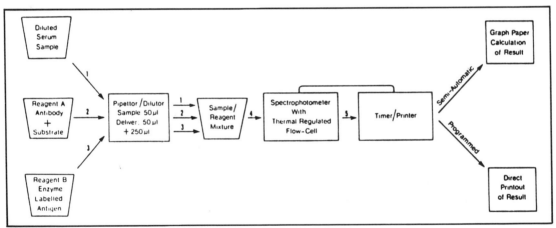

Figure 15-5. EMIT system. The serum sample, antibody-substrate, and enzyme-labeled drug are diluted and mixed before entering the spectrophotometer. The enzyme-substrate reaction is monitored by the timer-printer. Results are plotted on graph paper or calculated to give drug concentration in micrograms per milliliters. (Reproduced by permission of Syva Corp., Palo Alto, Calif.)

ter. The amount of light passing through the solution is recorded at 15 seconds and 45 seconds by a programmed calculator linked with the spectrophotometer. The drug concentration is calculated from the change in light concentration while NAD^+ is converted to NADH.

APPLICATIONS

EMIT reagents are available for six commonly used antiepileptic drugs—phenytoin, phenobarbital, primidone, carbamazepine, ethosuximide, and valproic acid. The assays are specific for the particular antiepileptic drug molecule, and there is virtually no cross reactivity with metabolites of the antiepileptic drug being assayed or with other antiepileptic drugs [37, 42]. Phenobarbital derived from primidone is not measured in the primidone assay but can be measured

separately by the phenobarbital assay. The physician must be careful to specify all antiepileptic drugs that are to be measured because laboratories utilizing the EMIT method test only for those requested. The EMIT method is not a general screening procedure as are many GC and LC methods.

A desirable feature of the EMIT microassay is the need for only 50 μl of serum or plasma to perform up to five tests. GC and LC methods often require several milliliters of blood. A finger- or heel-stick will fill several capillary tubes with enough blood to perform an EMIT assay.

The EMIT method can easily be used to measure the concentration of antiepileptic drug in CSF, saliva, or a protein-free filtrate (dialysate) of whole serum or plasma. The concentration of drug in these fluids is much lower than that in serum for drugs with considerable protein binding (see Chap. 14). In chromatography a large sample may be required to quantify low concentrations of antiepileptic drug, and sufficient quantities of CSF or plasma dialysate may not be available. The EMIT procedure can be modified to achieve a sixfold increase in drug concentration by omitting the preliminary dilution of the sample in buffer and performing the remainder of the assay as usual.

EMIT can also be used for rapid determinations in emergency situations. The speed of the EMIT system is advantageous in the outpatient clinic as well. Assays can be performed before the patient sees the physician, and the results will be ready for review during the visit.

SOURCES OF ERROR

Pipetter or Diluter
Sources of error include (1) use of nonrecommended pipetting and sample-handling apparatus, (2) inconsistent volumes, (3) leaks, and (4) air bubbles.

Spectrophotometer
Sources of error include (1) dirty flow cell, (2) leaking cuvette, (3) variation in absorbance characteristics of apparatus, (4) alteration of absorbance by serum that is icteric, hemolyzed, or lipemic, and (5) delay in entering the sample into the spectrophotometer after the enzyme has been added.

Quantitation
Sources of error include (1) testing a serum sample whose drug concentration is outside the range of the standard curve, (2) failure to determine the standard curve daily, and (3) failure to assay each serum sample in duplicate using a separate dilution each time.

Reagents
Sources of error include (1) decomposition and concentration (due to evaporation) of calibration standards with time, (2) improper reconstitution of lyophilized reagents, (3) variation from lot to lot, and (4) mixing reagents from different lots.

Other Immunoassay Techniques
Radioimmunoassay [30], rate nephelometric inhibition assay [32], and substrate-labeled fluorescent immunoassay [46] have all been used to determine

antiepileptic drug serum concentrations in some institutions.

Quality Control
Quality control (QC) measures consist of both routine checks done within a given laboratory (internal QC) and participation in local and national quality control programs (external QC). Internal QC checks should include frequent redetermination of standard curves and frequent checks of precision and accuracy. External QC programs involve checking the reliability of a laboratory's performance on unknown specimens supplied by an outside source.

INTERNAL QUALITY CONTROL MEASURES

Standard Curves
Standard curves for chromatographic methods are plots of the *ratio* of the drug peak area to the IS peak area obtained by using a fixed concentration of IS in several serum samples with different known concentrations of the drug. Standard curves for the EMIT method are obtained by measuring the change in substrate concentration during time with serum samples containing known amounts of drug. Standard curves are produced by assaying specimens with known drug serum concentrations (calibrators or standards) in the low, middle, and high portions of the therapeutic range of serum concentrations. The concentration of a drug in a clinical specimen is determined by plotting the ratio of the drug to the IS peak area (chromatography) or the change in substrate concentration produced by the specimen (EMIT) on the standard curve and reading across the standard curve to determine what the corresponding serum concentration should be. The slope of the standard curves can change from day to day, and such curves should be determined daily whether chromatographic or EMIT methods are employed.

Standard curves should not be extrapolated below or above the lowest or highest concentrations used to determine the curve because many methods do not have linear standard curves at very high and low drug concentrations and because very high or low concentrations of a drug may not be reliably measured by a method designed for a specific therapeutic range of values. Any patient sample that gives results outside the range of the standard curve should be repeated. Samples containing high drug concentrations should be diluted, and low concentration samples can be assayed with twice the usual volume of serum (on EMIT one dilution can be omitted).

Precision
The precision of antiepileptic drug assays is the agreement of repeated determinations of the same drug con-

centration, usually designated by the coefficient of variation. The coefficient of variation for most anti-epileptic drug methods is rarely less than 4 to 5 percent. Constantly checking the precision of a method will prevent reporting of inaccurate results if any series of determinations that does not fall within a reasonable coefficient of variation is repeated, and such checking will help the laboratory recognize problems due to human error or methodologic short-comings.

A reported drug concentration may vary within the range of the coefficient of variation. For example, a phenobarbital concentration of 20 $\mu g/ml$ may appear to rise or fall daily with reports ranging from 18 to 22 $\mu g/ml$, a ± 10 percent variation. The precision of most methods precludes the reporting of data other than in whole numbers; decimal point results are unrealistic (except for primidone and carbamazepine).

Accuracy

The accuracy of a given method refers to how close the drug serum concentration determination is to the actual concentration of the drug. A consistent error in methodology can produce results that are con-sistently reproducible (i.e., have a high "precision") and that produce linear standard curves. Nevertheless, the drug serum concentration determined by the method is far from the actual concentration (i.e., poor "accuracy"). Control samples other than calibrators with a known drug concentration are used to check the accuracy of a method.

EXTERNAL QUALITY CONTROL MEASURES

Several hundred laboratories throughout the country participate in a special QC program for antiepileptic drugs coordinated by the American Association of Clinical Chemistry. Samples containing six antiepi-leptic drugs are sent monthly to participants as unknown samples for assay. The laboratory receives the correct results only after sending its own results to the QC program. By this method the laboratory can evaluate its performance and resolve problems if they are discovered. Often the results for just one or two drugs are unreliable, suggesting problems with a specific method, or the results from nights or week-ends are less accurate than those from weekdays, suggesting poor technique.

ROLE OF PHYSICIAN IN QUALITY CONTROL

It is up to the physician to ask the laboratory what type of QC system is used. The coefficient of variation and performance on external QC tests should be queried for each drug being assayed. If no QC system is ap-parent, the physician should suggest one or send samples to another laboratory.

Comparison of All Methods

Statistically, the GC, LC, and EMIT methods compare well, with good correlation throughout the thera-peutic range for most drugs [5, 42]. The time and cost of analysis [8] vary according to the size of the batch. Preference for any single system depends on the instrument (cost, maintenance), reagents (cost, prepa-ration), operation (skill, time), and need for versa-tility (research, other chemical tests). Whereas the chromatographic systems use inexpensive chemicals and are versatile, they do require excellent technical skill in sample preparation and analysis as well as mechanical skill for repairs. The EMIT system is ex-pensive to run because reagents cost over $4.00 for each test. However, the semiautomated EMIT method can be operated reliably by a high school student. The time required to obtain a result during normal labora-tory operation must be considered. Chromatographic methods require considerable time for preparation and the chromatographic process. With chromato-graphic methods specimens are usually run in batches; only one batch can be run per day. Therefore, if a blood sample arrives in the laboratory late in the morning, it usually cannot be analyzed until the next day. When the EMIT system is used, routine samples can be added to the batch at any time while the instrument is in use. Emergency samples can be run by EMIT at any time of the day or night.

Cost to Patient

GC, LC, and EMIT are all relatively inexpensive methods. Nevertheless, many laboratories charge much more for antiepileptic drug serum concentra-tion determinations than for other chemical tests that have similar laboratory costs. In a survey sponsored by the Epilepsy Foundation of America in 1974, the total charge for determining the concentrations of four antiepileptic drugs in a serum specimen ranged from $10 to $105 [31].

Charging excessively high prices for antiepileptic drug serum concentration determinations creates an unacceptable hardship for patients with epilepsy be-cause (1) epilepsy is a chronic disease, and most patients will require many antiepileptic drug serum concentration determinations, (2) many patients are taking more than one antiepileptic drug, (3) many pa-tients are unemployed, and (4) patients with severe epilepsy are most likely to be unemployed, to require frequent drug serum concentration determinations, and to be taking multiple drugs. If antiepileptic drug serum concentration determinations are too expensive, the benefits of therapy guided by such determinations will not be available to many patients, especially those most in need of help. The physician must make certain that the laboratory he uses charges a reasonable fee for antiepileptic drug serum concentration determinations; if not, a change to another laboratory is in order.

References

1. Adams, R. F., and Vandemark, F. L. Simultaneous high pressure liquid chromatographic determination of some anticonvulsants in serum. *Clin. Chem.* 22:25, 1976.
2. Adams, R. F., Schmidt, G. J., and Vandemark, F. L. A micro-method for the determination of carbamazepine and the 10,11-epoxide metabolite in serum and urine by reverse phase liquid chromatography. *Chromatogr. Newsletter* 5:11, 1977.
3. Blackwell, B. The drug defaulter. *Clin. Pharmacol. Ther.* 13:841, 1972.
4. Blackwell, B. Drug therapy: Patient compliance. *N. Engl. J. Med.* 289:249, 1973.
5. Booker, H. E., and Darcey, B. A. Enzymatic immunoassay versus gas-liquid chromatographic determination of phenobarbital and phenytoin in serum. *Clin. Chem.* 21:1766, 1975.
6. Borofsky, L. G., Louis, S., and Kutt, H. Diphenylhydantoin in children: Pharmacology and efficacy. *Neurology* (Minneap.) 23:967, 1973.
7. Browne, T. R. et al. Applications of stable isotope methods to studying the clinical pharmacology of antiepileptic drugs in newborns, infants, children, and adolescents. *Ther. Drug Monit.* In press, 1983.
8. Chamberlain, R. T. et al. High pressure liquid chromatography and enzyme immunoassay compared with gas chromatography for determining phenytoin. *Clin. Chem.* 23:1764, 1977.
9. Chang, T., and Glazko, A. J. Quantitative assay of 5,5-diphenylhydantoin (Dilantin) and 5-(p-hydroxyphenyl)-5-phenyl hydantoin by gas-liquid chromatography. *J. Lab. Clin. Med.* 75:145, 1970.
10. Dawson, K. P., and Jamison, A. Value of blood phenytoin estimation in management of childhood epilepsy. *Arch. Child.* 46:386, 1971.
11. Desai, B. T. et al. Active noncompliance as a cause of uncontrolled seizures. *Epilepsia* 19:447, 1978.
12. DeSilva, J. A. et al. Determination of 1,4-benzodiazepines and -diazepin-2-ones in blood by electron capture gas-liquid chromatography. *Anal. Chem.* 48:10, 1976.
13. Dudley, K. H. et al. Gas chromatographic on-column methylation technique for simultaneous determination of antiepileptic drugs in blood. *Epilepsia* 18:259, 1977.
14. Gibberd, F. B. et al. Supervision of epileptic patients taking phenytoin. *Br. Med. J.* 1:247, 1970.
15. Glazko, A. J., and Chang, T. Diphenylhydantoin: Absorption, Distribution, Biotransformation, and Excretion. In D. M. Woodbury, J. K. Penry, and R. P. Schmidt (Eds.), *Antiepileptic Drugs.* New York: Raven Press, 1972.
16. Hansten, P. D. *Drug Interactions.* Philadelphia: Lea & Febiger, 1979.
17. Jenden, D. J., and Cho, A. K. Selected ion monitoring in pharmacology. *Biochem. Pharmacol.* 28:705, 1979.
18. Kabra, P. K., and Marton, L. J. High pressure liquid chromatographic determination of 5-(4-hydroxyphenyl)-5-phenylhydantoin in human urine. *Clin. Chem.* 22:1672, 1976.
19. Kabra, P. K., Stafford, B. E., and Marton, L. J. Simultaneous measurement of phenobarbital, phenytoin, primidone, ethosuximide, and carbamazepine in serum by high-pressure liquid chromatography. *Clin. Chem.* 23:1284, 1977.
20. Kupferberg, H. J. Quantitative estimation of diphenylhydantoin, primidone and phenobarbital in plasma by gas-liquid chromatography. *Clin. Chim. Acta* 29:283, 1970.
21. Kutt, H., and Penry, J. K. Usefulness of blood levels of antiepileptic drugs. *Arch. Neurol.* 21:283, 1974.
22. Kutt, H. et al. Insufficient parahydroxylation as a cause of diphenylhydantoin toxicity. *Neurology* (Minneap.) 14:542, 1964.
23. Lund, I. Anticonvulsant effect of diphenylhydantoin relative to plasma levels. *Arch. Neurol.* 31:289, 1974.
24. Mattson, R. H. et al. Valproic acid in epilepsy: Clinical and pharmacological effects. *Ann. Neurol.* 3:20, 1978.
25. Melikian, A. P. et al. Bioavailability of 11 phenytoin products. *J. Pharmacokinet. Biopharm.* 5:133, 1977.
26. Painter, M. J. et al. Phenobarbital and phenytoin in neonatal seizures: Metabolism and tissue distribution. *Neurology* (N.Y.) 31:1107, 1981.
27. Pentikainen, P. J., Neuvonen, P. J., and Elfving, S. M. Bioavailability of four brands of phenytoin tablets. *Eur. J. Clin. Pharmacol.* 9:213, 1975.
28. Perchalski, R. J., and Wilder, B. J. Determination of benzodiazepine anticonvulsants in plasma by high-performance liquid chromatography. *Anal. Chem.* 49:554, 1978.
29. Perucca, E., and Richens, A. General Principles: Biotransformation. In D. M. Woodbury, J. K. Penry,

and C. E. Pippenger (Eds.), *Antiepileptic Drugs.* New York: Raven Press, 1982. Pp. 31–56.

30. Pippenger, C. E., Penry, J. K., and Kutt, H. *Antiepileptic Drugs: Quantitative Analysis and Interpretation.* New York: Raven Press, 1978.

31. Pippenger, C. E. et al. Interlaboratory variability in determination of plasma antiepileptic drug concentrations. *Arch. Neurol.* 33:351, 1976.

32. Polito, A. J. Nephelometric assay. *Clin. Chem. News* 7(4):5, 1981.

33. Porter, A. M. W. Drug defaulting in general practice. *Br. Med. J.* 1:218, 1969.

34. Rail, L. Dilantin overdosage. *Med. J. Aust.* 2:339, 1968.

35. Sackett, D. L., and Haynes, R. B. (Eds.). *Compliance with Therapeutic Regimens.* Baltimore: Johns Hopkins Press, 1976.

36. Schmidt, G. J., and Slavin, W. Determination of dipropylacetic acid (sodium valproate) by liquid chromatography with pre-column labeling and ultraviolet detection. *Chromatogr. Newsletter* 6:22, 1978.

37. Schneider, R. S. et al. Homogeneous enzyme immunoassay for opiates in urine. *Clin. Chem.* 19:821, 1973.

38. Sherwin, A. L., Robb, J. P., and Lechter, M. Improved control of epilepsy by monitoring plasma ethosuximide. *Arch. Neurol.* 28:171, 1973.

39. Shope, J. et al. Correlates of antiepileptic drug compliance. *Epilepsia* 23:439, 1982.

40. Smith, D. L. Patient compliance with medical regimens. *Drug Intelligence Clin. Pharmacol.* 10:390, 1976.

41. Solow, E. G., and Green, J. B. The simultaneous determination of multiple anticonvulsant drug levels by gas-liquid chromatography. *Neurology* (Minneap.) 22:540, 1972.

42. Spiehler, V. et al. Radioimmunoassay, enzyme immunoassay, spectrophotometry, and gas-liquid chromatography compared for determination of phenobarbital and diphenylhydantoin. *Clin. Chem.* 22:749, 1976.

43. Szabo, G. K., and Browne, T. R. Improved isocratic liquid chromatographic simultaneous measurement of phenytoin, phenobarbital, primidone, carbamazepine, ethosuximide, and N-desmethylmethsuximide in serum. *Clin. Chem.* 28:100, 1982.

44. Tyrer, J. H. et al. Outbreak of anticonvulsant intoxication in an Australian city. *Br. Med. J.* 4:271, 1970.

45. Vasko, M. R. et al. Inheritance of phenytoin hypometabolism: A kinetic study of one family. *Clin. Pharmacol. Ther.* 27:96, 1980.

46. Wong, R. C. et al. Substrate-labeled fluorescent immunoassay for phenytoin in human serum. *Clin. Chem.* 25:686, 1979.

47. Zweig, G., and Sherma, J. *Handbook of Chromatography,* Vol. 2. Cleveland: CRC Press, 1972.

PHENYTOIN (DILANTIN) AND OTHER HYDANTOINS

16

Thomas R. Browne
Jonathan H. Pincus

Chemistry of Phenytoin

The structural formula of phenytoin (5,5-diphenyl-hydantoin, PHT, Dilantin) is shown in Table 16-1. Phenytoin is a weak acid with a molecular weight of 252.26 and a pK_a of 8.3 to 9.2 under different experimental conditions [22]. Because of its high pK_a, PHT is relatively insoluble in water at acid or physiologic pH but is quite soluble in water at alkaline pH. These relationships have important clinical consequences discussed below. The sodium salt of PHT has a molecular weight of 274.25 and contains the equivalent of 91.98 percent PHT acid [22].

In animal screening tests PHT has proved to be extremely effective against the tonic component of maximal electroshock seizures and to be inactive against seizures induced by pentylenetetrazol [59]. These results predict PHT should be effective in humans against tonic-clonic and complex partial seizures but not against absence seizures [59], and this has proven to be the case. A 5-phenyl substituent on the hydantoin ring appears to be necessary for activity against maximal electroshock seizures in animals and tonic-clonic seizures in humans. Alkyl substituents in position 5 increase the sedative effect and reduce the effect against maximal electroshock seizures.

Mechanism of Action of Phenytoin

INTRODUCTION

There have been many studies of the mechanism of action of PHT [2, 21], but at present the exact mechanism is unknown. What is known is how PHT affects certain aspects of normal and abnormal neuronal function. These effects will be reviewed, and when possible, attempts will be made to synthesize available information into possible mechanisms of action.

It is well established that the drug "stabilizes" the neuronal membrane in low external calcium concentrations, decreases post-tetanic hyperpolarization, and decreases post-tetanic potentiation. Interpretations of these basic observations, however, have not always been consistent.

LIMITATION OF PASSIVE SODIUM MOVEMENT DURING DEPOLARIZATION AND POSSIBLE ROLE OF CALCIUM

PHT has been unequivocally shown to decrease the inward sodium current in lobster axons, in voltage-

This work was supported in part by the Veterans Administration.

Table 16-1. Hydantoins

Substituents					
R_1	R_2	R_3	Generic Name	Trade Name	
H	C_6H_5*	C_6H_5*	Phenytoin	Dilantin	
CH_3	C_6H_5*	C_2H_5	Mephenytoin	Mesantoin	
C_2H_5	C_6H_5*	H	Ethotoin	Peganone	

*Phenyl ring

clamped squid axons, and in stimulated brain slices [36, 47]. The mechanism by which PHT reduces axonal sodium conductance is not known. Since it is believed that calcium ions may play a regulatory role in the movement of sodium across the nerve membrane, it is conceivable that PHT exerts its primary action upon calcium and indirectly suppresses sodium conductance. PHT has been found to reduce ^{45}Ca uptake and outflow in resting lobster nerves and to eliminate the increase in ^{45}Ca accumulation that normally occurs during stimulation. These experiments are consistent with the view that PHT might displace calcium from binding sites on the outer nerve membrane, thus reducing calcium movement across the membrane. Assuming that calcium has some role in the regulation of sodium movement across membranes, it is conceivable that PHT could block sodium conductance by occupying the calcium sites [27].

INHIBITION OF NEUROTRANSMITTER RELEASE
AND POSSIBLE ROLE OF CALCIUM
A major antiepileptic action of PHT is related to its reversal of post-tetanic potentiation (PTP). The phenomenon of PTP appears to be the result of increased transmitter release following repetitive stimulation. It is known that when the nerve impulse invades the presynaptic terminal, calcium (Ca^{2+}) entry into the presynaptic terminal is markedly increased, causing the release of transmitter quanta. PTP may be the result of increased calcium concentration in the presynaptic terminal due to repetitive stimulation.

Various agents known to interfere with calcium entry inhibit transmitter release. Moreover, the development of PTP requires the presence of calcium ions in the media. These factors suggest that one mode of action of PHT may be to decrease calcium accumulation in the presynaptic terminal during stimulation, resulting in decreased transmitter release.

This hypothesis was tested in a series of experiments in which rat brain slices were labeled with tritiated norepinephrine. The release of norepinephrine from the brain slices by stimulation was found to be calcium-dependent. PHT was found to inhibit both norepinephrine release and the uptake of ^{45}Ca into the brain slices [48]. Similarly, PHT has been shown to inhibit calcium uptake into isolated brain synaptosomes. With these observations in mind, it was clearly desirable to test the action of PHT on individual synapse.

The amount of release of transmitter with depolarization of the presynaptic terminal is highly dependent on the intracellular calcium concentration near the presynaptic membrane. This was proved by the observation that direct intracellular application of calcium in the giant synapse of the squid increases the rate of transmitter release [40]. Calcium levels in the axon terminal must be strictly and rapidly regulated. Most cells contain an appreciable amount of intracellular calcium, but very little is actually free in the cytoplasm. It is possible that the intracellular free calcium concentration is less than 10^{-6} M, whereas total tissue or serum calcium is in the range of 10^{-3} M. The low level of free calcium is maintained by three mechanisms: (1) mitochondria and endoplasmic reticulum actively accumulate calcium; (2) negatively charged macromolecules in the cell bind calcium; and (3) calcium is actively extruded by the axon membrane [1].

If PHT reduced the influx of calcium into the depolarized axon terminal, a depression in evoked neurosecretion would be expected. If PHT suppressed the intracellular calcium sequestration-extrusion mechanism, transmitter release would be facilitated, and the frequency of spontaneous release of individual transmitter packets would be increased. These predictions were tested on the frog neuromuscular synapse.

PHT was shown both to reduce quantal content (the number of transmitter packets released by an impulse) and to increase the frequency of miniature end-plate potentials (mepps), which represent individual packets of transmitter that are spontaneously released.

The PHT-induced reduction in quantal content in normal media may result from a decrease in Ca^{2+} influx into the presynaptic terminal during the nerve action potential [67]. The PHT-induced increase in mepps could be due to blockage of transport of calcium into intracellular binding sites or to blockage of calcium extrusion, causing an increase in resting internal calcium concentration and an increase in the rate of spontaneous mepp discharge. Supporting this hypothesis is the finding that the facilitatory action of PHT on mepp frequency does not require the presence of extracellular Ca^{2+} ions. Thus it is possible that PHT reduces calcium transport at the outer nerve membrane and at internal sites by blocking high-affinity binding sites for calcium [68].

REDUCED POTASSIUM CONDUCTANCE
AND POSSIBLE ROLE OF CALCIUM
In bursting pacemaker cells in Aplysia, a hyperpolarizing phase due to a slow increase in potassium conductance is reduced by PHT [2]. This effect is of special interest because the potassium conductance in question is activated by the influx of calcium during the preceding depolarizing phase. In other words, calcium enters the cell and changes the membrane potassium conductance. The change in potassium conductance caused by PHT in this cell may be related to its reduction of calcium entry.

REDUCED POSTSYNAPTIC MEMBRANE RESPONSE
PHT has also been shown to attenuate the effect of acetylcholine postsynaptically at the frog neuromuscular junction. The drug enhances the rate of postsynaptic receptor desensitization, reduces mepp amplitude, and reduces the half-time of recovery of end-plate potentials. The drug does not change membrane resistance, and it seems likely that it alters ionic conductances that are acetylcholine-dependent at the motor end-plate as do barbiturates and local anesthetics.

BLOCKAGE OF AXONAL CONDUCTION
Another action of PHT is blockage of the axonal conduction of nerve impulses, especially during repetitive stimulation at high rates [67, 68]. Epileptic cells are known to fire at high rates, and if PHT acts similarly on central neurons, this action would tend to limit the spread of epileptic discharge. The site of the block may be at terminal branching points, because such sites are known to have a low safety factor for impulse propagation. Interestingly, nerve conduction block has been seen in unpublished experiments with D600, a compound that blocks calcium movement across membranes.

MECHANISM OF REDUCTION OF CALCIUM INFLUX
It is not known exactly how PHT interacts with calcium. There is some evidence that cyclic AMP plays a role in regulating calcium influx into motor nerve terminals, and that PHT blocks this cyclic nucleotide-mediated calcium influx [19]. Also, calcium and PHT have antagonistic actions on the net level of endogenous phosphorylation of certain brain proteins that are present in synaptosomal preparations. The antagonistic actions of calcium and PHT on the phosphorylation of these proteins may in some way be related to the apparent actions of these agents on the release of neurotransmitter from the presynaptic terminal or on the sequestration of calcium within the cell [14].

ACTIVATION OF SODIUM-POTASSIUM ATPASE SYSTEM
The most important supporting data for the theory of Na-K ATPase activation involve observations in extraneural tissue. PHT has been shown to increase sodium transport in frog skin and guinea pig heart, kidney, and intestine. The evidence that PHT increases Na-K transport in neural tissue, however, is much more limited.

The drug has been shown to increase synaptosomal Na-K ATPase activity but only when the Na-K ratio is more than 30:1. At other Na-K ratios, PHT appears either to have no effect or to inhibit the Na-K ATPase enzyme. This enzyme is activated by intracellular sodium and extracellular potassium. It seems unlikely that the in vitro activation of this enzyme by PHT has very much to do with its antiepileptic effect in vivo because the specific relation of the activation of Na-K ATPase to the antiepileptic effect of PHT rests upon the assumption that in epileptic neurons the ratio of intracellular sodium to extracellular potassium exceeds 30:1. Much evidence has shown that this assumption is incorrect [2, 15].

In summary, there has never been a conclusive demonstration of PHT stimulation of active transport in a normally functioning neuron in vivo or in vitro [2, 15].

PHENYTOIN RECEPTORS
Binding of PHT at therapeutic concentrations to specific sites in brain synaptosomal fractions has recently been reported in rats and in humans [57]. Phenytoin binding is enhanced in the presence of chloride ions, and binding to phenytoin receptors may facilitate GABA-mediated chloride conductance in the postsynaptic membrane [57]. There is a good correlation for both phenytoin analogues and anti epileptic barbiturates between antiepileptic potency in the maximal electroshock model and affinity for the

phenytoin receptor site [57]. An endogenous compound with specific affinity for the PHT receptor site has been isolated from calf brains [57].

SUMMARY

PHT has been shown to decrease intracellular sodium in neuronal preparations. It seems likely that this is the result of its depression of sodium conductance rather than of its activation of a sodium pump. The mechanism by which the drug suppresses sodium conductance may depend upon its interaction with calcium. A large and growing body of evidence suggests that PHT depresses calcium conductance and that it interferes with such calcium-dependent processes as excitatory transmitter release and the activation of certain ionic conductances. Recent work suggests the presence of phenytoin receptors which may facilitate conductance in the postsynaptic membrane. As a result of its effect upon these ionic conductances, PHT increases inhibitory phenomena. In some preparations, the drug also causes a blockage of impulse transmission, particularly at high rates of stimulation, and this is mimicked by a drug that also blocks calcium movement. It is likely that these findings have an important bearing on the clinical usefulness of PHT as an antiepileptic drug.

Clinical Pharmacology of Phenytoin

ABSORPTION

Absorption by Oral Route

PHT is a weak acid with a pK_a of approximately 9.0 [22, 66]. At a pH of 1 to 2, PHT is less than 1 percent ionized and has a water solubility of 14 μg/ml. At a pH of 7.5, PHT is 3 percent ionized and has a water solubility of 100 μg/ml. Thus, only a small amount of PHT is absorbed in the stomach, and most PHT absorption takes place in the small intestine [66].

PHT has a solubility in intestinal fluid of approximately 100 μg/ml. This low solubility has several important consequences. Not all of an oral dose of PHT is absorbed, and some is lost in the feces. There are apparently considerable differences in the amount of PHT absorbed by different people, especially when the capsule form is used. Certain otherwise normal people require large doses of PHT to reach average drug serum concentrations, and these people are sometimes improperly accused of being noncompliant. Altered PHT absorption is also associated with certain physiologic states. Pregnancy reduces absorption of PHT, and pregnant women may require very large doses of PHT to maintain a therapeutic serum concentration [50]. Neonates absorb oral PHT incompletely and erratically [7, 43]. A final consequence of the

marginal intestinal solubility of PHT is that any substance that interferes with the dissolution of PHT or adsorbs PHT in intestinal fluids (e.g., nasogastric feedings, antacids, certain foods, and certain other drugs) will inhibit its absorption [5].

Peak serum concentration of PHT is usually reached 4 to 8 hours after an oral dose, although the peak may be reached as early as 3 hours or as late as 12 hours [54, 65, 66].

Bioavailability of Generic Oral Preparations

There are substantial differences in bioavailability of different generic forms of PHT [8, 11, 45, 54]. This is not surprising in view of PHT's marginal solubility and the effects that formulation (especially particle size) can have on solubility. Care must be taken always to prescribe the same generic form of PHT for a given patient. Increased seizure frequency and drug toxicity have been reported when the brand of PHT capsule used by a group of patients was changed [8, 54, 66]. The oral suspension of PHT has greater bioavailability than many capsule preparations [45]. Patients who do not absorb PHT capsules well may have a considerable increase in serum PHT concentration when they are given the same dose in oral suspension form.

Absorption by Intramuscular Route

To dissolve PHT in a small volume of liquid for parenteral administration, the marketed solution is prepared with a pH of 12. When this preparation is injected intramuscularly (i.e., into a medium with a pH of about 7.4), the water solubility of the drug decreases substantially, PHT crystals precipitate in the muscle [8], and the drug is absorbed very slowly [8, 30].

Peak serum PHT concentrations occur approximately 24 hours after a single intramuscular injection and are considerably less than the peak levels produced by the same dose given by rapid intravenous infusion [30]. PHT should not be given via the intramuscular route in emergency situations (e.g., status epilepticus) because of the slowness of absorption and the relatively low peak serum concentrations produced by that route.

Use of the intramuscular route for administration of maintenance doses of PHT remains controversial. Eventually, almost all of an intramuscular injection of PHT is absorbed, and regimens for administration of maintenance doses of intramuscular PHT have been published [8]. However, peak PHT serum concentrations occur 24 hours after an intramuscular injection and are variable [30]. Further, serum concentrations may fall below therapeutic levels shortly after switching to the intramuscular route from the oral or intravenous route and may ascend into the toxic range because of accumulation after switching back from the intramuscular to the oral route [8]. In most situations maintenance doses of PHT should not be given by the intramuscular route because of the slowness and variability of absorption, and because of the danger of over- and undermedication when switching to and from other routes of administration.

DISTRIBUTION

Protein Binding
PHT is 69 to 96 percent protein bound. This protein binding has several clinically important consequences, which are discussed in Chapter 14.

Distribution to Brain
The concentration of PHT in brain parenchyma and cerebrospinal fluid (CSF) may not reach peak levels until an hour or more after intravenous injection in humans [64]. However, the brain parenchyma concentration of PHT remains greater than the serum concentration of free PHT once steady state serum concentrations are reached, presumably because of binding by proteins and phospholipids [8].

Distribution to Transcellular Fluids: CSF and Saliva
The concentrations of PHT in CSF and in saliva are essentially identical to the concentrations of free (nonprotein-bound) PHT in plasma (see Chap. 14).

Distribution to Fetus and Breast Milk
PHT freely crosses the placenta [66]. It enters breast milk with the milk: serum PHT concentration ratio being about 0.2 [54].

Distribution of PHT to Other Tissues
This topic is reviewed elsewhere [66].

BIOTRANSFORMATION AND EXCRETION

Normal Pathways
The major route of biotransformation of PHT is para-hydroxylation of a phenyl ring by the liver cytochrome oxidase system to form 5-(*p*-hydroxyphenyl)-5-phenylhydantoin (*p*-HPPH) [10]. HPPH has little antiepileptic effect. Thus, PHT does not have active metabolites, and measurement of serum PHT concentration measures the total active drug in the serum.

PHT is excreted in the urine and feces mainly as its metabolites. Less than 5 percent is excreted unmetabolized [10, 66]. Over 60 percent of PHT is excreted as *p*-HPPH, the majority of which is conjugated with glucuronide [10, 66]. Minor metabolites include meta-HPPH; a dihydrodiol derivative; diphenylhydantoic

acid; 5,5-bis(4-hydroxyphenyl)hydantoin; 5-(3,4-di-hydroxyphenyl)-5-phenylhydantoin, and 5-(3-methoxy-4-hydroxyphenyl)-5-phenylhydantoin [10, 66].

Dose-Dependence of PHT Elimination
Using stable isotope tracer methods, Browne et al. [9] have definitely established that PHT inhibits its own biotransformation to HPPH in a dose-dependent manner at therapeutic serum concentrations. When a patient begins PHT therapy, the PHT serum concentration rises, which in turn inhibits PHT biotransformation, which in turn causes the PHT serum concentration to rise further. This self-propagating cycle results in a progressive increase in PHT elimination half-life and serum concentration during the first 4 to 12 weeks of PHT therapy [9]. Thus, PHT can require 4 to 12 weeks to come to a steady-state serum concentration rather than the 5 days (5 elimination half-lives) predicted by a model with simple first-order elimination kinetics [9] (see Chap. 14). Furthermore, the enzyme system eliminating PHT can be completely saturated with usual therapeutic doses of PHT, resulting in zero order elimination kinetics [8, 18, 54]. The human body can eliminate only 3.8 to 31.8 mg/kg/day of PHT, and for most people the maximum rate of elimination of PHT is 4 to 12 mg/kg/day [8, 18, 54]. When the dosage exceeds 4 to 12 mg/kg/day, a small increase in dosage may produce a large increase in PHT serum concentration, a further increase in the apparent elimination half-life, and unexpected drug toxicity [8, 18, 54].

Effect of Age on PHT Elimination
Neonates eliminate PHT more slowly than adults or children (see below). Young children metabolize PHT more rapidly than older children and adults; they require higher milligram-per-kilogram doses of PHT to achieve a given serum concentration and sometimes cannot maintain therapeutic serum concentrations with once daily administration [8, 18, 54]. Serum PHT concentrations for a given daily dose are higher in the elderly than in young adults [4, 54].

Effects of Pregnancy, Renal Failure, and Hepatic Failure
These topics are discussed in Chapters 14, 15, and 29.

CLINICAL PHARMACOKINETICS

Elimination Half-Life
The elimination half-life of PHT in adults ranges from 10 to 34 hours, with an average value of approximately 22 hours [8, 9]. In children the elimination half-life appears to be considerably less, on the order of 5 to 18

hours [8, 17]. The elimination half-life in premature infants is quite long and variable (75.4 ± 64.5 hours) [37]. In full-term infants the elimination half-life is longer (20 to 60 hours) than it is in older children for about the first week of life [7, 37].

Time to Reach Steady State

The time needed to reach steady state serum concentration may be 2 to 12 weeks in a patient given a dose yielding a therapeutic concentration [9, 54] (see Dose-Dependence of PHT Elimination above).

DRUG INTERACTIONS

Many drugs have been reported to increase the PHT serum concentration, presumably by interfering with the metabolism of PHT. Proceeding from most likely to least likely, the list includes: disulfiram, sulthiame, isoniazid, dicumarol, phenyramidol, carbamazepine, phenobarbital, primidone, chloramphenicol, methylphenidate, diazepam, sulfamethizole, phenylbutazone, sulfhaphenazone, ethosuximide, chlorpromazine, prochlorperazine, chlordiazepoxide, and propoxyphene [8, 23, 32, 54, 63].

The following drugs have been reported to lower total PHT serum concentration either by displacing it from protein-binding sites or by increased metabolism: valproic acid, ethanol, phenobarbital, phenylbutazone, and salicylates [8, 32, 42, 54, 63].

PHT has been reported to lower the levels of the following drugs either by enhanced metabolism or by displacing the drug from its protein-binding sites: digitoxin, bishydroxycoumarin, metyrapone, DDT, dexamethasone, cortisol, contraceptive steroids, 25-hydroxycholecalciferol, and thyroxine [32, 63].

Coadministration of PHT has been reported to raise the serum concentration of phenobarbital, phenobarbital derived from primidone, and N-desmethyl-methsuximide derived from methsuximide [8, 34] (see Chaps. 14 and 19). The presumed mechanism of this effect is competitive inhibition of hydroxylation of the phenyl ring.

BLOOD LEVELS

Methods of Determination

Reliable methods for determining the concentration of PHT in biologic fluids have been reported employing gas-liquid chromatography, high-performance liquid chromatography, and enzyme-multiplied immunoassay technique (see Chap. 15).

Relationship of Dosage to Serum Concentration

Drug serum concentration generally tends to increase with increasing dosage in patients of the same age

[33]. The average dosage (in milligrams per kilograms) required to achieve a given serum concentration is greater in children than in adults [8, 33]. However, the serum concentration produced by a given dose of PHT varies so much that it is impossible to predict a given patient's drug serum concentration from the dosage [33]. Laboratory tests are the only assured method of determining a patient's drug serum concentration.

Therapeutic Range of Serum Concentration

The therapeutic range for PHT serum concentration is usually set at 10 to 20 μg/ml (see Chap. 14). The lower limit of 10 μg/ml is determined by the observation that the majority of patients with PHT serum concentrations of less than 10 μg/ml do not achieve good seizure control [8, 33]. The upper limit of 20 μg/ml is determined by the observation that the majority of patients will show some signs or symptoms of PHT intoxication with serum concentrations above this value [8, 33]. There is some evidence that patients whose seizures are not controlled by serum concentrations in the lower part of the therapeutic range may achieve good seizure control with serum concentrations in the upper part of the therapeutic range [38]. The therapeutic range of PHT serum concentration just cited represents values indicative of the majority but not all patients (see Chap. 15).

DOSAGE AND ADMINISTRATION

Initial Dosage

The initial dosage in adults is 300 mg/day. The initial dosage in children is 5 mg/kg/day. Because of the very slow metabolism of PHT in premature and term infants, the usual doses of PHT can produce toxic serum concentrations in these infants [37]. It is often impossible to predict the proper dosage of PHT in such patients, and the dosage must be adjusted by frequent monitoring of PHT serum concentration.

Procedure for Raising Dosage

The usual daily dose of 300 mg/day does not produce good seizure control or high therapeutic serum concentrations in many patients. In such patients the dosage of PHT must be raised until good seizure control is obtained, a high therapeutic serum concentration is reached, or toxicity precludes further increases. In raising the dosage of PHT, one is faced with two conflicting considerations. In some patients, a small increase in PHT dosage will result in an unexpectedly great increase in serum concentration and drug toxicity owing to the phenomenon of dose-dependent metabolism. This result argues for increasing the dosage in small increments. Other patients absorb PHT poorly and require large increases in dosage to achieve therapeutic drug serum concentrations. This would argue for increasing dosage in large increments. One workable compromise is to increase PHT dosage in 100 mg/day increments until a serum concentration of 10 μg/ml is reached. After that, further increments of 50 mg/day or less can be added. Only one increment should be added every 4 weeks or longer because it takes that much time to reach a steady-state serum concentration and to discern the full therapeutic and toxic effects of the dosage regimen.

As noted above, some patients who do not absorb PHT capsules well will absorb the oral suspension form of the drug much better. If a patient is taking a dose of 600 mg/day and does not have a therapeutic serum concentration, and if noncompliance has been excluded, it may be helpful to switch from the capsule form to the oral suspension form. This often results in therapeutic (and sometimes toxic) drug serum concentrations. PHT oral suspension must be shaken well before each dose to prevent the drug from settling in the bottom of the bottle, resulting in undermedication when the suspension is taken from the top of the bottle and overmedication when it is taken from the bottom of the bottle.

Divided Dose Versus Single Dose
Several groups have shown that once-daily administration of PHT will maintain therapeutic serum concentrations in the majority of adults, although there is a twofold difference between maximum and minimum PHT serum concentrations because PHT has an elimination half-life of approximately 1 day [8, 33, 65]. Because once-daily administration is the most convenient dosage schedule for many patients, it probably encourages increased compliance (see Chap. 14). However, there are three groups of patients who probably should receive PHT in two divided doses. The first group is adults who have side effects associated with peak serum concentrations after once-daily administration. The second group includes patients of any age with poorly controlled seizures. Dividing the dose of PHT will result in a smaller fall in PHT serum concentration at times of minimum drug serum concentration. The third group is children, since children metabolize PHT more rapidly than adults and cannot always maintain a therapeutic serum concentration with once daily administration [8, 17, 37]. Even with their more rapid rate of elimination of PHT, children can maintain therapeutic plasma levels with twice-daily administration [17].

Administration of PHT in three or four divided doses is almost never necessary and should be avoided.

Patients often omit doses of drugs that must be taken at school or work, and tid and qid regimens often lead to increased noncompliance [8].

The largest dose of PHT is usually given at bedtime. This reduces drowsiness, ataxia, and other side effects that can be associated with peak PHT serum concentrations.

Loading Dose
It can take several weeks to reach a steady-state serum concentration when PHT therapy is initiated with the usual maintenance doses. To achieve a serum concentration in the therapeutic range rapidly it is necessary to give a loading dose (see Chap. 14). Therapeutic serum concentrations can be achieved very quickly with an intravenous loading dose in emergency situations. The intravenous loading dose of PHT is 13 to 14 mg/kg in adults and 15 to 20 mg/kg in neonates (see Chap. 30).

Administration of an oral loading dose of PHT is less rapid but less dangerous than intravenous loading. In adults, administration of 400 mg followed in 4 hours with 300 mg followed in 4 hours with a final 300-mg dose will result in therapeutic PHT serum concentrations 14 to 20 hours after the first dose and steady state serum concentrations 36 to 40 hours after the first dose [65]. More rapid administration of oral PHT in alert patients may result in gastrointestinal upset, drowsiness, and "spacy" feelings.

In children, oral loading with PHT can be accomplished by administering four doses of 5 to 6 mg/kg at 8-hour intervals (see Chap. 30). With this regimen serum concentrations of 10 μg/ml or more are reached 16 to 38 hours after the first dose.

Indications for Phenytoin
Tonic-clonic and complex partial seizures are the only FDA-approved indications for oral PHT, and tonic-clonic status epilepticus is the only FDA-approved indication for parenteral PHT. Phenytoin monotherapy is effective for the majority of patients with these conditions if therapeutic plasma concentrations are maintained (see refs. 24 and 53, and Chap. 14).

TONIC-CLONIC SEIZURES
Animal studies indicate that PHT reduces the spread of abnormal discharge from seizure foci, inhibits post-tetanic potentiation, and inhibits the tonic phase of electrically induced seizures (see above). These findings predict PHT should be effective against tonic-clonic seizures. Coatsworth's extensive review [12] found that two of two clinical trials and 9 of 11 case report studies of PHT for tonic-clonic seizures reported

seizures to be "greatly or totally improved" in the majority of patients studied.

COMPLEX PARTIAL SEIZURES
In Coatsworth's review [12] of PHT for complex partial seizures, five of six studies reported that seizures were "greatly or totally improved" in the majority of patients studied.

STATUS EPILEPTICUS
See Chapter 30.

SIMPLE PARTIAL SEIZURES
PHT has not been extensively studied for use in patients with simple partial seizures, although some case reports indicate that it may be effective [12]. Animal studies indicate that PHT usually does not completely suppress seizure foci, although partial suppression of a focus and of the spread of abnormal electrical activity to adjacent normal brain may be sufficient to prevent a clinical seizure.

In patients with simple partial and secondarily generalized tonic-clonic seizures, it is best to begin therapy with PHT. If the simple partial seizures are not controlled, phenobarbital or carbamazepine can be added later for control of simple partial seizures.

ABSENCE SEIZURES
Animal models predict that PHT should not be effective for controlling absence seizures, and clinical experience has shown this prediction to be correct.

OTHER INDICATIONS
PHT has been investigated for use in many other conditions. At present the drug appears promising in the treatment of digitalis-induced cardiac arrhythmias, behavior disorders (episodic impulsivity, aggression, or other antisocial acts), and trigeminal neuralgia [46]. PHT controls trigeminal neuralgia in a smaller percentage of patients than carbamazepine but probably does not cause bone marrow depression as often as carbamazepine. The combined use of PHT and carbamazepine for trigeminal neuralgia is sometimes more effective than carbamazepine alone [46].

PHT has been suggested as a therapy for a wide variety of organic and functional diseases of the nervous and cardiovascular systems as well as for other conditions including asthma, hypoglycemia, hyperthyroidism, and periodontal disease [6]. These uses have been reviewed in a volume widely distributed to physicians [6]. Although this volume contains many useful references, the reader is cautioned that many of the studies quoted are uncontrolled, that the

authors are rather enthusiastic in their promotion of PHT, and that epilepsy is the only FDA-approved indication for the drug.

Toxicity of Phenytoin

DOSE-DEPENDENT SIDE EFFECTS
The usual dose-dependent side effects of PHT include nystagmus, ataxia, drowsiness, and tremor [13]. Nystagmus is usually horizontal but can be vertical as well with high drug serum concentrations. The ataxia involves station and gait more than fine motor movements. There is an approximate correlation of signs of PHT intoxication with drug serum concentration. In the majority of patients, nystagmus appears with drug serum levels of about 20 μg/ml, ataxia with levels of about 30 μg/ml, and drowsiness with levels of more than 40 μg/ml [33]. On rare occasions patients may experience an excited delirium rather than sedation with therapeutic and toxic PHT serum concentrations [13].

PHT can cause nausea, vomiting, or constipation. Administration with or immediately after meals can reduce gastrointestinal discomfort.

A reversible syndrome of "PHT encephalopathy" has been described as a complication of chronic PHT therapy, usually with PHT serum concentrations in the toxic range [13, 52]. The syndrome is characterized by mental changes, increased slowing and increased paroxysmal activity on electroencephalograms (EEG), increased seizure frequency, and a change in seizure pattern involving development of more tonic components. The mental changes may include drowsiness, progressive decline in higher intellectual function, depression, or euphoria. Focal neurologic signs such as hemiparesis and hemisensory defects may occur. Ataxia and nystagmus may be present or absent, and the CSF protein value may be elevated. All these features generally disappear when PHT is discontinued.

Movement disorders (usually choreoathetosis and oro-facial dyskinesia, rarely asterixis, ballismus, hyperkinesia, external ophthalmoplegia, periodic alternating nystagmus, or downbeat nystagmus) have been reportedly caused by PHT [13, 51]. These disorders usually occur only with toxic PHT serum concentrations but may occur with "therapeutic" serum concentrations in a smaller number of patients [13, 46].

IDIOSYNCRATIC SIDE EFFECTS
A variety of signs and symptoms in various combinations may occur as a result of PHT hypersensitivity reactions (Table 16-2). The majority of such reactions

Table 16-2. Signs and Symptoms in 38 Cases of
Phenytoin Hypersensitivity Reaction

Sign or Symptom	Percent of Patients
Rash	
Morbilliform or licheniform	66
Erythema multiform	18
Stevens-Johnson Syndrome	13
Total	74
Fever	13
Abnormal liver function tests	29
Lymphoid hyperplasia	24
Eosinophilia	21
Blood dyscrasias	
Leukopenia	16
Thrombocytopenia	5
Anemia	16
Increased atypical lymphocytes	3
Total	31
Serum sickness	5
Albuminuria	5
Renal failure	3

Source: Modified from Haruda [26].

(92%) occur during the first 2 months of PHT therapy [26].

Rashes, which are most common in children and young adults, usually occur within the first 10 days of PHT therapy and may be accompanied by fever, leukopenia, or lymphadenopathy [13]. These symptoms disappear when the drug is discontinued and reappear with readministration of PHT [13]. More serious dermatologic disorders that can be rare side effects of PHT include erythema multiforme, exfoliative dermatitis, and Stevens-Johnson syndrome [13].

A "serum sickness"-like illness with rash, fever, arthralgias, and atypical lymphocytes may occur with PHT administration [13]. In addition to discontinuing PHT, adrenal steroids may be helpful in treating this disorder [13].

Hepatitis (hepatic necrosis, inflammation, cholangitis) is a rare but serious complication that usually occurs during the first 6 weeks of PHT therapy [13, 44]. It usually occurs in association with other symptoms of hypersensitivity such as rash (100%), fever (90%), lymphadenopathy (75%), or blood dyscrasias [13, 44].

Systemic lupus erythematosus (SLE) has been reported in association with PHT therapy [13]. In some cases SLE appears to result from PHT administration, but in other cases preexisting SLE probably caused a seizure disorder that caused PHT to be prescribed [13].

Although lymphadenopathy is not uncommon with PHT therapy, the question of whether PHT can cause malignant lymphomas remains controversial [49, 55]. Cases with features such as lymphadenopathy, fever, eosinophilia, hepatomegaly, splenomegaly, and certain malignant-appearing features on lymph node biopsy that remitted when PHT was stopped have been reported [13, 49]. A smaller number of cases of persistent malignant lymphoma after PHT was discontinued have been reported [13, 49]. It is difficult to know whether such symptoms are due to PHT, other drugs, or the spontaneous appearance of malignant lymphoma. Nevertheless, it is prudent to discontinue PHT in any patient with lymphadenopathy.

One case of fatal allergic interstitial nephritis in association with PHT therapy has been reported [39].

PHT has been reported to precipitate autoimmune myasthenia gravis in patients not known to have the disease and to exacerbate the disease in patients known to have it [20, 56].

SIDE EFFECTS OF CHRONIC ADMINISTRATION

Gingival hyperplasia occurs in at least 40 percent of patients on PHT and in up to 60 to 70 percent of children taking the drug [52]. It usually becomes apparent within 2 to 3 months after commencing PHT therapy and reaches a maximum in 9 to 12 months [52]. The disfigurement can be a serious problem, especially to young women. Gingival hyperplasia can be reduced by good oral hygiene. Periodic gingivectomy can remove the excess tissue and improve cosmetic appearance. Discontinuing PHT will result in regression of the gingival changes in 3 to 6 months [52]. The most striking histologic finding in specimens of hypertrophied gingival tissue is an increase in the number of fibroblasts and in the amount of connective tissue [29], possibly as a result of decreased collagenase activity [3]. The effects of PHT on connective tissue and possible pathogenic mechanisms for production of gingival hyperplasia have been reviewed elsewhere [3, 28, 29, 52].

Enlargement of the lips and nose, coarsening of the facial features, hirsutism, cholasmalike pigmentation, and acne all occur in a significant percentage of patients on chronic PHT therapy [52]. The cause of these side effects is unknown but may be related to the effects of PHT on connective tissue or endocrine systems [29, 52].

Certain authors have reported a loss of cerebellar Purkinje cells in association with PHT therapy [13, 52]. However, loss of Purkinje cells is a common finding in patients with epilepsy, whether or not they take antiepileptic drugs. Dam [13] recently reviewed the human and animal data on the effects of PHT on Purkinje cells and concluded that PHT in therapeutic doses does not lead to changes in the density or substructure of Purkinje cells. Reynolds [52] concluded that although much of the data on this topic is controversial, there are several convincing clinical reports of chronic cerebellar dysfunction following acute PHT intoxication. This permanent dysfunction is a very rare complication of PHT intoxication and may be related to the duration of acute PHT toxicity or to preexisting pathologic damage in the cerebellum due to seizures or other causes [52].

Perhaps the most important questions about PHT toxicity are concerned with what, if any, effects the drug has on behavior and cognitive functions at therapeutic blood levels. A small but growing body of evidence indicates that PHT may impair cognitive function (e.g., attention, problem solving) and that withdrawal of PHT may result in improved cognitive performance [16, 52, 60]. PHT appears to have little effect on behavior in most people [60].

The determination of whether PHT impairs cognitive function and, if it does, the relative cognitive toxicity of PHT, phenobarbital, primidone, and carbamazepine will be crucial information in establishing drugs of choice for epilepsy. The Veterans Administration is conducting a multicenter cooperative study to answer this question (see Chap. 14).

Chronic PHT administration may lead to a bilateral peripheral neuropathy characterized by decreased reflexes and decreased nerve conduction velocities (especially motor), and sensory deficits [13, 52, 56]. Most patients are asymptomatic, although a minority complain of weakness or dysesthesia. The occurrence of this complication correlates with the duration of PHT therapy. The neuropathy does not seem to be related to folate level, vitamin B_{12} level, hemoglobin, blood cell counts, or blood sugar. Administration of folic acid or withdrawal of PHT does not seem to improve the neuropathy.

There is some controversial evidence that PHT may suppress both humoral and cellular immune mechanisms [28, 52].

ENDOCRINE SIDE EFFECTS
PHT initially causes an increase in circulating ACTH and corticol, but levels of these hormones subsequently decline to below normal concentrations [52]. Chronic PHT administration enhances hydroxylation of cortisol and increases urinary excretion of 6-hydroxycortisol [52].

PHT depresses the release of antidiuretic hormone and oxytocin [52], and it can displace thyroxine from thyroxine-binding globulin [13, 52], which can result in reduced protein-bound iodine and increased T_3 uptake. Therapeutic serum levels of PHT decrease the insulin secretory response of the pancreas to glucose [52]. This can result in hyperglycemia [13, 52, 58].

Hypocalcemia, usually minor, occurs in 0 to 30 percent of patients on chronic antiepileptic drug therapy, including PHT [52]. Radiologic evidence of osteomalacia can be found in 15 to 46 percent of such patients [52]; however, clinical rickets is extremely rare [52]. Some evidence suggests that the hypocalcemia and osteomalacia result from accelerated vitamin D metabolism due to induction of enzymes metabolizing vitamin D by antiepileptic drugs [52, 69]. Other possible mechanisms are reviewed elsewhere [52, 69].

The effects of PHT on sex hormones are reviewed in Chapter 29.

HEMATOLOGIC SIDE EFFECTS
Aplastic anemia, leukopenia, thrombocytopenia, erythroid aplasia, and pancytopenia have all been associated with PHT therapy [49]. These side effects are very rare, usually occur during the first few months of therapy, are unrelated to dosage, and are often associated with other evidence of hypersensitivity phenomena [49].

Macrocytosis is found in 0 to 36 percent of patients on chronic PHT therapy [52]. Subnormal serum folate levels are found in 27 to 91 percent of patients on chronic PHT therapy, and subnormal CSF folate levels are found in 0 to 45 percent of such patients [52]. The mechanism of producing low serum folate levels is not known for certain; possible mechanisms have been reviewed by Reynolds [52]. Despite the high incidence of macrocytosis and folate deficiency in patients on PHT, only 0.15 to 0.75 percent of patients develop megaloblastic anemia [52]. Subnormal serum vitamin B_{12} levels are found in 0 to 11 percent of patients on chronic PHT therapy, probably because of malabsorption of vitamin B_{12} as a secondary effect of low serum folate levels [52].

The clinical importance of these findings is controversial. Megaloblastic anemia that is reversible with folate can occur with PHT, and there is highly controversial evidence that folate deficiency may lead to psychiatric disturbances in patients on PHT that are reversible with folate [52]. These considerations favor routine detection and treatment of folate deficiency in patients on PHT. On the other hand, animal work indicates that folate antagonizes the antiepileptic effect of PHT, and there is conflicting clinical evidence that administration of folate may increase seizure frequency in patients taking PHT [52]. Folate levels are an expensive laboratory test. Indications for folate treatment, the dose and duration of therapy, and the question of whether to give vitamin B_{12} as well as folate all remain to be clarified [52].

TERATOGENICITY

The absolute and relative teratogenic risks of antiepileptic drugs are reviewed in Chapter 29. The most frequent malformations in infants born to mothers taking PHT are cleft lip, cleft palate, and congenital heart disease. Cleft palate is due to decreased growth of the lateral nasal process, possibly because PHT and its metabolites bind to critical macromolecules [28].

A "fetal hydantoin syndrome" has been reported in the infants of a small number of mothers taking PHT. This syndrome consists of craniofacial anomalies, nail and digit hypoplasia, prenatal onset of growth deficiency, mental deficiency, and neuroblastoma in various combinations [25].

NEONATAL HEMORRHAGE

See Chapter 29.

Mephenytoin (Mesantoin)

CHEMISTRY AND MECHANISM OF ACTION

The chemical structure of mephenytoin is shown in Table 16-1. The N-methylation at position 3 in the hydantoin ring and the substitution of an ethyl for one phenyl group at position 5 provide a broader spectrum of action in animal screening tests for antiepileptic drugs than PHT. Mephenytoin has some protective effect against pentylenetetrazol seizures, whereas PHT does not [31, 41]. However, these structural changes in mephenytoin also result in increased neurotoxicity and a decreased potency and protective index against maximal electroshock seizures when compared with PHT [31, 41].

CLINICAL PHARMACOLOGY

Absorption, Biotransformation, and Excretion

Peak plasma concentrations of mephenytoin occur 45 to 120 minutes after an oral dose [31, 61]. Mephenytoin is rapidly demethylated to the active metabolite nirvanol (5-ethyl-5-phenylhydantoin) [31, 61, 62]. Nirvanol is further metabolized by *p*-hydroxylation and/or glucuronide formation and then excreted in the urine [31]. A number of other minor metabolic pathways of mephenytoin have been reported [31]. The protein binding of mephenytoin and nirvanol is 39 percent and 29 percent, respectively [61].

Clinical Pharmacokinetics

The elimination half-lives of mephenytoin and nirvanol are 7 and 96 hours, respectively [31, 61, 62]. Nirvanol constitutes over 90 percent of the active antiepileptic drug in serum at steady state [31, 61, 62]. Because of the long elimination half-life of nirvanol, mephenytoin needs to be given only once or twice a day, and steady state plasma concentrations will be reached in approximately 3 weeks [62].

Blood Levels

Total combined mephenytoin plus nirvanol plasma concentration must be determined for therapeutic drug monitoring [62]. Total concentrations of 10 to 35 μg/ml are required for seizure control [62].

Drug Interactions

The drug interactions of mephenytoin are numerous and complex [61, 62]. Autoinduction of metabolism of mephenytoin and nirvanol occurs, leading to an eventual downward drift of serum concentration of both drugs with chronic administration. Also, mutual induction of metabolism occurs when mephenytoin is coadministered with carbamazepine, barbiturates, or benzodiazepines. Mephenytoin and nirvanol are metabolized by the same saturable enzyme system that metabolizes PHT. At low plasma concentrations of mephenytoin-nirvanol and PHT there is mutual induction of biotransformation (with a fall in drug plasma concentrations), whereas at high plasma concentrations there is mutual inhibition of biotransformation (with an increase in drug plasma concentrations).

Dosage and Administration

The initial dosage is 50 or 100 mg/day during the first week. The daily dosage is then increased by 50 or 100 mg at weekly intervals until seizure control is obtained or toxicity precludes further increases. Increases in dosage should not be made more often than once a week. Because of the toxicity of mephenytoin, one should attempt to control seizures with the smallest possible dose. The average daily dose required is 200 to 600 mg in adults and 100 to 400 mg in children.

INDICATIONS

Mephenytoin is approved by the FDA for treatment of tonic-clonic, simple partial, and complex partial seizures in patients who have been refractory to less toxic antiepileptic drugs. There have been no controlled clinical trials of mephenytoin. Uncontrolled trials indicate that a majority of patients with tonic-clonic or simple partial seizures will experience a consider-

Table 16-3. Comparative Toxicity of Hydantoins

Side Effect	PHT	Mephenytoin	Ethotoin
Drowsiness	±	++ (16%)	±
Skin rash	++ (5–10%)	++ (9%)	± (2%)
Adenopathy	++	++ (6%)	−
Vomiting	+	±	± (3%)
Gum swelling	++	+ (3%)	−
Hirsutism	+	±	−
Leukopenia	Rare	++ (23%)	−
Aplastic anemia	Rare	++	−
Hepatitis	Rare	+	−
Fatal reactions	+	+	−

Source: Modified from J. G. Millichap. Other Hydantoins: Mephenytoin, Ethotoin, and Albutoin. In D. M. Woodbury, J. K. Penry, and R. P. Schmidt (Eds.), *Antiepileptic Drugs.* New York: Raven Press, 1972. By permission of Raven Press.

able reduction in seizure frequency with mephenytoin, whereas only a minority of patients with complex partial seizures respond favorably [12, 31, 41]. Absence seizures do not seem to respond to the drug [12, 41].

TOXICITY

The relative toxicity of hydantoins is summarized in Table 16-3. Compared with PHT, mephenytoin causes less nausea and vomiting, less ataxia, and less gingival hyperplasia [41]. These advantages are offset by a greater incidence of drowsiness, serious dermatitis, agranulocytosis, aplastic anemia, and hepatitis [41, 62]. The incidence of fatalities from these serious side effects appears to be greater with mephenytoin than with PHT [41, 62]. In view of the relatively high incidence of serious side effects with mephenytoin, the drug is indicated only for patients with severe seizure disorders that are resistant to less toxic drugs. Physical and laboratory examinations should be performed every 2 weeks at the initiation of therapy and monthly thereafter. The patient should be warned to report immediately to his physician if skin rash, jaundice, nausea, or bleeding occur.

Ethotoin (Peganone)

CHEMISTRY AND MECHANISM OF ACTION

The chemical structure of ethotoin is shown in Table 16-1. The addition of an ethyl group in position 3 and the deletion of one phenyl group from position 5 in the hydantoin ring result in a compound that is both less potent against maximal electroshock seizures in animals and less toxic than PHT [31, 41]. Ethotoin has some activity against pentylenetetrazol seizures in

animals but has proved to have little effect on absence seizures in patients [12, 31, 41].

CLINICAL PHARMACOLOGY

Clinical Pharmacokinetics
Peak plasma concentrations of ethotoin occur 2 to 4 hours after oral doses [31, 61]. Ethotoin is 46 percent protein bound [61]. The elimination half-life of the drug is 5 hours, and the drug has no active metabolites [31, 61]. Therefore, ethotoin must be given in four or more divided doses to keep fluctuations between peak and trough plasma concentrations under 100 percent [61].

Blood Levels
The therapeutic range of ethotoin plasma concentration is 15 to 50 μg/ml [35, 62].

Dosage and Administration
In adults, the initial dose should be 1,000 mg/day or less. Dosage is then gradually increased for several days until the optimal dosage is reached. Most adults require 2,000 to 3,000 mg daily. Doses of less than 2,000 mg/day are seldom effective.

In children, the initial dose should be 750 mg/day or less. The usual maintenance dose is 500 to 1,000 mg/day, although daily doses of up to 3,000 mg are sometimes necessary.

Ethotoin is administered in four to six divided doses daily. The drug should be taken after meals, and the doses should be divided as evenly as possible.

INDICATIONS

Ethotoin is approved by the FDA for the treatment of tonic-clonic and complex partial seizures. There are no controlled trials of ethotoin. Uncontrolled studies indicate that ethotoin has some efficacy against tonic-clonic and complex partial seizures but probably does not control such seizures as frequently as PHT [12, 41]. The lack of efficacy of ethotoin may be related in part to the large doses necessary to obtain seizure control and to the necessity to administer the drug in four to six divided doses daily. The drug has little efficacy against simple partial and absence seizures [12, 41]. Several authors have suggested ethotoin for the treatment of patients, particularly children, with mild tonic-clonic seizure disorders and hypersensitivity to more potent agents [41].

TOXICITY

The toxicity of ethotoin is summarized in Table 16-3. Side effects occur less frequently than with PHT. Side effects include skin rash (2%), anorexia and vomiting (3%), drowsiness, nystagmus, and occasionally lymphadenopathy [41]. Ataxia occurs only with large doses, and gingival hyperplasia and hirsutism have not been reported [41].

References

1. Alnaes, E., and Rahamimoff, R. On the role of mitochondria in transmitter release from motor nerve terminals. *J. Physiol.* 248:285, 1975.
2. Ayala, G. F., and Johnston, D. The influence of phenytoin on the fundamental electrical properties of simple neural systems. *Epilepsia* 18:299, 1977.
3. Bauer, E. A. et al. Phenytoin therapy of recessive dystrophic epidermolysis bullosa: Clinical trial and proposed mechanism of action on collagenase. *N. Engl. J. Med.* 303:776, 1980.
4. Bauer, L. A., and Blouin, R. A. Age and phenytoin kinetics in adult epileptics. *Clin. Pharmacol. Ther.* 31:301, 1982.
5. Bauer, L. A. Interference of oral phenytoin absorption by continuous nasogastric feedings. *Neurology* (N.Y.) 32:570, 1982.
6. Bogoch, S., and Dreyfus, J. *DPH 1975: Bibliography and Review.* New York: Dreyfus Medical Foundation, 1975.
7. Bourgeois, B. F. D., and Dodson, W. E. Phenytoin bioavailability and kinetics in newborns. *Epilepsia* 23:436, 1982.
8. Browne, T. R. Clinical pharmacology of antiepileptic drugs. *Drug. Ther. Rev.* 2:469, 1979.
9. Browne, T. R. et al. Applications of Stable Isotopes to Human Drug Interaction Studies. In A. B. Susan (Ed.), *Proceedings of the International Symposium on the Synthesis and Applications of Isotopically Labeled Compounds.* Amsterdam: Elsevier. In press, 1983.
10. Chang, T., and Glazko, A. J. Phenytoin: Biotransformation. In D. M. Woodbury, J. K. Penry, and C. E. Pippenger (Eds.), *Antiepileptic Drugs.* New York: Raven Press, 1982.
11. Chen, S. S. et al. Comparative bioavailability of phenytoin from generic formulations in the United Kingdom. *Epilepsia* 23:149, 1982.
12. Coatsworth, J. J. *Studies on the Clinical Efficacy of Marketed Antiepileptic Drugs.* Washington, D.C.: U.S. Government Printing Office, 1971.
13. Dam, M. Phenytoin: Toxicity. In D. M. Woodbury, J. K. Penry, and C. E. Pippenger (Eds.), *Antiepileptic Drugs.* New York: Raven Press, 1982.
14. DeLorenzo, R. J. Possible role of calcium-dependent protein phosphorylation in mediating neurotransmitter release and anticonvulsant action. *Epilepsia* 17:357, 1977.
15. Deupree, J. D. The role or non-role of ATPase activation by phenytoin in the stabilization of excitable membranes. *Epilepsia* 18:309, 1977.
16. Dodrill, C. B., and Troupin, A. S. Psychotropic effects of carbamazepine in epilepsy: Comparison with phenytoin. *Neurology* (Minneap.) 27:1023, 1977.
17. Dodson, W. E. Phenytoin elimination in childhood: Effect of concentration-dependent kinetics. *Neurology* (N.Y.) 30:196, 1980.
18. Dodson, W. E. Nonlinear kinetics of phenytoin in children. *Neurology* (N.Y.) 32:42, 1982.
19. Dretchen, K. L., Standaert, F. G., and Raines, A. Effects of phenytoin on the cyclic nucleotide system in the motor nerve terminal. *Epilepsia* 18:337, 1977.
20. Franco, L. F., and Festoff, B. W. Phenytoin and the "safety margin" of neuromuscular transmission. *Ann. Neurol.* 8:95, 1980.
21. Glaser, G. H., Penry, J. K., and Woodbury, D. M. *Antiepileptic Drugs: Mechanisms of Action.* New York: Raven Press, 1980.
22. Glazko, A. J. Phenytoin: Chemistry and Methods of Determination. In D. M. Woodbury, J. K. Penry, and C. E. Pippenger (Eds.), *Antiepileptic Drugs.* New York: Raven Press, 1982.
23. Gratz, E. J. et al. Effect of carbamazepine on phenytoin clearance in patients with complex partial seizures. *Neurology* (N.Y.) 32:A223, 1982.
24. Hakkarainen, H. Carbamazepine vs. diphenylhydantoin vs. their combination in adult epilepsy. *Neurology* (N.Y.) 30:354, 1980.
25. Hanson, J. W., and Smith, D. W. The fetal hydantoin syndrome. *J. Pediatr.* 87:285, 1975.

26. Haruda, F. Phenytoin hypersensitivity: 38 cases. *Neurology* (N.Y.) 29:1480, 1979.

27. Hasbani, M., Pincus, J. H., and Lee, S. H. Diphenyl-hydantoin and calcium movement in lobster nerves. *Arch. Neurol.* 31:250, 1974.

28. Hassell, T. M. et al. Summary of an International Symposium on phenytoin-induced teratology and gingival pathology. *J. Am. Dent. Assoc.* 99:652, 1979.

29. Keith, D. A. Side effects of diphenylhydantoin: A review. *J. Oral Surg.* 36:206, 1978.

30. Kostenbauder, H. B. et al. Bioavailability and single-dose pharmacokinetics of intramuscular phenytoin. *Clin. Pharmacol. Ther.* 18:449, 1975.

31. Kupferberg, H. J. Other Hydantoins: Mephenytoin and Ethotoin. In D. M. Woodbury, J. K. Penry, and C. E. Pippenger (Eds.), *Antiepileptic Drugs.* New York: Raven Press, 1982.

32. Kutt, H. Phenytoin: Interaction with Other Drugs. In D. M. Woodbury, J. K. Penry, and C. E. Pippenger (Eds.), *Antiepileptic Drugs.* New York: Raven Press, 1982.

33. Kutt, H. Phenytoin: Relation of Plasma Concentration to Seizure Control. In D. M. Woodbury, J. K. Penry, and C. E. Pippenger (Eds.), *Antiepileptic Drugs.* New York: Raven Press, 1982.

34. Lambie, D. G., and Johnson, R. H. The effects of phenytoin on phenobarbital and primidone metabolism. *J. Neurol. Neurosurg. Psychiatr.* 44:148, 1981.

35. Larson, N. E., and Naestoft, J. Quantitative determination of ethotoin in serum by gas chromatography. *J. Chromatogr.* 92:157, 1974.

36. Lipicky, R. J., Gilbert, D. C., and Stillman, I. M. Diphenylhydantoin inhibition of sodium conductance in squid giant axon. *Proc. Natl. Acad. Sci. USA* 69:1758, 1972.

37. Loughman, P. M. et al. Pharmacokinetic observations of phenytoin disposition in the newborn and young infant. *Arch. Dis. Child.* 52:302, 1977.

38. Lund, L. Anticonvulsive effect of diphenylhydantoin relative to plasma levels. *Arch. Neurol.* 31:289, 1974.

39. McCarthy, L. J., and Aguilar, J. C. Fatal benign phenytoin hypersensitivity. *Lancet* 2:932, 1977.

40. Mildei, R. Transmitter release induced by injection of calcium ions into nerve terminals. *Proc. R. Soc. Bio.* 183:421, 1973.

41. Millichap, J. G. Other Hydantoins: Mephenytoin, Ethotoin, and Albutoin. In D. M. Woodbury, J. K. Penry, and R. P. Schmidt (Eds.), *Antiepileptic Drugs.* New York: Raven Press, 1972.

42. Oldnow, C. W., Finn, A. L., and Prussak, C. The effects of salicylate on the pharmacokinetics of phenytoin. *Neurology* (N.Y.) 31:341, 1981.

43. Painter, M. J. et al. Phenobarbital and phenytoin in neonatal seizures: Metabolism and tissue distribution. *Neurology* (N.Y.) 31:1107, 1981.

44. Parker, W. A., and Shearer, C. A. Phenytoin hepatotoxicity: A case report and review. *Neurology* (N.Y.) 29:175, 1979.

45. Pentikainen, P. J., Neuvonen, P. J., and Elfving, S. M. Bioavailability of four brands of phenytoin tablets. *Eur. J. Clin. Pharmacol.* 9:213, 1975.

46. Phenytoin (Diphenylhydantoin). *Med. Lett. Drugs Ther.* 18:23, 1976.

47. Pincus, J. H. Diphenylhydantoin and ion flux in lobster nerves. *Arch. Neurol.* 26:4, 1972.

48. Pincus, J. H., and Lee, S. H. Diphenylhydantoin and calcium: Relation to norepinephrine release from brain slices. *Arch. Neurol.* 29:239, 1973.

49. Pisciotta, A. V. Phenytoin: Hematologic Toxicity. In D. M. Woodbury, J. K. Penry, and C. E. Pippenger (Eds.), *Antiepileptic Drugs.* New York: Raven Press, 1982.

50. Ramsay, E. R. et al. Status epilepticus in pregnancy: Effect of phenytoin malabsorption on seizure control. *Neurology* (N.Y.) 28:85, 1978.

51. Rasmussen, S., and Kristensen, M. Choreoathetosis during phenytoin treatment. *Acta Med. Scand.* 201(3):239, 1977.

52. Reynolds, E. H. Chronic antiepileptic toxicity: A review. *Epilepsia* 16:319, 1975.

53. Reynolds, E. H. et al. Phenytoin monotherapy for epilepsy: A long-term prospective study assisted by serum level monitoring in previously untreated patients. *Epilepsia* 22:475, 1981.

54. Richens, A. Clinical pharmacokinetics of phenytoin. *Clin. Pharmacokinet.* 4:154, 1979.

55. Scoville, B., and White, B. G. The carcinogenicity of hydantoins: History, data, hypotheses, and public policy. *Acta Neurol. Scand.* 62 (Suppl. 79): 89, 1980.

56. So, E. L., and Penry, J. K. Adverse effects of phenytoin on peripheral nerve and neuromuscular junction: A review. *Epilepsia* 22:467, 1982.

57. Spero, L. Neurotransmitters and CNS disease: Epilepsy. *Lancet* 2:1319, 1982.

58. Stansell, P. E. et al. Pediatric review: Transient diabetes mellitus secondary to diphenylhydantoin intoxication. *J. Arkansas Med. Soc.* 76:209, 1979.

59. Swinyard, E. A. Laboratory evaluation of antiepileptic drugs: Review of laboratory methods. *Epilepsia* 10:107, 1969.

60. Thompson, P. Effect of Antiepileptic Drugs on Psychosocial Development: Phenytoin. In P. L. Morselli, J. K. Penry, and R. P. Schmidt (Eds.), *Antiepileptic Drug Therapy in Pediatrics*. New York: Raven Press, 1982.

61. Troupin, A. S. et al. Clinical pharmacology of mephenytoin and ethotoin. *Ann. Neurol.* 6:410, 1979.

62. Troupin, A. S., Ojemann, L. M., and Dodrill, C. B. Mephenytoin (Mesantoin): A reappraisal. *Epilepsia* 17:403, 1976.

63. Wilder, B. J. Anticonvulsant drug interactions. Veterans Administration Epilepsy Workshop, Durham, N.C., March 31, 1978.

64. Wilder, B. J. et al. Efficacy of intravenous phenytoin in the treatment of status epilepticus: Kinetics of central nervous system penetration. *Ann. Neurol.* 1:511, 1977.

65. Wilder, B. J., Streiff, R. R., and Hammer, R. H. Di-phenylhydantoin: Absorption, Distribution, and Excretion: Clinical Studies. In D. M. Woodbury, J. K. Penry, and R. P. Schmidt (Eds.), *Antiepileptic Drugs*. New York: Raven Press, 1972.

66. Woodbury, D. M. Phenytoin: Absorption, Distribution, and Excretion. In D. M. Woodbury, J. K. Penry, and C. E. Pippenger (Eds.), *Antiepileptic Drugs*. New York: Raven Press, 1982.

67. Yaari, Y., Pincus, J. H., and Argov, Z. Depression of synaptic transmission by diphenylhydantoin. *Ann. Neurol.* 1:334, 1977.

68. Yaari, Y., Pincus, J. H., and Argov, Z. Phenytoin and transmitter release at the neuromuscular junction of the frog. *Brain Res.* 160:479, 1979.

69. Zerwekh, J. E. et al. Decreased serum 24,25-dihydroxyvitamin D concentration during long-term anticonvulsant therapy in adult epileptics. *Ann. Neurol.* 12:184, 1982.

PHENOBARBITAL, PRIMIDONE (MYSOLINE), AND MEPHOBARBITAL (MEBARAL)

17

Richard H. Mattson

The first clinical use of phenobarbital in the treatment of seizures was reported in 1912 by Hauptmann [33]. Its introduction revolutionized the treatment of seizures. The remarkable qualities of phenobarbital are evident in the fact that more than two thirds of a century later it continues to be one of the primary antiepileptic drugs in current use. This unique compound possesses a broad spectrum of antiepileptic activity yet causes few serious side effects. However, annoying neurotoxicity makes it less than an ideal drug. Many analogs of phenobarbital have been synthesized in an attempt to obtain comparable or superior efficacy with less hypnotic side effects. Most of these have proved to have lesser efficacy or, at most, equal benefit and similar sedative effects. Primidone and mephobarbital are two drugs that continue to be widely used.

Phenobarbital

CHEMISTRY

Phenobarbital (5-ethyl-5-phenylbarbituric acid, Fig. 17-1) is a white crystalline substance poorly soluble in water but soluble in organic solvents including ethanol, propylene glycol, ether, and chloroform. The sodium salt is more freely soluble in water. Phenobarbital is a weakly acidic compound with a pK_a of 7.3; at a serum pH of 7.4, approximately 40 percent of the drug is un-ionized. Changes in blood or urine pH alter the extent of ionization of phenobarbital and affect its pharmacokinetics substantially. The drug is available in tablets and as a sodium salt elixir. Generic formulations of the tablets from various manufacturers are equivalent. Preparations for parenteral use are available in ampules containing propylene glycol with 120 mg/ml of phenobarbital or in powder form to be reconstituted with water at the time of administration.

MECHANISM OF ACTION

The mechanism of action by which phenobarbital exerts an antiepileptic effect remains unknown. Like phenytoin, it inhibits the spread of seizure activity [1], but unlike phenytoin, phenobarbital also elevates the seizure threshold [3, 68]. Animal experimental studies suggest that phenobarbital may act by potentiating gamma-aminobutyric acid effects (see Chaps.

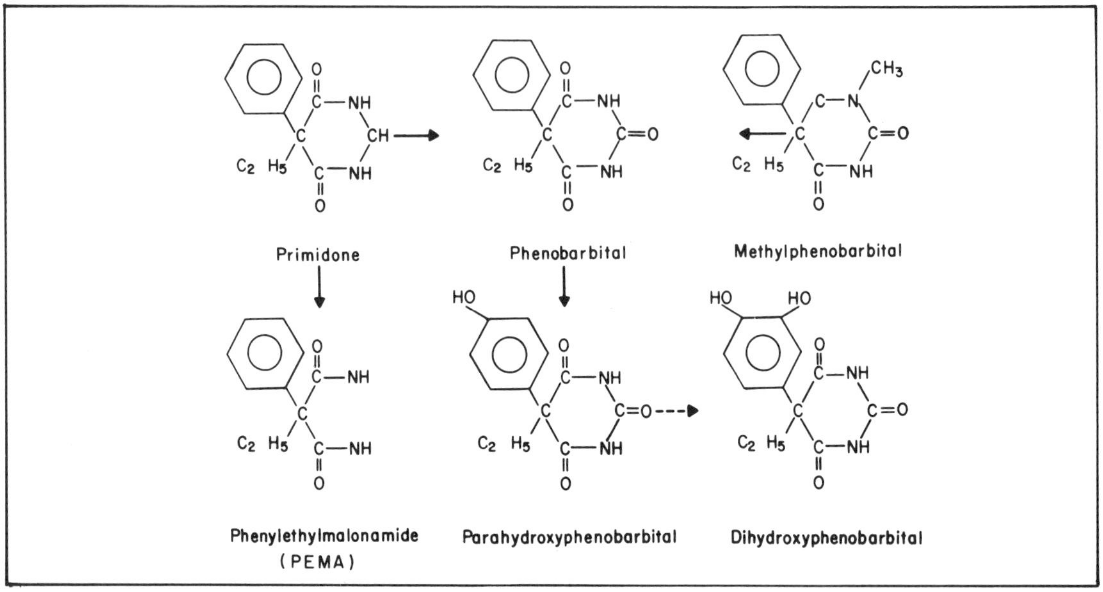

192

Figure 17-1. Structural formulas of antiepileptic barbiturates and their metabolic products.

2, 16, and 21) and by blocking some transmitters of postsynaptic excitability [62].

CLINICAL PHARMACOLOGY

Despite the fact that phenobarbital is the oldest antiepileptic drug, fewer pharmacokinetic studies of it have been performed than of drugs only recently introduced. Nonetheless, generations of clinical experience have confirmed the careful original studies by Butler and colleagues of the pharmacokinetics of phenobarbital [12, 14, 15, 77].

Absorption and Distribution

Phenobarbital is well absorbed from the gastrointestinal tract. Lous [47] found peak serum levels as late as 18 hours after oral intake of 750 mg of phenobarbital. In contrast, a serum peak 2 hours after oral administration of a 30-mg dose was found by Viswanathan et al. [75]. These studies, as well as those of others, provide indirect evidence [11, 14] of complete absorption after oral intake. Whyte and Dekaban [79] confirmed this assumption when they found no phenobarbital in the feces of 4 patients receiving phenobarbital. After entering the circulation, 40 to 60 percent of the drug is protein bound; accordingly, the concentration of phenobarbital in CSF has been found to be approximately half that in serum [63]. Because serum protein binding is not high, alterations in serum protein binding do not significantly alter the distribution or therapeutic effects of the drug.

Biotransformation and Excretion

Phenobarbital is metabolized in the liver by the mixed function oxidase enzyme systems. A primary metabolite is the parahydroxy compound as well as small amounts of dihydroxy or catechol compounds, all of which are subsequently conjugated and excreted as glucuronides or sulfates (Fig. 17-1) and account for about 30 to 50 percent of the dose [15, 54]. Approximately 25 percent of the drug is excreted in the urine unchanged. An unconfirmed report by Tang et al. [71] on the metabolic fate of phenobarbital in two patients identified 30 and 24 percent, respectively, of the phenobarbital excreted as the N-glucopyranoside.

Pharmakokinetics

Phenobarbital has an elimination half-life in adults of 46 to 136 hours (average, approximately 4 days), the longest of any antiepileptic drug (see Chap. 14). The value can vary considerably among patients, and the dosage may need to be modified accordingly. Approximately 15 percent of phenobarbital is cleared from the body daily, so that after initiation of daily oral intake there is accumulation for 2 to 3 weeks before steady state is reached (see Chap. 14).

The elimination half-life is shorter in children than in adults (37 to 73 hours; average, approximately 2 days), and children require a larger dose of phenobarbital (on a milligram per kilogram basis) to maintain a given plasma concentration [30, 34, 59, 70]. The elimination half-life is longer in neonates than in either children or adults (61 to 173 hours) [34, 35, 45, 60].

pH Effects
Waddell and Butler [77] performed studies demonstrating that changes in serum or urinary pH can alter phenobarbital concentration, causing clinically important effects on distribution and renal clearance. At pH 7.4, 60 percent of the drug is ionized. This polar compound crosses cellular membranes poorly. Penetration into and out of tissue is possible for the 40 percent of the drug that is not ionized, and changes in serum pH produce shifts in the percentage of un-ionized phenobarbital. When acidosis occurs, a higher percentage of phenobarbital is un-ionized, allowing passage into the intercellular space. This effectively increases tissue concentrations without producing any change in the total body amount of phenobarbital. Alkalosis has an opposite effect and leads to movement of phenobarbital out of brain and other tissues. Similarly, shifts in urinary pH can greatly modify the rate of phenobarbital clearance. Phenobarbital is excreted from the kidney into the urine, largely in the un-ionized form at the usual acid pH. It is readily reabsorbed from the kidney tubule back into the circulation. In alkaline urine the excreted phenobarbital becomes ionized and is not reabsorbed. Alkalinization of the urine, particularly with forced diuresis, can appreciably increase excretion and clearance of phenobarbital from the body. The effect of alkalinization has been utilized in the treatment of phenobarbital overdose because it facilitates movement from the brain to the extracellular space and hastens renal clearance [77].

Blood Levels
Reliable methods for determination of phenobarbital serum concentration are widely available using gas chromatography, liquid chromatography, or enzyme multiplied immunoassay technique methods, although some technical problems may give misleading values (see Chap. 15). Due to the drug's long half-life, serum levels are usually constant and independent of the time of administration. Even a random blood sample should provide a reliable measure of the serum concentration throughout the day. The therapeutic levels expected to provide an antiepileptic effect without side effects are 15 to 40 mg/ml [7, 11]. However, the correlation between serum levels, seizure control, and side effects are less clear than with phenytoin therapy [7].

Drug Interactions
Phenobarbital induces enzymatic metabolism of other antiepileptic drugs used concurrently. These drugs are

metabolized by the same enzyme systems and can be affected by a phenobarbital-induced increased rate of biotransformation (see Chap. 14).

The increased metabolism may be offset by competition for the same enzymes for hydroxylation. For example, there is evidence that the addition of phenytoin, valproic acid, or methsuximide may increase the serum levels of phenobarbital owing to a decreased rate of p-hydroxylation [39, 40, 41] (see Chaps. 14, 16, and 19).

Dosage and Administration
Phenobarbital is usually prescribed in doses of 2 to 3 mg/kg in adults. Once-daily dosing is sufficient owing to the slow elimination of the drug. Administration before bedtime allows any peak sedative effect to occur during sleep. Easily swallowed small tablets are available in a wide range of strengths (15, 30, 60 and 100 mg), simplifying individualization of dosage. A rather unpalatable elixir containing 20 mg per 5 ml can be given to children or others if tablets are not acceptable. When therapeutic serum concentrations need to be reached fairly quickly, loading doses of 2 times the usual daily maintenance dose should be given for 4 days, and this will bring the serum concentration up to the steady state value within 3 days [69]. In the drug-naive patient, the more rapidly therapeutic concentrations are achieved, the more likely the drug will exert a sedative effect, since sufficient time will not have passed to allow tolerance to develop. Whether patients have been given a loading dose or a maintenance dose, they should be encouraged to accept some sedative effect for several weeks because tolerance will develop in most patients. When phenobarbital is added as an adjunct to another antiepileptic drug, the more gradual build-up is probably preferable.

When phenobarbital is to be discontinued, the dosage should be gradually reduced or tapered for a period of several weeks when practical. There is evidence that sudden discontinuation of phenobarbital therapy in patients with epilepsy may be accompanied by withdrawal seizures [11] in addition to the seizures that may be reexacerbated as a result of the termination of any antiepileptic drug.

When administered parenterally for the treatment of acute seizures or status epilepticus, phenobarbital must be given in sufficient quantities to obtain a therapeutic concentration rapidly. In neonates, a loading dose of 8 to 20 mg/kg is necessary (see Chap. 30). In adults, the loading dose is not well established but may be similar to the loading dose in neonates (see Chap. 30). Although respiratory depression may accompany high concentrations of phenobarbital in the brain, the relatively slow penetration into the CNS, even following intravenous administration, minimizes this effect. More cautious use or lesser amounts should be given when other antiepileptic drugs with respiratory depressant effects, such as diazepam or paraldehyde, have been given prior to the phenobarbital.

The lengthy half-life of phenobarbital offers an advantage in the management of epilepsy, because once-daily doses produce relatively constant serum levels. An occasional missed dose can be expected to have comparatively little adverse effect on steady-state tissue concentrations and seizure control. On the other hand, the long half-life is a disadvantage in patients with toxic reactions or when serum concentrations inadvertently have become too high (e.g., following accidental or purposeful overdose) because the drug is cleared very slowly from the body. Clearance can be accelerated fivefold by alkalinization of serum and urine by administration of sodium bicarbonate coupled with forced diuresis [77]. Phenobarbital clearance can also be accelerated by administration of oral activated charcoal [5].

INDICATIONS

Animal Studies

Studies in animals indicate that phenobarbital has a broad spectrum of antiepileptic activity with efficacy against maximal electroshock, minimal electroshock, kindling, strychnine, and photic-sensitive seizures; it also has a lesser effect on subcutaneous pentylenetetrazol seizure threshold [76, 83]. The broad spectrum of efficacy of phenobarbital is reflected in its clinical usage.

Chronic Preventive Antiepileptic Drug Therapy

Phenobarbital remains one of the primary antiepileptic drugs in use today; an eloquent testimony to its effectiveness. It was the sole significant antiepileptic drug for prevention of seizures for a quarter of a century until the introduction of phenytoin in 1938 [57]. Phenobarbital proved valuable in the treatment of tonic-clonic, simple partial, and complex partial seizures, although its efficacy was minimal in the prevention of absence, myoclonic, and related seizure types. After the introduction of phenytoin, a number of studies suggested that the new drug was more effective. Later retrospective analyses failed to show convincing evidence of the superiority of either phenobarbital or phenytoin in controlling seizures [37]. Phenobarbital continued to be a drug of choice, particularly for children in whom the dysmorphic side effects of gum hypertrophy and hirsutism caused by phenytoin were undesirable [44]. The introduction of primidone and carbamazepine failed to show evidence in controlled clinical trials of a superiority in efficacy of either of these agents [17, 58]. Early trials are inadequate by current standards because drug serum concentration determinations, precise seizure classification, and careful experimental design with statistical analyses were rarely employed [50].

At present, the evidence suggests that phenobarbital is equivalent in efficacy to these other drugs, although it may not always be the drug of choice owing to its side effects (Table 17-1). In any given patient, phenobarbital may prove most (or least) effective compared with the other widely used medications (phenytoin, carbamazepine, and primidone). If not used as a primary antiepileptic drug, phenobarbital is often used in combination with another drug in patients whose seizure control is difficult. Yahr et al. [84] demonstrated that phenytoin in combination with phenobarbital was more effective than either drug alone. Phenobarbital in combination with carbamazepine also can be expected to improve seizure control. Since primidone is metabolized to phenobarbital and both cause similar sedative side effects, there is little justification for using these two drugs in combination. Finally, phenobarbital is often used with ethosuximide or valproic acid to control mixed absence and tonic-clonic seizures.

Status Epilepticus

Phenobarbital is especially useful for the treatment of acute, frequently repetitive seizures or for status epilepticus. Unlike primidone and carbamazepine, which can be given only by the oral route, phenobarbital is readily available in soluble form and can be given by intravenous or intramuscular administration.

Its gradual onset of action, even when administered intravenously, is a disadvantage of phenobarbital in treating status epilepticus. The low lipid solubility and extensive ionization at blood pH results in a relatively slow passage across the blood-brain barrier. Peak brain levels and antiepileptic activity may not be achieved for 20 to 90 minutes (see Chap. 30) [12]. Diazepam penetrates the blood-brain barrier and exerts an effect much more rapidly and is preferred if immediate cessation of an attack is necessary (see Chap. 30). However, diazepam has only a short duration of peak effect, whereas phenobarbital, due to its very slow elimination, provides long-lasting protection. Intravenous phenytoin provides effective, rapid, long-lasting control of tonic-clonic status epilepticus (see Chap. 30) [80], but phenobarbital possesses a broader spectrum of action and may be more effective if seizures are caused by toxic, metabolic, or withdrawal states [1, 22, 23, 55, 81, 83].

Table 17-1. Advantages and Disadvantages of Phenobarbital Relative to Other Antiepileptic Drugs

Advantages	Disadvantages
Long history of usage with few serious systemic and no dysmorphic side effects	Annoying sedative effects in many patients even within therapeutic range
Inexpensive and widely available	Significant disturbance of cognitive function, mood, or behavior in some, especially children and elderly
Can be used both orally and parenterally	
Long elimination half-life, allowing simple single daily administration; missed doses have little clinical effect	Rapid manipulation to raise or lower serum levels somewhat difficult due to slow accumulation and elimination
Broad-spectrum antiepileptic properties; useful for febrile, toxic metabolic, and withdrawal seizures	Accidental or purposeful overdose may be lethal
Teratogenicity risk less than with phenytoin	

Other Indications

Its broad spectrum of antiepileptic activity suggests that phenobarbital may be more effective than other antiepileptic drugs in selected circumstances. Phenobarbital has been found to be superior to phenytoin in a number of animal models and clinical seizure types [1].

In controlled trials continuous phenobarbital therapy has proved effective in preventing the recurrence of febrile seizures [23, 81], whereas phenytoin has proved ineffective [55]. Insufficient evidence is available to decide whether primidone, carbamazepine, or valproic acid are as effective. In the baboon (*Papio papio*) model of primarily generalized photic-sensitive epilepsy, seizures are more completely prevented by phenobarbital than by phenytoin [67]. Withdrawal seizures are prevented or controlled more effectively by phenobarbital than by phenytoin [22]. Phenytoin, unlike phenobarbital, is quite ineffective in preventing chemically induced seizures, and in neonates it may actually lower the seizure threshold [83]. Finally, the evidence that phenobarbital, but not phenytoin, prevents or limits kindling in experimental animals [76] suggests that it may be the best drug to prevent development of seizures after head trauma or brain abscess.

TOXICITY

Systemic Toxicity

Phenobarbital causes very few serious systemic side effects. The most frequent is a morbilliform rash that is often transient and may not require discontinuation of the drug. However, this complication may be persistent and more severe, requiring substitution of another antiepileptic drug. Very rarely, there may be associated bone marrow depression, hepatitis, or lupus erythematosus [2, 53, 56, 78]. As with other antiepileptic drugs, blood and CSF folate levels may be depressed after chronic administration of phenobarbital, but this is of doubtful clinical significance [53].

Neurotoxicity

Although serious and important systemic side effects are very uncommon, neurotoxicity is a major problem accompanying the use of phenobarbital. Although its sedative effects are minimal compared with other barbiturates, it still possesses sufficient hypnotic effects to interfere with everyday function in a significant percentage of patients [73, 74]. The presence and persistence of side effects are extremely variable. Some patients may have phenobarbital serum concentrations as high as 50 to 60 μg/ml without complaint, whereas others have difficulty tolerating serum concentrations as low as 15 μg/ml [53]. The side effects are particularly prominent during the initiation of phenobarbital therapy, although most patients develop tolerance after several weeks. Butler et al. [14] described patients who reported sedation at the onset of treatment when serum levels were only 5 μg/ml. Two weeks later there were far fewer complaints despite the fact that serum levels were 5 times higher

Although the subjective complaints of sedation can be annoying and may result in discontinuation of phenobarbital therapy, equally serious side effects may affect behavior or cognitive functioning in ways that are not always recognizable [73, 74]. Hyperactivity or sleeplessness, particularly in children, and excitement, agitation, or confusion in the elderly may appear as seemingly paradoxical side effects. The presence of organic brain disease increases the likelihood of such side effects [73, 82]. Disturbances in cognitive function may be subtle and are manifest as a modest but important decline in school performance [73, 74]. Documentation of this cognitive impairment may be quantifiable by psychometric testing [36, 73, 74].

Such disturbances may be most apparent when improvement results from a change from phenobarbital to carbamazepine therapy [38]. Affective changes are most commonly characterized by depression and lack of interest or ambition. These changes are sometimes more obvious to family and friends than to the patient. Closely related to this problem may be an associated decrease in libido and potency.

Primidone

Primidone (2-deoxy-phenobarbital, Mysoline), a congener of phenobarbital, was synthesized in 1949 [6], and the results of animal studies were reported first in 1952 by Handley and Stewart [32]. Primidone has been used extensively since then as a major antiepileptic drug, although controversy exists about whether primidone possesses any independent or superior properties when compared with phenobarbital.

CHEMISTRY

The chemical name of primidone is 5-phenyl-5-ethylhexahydroprimidine-4:6-dione (see Fig. 17-1). The white, crystalline powder is minimally soluble in water and alcohol.

CLINICAL PHARMACOLOGY

Absorption and Distribution
Primidone is well absorbed, with peak levels appearing 1 to 3 hours after an oral dose [8, 27, 64]. Primidone is minimally protein bound [10, 49, 63]. The protein binding of primidone varies considerably during the day and appears to correlate with the total primidone serum concentration (i.e., the greatest binding occurs at the time of highest total serum primidone concentration [49, 64]. The concentration of primidone in the cerebrospinal fluid is essentially identical to the concentration of free drug in the serum [10, 64]. The lipid solubility of primidone appears to be similar to that of phenobarbital [64].

Elimination and Elimination Half-Life
Primidone is metabolized through oxidation to phenobarbital [16, 64] and splitting of the ring to form phenylethylmalonamide (PEMA) [4, 27, 64] (Fig. 17-1). Primidone is excreted unchanged by the kidney, and crystals can form in the urine when high serum levels have followed inadvertent or suicidal overdosage [9]. The metabolically-derived phenobarbital is assumed to follow the usual process of further biotransformation and excretion as described earlier. PEMA is largely excreted unchanged in the urine [18].

The elimination half-life of primidone is 5 to 18

hours [10, 64]. The elimination half-life of phenobarbital is 46 to 136 hours, and that of PEMA is 10 to 36 hours [4, 18].

Blood Levels
The patient on primidone monotherapy actually has three active antiepileptic drugs in his blood—primidone, phenobarbital, and PEMA. The primidone serum concentration tends to vary widely during the day because of the drug's short half-life, while phenobarbital and PEMA serum concentrations remain more stable. When monitoring the serum concentrations of a patient on primidone, determinations of at least the primidone and phenobarbital serum concentrations must be ordered to know the amount of active barbiturate in the blood.

Fincham et al. [24] reported that patients given 10 mg/kg of primidone alone had mean primidone serum levels of 13.15 μg/ml and metabolically derived phenobarbital levels of 17.34 μg/ml. Patients receiving a similar dose of primidone in addition to phenytoin were found to have mean primidone levels of 8.1 μg/ml and phenobarbital levels of 27.2 μg/ml. Other studies confirm that in patients taking primidone and phenytoin, the usual recommended dose of 15 mg/kg will produce serum phenobarbital levels of 20 to 40 μg/ml at steady state [8, 24, 58, 61, 63].

Early studies reported that the therapeutic range of primidone serum concentration was 4 to 12 μg/ml and that there was a high incidence of side effects with serum concentrations of above 12 μg/ml. These studies usually involved patients who were also receiving other antiepileptic drugs and therefore had higher concentrations of derived phenobarbital in their serum than patients on primidone monotherapy. More recent studies with primidone monotherapy indicate that the usual daily doses of 10 to 15 mg/kg/day produce primidone serum concentrations of 15 to 20 μg/ml and that these concentrations produce no signs or symptoms of neurotoxicity during chronic therapy [25, 49, 65].

Dosage and Administration
Primidone is supplied as scored tablets of 50 mg or 250 mg and as a suspension containing 250 mg/5 ml. Because of the neurotoxicity often associated with the initiation of therapy (see Toxicity below), dosage must be slowly built up. The manufacturer recommends the following regimen for patients 8 years of age and over: days 1 to 3, 100 to 125 mg hs; days 4 to 6, 100 to 125 mg bid; days 7 to 9, 100 to 125 mg tid; day 10, 250 mg tid. The usual maintenance dose is 750 to 1,000 mg per day in 3 or 4 divided doses. Cross-tolerance allows

maintenance doses of primidone to be substituted for phenobarbital (and vice versa) without crossover.

INDICATIONS

Animal Studies

Primidone possesses antiepileptic efficacy in experimental animal models of tonic-clonic and partial seizures but only minimal potency in protecting against absence seizure models [6, 31]. It is very difficult to define the exact antiseizure effect produced by primidone independent of its derived metabolic products, specifically phenobarbital. Gallagher et al. [29] found that the threshold for tonic-clonic seizures was higher in a group of rats treated with primidone than in a control group treated with phenobarbital when both groups of animals had comparable phenobarbital levels. Early animal studies [26, 31] in rats and mice showed considerable antiepileptic activity within 3 hours of primidone administration. Although serum levels of phenobarbital were not determined in those studies, a later report [29] has indicated that substantial levels of derived phenobarbital were not found until 6 hours after a dose of primidone. It can be inferred that primidone itself provided the antiepileptic effect in these earlier experiments.

Clinical Efficacy

Since the initial report of Handley and Stewart [32], further clinical trials have indicated that primidone is unequivocally effective in the prevention of tonic-clonic and partial seizures. Unfortunately, investigators in most of the early trials did not obtain blood levels for phenobarbital. Olesen and Dam [58] concluded on the basis of their controlled study that patients receiving primidone were no more protected than a control group using phenobarbital when comparable blood levels of phenobarbital were obtained. They postulated that the superior efficacy of primidone compared with phenobarbital in earlier reports was due to higher derived phenobarbital levels [58]. Recent studies by Fincham et al. [24] utilized primidone as the sole drug, with resulting "subtherapeutic" concentrations of derived phenobarbital. These patients had better seizure control with primidone than with phenobarbital therapy with higher serum phenobarbital levels.

Many of the early reports of superior efficacy and minimal long term primidone side effects were based on the use of primidone as the sole drug therapy [32, 43, 48]. It may be inferred that optimal efficacy of primidone with minimal side effects of phenobarbital will be obtained when primidone is used alone. Greater phenobarbital toxicity can be expected when primidone is used in combination with phenytoin because of its increased conversion to phenobarbital. At present, there is no convincing proof of the superior efficacy of primidone therapy compared with phenobarbital or other drugs. However, for a given patient, primidone may give superior control of tonic-clonic or partial seizures compared with other primary antiepileptic drugs (phenytoin, phenobarbital, carbamazepine); its use as an alternate sole drug should be considered. Most often, primidone is given as an adjunctive medication in patients whose seizures are uncontrolled on phenytoin or carbamazepine therapy. As previously noted, there is little reason for the combined use of primidone and phenobarbital in the treatment of epilepsy.

TOXICITY

Although there is disagreement about the efficacy of primidone independent of its metabolically derived phenobarbital, convincing evidence exists that primidone itself produces neurotoxicity. As early as 1955, Timberlake et al. [72] advised a very cautious initiation of therapy with 125 mg of primidone daily at bedtime followed by slow weekly increments. Indeed, the first report of Handley and Stewart [32] advised caution and gradual initiation of treatment to avoid sedation, dizziness, and incoordination. Sciarra et al. [66] reported that side effects occur in 82 percent of patients taking primidone.

The report of Gallagher et al. [28] established that the acute side effects that occurred in patients on initiation of primidone therapy were due to primidone itself rather than to derived phenobarbital or PEMA. Serum levels of the metabolites were very low when symptoms appeared. Similarly, Brillman et al. [9] reported a patient who was comatose following an overdose of primidone. Clearing of consciousness occurred simultaneously with falling primidone levels at a time when the derived phenobarbital concentration had decreased very little.

Tolerance develops within a few days or weeks, and most patients have much fewer side effects with long-term use. This tolerance contrasts with the chronic complaints of sedation in patients taking primidone and phenytoin, in whom moderately high serum phenobarbital levels are found [8, 65, 66].

In addition to the acute toxic effects described above, primidone may produce some or all of the side effects associated with the use of phenobarbital, including chronic neurotixicity [42, 73]. A number of reports have also mentioned occasional drug psychoses with this drug [42]. Impaired sexual potency has been an important complaint in some patients [66, 72].

Serious systemic toxicity to primidone has been rare [42]. Transient drug rashes have been observed infrequently, and a very few idiosyncratic cases of lupus erythematosus have been reported [2].

Mephobarbital

Mephobarbital has been used since 1932, particularly in patients who seem to lack tolerance to the neurotoxic side effects of phenobarbital.

CHEMISTRY

Mephobarbital (5-ethyl-1-methyl-barbituric acid, methylphenobarbital, Mebaral; see Fig. 17-1) is the N-1 methyl analog of phenobarbital and is a relatively water-insoluble substance with a pK_a of 7.8. Mephobarbital is more lipid-soluble than phenobarbital [20].

CLINICAL PHARMACOLOGY

The oral bioavailability of mephobarbital is 50 to 75 percent [13, 20]. The drug is biotransformed by demethylation to phenobarbital [20]. There may also be an epoxide metabolite [20]. The elimination half-life of mephobarbital is 12 to 24 hours during chronic therapy [20]. It is assumed, but unproved, that the derived phenobarbital is further metabolized and excreted as previously described (Fig. 17-1). At steady state, the serum concentration of derived phenobarbital is 7 to 20 times that of mephobarbital, and it is probably sufficient to merely determine the serum concentration of phenobarbital for routine therapeutic drug monitoring [20].

INDICATIONS AND TOXICITY

Mephobarbital has the same clinical indications as phenobarbital and is used as an alternative drug. Daily doses of 4 mg/kg produce serum concentrations of phenobarbital comparable to those obtained when phenobarbital doses of 2 mg/kg are taken on a regular basis.

No controlled trials have provided evidence that the efficacy of mephobarbital is not the result of metabolically derived phenobarbital, although animal studies have shown that mephobarbital itself possesses some independent antiepileptic properties [19]. Mephobarbital continues to be used primarily because of anecdotal reports that it causes less hyperactivity and sedation than phenobarbital. It has been postulated that mephobarbital decreases these side effects by competition with phenobarbital for sites of action in the CNS. No controlled studies have been done comparing side effects of mephobarbital and phenobarbital with equivalent serum levels of phenobarbital. In fact, Eadie [21] observed marked sedation

in one patient with moderate mephobarbital and low phenobarbital levels.

References

1. Aird, R. B., and Woodbury, D. M. *The Management of Epilepsy.* Springfield, Ill.: Thomas, 1974.
2. Alarcon-Segovia, D. Drug-induced lupus syndrome. *Mayo Clin. Proc.* 44:664, 1969.
3. Aston, R., and Domino, E. I. Differential effects of phenobarbital, pentobarbital, and diphenylhydantoin on motor-cortical and reticular thresholds in the Rhesus monkey. *Psychopharmacol.* 2:304, 1961.
4. Baumel, I. P., Gallagher, B. B., and Mattson, R. H. Phenylethylmalonamide (PEMA) an important metabolite of primidone. *Arch. Neurol.* 27:34, 1972.
5. Berg, M. J. et al. Acceleration of body clearance of phenobarbital by activated charcoal. *N. Engl. J. Med.* 307:642, 1982.
6. Bogue, J. T., and Carrington, H. C. The evaluation of "Mysoline" a new anticonvulsant drug. *Br. J. Pharmacol.* 8:230, 1953.
7. Booker, H. E. Phenobarbital: Relation of Plasma Concentration to Seizure Control. In D. M. Woodbury, J. K. Penry, and C. E. Pippenger (Eds.), *Antiepileptic Drugs.* New York: Raven Press, 1982.
8. Booker, H. E. et al. A clinical study of serum primidone levels. *Epilepsia* 11:395, 1970.
9. Brillman, J., Gallagher, B. B., and Mattson, R. H. Acute primidone intoxication. *Arch. Neurol.* 30: 255, 1974.
10. Browne, T. R. Clinical pharmacology of antiepileptic drugs. *Drug Ther. Rev.* 2:469, 1979.
11. Buchthal, F., Svensmark, O., and Simonson, H. Relation of EEG and seizures to phenobarbital in serum. *Arch. Neurol.* 19:362, 1968.
12. Butler, T. C. The delay of onset of action of intravenously injected anesthetics. *J. Pharmacol. Exp. Ther.* 74:118, 1942.
13. Butler, T. C. Quantitative studies of the metabolic rate of mephobarbital (N-methyl-phenobarbital). *J. Pharmacol. Exp. Ther.* 106:235, 1952.
14. Butler, T. C., Mehafee, O., and Waddell, W. J. Phenobarbital: Studies of elimination, accumulation, tolerance, and dosage schedules. *J. Pharmacol. Exp. Ther.* 11:425, 1954.
15. Butler, T. C. The metabolic hydroxylation of phenobarbital. *J. Pharmacol. Exp. Ther.* 116:326, 1956.
16. Butler, T. C., and Waddell, W. J. Metabolic conversion of primidone (Mysoline) to phenobarbital. *Proc. Soc. Exp. Biol. Med.* 93:544, 1956.

17. Cereghino, J. J. et al. Carbamazepine for epilepsy. *Neurology* (Minneap.) 24:401, 1974.
18. Cottrell, P. R. et al. Pharmacokinetics of phenylethylmalonamide (PEMA) in normal subjects and in patients treated with antiepileptic drugs. *Epilepsia* 23:307, 1982.
19. Craig, C. R., and Schideman, F. E. Metabolism and anticonvulsant properties of mephobarbital and phenobarbital in rats. *J. Pharmacol. Exp. Ther.* 176:33, 1971.
20. Eadie, M. J. Methylphenobarbital and Metharbital. In D. M. Woodbury, J. K. Penry, and C. E. Pippenger (Eds.), *Antiepileptic Drugs*. New York: Raven Press, 1982.
21. Eadie, N. J., and Tyre, J. H. *Anticonvulsant Therapy*. London: Livingston, 1980.
22. Essig, C. F., and Carter, W. C. Failure of diphenylhydantoin in preventing barbiturate withdrawal convulsions in the dog. *Neurology* (Minneap.) 12:481, 1962.
23. Faero, O. et al. Successful prophylaxis of febrile convulsions with phenobarbital. *Epilepsia* 13:271, 1972.
24. Fincham, R. W., and Schottelius, D. D. Primidone: Interactions with Other Drugs. In D. M. Woodbury, J. K. Penry, and C. E. Pippenger (Eds.), *Antiepileptic Drugs*. New York: Raven Press, 1982.
25. Fincham, R. W., and Schottelins, D. D. Primidone: Relation of Plasma Concentration to Seizure Control. In D. M. Woodbury, J. K. Penry, and C. E. Pippenger (Eds.), *Antiepileptic Drugs*. New York: Raven Press, 1982.
26. Frey, H. H., and Hahn, L. Untersuchungen über die Bedeutung der durch Biotransformation gebildeten Phenobarbital für die antikonvulsive Wirkung von Primidon. *Arch. Int. Pharmacodyn. Ther.* 12:281, 1960.
27. Gallagher, B. B., Baumel, I. P., and Mattson, R. H. Metabolic disposition of primidone and its metabolites in epileptic subjects after single and repeated administration. *Neurology* (Minneap.) 22:1186, 1972.
28. Gallagher, B. B. et al. Primidone, diphenylhydantoin and phenobarbital: Aspects of acute and chronic toxicity. *Neurology* (Minneap.) 23:145, 1973.
29. Gallagher, B. B., Smith, D. B., and Mattson, R. H. The relationship of the anticonvulsant properties of primidone to phenobarbital. *Epilepsia* 11:293, 1970.
30. Garretson, L. K., and Dayton, P. G. Disappearance of phenobarbital and diphenylhydantoin from serum of children. *Clin. Pharmacol. Ther.* 11:674, 1970.
31. Goodman, L. S. et al. Anticonvulsant properties of 5-phenyl-5-ethylhexahydro-pyrimidone-4-6 dione (Mysoline), a new antiepileptic drug. *J. Pharmacol. Exp. Ther.* 108:428, 1953.
32. Handley, R., and Stewart, A. S. R. Mysoline®, a new drug in the treatment of epilepsy. *Lancet* 262:742, 1952.
33. Hauptmann, A. Luminal bie Epilepsia. *Münch. Med. Wochenschr.* 59:1907, 1912.
34. Heimann, G., and Gladthe, E. Pharmacokinetics of phenobarbital in childhood. *Eur. J. Clin. Pharmacol.* 12:305, 1977.
35. Horning, M. G. et al. Drug metabolism in the human neonate. *Life Sci.* 16:651, 1975.
36. Hutt, S. J. et al. Perceptual motor behavior in relation to blood phenobarbital level: A preliminary report. *Develop. Med. Child. Neurol.* 10:626, 1968.
37. Ives, E. R. Comparison of efficacy of various drugs in treatment of epilepsy. *J.A.M.A.* 147:1332, 1951.
38. Jacobides, G. M. Alertness and Scholastic Achievement in Young Epileptics Treated with Carbamazepine (Tegretol). In H. Meindardi, and A. J. Rowan (Eds.), *Advances in Epileptology*. Amsterdam: Swets and Zeitlinger, 1978.
39. Kapetanovic, I. et al. Valproic Acid-Phenobarbital Interaction: A Systemic Study Using Stable Isotopically Labeled Phenobarbital in an Epileptic Patient. In *Proc. WODADIBF IV*, Voksenasen, Norway. New York: Raven Press, 1980.
40. Kutt, H., and Paris-Kutt, H. Phenobarbital: Interactions with Other Drugs. In D. M. Woodbury, J. K. Penry, and C. E. Pippenger (Eds.), *Antiepileptic Drugs*. New York: Raven Press, 1982.
41. Lambie, D. G., and Johnson, R. H. The effects of phenytoin on phenobarbitone and primidone metabolism. *J. Neurol. Neurosurg. Psychiat.* 44:148, 1981.
42. Leppik, I. E., and Cloyd, J. C. Primidone: Toxicity. In D. M. Woodbury, J. K. Penry, and C. E. Pippenger (Eds.), *Antiepileptic Drugs*. New York: Raven Press, 1982.
43. Livingston, S., and Petersen, D. Primidone (Mysoline) in the treatment of epilepsy. *N. Engl. J. Med.* 254:327, 1956.
44. Livingston, S., and Pauli, L. L. Treatment of grand mal epilepsy: Phenobarbital versus diphenylhydantoin sodium. *Clin. Ped.* 7:444, 1968.
45. Lockman, L. et al. Phenobarbital dosage of control of neonatal seizures. *Neurology* (N.Y.) 29:145, 1979.

46. Lous, P. Barbituric acid concentration in serum from patients with severe acute poisoning. *Acta Pharmacol. Toxicol.* 10:261, 1954.

47. Lous, P. Plasma levels and urinary excretion of three barbituric acids after oral administration to man. *Acta Pharmacol. Toxicol.* 10:147, 1954.

48. Lyons, J. B., and Liversedge, L. A. Primidone in the treatment of epilepsy. *Br. Med. J.* 2:625, 1954.

49. Mattson, R. H. Unpublished data, 1982.

50. Mattson, R. H. et al. Prospective Study of the Relative Efficacy and Toxicity of Anti-Epileptic Drugs on Well-Defined Types of Seizures. In J. Wada, and J. K. Penry (Eds.), *Advances in Epileptology, Xth Epilepsy International Symposium.* New York: Raven Press, 1980.

51. Mattson, R. H. et al. Folate therapy in epilepsy. A controlled study. *Arch. Neurol.* 29:78, 1973.

52. Mattson, R. H., Williamson, P. D., and Hanahan, E. Eterobarb therapy in epilepsy. *Neurology* (Minneap.) 26:1014, 1976.

53. Mattson, R. H., and Cramer, J. A. Phenobarbital: Toxicity. In D. M. Woodbury, J. K. Penry, and C. E. Pippenger (Eds.), *Antiepileptic Drugs* (2nd ed.). New York: Raven Press, 1982.

54. Maynert, E. W. Phenobarbital: Absorption, Distribution, and Excretion. In D. M. Woodbury, J. K. Penry, and C. E. Pippenger (Eds.), *Antiepileptic Drugs.* New York: Raven Press, 1982.

55. Melchior, J. C., Buchthal, F., and Lennox-Buchthal, M. The ineffectiveness of diphenylhydantoin in preventing febrile seizures in the age of greatest risks under three years. *Epilepsia* 12:55, 1971.

56. McGeachy, T. E., and Bloomer, W. E. The phenobarbital sensitivity syndrome. *Am. J. Med.* 14:600, 1953.

57. Merritt, H. H., and Putnam, T. J. Further experiences with the salt of sodium diphenyl hydantoinate in the treatment of convulsive disorders. *Am. J. Psych.* Mar. 1023, 1940.

58. Oleson, O. V., and Dam, M. The conversion of primidone to phenibarbitone in patients under long term treatment. *Arch. Neurol. Scand.* 43:348, 1967.

59. Plaa, G. L., and Hine, C. H. Hydantoin and barbiturate levels observed in epileptics. *Arch. Int. Pharmacodyn. Ther.* 128:375, 1960.

60. Plowman, L., and Persson, B. H. On the transfer of barbiturates to the human fetus and their accumulation in some of the vital organs. *J. Obstet. Gynecol. Br. Common.* 64:706, 1957.

61. Porro, M. G. et al. Phenytoin: A competitive inhibitor and inducer of metabolism in patients with seizures. *Epilepsia.* In press, 1983.

62. Prichard, J. W. Phenobarbital: Mechanisms of Action. In D. M. Woodbury, J. K. Penry, and C. E. Pippenger (Eds.), *Antiepileptic Drugs.* New York: Raven Press, 1982.

63. Reynolds, E. H., Mattson, R. H., and Gallagher, B. B. Relationship between serum and cerebrospinal fluid anticonvulsant drug and folic acid concentrations in epileptic patients. *Neurology* (Minneap.) 22:841, 1972.

64. Schottelius, D. D. Primidone: Absorption, Distribution, and Excretion. In D. M. Woodbury, J. K. Penry, and C. E. Pippenger (Eds.), *Antiepileptic Drugs.* New York: Raven Press, 1982.

65. Schottelius, D. D., and Fincham, R. W. Clinical effectiveness of primidone as a single antiepileptic medication. *Neurology* (Minneap.) 28:409, 1978.

66. Sciarra, D. et al. Clinical evaluation of primidone (Mysoline), new anticonvulsant drug. *J.A.M.A.* 154:824, 1954.

67. Stark, L. G., Killam, K. F., and Killam, E. K. The anticonvulsant effects of phenobarbital diphenylhydantoin and two benzodiazepines in the baboon, *Papio papio. J. Pharmacol. Exp. Ther.* 173:125, 1970.

68. Strobos, R. R. J., and Spudis, E. V. Effect of anticonvulsant drugs on cortical and subcortical seizure discharges in cats. *Arch. Neurol.* 2:399, 1960.

69. Svensmark, O., and Buchthal, F. Accumulation of phenobarbital in man. *Epilepsia* 4:199, 1963.

70. Svensmark, O., and Buchthal, F. Diphenylhydantoin and phenobarbital. Serum levels in children. *Am. J. Dis. Child.* 108:82, 1964.

71. Tang, B. K., Kalow, W., and Grey, A. A. Metabolic fate of phenobarbital in man. N-Glucoside formation. *Drug Metab. Dispos.* 7:315, 1979.

72. Timberlake, W. H., Abbott, J. A., and Schwab, R. S. An effective anticonvulsant with initial problems of adjustment. *N. Engl. J. Med.* 252:304, 1955.

73. Trimble, M. Effect of Antiepileptic Drugs on Psychosocial Development: Phenobarbital and Primidone. In P. L. Morselli, J. K. Penry, and C. E. Pippenger (Eds.), *Antiepileptic Drug Therapy in Pediatrics.* New York: Raven Press, 1982.

74. Vining, E. P. G. et al. Effects of phenobarbital and valproic acid on neuropsychological function. *Epilepsia.* In press, 1983.

75. Viswanathan, C. T., Booker, H. E., and Welling, P. G. Bioavailability of oral and intramuscular phenobarbital. *J. Clin. Pharmacol.* 18:100, 1978.

76. Wada, J. A. et al. Prophylactic effects of phenytoin, phenobarbital, and carbamazepine examined in

kindling cat preparations. *Arch. Neurol.* 33:426, 1976.

77. Waddell, W. J., and Butler, T. C. The distribution and excretion of phenobarbital. *J. Clin. Invest.* 36:1217, 1957.

78. Welton, D. G. Exfoliative dermatitis and hepatitis due to phenobarbital. *J.A.M.A.* 143:232, 1950.

79. Whyte, M. P., and Dekaban, A. S. Metabolic fate of phenobarbital. A quantitative study of p-hydroxy-phenobarbital in man. *Drug Metab. Dispos.* 5:63, 1977.

80. Wilder, B. J. et al. Efficacy of intravenous phenytoin in the treatment of status epilepticus: Kinetics of central nervous system penetration. *Ann. Neurol.* 1:511, 1977.

81. Wolf, S. M. et al. The value of phenobarbital in the child who has had a single febrile seizure: A controlled prospective study. *Pediatric* 59:378, 1977.

82. Wolf, S. M., and Forsythe, A. Behavior Disturbance, Phenobarbital and Febrile Seizures. In H. Meindardi, and A. J. Rowan (Eds.), *Advances in Epileptology.* Amsterdam: Swets and Zeitlinger, 1978.

83. Woodbury, D. M. Applications to Drug Evaluation. In D. P. Purpura et al. (Eds.), *Experimental Models of Epilepsy.* New York: Raven Press, 1972.

84. Yahr, M. D. et al. Evaluation of standard anticonvulsant therapy in 319 patients. *J.A.M.A.* 150:663, 1952.

CARBAMAZEPINE (TEGRETOL)

18

Ernst A. Rodin

Chemistry

Carbamazepine (CBZ; 5-carbamyl-5H-dibenz[b, f]aze-pine; 5H-dibenz[b, f]azepine-5-carboxamide; Tegre-tol) is a derivative of iminostilbene and is chemically re-lated to the tricyclic antidepressants, especially imi-pramine. CBZ has a molecular weight of 236.26, and its structural formula is shown in Figure 18-1. CBZ is a white crystalline compound that is poorly soluble in water but is readily soluble in ethanol, acetone, and propylene glycol. The poor water solubility must be kept in mind when the drug is administered in tablet form, as is usual in the United States, because part of the compound is excreted unchanged in feces. There are published methods for determination of serum levels of CBZ by gas-liquid chromatography, high-pressure liquid chromatography, and enzyme mul-tiplied immunoassay technique (see Chap. 15). The chemistry and methods of determination of CBZ have been extensively reviewed by Kutt [32] and by Gagneux [17].

Mechanism of Action

The literature dealing with the mechanisms of action of CBZ is fragmentary [29]. The following comments summarize the findings. An attempt will be made here to relate some of these aspects to clinical observations in patients.

EFFECTS IN ANTIEPILEPTIC DRUG SCREENING TESTS

CBZ affords greater protection against electroshock (ES) than against pentylenetetrazol (PTZ)-induced seizures. This is of clinical interest because drugs that raise the ES rather than the PTZ threshold tend to be more effective against tonic-clonic and partial seizures than against absence seizures.

EFFECTS ON AXONS

Using the voltage clamp technique, no effect on any parameter of the membrane of an axon could be demonstrated with CBZ levels of 23.6 μg/ml. At levels of 118 μg/ml, sodium and potassium conductance were decreased by 50 percent and 40 percent, respec-tively. These are exceedingly toxic levels and are not relevant to the clinical action of the compound. No effect on electrical excitability or conduction velocity of myelinated or unmyelinated fibers at levels of 5 to 20 μg/ml were noted in the sciatic nerve of the frog.

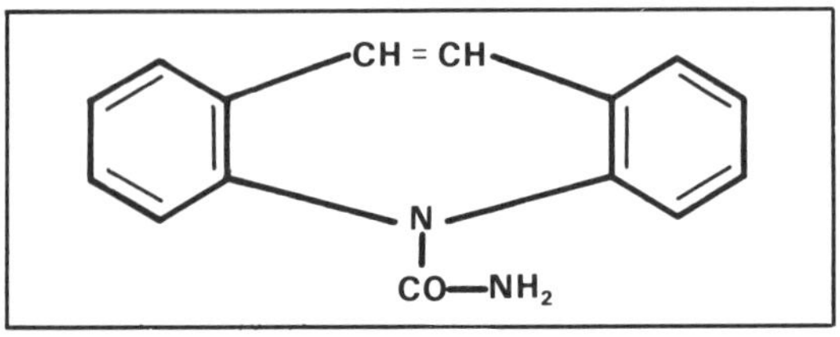

Figure 18-1. Structural formula of carbamazepine.

EFFECTS ON POST-TETANIC POTENTIATION

In the spinal cord of the cat, a slight depressant action on post-tetanic potentiation (PTP) was reported after doses of 10 mg/kg IV, and greater depression (40 to 50 percent) was found after 30 mg/kg IV. Since the latter dose is above that usually administered to patients, its clinical relevance is unclear. No effect on spinal cord PTP was found with therapeutic doses of 10 to 20 mg/kg given intraperitoneally (producing drug plasma levels of 3.5 to 10 μg/ml), and doses of 30 to 40 mg/kg were needed to demonstrate an effect.

EFFECTS ON SYNAPTIC TRANSMISSION

A depression of synaptic transmission in the spinal trigeminal nucleus at IV CBZ doses of 6 mg/kg has been observed. Because this amount is comparable to the lowest effective clinical dose, it might well be related to the drug's usefulness in patients with trigeminal neuralgia.

EFFECTS ON THALAMIC PATHWAYS

Conflicting results have been reported in studies of the effects of CBZ at the thalamic level. One group demonstrated depression of synaptic transmission of trigeminal pain impulses, especially in the nucleus centrum medianum (at doses of 15 mg/kg), but Dolce [14] found no significant effect on recruitment responses elicited by stimulation of the centrum medianum after 5 mg/kg doses. Whether or not the marked difference in the amount of the drug dose would explain this discrepancy cannot be decided at this time. The effect on the nucleus ventralis anterior, which has been implicated in the generalization of epileptiform discharges, was investigated in encephale isole cats. It was observed that with levels of 5 to 9 μg/ml a rather specific depression of activity occurred in the nucleus ventralis anterior. This was not present at these dose levels in the nucleus ventralis medialis, reticular formation, amygdala, hippocampus, caudate, or pallidum. Dolce's extensive study [14] in cats given 2 to 10 mg/kg of CBZ can be summarized as follows: (1) Electrical stimulation of basolateral amygdala did not produce cortical after-discharges; (2) The alerting reaction from electrical stimulation of the

midbrain reticular formation was not markedly influenced; (3) Recruiting responses in the sensory-motor cortex resulting from stimulation of the nucleus centralis medialis were unaffected; (4) There was no appreciable change in the bulbar or midbrain reticular formation after sciatic stimulation; (5) There was an increase in amplitude of the electroretinogram as well as various components of the visual evoked potential at the level of the lateral geniculate body and striate cortex but not at the chiasm.

EFFECTS ON KINDLING

Kindling experiments involving amygdaloid electrical stimulation were inconclusive because of the small numbers of animals investigated. In the hippocampus, electrically induced after-discharges were significantly shortened in duration. Motor responses and generalized seizures, which tend to occur after repeated stimulation, were also suppressed.

EFFECTS ON CORTICAL FOCI

CBZ virtually abolished sustained epileptiform discharges resulting from subpial penicillin injections in doses of 5 mg/kg but left focal spiking intact. A much lesser effect was noted when conjugated estrogen was used to produce epileptiform discharges [29]. Because the latter compound is regarded as a model for absence seizures and the former as one for focal motor attacks, this difference is certainly of interest. Threshold after-discharge voltages of the midsupra sylvian cortex were lowered, and the duration of prolonged after-discharge episodes was shortened by CBZ [14].

The effect on alumina cream foci was also striking in three monkeys. Behavioral and electrographic seizures were suppressed in all animals at CBZ plasma levels of 4 to 8 μg/ml [29]. Seizure activity returned within 10 to 16 days after cessation of CBZ treatment. These findings agree with those of David and Grewal [12], who placed alumina cream foci in the motor cortex and hippocampus of monkeys. Clinical seizures were abolished, electroencephalographic (EEG) spikes were reduced, and the threshold to PTZ was elevated. In addition, aggression was markedly reduced during CBZ treatment in the animals that had hippocampal foci. The latter finding is of considerable interest because of the drug's reputed psychotropic effect (see below).

EFFECTS ON CEREBELLAR PATHWAYS

Julien [29] noted no change in the Purkinje cell discharge rate when a sensory-motor cortical penicillin focus was treated with CBZ. This result contrasts with studies of phenytoin (PHT), in which disappearance of cortical seizure discharges is accompanied by increased Purkinje cell discharges. With CBZ, only the focus disappeared, and there was no change in the Purkinje cell discharge rate, suggesting that the antiepileptic properties of CBZ do not utilize cerebellar pathways.

EFFECTS ON SLEEP

Slow-wave sleep is increased, but REM sleep is not shortened with chronic CBZ administration. The increase of slow-wave sleep is related to fewer waking portions during the night. Withdrawal of CBZ does not lead to a rebound phenomenon but merely restores the pretreatment sleep pattern.

EFFECTS ON ENDOCRINE SYSTEMS

Lühdorf et al. [39] reported that follicle-stimulating hormone, luteinizing hormone, and testosterone levels remained unchanged in the serum, but there was a significant decrease in the free T_3 and T_4 index. These findings were similar to those obtained with PHT. In addition, it was noted that 17-ketosteroid excretion decreased, but there was a significant increase in urine cortisol excretion. This latter finding may not be real, however, because a false increase in fluorescence during cortisol determinations may occur as a side effect of CBZ.

EFFECT ON NEUROTRANSMITTERS

Monaco et al. [43], who determined free amino acid levels in the blood of 6 epileptic paients after 7 days of CBZ treatment, reported an increase in taurine and a decrease in glutamate. Since taurine has recently received considerable attention as having antiepileptic properties, this finding may be of clinical importance if confirmed. There is no information available on the effect of other neurotransmitters in humans, but Consolo et al. [8] found a selective increase in striatal acetylcholine resulting from CBZ administration in rats. Although this finding is difficult to integrate with the usual human clinical data, it may be of value in understanding some of the toxic effects resulting from overdosage (see below).

CONCLUSION

The many discrepancies reported in this section indicate that much more work needs to be done to delineate the most important mechanisms of action of CBZ. At this time, only fragmentary evidence can be presented that does not lend itself to a holistic theory.

Clinical Pharmacology

ABSORPTION

CBZ is poorly soluble in water. As a result, part of it is not absorbed in humans but instead is excreted in the feces (oral bioavailability = 75 to 85 percent [44]). Its solubility can be enhanced by taking the drug with meals, thereby increasing gastrointestinal secretions. Peak plasma levels are reached approximately 6 hours after an oral dose (range, 2 to 12 hours) [33, 44].

DISTRIBUTION

Tissue Binding

High levels of CBZ were found in the liver, bile, kidney, urine, and intestinal contents in animal studies. Although these observations are understandable on the basis of excretion mechanisms, the additional findings of high levels in the yellow ligaments and uveal layers of the eyes are puzzling. Although corneal opacities have been reported in the human as a side effect of the drug, there are no known cases of uveal pathology. Also contrary to expectations, the highest levels in the brain in animals and humans were found in white matter rather than in gray matter. High levels were also found in the peripheral nerves. This observation is especially unexpected because the literature on drug action involving peripheral nerves states that there is no effect on myelinated or unmyelinated fibers and no effect on axon membrane properties.

Protein Binding

About 70 to 80 percent of CBZ in plasma is protein-bound, and about 25 percent remains free [5, 28, 33, 44]. Whether the drug binds mainly to albumin has been debated by Di Salle et al. [13].

Distribution to Fetus and to Breast Milk

CBZ passes the placental barrier into the newborn, who promptly eliminates the compound [57]. The drug can be passed on through breast feeding to the baby [44, 45]. No difference in the half-life between newborns and adults has been found [5, 44, 45].

BIOTRANSFORMATION AND EXCRETION

The double bond of the CBZ molecule between positions 10 and 11 is somewhat unstable and provides the major route of biotransformation. The main breakdown product of the drug is its 10,11-epoxide, which is further metabolized, mostly to 10,11-dihydroxide [15, 44]. Two thirds of the 10,11-dihydroxide is eliminated in free form in the urine, and the rest is conjugated with glucuronic acid [15, 44]. Iminostilbene can also be recovered in the urine as a further minor metabolite [15, 44]. The end product of pyrolytic breakdown of CBZ is 9-methyl acridine. The data on elimination of CBZ as well as its breakdown products are incomplete. Up to 1 percent appears as the parent compound in the urine, 1 to 2 percent as the 10,11-epoxide, about 20 percent as the 10,11-dihydroxy-epoxide, and less than 1 percent as iminostilbene [15, 33, 44]. Another 10 to 20 percent is excreted in feces, partly as parent drug and partly as metabolites, leaving more than half of the compound unaccounted for [15, 33, 44]. The literature agrees that the 10,11-epoxide is the main metabolic breakdown product of CBZ and that the amount of 10,11-epoxide correlates well with plasma levels of CBZ. However, there is still argument about the antiepileptic and toxic properties of 10,11-epoxide [11, 15, 44]. The metabolism of CBZ has been extensively reviewed elsewhere [15, 33, 44].

BLOOD LEVELS AND ELIMINATION HALF-LIFE

Therapeutic Range of Blood Levels
Early reports indicated that therapeutic plasma levels of CBZ ranged from 4 to 7 μg/ml. This estimate has been revised upward to 6 to 10 μg/ml [5, 6, 33]. Levels above 10 μg/ml need not be alarming if they are not accompanied by side effects. In general, side effects can be anticipated if blood levels are above 9 μg/ml: Levels of 30 μg/ml or more are likely to be a result of laboratory error.

Relationships of Dosage, Plasma Level, and Elimination Half-Life
Plasma levels frequently do not correspond exactly to milligram-per kilogram intake, even in hospitalized patients in whom compliance is not a factor [6, 19, 28]. Virtually all investigators of the pharmacokinetics of CBZ have noted not only considerable interindividual differences but also intraindividual differences in absorption and breakdown. Nevertheless, a certain concensus does emerge from a review of the literature.

The highest levels and longest half-lives with the least amount of drug are achieved either with single-dose acute administration or with short-term administration over a period of a few weeks to healthy volunteers. Under these conditions, the elimination half-life of CBZ is usually 30 to 40 hours [15, 44, 56]. The half-life reported for patients with epilepsy who take CBZ chronically is, on the average, 20 hours or less [1, 5, 15, 33, 44]. A progressive decrease in CBZ elimination half-life and a progressive increase in CBZ clearance have been demonstrated by serial stable isotope tracer dose studies in patients beginning chronic CBZ monotherapy [1].

The highest blood levels with the lowest dosages are encountered when the drug is used alone [68]. Levels drop when CBZ is administered in combination with PHT, phenobarbital (PB), or primidone [5, 35, 67, 68]. The lowest levels at high dosages are observed in brain damaged institutionalized patients

[62]. The half-life is reportedly shorter and the clearance faster in children than in adults, although considering the variability encountered in half-lives and clearance rates, this finding may not be statistically significant [5, 44, 56]. The average value for the half-life of CBZ upon chronic administration is approximately 20 hours [5, 15, 33, 44]. Because there are marked individual differences, this figure has more theoretical than practical value and cannot be directly translated into the frequency with which the compound should be administered to a given patient.

DRUG INTERACTIONS
The addition of PHT, PB, or primidone may cause a decrease in CBZ plasma concentration [5, 35, 67]. Clonazepam appears to have no effect on CBZ levels [5]. Addition of CBZ decreases PHT clearance and increases the plasma concentration of PHT [22]. Addition of CBZ does not appear to change the plasma concentration of PB [5, 35, 67], although CBZ may cause an increase in the plasma concentration of PB derived from primidone [5, 35]. Addition of CBZ reduces the plasma concentration and increases the clearance of ethosuximide [35, 71] and valproic acid [4, 5, 10, 35], and it reduces the plasma concentration and elimination half-life of clonazepam [34, 35]. CBZ accelerates the metabolism of warfarin and tetracycline. CBZ may also increase or induce bradycardia resulting from digitalis. Finally, on theoretical grounds an interaction would be expected to occur between CBZ and monoamine oxidase inhibitors, but actual case reports have not been found.

DOSAGE AND ADMINISTRATION
The initial dose for patients over 12 years of age is 200 mg bid. The dosage is then gradually increased by adding up to 200 mg/day until the best response is obtained. The usual maintenance dose is 800 to 1200 mg daily.

In children 6 to 12 years of age the initial dose is 100 mg bid. The dosage is then gradually increased by adding up to 100 mg/day until the best response is obtained. The usual maintenance dose in children is 400 to 800 mg daily.

The maximum daily dosage recommended by the manufacturer is 1000 mg for patients up to 15 years of age and 1200 mg for patients over 15 years of age. Larger doses have been used in some instances.

No concensus exists in the literature about the best regimen for CBZ administration. Suggestions range from twice a day doses to six daily doses. The manufacturer recommends a regimen of three or four doses per day. Schneider [62] reported that with three

400-mg doses the highest blood levels are achieved at 10 P.M., the trough occurring around 6 A.M. Strandjord [67] found that the trough occurred 1 hour after the morning dose, and blood levels rose thereafter fairly uniformly throughout the next 8 hours. Keeping the slow absorption rate of the tablet in mind, it would seem reasonable to take the time of occurrence of the patient's seizures into account in deciding upon the dosage schedule so that the patient can be given maximum protection when it is most needed.

CBZ is marketed in the United States as a 200-mg scored tablet and as a 100-mg chewable scored tablet. A pediatric suspension is currently undergoing investigation and may soon be marketed.

FURTHER READING
Further detailed information on the pharmacology of CBZ can be found in several recent publications [5, 46, 50, 51, 53, 63, 73].

Indications

FDA-APPROVED INDICATIONS
CBZ is approved by the FDA for treatment of patients 6 years of age or older with the following seizure conditions that have not responded favorably to other agents such as PHT, PB, or primidone: (1) complex partial seizures, (2) tonic-clonic seizures, (3) mixed seizure patterns that include complex partial, tonic-clonic, other partial, or other generalized seizures. Trigeminal neuralgia is also an FDA-approved indication for CBZ. Absence seizures do not appear to respond to CBZ. Note that CBZ is not approved by the FDA as an initial therapy for epilepsy. However, there is much reported evidence that CBZ is effective as an initial therapy. Further testing is in progress, and CBZ may be approved for initial therapy for epilepsy in the near future.

It would serve no useful purpose here to cite the numerous references testifying to the efficacy of CBZ as an antiepileptic drug and its relative lack of side effects when therapy is instituted gradually. As of 1977 there were more than 7500 published case reports [65], and there are excellent summaries in print [46, 50, 51, 72]. This review will therefore limit itself to six areas: (1) early studies, (2) reports by investigators who have long-term experience with the compound, (3) double-blind studies, (4) psychotropic properties, (5) effectiveness in children, and (6) indications other than epilepsy.

EARLY STUDIES
In 1963 and 1964, Bonduelle et al. [3] and Lorgé [37] reported independently on the effectiveness of CBZ

as an antiepileptic agent. These early reports are important because they foreshadowed subsequent experiences. Bonduelle et al. concluded that in 69 percent of patients good results were achieved with the compound when compared with previous therapies, and in 26 percent of these patients the result was excellent. There was only an inconstant effect on absence seizures. Also, CBZ was no more effective than PB in patients who had only infrequent seizures that were quite well controlled by other drugs. Its major effectiveness was in patients who were poorly controlled with conventional medications, especially those who suffered from frequent complex partial seizures. It was also stated that the drug merits systematic utilization in patients who have additional psychiatric symptoms. Remarkable effectiveness was noted in patients who suffered from trigeminal neuralgia.

Lorgé [37], who had used the preparation in 132 institutionalized patients for a 3½ year period, noted that nearly 75 percent of the patients had improved as a result of the drug, and 25 percent of the improved patients had become seizure-free. He found that all seizure types apart from absence seizures were influenced positively. In addition, he noted that the mental state of 101 patients who had definite mental changes improved markedly in 30 percent and moderately in 20 percent.

LONG-TERM STUDIES
Hassan and Parsonage [26] reported on 254 patients treated for 1 to 12 years. Reduction of seizure frequency by more than 50 percent occurred in 62 percent of patients with partial seizures and 56 percent of patients with tonic-clonic seizures. Side effects necessitating withdrawal of the drug occurred in 6 patients, and the drug was withdrawn in 21 other patients because of lack of improvement or worsening of the clinical state. In 1972, Bonduelle presented data comparing the results of the initial study with those of an 8- to 11-year follow-up [2]. Fifty-eight of the original 89 cases were available. Satisfactory seizure reduction of more than 50 percent of seizures was encountered in 71 percent of the patients, which compared favorably with such improvement in 69 percent of the original group. Psychiatric problems had improved in 76 percent of the patients at the time of follow-up and in 70 percent during the initial study. The findings indicate that the effectiveness of the compound does not decrease with lapse of time.

DOUBLE-BLIND STUDIES
The first double-blind studies were carried out by Cereghino et al. [6, 7] on institutionalized patients.

Initially, no superiority in seizure control over PHT or PB could be demonstrated if the drugs were used singly rather than in combination. Side effects were minimal. In a subsequent double-blind study [7], the effectiveness of the drug was enhanced when it was combined with either PB or PHT, and a combination of all three drugs gave the best results. Under these circumstances, however, the CBZ blood levels were lower than when the drug was used as the sole anti-epileptic agent [7]. These findings agree with the subsequent studies of Rodin et al. [59], who compared the effectiveness of PHT, PB, and placebo versus PHT, PB, and CBZ in a double-blind, single cross-over design. Thirty-six patients who had severe, intractable complex partial seizures with intermittent tonic-clonic seizures were treated in this manner. A reduction of 83 percent of complex partial seizures and 55 percent of tonic-clonic seizures was found when CBZ was added to the PHT-PB combinations. According to the study design, patients were suddenly changed from CBZ to placebo and vice versa. The discontinuation of CBZ led to an exacerbation (mostly of complex partial seizures) in 7 cases during the first 3 to 4 days, suggesting that the drug should be discontinued gradually and only when therapeutic doses of the compound replacing it have been achieved. The EEG during CBZ therapy showed an insignificant decrease in focal spike activity, at times a change of spikes into random slow waves, slowing of background rhythms, and occasional occurrence of diffuse paroxysmal events. These findings agree with those in the literature [72], and it is evident that the EEG cannot be used to predict the clinical course.

Three double-blind comparisons of PHT versus CBZ monotherapy have failed to establish a significant difference in either the efficacy or the toxicity of the two drugs in managing simple partial, complex partial, or tonic-clonic seizures [28, 64, 70]. One comparison of PHT with CBZ showed fewer objective side effects with CBZ [70], but at the conclusion of the double-blind study, the patients were about evenly divided in their preference for continued treatment of indefinite length. The patients' decisions were based not only on seizure control but also on the discomfort associated with subjective side effects. The suggestion by Simonsen et al. [64] that PHT and CBZ should be tried separately before they are combined is therefore reasonable.

When the relative efficacy of CBZ and primidone on seizure control was compared in patients with complex partial seizures, secondarily generalized seizures, and primarily generalized seizures in a single-blind study on outpatients, no significant difference between the two compounds could be demonstrated in seizure frequency [61]. Although this study showed more subjective side effects with CBZ than with primidone, there was no difference in objective side effects such as rash or decreased white blood cell or platelet counts.

PSYCHOTROPIC ACTIONS

Psychotropic actions were initially reported by Lorge [37] as well as by Bonduelle [3], but the finding has remained controversial [9, 40]. Since most reports deal with subjective impressions in relatively few patients who tend to be on complex medication regimens, caution is obviously indicated in interpretating the results. Our own acute, double-blind study [59] failed to demonstrate a psychotropic effect when a large variety of behavioral and neuropsychologic scales was used. This study had, however, two potential drawbacks. One is that it lasted for only 3 weeks, which may have been an inadequate amount of time in which to demonstrate significant objective behavioral changes. The other is that CBZ was merely added to PHT and PB rather than simultaneously withdrawing one of the other two compounds. Although statistical evaluation did not bear out the presence of psychotropic effects, several patients were clearly improved on CBZ, as case report No. 7 in reference 60 demonstrates. This particular patient is still being followed on an outpatient basis and is doing quite well on CBZ. It is important to point out a case of this type because even if the number of psychiatrically improved patients is too small to be statistically significant, the improvement in a few can make a great deal of difference to the individual patient and the family.

Although the statistics favoring the drug's reputed psychotropic effect are not as marked as would be desirable, statistical evaluations dealing with cognitive and behavioral functions of the patient while on CBZ are available, and they are encouraging. Only the double-blind studies will be reported here. Although the CBZ-primidone comparison study by Rodin et al. [61] was conducted in a single-blind manner as far as the physicians in charge of the patients' treatment were concerned, it was kept double-blind for the electroencephalographer and psychologists evaluating the test results. It was found that patients scored higher on the psychopathic deviate scale while taking primidone than while taking CBZ ($p < 0.01$). There was also significantly greater impairment in repeatable cognitive perceptual motor tests with primidone than with CBZ. Troupin et al. [70] reported fewer errors on tasks requiring attention and problem-solving when patients were taking CBZ rather than PHT. On the MMPI, all scales improved slightly with CBZ, but only the F scale was affected to a statistically significant

study with emphasis on untoward reac-
. *Nerv. Syst.* 35:103, 1974.

M. Klinische Erfahrungen mit einem
ntiepilepticum, Tegretol (G 32.883), mit
er Wirkung auf die epileptische Wesens-
rung. *Schweiz. Med. Wochenschr.* 93:
63.

Some Aspects of Clinical Tolerance of
In C. A. S. Wink (Ed.), *Tegretol in Epi-*
port of an International Clinical Sympo-
anchester, Eng.: C. Nicholls, 1972. Pp.

K. et al. The Influence of Phenytoin and
zepine on Endocrine Function: Pre-
Results. In J. K. Penry (Ed.), *Epilepsy: The*
ternational Symposium. New York: Raven
77.

R. L. Carbamazepine: Neurotoxicity. In
oodbury, J. K. Penry, and C. E. Pippenger
Antiepileptic Drugs. New York: Raven
82.

on, P. R., and Sullivan, F. M. Comparative
icity of six antiepileptic drugs in the
Br. J. Pharmacol. 59:494, 1977.

G. The teratological effects of anticon-
and the effects on pregnancy and birth.
urol. 10:179, 1973.

F. et al. Free amino acid plasma levels in
patients treated with carbamazepine:
ary results. (Italian) *Acta Neurol.* 30:608,

P. L., and Bossi, L. Carbamazepine: Ab-
, Distribution, and Excretion. In D. M.
ry, J. K. Penry, and C. E. Pippenger (Eds.),
ptic Drugs. New York: Raven Press, 1982.
P. L. Clinical pharmacokinetics in neo-
lin. Pharmacokinet. 1:81, 1976.

P. L., Penry, J. K., and Pippenger, C. E.
ptic Drug Therapy in Pediatrics. New
ven Press, 1982.

W. J. Carbamazepine-induced opthal-
a. *Arch. Neurol.* 39:64, 1982.

R. et al. Carbamazepine levels in preg-
d lactation. *Obstet. Gynecol.* 53:139, 1979.
R. B., Paulson, G. W., and Jreissaty, S.
in and carbamazepine in production of
ates in mice: Comparison of teratogenic
Arch. Neurol. 36:832, 1979.

K., and Daly, D. D. (Eds.). *Advances in*
gy, Vol. 11, *Complex Partial Seizures and*
eatment. New York: Raven Press, 1975.
K. (Ed.). *Epilepsy: The Eighth International*
um. New York: Raven Press, 1977.

52. Perucca, E., and Richens, A. Water intoxication
produced by carbamazepine and its reversal by
phenytoin. *Br. J. Clin. Pharmacol.* 9:302P, 1980.

53. Pippenger, C. E., Penry, J. K., and Kutt, H. (Eds.),
Antiepileptic Drugs: Quantitative Analysis and
Interpretation. New York: Raven Press, 1978.

54. Pisciotta, A. V. Carbamazepine: Hematological
Toxicity. In D. M. Woodbury, J. K. Penry, and C. E.
Pippenger (Eds.), *Antiepileptic Drugs.* New York:
Raven Press, 1982.

55. Puente, R. M. The Use of Carbamazepine in the
Treatment of Behavioral Disorders in Children.
In W. Birkmayer (Ed.), *Epileptic Seizures—Be-*
haviour—Pain. Berne: Hans Huber, 1976. Pp.
243–247.

56. Phynnonen, S. et al. Elimination of Carbamazepine
in Children After Single and Multiple Doses. In
J. K. Penry (Ed.), *Epilepsy: The Eighth International*
Symposium. New York: Raven Press, 1977.

57. Rane, A., Bertilsson, L., and Palmer, L. Disposition
of placentally transferred carbamazepine (Tegretol) in the newborn. *Eur. J. Clin. Pharmacol.*
8:283, 1975.

58. Reynolds, E. H. Neurotoxicity of Carbamazepine.
In J. K. Penry, and D. D. Daly (Eds.), *Advances in*
Neurology, Vol. 11, *Complex Partial Seizures and*
Their Treatment. New York: Raven Press, 1975.

59. Rodin, E. A., Rim, C. S., and Rennick, P. M. The
effects of carbamazepine on patients with psychomotor epilepsy: Results of a double-blind study.
Epilepsia 15:547, 1974.

60. Rodin, E. A. Psychosocial Management of Patients
with Complex Partial Seizures. In J. K. Penry, and
D. D. Daly (Eds.), *Advances in Neurology,* Vol. 11,
Complex Partial Seizures and Their Treatment.
New York: Raven Press, 1975.

61. Rodin, E. A. et al. A comparison of the effectiveness
of primidone versus carbamazepine in epileptic
outpatients. *J. Nerv. Ment. Dis.* 163:41, 1976.

62. Schneider, H. Carbamazepine: An Attempt to Cor-
relate Serum Levels with Anti-epileptic and Side
Effects. In H. Schneider et al. (Eds.), *Clinical*
Pharmacology of Antiepileptic Drugs. Berlin-
Heidelberg: Springer Verlag, 1975.

63. Schneider, H. et al. (Eds.). *Clinical Pharmacology*
of Antiepileptic Drugs. Berlin-Heidelberg: Springer
Verlag, 1975.

64. Simonsen, N. et al. A comparative controlled study
between carbamazepine and diphenylhydantoin
in psychomotor epilepsy. *Epilepsia* 17:169, 1976.

65. Singh, A. N., Saxena, B. M., and Germain, M. Anticonvulsive and Psychotropic Effects of Carbamazepine in Hospitalized Epileptic Patients: A Long-

degree. Groh's study [23] in children showed effectiveness mostly on increase in drive level and mood
improvement. Puente [55] also reported "considerable reduction in the signs and symptoms of children
with behavioral disorders, thereby improving their
performance at school, their family relationships, and
their adaptation to their environment and to society
in general."

EFFECTIVENESS IN CHILDREN

The use of CBZ in children was reviewed by Gamstorp
[18], who has had experience with the drug for more
than 10 years. Two-thirds of her patients with focal
seizures, including complex partial seizures, became
seizure-free or were greatly improved. Tonic-clonic
seizures also responded at times, but absences rarely
did. Only one case of bone marrow depression and
one case of hepatic dysfunction were encountered.
One patient developed psychotic symptoms. None of
these side effects were irreversible. Considering the
fact that this study covers a 10-year observation period,
it must be concluded that this is a remarkable track
record for any drug.

Apart from Gamstorp's experience [18], the consensus of the literature is that the compound is most
useful in children who have partial and secondarily
generalized seizures. It is usually not effective in
febrile seizures, infantile spasms, atonic seizures,
myoclonic seizures, or absences. Its effect in primary
generalized tonic-clonic seizures is variable.

INDICATIONS OTHER THAN EPILEPSY

CBZ is an FDA-approved therapy for trigeminal neuralgia. Other indications (not yet FDA-approved) for
which there is evidence that CBZ may be effective include (1) hemifacial spasm, (2) prevention of seizures
after severe head injuries, (3) childhood behavior
disorders, especially when episodic, (4) episodic nocturnal events not clearly epileptic in nature, (5) episodic phenomena in multiple sclerosis, (6) episodic
events occurring by themselves rather than as part of
another illness, (7) central diabetes insipidus, and
(8) dystonia.

Toxicity

A long list of side effects associated with CBZ therapy
appears on the package insert and is reviewed in detail elsewhere [20, 24, 31, 36, 38, 40, 46, 54, 58]. This
section will limit itself to those side effects that are
encountered most commonly. A useful classification
of drug toxicity would be one that could be called
dose-related versus idiosyncratic. It cannot be put completely into practice because the literature frequently
leaves the clinician in doubt about whether a given

symptom disappeared with dose reduction or with
discontinuation of the drug. Nevertheless, an attempt
of this type will be made here by starting from the opposite extreme—namely, massive ingestion of CBZ by
patients with suicidal intent.

OVERDOSAGE

The signs and symptoms of acute massive overdosage
with CBZ may include coma, respiratory depression,
seizures, myoclonus, nystagmus, tremor, rigidity,
ballistic movements, orofacial dyskinesia, hyperreflexia, hyporeflexia, delayed gastric emptying with
cyclic coma, ataxia, sinus tachycardia, atrioventricular
conduction delay, opthalmoplegia, and dilated pupils
[40, 47, 69]. During recovery there may be agitation,
blurred vision, ataxia, and nystagmus (horizontal or
downbeat) [40, 69]. Cardiac arrhythmias and conduction defects like those occurring with overdosage
of other tricyclics have not been described with CBZ
overdose [69]. To date, there are no reported fatalities
from overdosage.

DOSE-DEPENDENT SIDE EFFECTS

Reviewing the symptoms of overdosage in reverse, one
can conclude that dose-related symptoms and signs
within the therapeutic range are likely to consist in
the following: subjective dizziness that may be related
to accommodation problems (frequently referred to
as diplopia) or may be cerebellovestibular in nature;
drowsiness, ataxia, and nystagmus; and possibly irritability or hyperactivity [20, 24, 29, 31, 36, 38, 40, 58].
The toxic symptoms of ballistic movements, rigidity,
and oculogyric crisis that have been reported are
interesting in regard to the animal studies described
earlier (see Mechanisms of Action, above), where it
was mentioned that the most marked cholinergic effect
was on the striatum. A cholinergic effect could also
account for the problems seen with accommodation.

Decreased plasma sodium concentration, decreased
plasma osmolality, and decreased ability to handle a
water load occur in a minority of patients taking CBZ
[40, 52]. This phenomenon varies directly with CBZ
plasma concentration in patients who experience it
[40, 52]. Hyponatremia is more likely to occur in patients taking CBZ alone than in patients taking CBZ
and PHT in combination because PHT lowers CBZ
plasma concentrations [52].

IDIOSYNCRATIC REACTIONS

Range of Reactions

The following reactions to CBZ are likely to be idiosyncratic: exfoliative dermatitis, jaundice, lymphatic
hyperplasia, lenticular opacities, aplastic anemia,

thrombocytopenia, and pancytopenia [20, 24, 28, 31, 36, 54]. The following side effects may be either idiosyncratic or dose-related: an urticarial type of rash and depression of one or more values of cellular or humoral immune responses.

Hematopoietic Side Effects

Several early reports of serious bone marrow depression in association with CBZ therapy led to a special bold-print warning on the package insert and the recommendation that frequent blood cell counts be obtained. Recent comprehensive reviews of all available data indicate the hematopoietic toxicity of CBZ is much less than originally feared [25, 54]. Hart and Easton [25] tabulated the prevalence of CBZ-hematologic toxicity as follows: aplastic anemia—< 1/50,000 (a total of 20 cases), transient leukopenia—10 percent, persistent leukopenia—2 percent, thrombocytopenia—2 percent (average change 0–20,000/mm^3), and anemia—< 5 percent (average change 0–0.5 gm Hb/dl). Pisciotta [54] calculated similar risks and pointed out that in many of the reported cases of CBZ-hematopoietic toxicity, the patient was taking other drugs that either have hematopoietic side effects of their own or may potentiate latent ones.

CHROMOSOMAL CHANGES

The question of chromosomal changes has been raised by one report of an increase in chromatid dislocations with CBZ.

TERATOGENICITY

A review of 99 pregnancies, during which CBZ was taken for at least the first 3 months, revealed 96 normal offspring, 2 abortions in the third month, and 1 child born with atresia of the arms [48]. Meyer [42] found an association with cleft palate and harelip in offspring of epileptic mothers who were treated with PHT and PB but not with CBZ. However, a recent prospective study reported a statistically significant decrease in head circumference of neonates born to mothers taking CBZ that was not present in neonates born to mothers taking PHT or PB monotherapy [27].

Several animal studies performed without blood-level monitoring have reported higher rates of congenital malformations with PHT and PB than with CBZ [16, 41]. These results may be misleading because CBZ has a very rapid metabolism and poor oral absorption in animals [49]. In a mouse study done with blood-level control, PHT and CBZ at low therapeutic serum concentrations did not produce a statistically significant increase in congenital malformations, but PHT at high therapeutic and toxic serum concentra-

tions did produce a significant increase [49]. CBZ blood levels above a low therapeutic level (4.3 µg/ml) could not be obtained even with massive daily doses of CBZ (1,600 mg/kg).

The teratogenicity of antiepileptic drugs is reviewed in more detail in Chap. 29.

CONCLUSION

CBZ, like any other effective drug, can produce side effects. These are usually subjective unless they are idiosyncratic or due to overdose. They rarely necessitate the discontinuation of the drug. Our own experience agrees with that of Reynolds [58] that less than 5 percent of patients develop disabling symptoms that necessitate reduction or cessation of the drug when it is used prudently.

References*

1. Bertilsson, L. et al. Autoinduction of carbamazepine metabolism in children examined by a stable isotope technique. *Clin. Pharmacol. Ther.* 27:83, 1980.
2. Bonduelle, M. My study of Tegretol in the treatment of epilepsy. In C. A. S. Wink (Ed.), *Tegretol in Epilepsy: Report of an International Clinical Symposium.* Manchester: C. Nicholls, 1972. Pp. 80–88.
3. Bonduelle, M., Bouygues, P., Sallou, C. et al. Expérimentation clinique de l'antiépiletique G 32.883 (Tegretol): Résultats portant sur 100 cas observés en trois ans. *Revue Neurol.* 110:209, 1964.
4. Bowdle, T. A., Levy, R. H., and Cutler, R. E. Effects of carbamazepine on valproic acid kinetics in normal subjects. *Clin. Pharmacol. Ther.* 26:629, 1979.
5. Browne, T. R. Clinical pharmacology of antiepileptic drugs. *Drug Ther. Rev.* 2:469, 1979.
6. Cereghino, J. J. Carbamazepine: Relation of Plasma Concentration to Seizure Control. In D. M. Woodbury, J. K. Penry, and C. E. Pippenger (Eds.), *Antiepileptic Drugs.* New York: Raven Press, 1982.
7. Cereghino, J. J. et al. The efficacy of carbamazepine combinations in epilepsy. *Clin. Pharmacol. Ther.* 18:733, 1975.
8. Consolo, S., Bianchi, S., and Ladinsky, H. Effect of carbamazepine on cholinergic parameters in rat brain areas. *Neuropharmacol.* 15:653, 1976.
9. Dalby, M. A. Behavioral Effects of Carbamazepine. In J. K. Penry, and D. D. Daly (Eds.), *Advances in Neurology,* Vol. 11. *Complex Partial Seizures and Their Treatment.* New York: Raven Press, 1975.
10. Dalby, M. A. Interaction carbamazepine-dipropylacetate. *Acta Neurol. Scand.* 62 [Suppl. 79]:101, 1980.
11. Dam, M., Jensen, A., and Christiansen, J. Plasma level and effect of carbamazepine in grand mal and psychomotor epilepsy. *Acta Neurol. Scand.* 60: 33, 1975.
12. David, J., and Grewal, R. S. Effect of carbamazepine (Tegretol) on seizure and EEG patterns in monkeys with alumina-induced focal motor and hippocampal foci. *Epilepsia* 17:415, 1976.
13. Di Salle, E., Pacifici, G. M., and Morselli, P. L. Studies on plasma protein binding of carbamazepine. *Pharmacolog. Research Commun.* 6:193, 1974.
14. Dolce, G. Uber den antiepileptischen Aktionsmechanismus von 5-Carbamyl-5H-dibenzo(b, f)-azepin. *Arzneimittelforschung* 19:1257, 1969.
15. Faigle, J. W., and Feldmann, K. F. Carbamazepine: Biotransformation. In D. M. Woodbury, J. K. Penry, and C. E. Pippenger (Eds.), *Antiepileptic Drugs.* New York: Raven Press, 1982.
16. Fritz, H., Muller, D., and Hess, R. Comparative study of the teratogenicity of phenobarbitone, diphenylhydantoin and carbamazepine in mice. *Toxicology* 6:323, 1976.
17. Gagneux, A. R. The Chemistry of Carbamazepine. In W. Birkmayer (Ed.), *Epileptic Seizures—Behaviour—Pain.* Berne: Hans Huber, 1976.
18. Gamstorp, I. Treatment with Carbamazepine: Children. In J. K. Penry, and D. D. Daly (Eds.), *Advances in Neurology,* Vol. 11. *Complex Partial Seizures and Their Treatment.* New York: Raven Press, 1975.
19. Gardner-Thorpe, C., Parsonage, M. J., Smethurst, P. F. et al. Antiepileptic drug concentrations in plasma: Clinical evaluation of 321 estimations in 237 unselected patients. *Acta Neurol. Scand.* 48:213, 1972.
20. Gayford, J. J., and Redpath, T. H. The side effects of carbamazepine. *Proc. R. Soc. Med.* 6:615, 1969.
21. Grant, R. H. E. The Use of Carbamazepine (Tegretol) in Patients with Epilepsy and Multiple Handicaps. In C. A. S. Wink (Ed.), *Tegretol in Epilepsy: Report of an International Clinical Symposium.* Manchester: C. Nicholls, 1972.
22. Gratz, E. S. et al. Effect of carbamazepine on phenytoin clearance in patients with complex partial seizures. *Neurology* (N.Y.) 32:A223, 1982.
23. Groh, C. The Psychotropic Effect of Tegretol in Non-Epileptic Children with Particular Reference

*The references given here are highly selective, and a complete bibliography dealing with statements appearing in this chapter can be obtained from the author.

to the Drug's
Epileptic Seizu
Hans Huber, 1

24. Hanke, N. F. J.
C. A. S. Wink (
an Internation
C. Nicholls, 19
25. Hart, R. G., an
hematological
1982.
26. Hassan, M. N.,
the Long-Term
in the Treatme
Epilepsy: The
New York: Rav
27. Iivanainen, M.
Human Body
Penry, and C.
Drug Therapy
Press, 1982.
28. Johannessen, S
tration of carba
in cerebrospin
Epilepsia 14:37
29. Julien, R. M.
Action. In D. M
Pippenger (Eds
Raven Press, 19
30. Kosteljanetz, M
epileptic
Prelimin
generalized epi
1975.
31. Kugler, J. Side-E
Wink (Ed.), *Te*
ternational Clin
C. Nicholls, 197
32. Kutt, H., and Par
istry and Meth
Woodbury, J. K.
Antiepileptic Dr
33. Kutt, H. Clinical
In C. E. Pippeng
Antiepileptic D
York: R
34. Lai, A. A., Levy, F
of interaction b
nazepam in nor
24:316, 1978.
35. Levy, R. H.; and
Interactions with
J. K. Penry, and
leptic Drugs. Ne

follow-u
tions. *D*
37. Lorgé, V
neuen A
besonde
veraend
1042, 19
38. Lorgé, M
Tegretol
lepsy: R
sium. M
107–109
39. Lühdorf,
Carbam
liminary
Eighth I
Press, 19
40. Masland
D. M. W
(Eds.),
Press, 19
41. McElhat
teratoge
mouse.
42. Meyer, J
vulsants
Eur. Ne
43. Monaco
epileptic
Prelimi
1975.
44. Morselli
sorption
Woodbu
Antiepi
45. Morselli
nates. *C*
46. Morselli
Antiepi
York: R
47. Mullally
moplegi
Interpretation. N
48. Niebyl,
nancy a
49. Paulson
Phenyto
cleft pa
effects.
50. Penry, J
Neurol
Their T
51. Penry, J
Sympos

Neurology, Vol. 11. *Complex Partial Seizures and Their Treatment.* New York: Raven Press, 1975.
36. Livingston, S., P
bamazepine (T

Term Study. In J. K. Penry (Ed.), *Epilepsy: The Eighth International Symposium.* New York: Raven Press, 1977.

66. Smith, G. A. et al. Factors influencing plasma concentrations of ethosuximide. *Clin. Pharmacokinet.* 4:38, 1979.

67. Strandjord, R. E., and Johannessen, S. I. A Preliminary Study of Serum Carbamazepine Levels in Healthy Subjects and in Patients with Epilepsy. In H. Schneider et al. (Eds.), *Clinical Pharmacology of Antiepileptic Drugs.* Berlin-Heidelberg: Springer Verlag, 1975.

68. Strandjord, R. E., and Johannessen, S. I. Single-drug therapy with carbamazepine in patients with epilepsy: Serum levels and clinical effect. *Epilepsia* 21:655, 1980.

69. Sullivan, J. B., Rumack, B. H., and Peterson, R. G. Acute carbamazepine toxicity resulting from overdose. *Neurology* (N.Y.) 31:621, 1981.

70. Troupin, A. et al. Carbamazepine—A double-blind comparison with phenytoin. *Neurology* 27:511, 1977.

71. Warren, J. W. et al. Kinetics of carbamazepine-ethosuximide interaction. *Clin. Pharmacol. Ther.* 28:646, 1980.

72. Wink, C. A. S. (Ed.). *Tegretol in Epilepsy: Report of an International Clinical Symposium.* Manchester, Eng.: C. Nicholls, 1972.

73. Woodbury, D. M., Penry, J. K., and Pippenger, C. E. (Eds.), *Antiepileptic Drugs.* New York: Raven Press, 1982.

degree. Groh's study [23] in children showed effectiveness mostly on increase in drive level and mood improvement. Puente [55] also reported "considerable reduction in the signs and symptoms of children with behavioral disorders, thereby improving their performance at school, their family relationships, and their adaptation to their environment and to society in general."

Effectiveness in Children

The use of CBZ in children was reviewed by Gamstorp [18], who has had experience with the drug for more than 10 years. Two-thirds of her patients with focal seizures, including complex partial seizures, became seizure-free or were greatly improved. Tonic-clonic seizures also responded at times, but absences rarely did. Only one case of bone marrow depression and one case of hepatic dysfunction were encountered. One patient developed psychotic symptoms. None of these side effects were irreversible. Considering the fact that this study covers a 10-year observation period, it must be concluded that this is a remarkable track record for any drug.

Apart from Gamstorp's experience [18], the consensus of the literature is that the compound is most useful in children who have partial and secondarily generalized seizures. It is usually not effective in febrile seizures, infantile spasms, atonic seizures, myoclonic seizures, or absences. Its effect in primary generalized tonic-clonic seizures is variable.

Indications Other Than Epilepsy

CBZ is an FDA-approved therapy for trigeminal neuralgia. Other indications (not yet FDA-approved) for which there is evidence that CBZ may be effective include (1) hemifacial spasm, (2) prevention of seizures after severe head injuries, (3) childhood behavior disorders, especially when episodic, (4) episodic nocturnal events not clearly epileptic in nature, (5) episodic phenomena in multiple sclerosis, (6) episodic events occurring by themselves rather than as part of another illness, (7) central diabetes insipidus, and (8) dystonia.

Toxicity

A long list of side effects associated with CBZ therapy appears on the package insert and is reviewed in detail elsewhere [20, 24, 31, 36, 38, 40, 46, 54, 58]. This section will limit itself to those side effects that are encountered most commonly. A useful classification of drug toxicity would be one that could be called dose-related versus idiosyncratic. It cannot be put completely into practice because the literature frequently leaves the clinician in doubt about whether a given symptom disappeared with dose reduction or with discontinuation of the drug. Nevertheless, an attempt of this type will be made here by starting from the opposite extreme—namely, massive ingestion of CBZ by patients with suicidal intent.

Overdosage

The signs and symptoms of acute massive overdosage with CBZ may include coma, respiratory depression, seizures, myoclonus, nystagmus, tremor, rigidity, ballistic movements, orofacial dyskinesia, hyperreflexia, hyporeflexia, delayed gastric emptying with cyclic coma, ataxia, sinus tachycardia, atrioventricular conduction delay, opthalmoplegia, and dilated pupils [40, 47, 69]. During recovery there may be agitation, blurred vision, ataxia, and nystagmus (horizontal or downbeat) [40, 69]. Cardiac arrhythmias and conduction defects like those occurring with overdosage of other tricyclics have not been described with CBZ overdose [69]. To date, there are no reported fatalities from overdosage.

Dose-Dependent Side Effects

Reviewing the symptoms of overdosage in reverse, one can conclude that dose-related symptoms and signs within the therapeutic range are likely to consist in the following: subjective dizziness that may be related to accommodation problems (frequently referred to as diplopia) or may be cerebellovestibular in nature; drowsiness, ataxia, and nystagmus; and possibly irritability or hyperactivity [20, 24, 29, 31, 36, 38, 40, 58]. The toxic symptoms of ballistic movements, rigidity, and oculogyric crisis that have been reported are interesting in regard to the animal studies described earlier (see Mechanisms of Action, above), where it was mentioned that the most marked cholinergic effect was on the striatum. A cholinergic effect could also account for the problems seen with accommodation.

Decreased plasma sodium concentration, decreased plasma osmolality, and decreased ability to handle a water load occur in a minority of patients taking CBZ [40, 52]. This phenomenon varies directly with CBZ plasma concentration in patients who experience it [40, 52]. Hyponatremia is more likely to occur in patients taking CBZ alone than in patients taking CBZ and PHT in combination because PHT lowers CBZ plasma concentrations [52].

Idiosyncratic Reactions

Range of Reactions

The following reactions to CBZ are likely to be idiosyncratic: exfoliative dermatitis, jaundice, lymphatic hyperplasia, lenticular opacities, aplastic anemia, thrombocytopenia, and pancytopenia [20, 24, 28, 31, 36, 54]. The following side effects may be either idiosyncratic or dose-related: an urticarial type of rash and depression of one or more values of cellular or humoral immune responses.

Hematopoietic Side Effects
Several early reports of serious bone marrow depression in association with CBZ therapy led to a special bold-print warning on the package insert and the recommendation that frequent blood cell counts be obtained. Recent comprehensive reviews of all available data indicate the hematopoietic toxicity of CBZ is much less than originally feared [25, 54]. Hart and Easton [25] tabulated the prevalence of CBZ-hematologic toxicity as follows: aplastic anemia—< 1/50,000 (a total of 20 cases), transient leukopenia—10 percent, persistent leukopenia—2 percent, thrombocytopenia—2 percent (average change 0–20,000/mm^3), and anemia—< 5 percent (average change 0–0.5 gm Hb/dl). Pisciotta [54] calculated similar risks and pointed out that in many of the reported cases of CBZ-hematopoietic toxicity, the patient was taking other drugs that either have hematopoietic side effects of their own or may potentiate latent ones.

CHROMOSOMAL CHANGES
The question of chromosomal changes has been raised by one report of an increase in chromatid dislocations with CBZ.

TERATOGENICITY
A review of 99 pregnancies, during which CBZ was taken for at least the first 3 months, revealed 96 normal offspring, 2 abortions in the third month, and 1 child born with atresia of the arms [48]. Meyer [42] found an association with cleft palate and harelip in offspring of epileptic mothers who were treated with PHT and PB but not with CBZ. However, a recent prospective study reported a statistically significant decrease in head circumference of neonates born to mothers taking CBZ that was not present in neonates born to mothers taking PHT or PB monotherapy [27].

Several animal studies performed without blood-level monitoring have reported higher rates of congenital malformations with PHT and PB than with CBZ [16, 41]. These results may be misleading because CBZ has a very rapid metabolism and poor oral absorption in animals [49]. In a mouse study done with blood-level control, PHT and CBZ at low therapeutic serum concentrations did not produce a statistically significant increase in congenital malformations, but PHT at high therapeutic and toxic serum concentra-

tions did produce a significant increase [49]. CBZ blood levels above a low therapeutic level (4.3 μg/ml) could not be obtained even with massive daily doses of CBZ (1,600 mg/kg).

The teratogenicity of antiepileptic drugs is reviewed in more detail in Chap. 29.

CONCLUSION
CBZ, like any other effective drug, can produce side effects. These are usually subjective unless they are idiosyncratic or due to overdose. They rarely necessitate the discontinuation of the drug. Our own experience agrees with that of Reynolds [58] that less than 5 percent of patients develop disabling symptoms that necessitate reduction or cessation of the drug when it is used prudently.

References*
1. Bertilsson, L. et al. Autoinduction of carbamazepine metabolism in children examined by a stable isotope technique. *Clin. Pharmacol. Ther.* 27:83, 1980.
2. Bonduelle, M. My study of Tegretol in the treatment of epilepsy. In C. A. S. Wink (Ed.), *Tegretol in Epilepsy: Report of an International Clinical Symposium.* Manchester: C. Nicholls, 1972. Pp. 80–88.
3. Bonduelle, M., Bouygues, P., Sallou, C. et al. Expérimentation clinique de l'antiépiletique G 32.883 (Tegretol): Résultats portant sur 100 cas observés en trois ans. *Revue Neurol.* 110:209, 1964.
4. Bowdle, T. A., Levy, R. H., and Cutler, R. E. Effects of carbamazepine on valproic acid kinetics in normal subjects. *Clin. Pharmacol. Ther.* 26:629, 1979.
5. Browne, T. R. Clinical pharmacology of antiepileptic drugs. *Drug Ther. Rev.* 2:469, 1979.
6. Cereghino, J. J. Carbamazepine: Relation of Plasma Concentration to Seizure Control. In D. M. Woodbury, J. K. Penry, and C. E. Pippenger (Eds.), *Antiepileptic Drugs.* New York: Raven Press, 1982.
7. Cereghino, J. J. et al. The efficacy of carbamazepine combinations in epilepsy. *Clin. Pharmacol. Ther.* 18:733, 1975.
8. Consolo, S., Bianchi, S., and Ladinsky, H. Effect of carbamazepine on cholinergic parameters in rat brain areas. *Neuropharmacol.* 15:653, 1976.
9. Dalby, M. A. Behavioral Effects of Carbamazepine. In J. K. Penry, and D. D. Daly (Eds.), *Advances in*

*The references given here are highly selective, and a complete bibliography dealing with statements appearing in this chapter can be obtained from the author.

Neurology, Vol. 11. *Complex Partial Seizures and Their Treatment.* New York: Raven Press, 1975.

10. Dalby, M. A. Interaction carbamazepine-dipropyl-acetate. *Acta Neurol. Scand.* 62 [Suppl. 79]:101, 1980.

11. Dam, M., Jensen, A., and Christiansen, J. Plasma level and effect of carbamazepine in grand mal and psychomotor epilepsy. *Acta Neurol. Scand.* 60: 33, 1975.

12. David, J., and Grewal, R. S. Effect of carbamazepine (Tegretol) on seizure and EEG patterns in monkeys with alumina-induced focal motor and hippocampal foci. *Epilepsia* 17:415, 1976.

13. Di Salle, E., Pacifici, G. M., and Morselli, P. L. Studies on plasma protein binding of carbamazepine. *Pharmacolog. Research Commun.* 6:193, 1974.

14. Dolce, G. Uber den antiepileptischen Aktionsmechanismus von 5-Carbamyl-5*H*-dibenzo(*b, f*)-azepin. *Arzneimittelforschung* 19:1257, 1969.

15. Faigle, J. W., and Feldmann, K. F. Carbamazepine: Biotransformation. In D. M. Woodbury, J. K. Penry, and C. E. Pippenger (Eds.), *Antiepileptic Drugs.* New York: Raven Press, 1982.

16. Fritz, H., Muller, D., and Hess, R. Comparative study of the teratogenicity of phenobarbitone, diphenylhydantoin and carbamazepine in mice. *Toxicology* 6:323, 1976.

17. Gagneux, A. R. The Chemistry of Carbamazepine. In W. Birkmayer (Ed.), *Epileptic Seizures—Behaviour—Pain.* Berne: Hans Huber, 1976.

18. Gamstorp, I. Treatment with Carbamazepine: Children. In J. K. Penry, and D. D. Daly (Eds.), *Advances in Neurology,* Vol. 11. *Complex Partial Seizures and Their Treatment.* New York: Raven Press, 1975.

19. Gardner-Thorpe, C., Parsonage, M. J., Smethurst, P. F. et al. Antiepileptic drug concentrations in plasma· Clinical evaluation of 321 estimations in 237 unselected patients. *Acta Neurol. Scand.* 48:213, 1972.

20. Gayford, J. J., and Redpath, T. H. The side effects of carbamazepine. *Proc. R. Soc. Med.* 6:615, 1969.

21. Grant, R. H. E. The Use of Carbamazepine (Tegretol) in Patients with Epilepsy and Multiple Handicaps. In C. A. S. Wink (Ed.), *Tegretol in Epilepsy: Report of an International Clinical Symposium.* Manchester: C. Nicholls, 1972.

22. Gratz, E. S. et al. Effect of carbamazepine on phenytoin clearance in patients with complex partial seizures. *Neurology* (N.Y.) 32:A223, 1982.

23. Groh, C. The Psychotropic Effect of Tegretol in Non-Epileptic Children with Particular Reference to the Drug's Indications. In W. Birkmayer (Ed.), *Epileptic Seizures—Behaviour—Pain.* Berne: Hans Huber, 1976.

24. Hanke, N. F. J. Clinical Tolerance of Tegretol. In C. A. S. Wink (Ed.), *Tegretol in Epilepsy: Report of an International Clinical Symposium.* Manchester: C. Nicholls, 1972.

25. Hart, R. G., and Easton, J. D. Carbamazepine and hematological monitering. *Ann. Neurol.* 11:309, 1982.

26. Hassan, M. N., and Parsonage, M. J. Experience in the Long-Term Use of Carbamazepine (Tegretol) in the Treatment of Epilepsy. In J. K. Penry (Ed.), *Epilepsy: The Eighth International Symposium.* New York: Raven Press, 1977.

27. Iivanainen, M. Effect of Antiepileptic Drugs on Human Body Maturation. In P. L. Morselli, J. K. Penry, and C. E. Pippenger (Eds.), *Antiepileptic Drug Therapy in Pediatrics.* New York: Raven Press, 1982.

28. Johannessen, S. I., and Strandjord, R. E. Concentration of carbamazepine (Tegretol) in serum and in cerebrospinal fluid in patients with epilepsy. *Epilepsia* 14:373, 1973.

29. Julien, R. M. Carbamazepine: Mechanisms of Action. In D. M. Woodbury, J. K. Penry, and C. E. Pippenger (Eds.), *Antiepileptic Drugs.* New York: Raven Press, 1982.

30. Kosteljanetz, M. et al. Carbamazepine vs. phenytoin: A controlled clinical trial in focal motor and generalized epilepsy. *Arch. Neurol.* 36:22, 1979.

31. Kugler, J. Side-Effects of Carbamazepine. In C. A. S. Wink (Ed.), *Tegretol in Epilepsy: Report of an International Clinical Symposium.* Manchester, Eng.: C. Nicholls, 1972.

32. Kutt, H., and Paris-Kutt, H. Carbamazepine: Chemistry and Methods of Determination. In D. M. Woodbury, J. K. Penry, and C. E. Pippenger (Eds.), *Antiepileptic Drugs.* New York: Raven Press, 1982.

33. Kutt, H. Clinical Pharmacology of Carbamazepine. In C. E. Pippenger, J. K. Penry, and H. Kutt (Eds.), *Antiepileptic Drugs: Quantitative Analysis and Interpretation.* New York: Raven Press, 1978.

34. Lai, A. A., Levy, R. H., and Cutler, R. E. Time course of interaction between carbamazepine and clonazepam in normal man. *Clin. Pharmacol. Ther.* 24:316, 1978.

35. Levy, R. H.; and Pitlick, W. H. Carbamazepine: Interactions with Other Drugs. In D. M. Woodbury, J. K. Penry, and C. E. Pippenger (Eds.), *Antiepileptic Drugs.* New York: Raven Press, 1982.

36. Livingston, S., Pauli, L. L., and Berman, W. Carbamazepine (Tegretol) in epilepsy: Nine-year

212

follow-up study with emphasis on untoward reactions. *Dis. Nerv. Syst.* 35:103, 1974.

37. Lorgé, V. M. Klinische Erfahrungen mit einem neuen Antiepilepticum, Tegretol (G 32.883), mit besonderer Wirkung auf die epileptische Wesensveraenderung. *Schweiz. Med. Wochenschr.* 93:1042, 1963.

38. Lorgé, M. Some Aspects of Clinical Tolerance of Tegretol. In C. A. S. Wink (Ed.), *Tegretol in Epilepsy: Report of an International Clinical Symposium.* Manchester, Eng.: C. Nicholls, 1972. Pp. 107–109.

39. Lühdorf, K. et al. The Influence of Phenytoin and Carbamazepine on Endocrine Function: Preliminary Results. In J. K. Penry (Ed.), *Epilepsy: The Eighth International Symposium.* New York: Raven Press, 1977.

40. Masland, R. L. Carbamazepine: Neurotoxicity. In D. M. Woodbury, J. K. Penry, and C. E. Pippenger (Eds.), *Antiepileptic Drugs.* New York: Raven Press, 1982.

41. McElhatton, P. R., and Sullivan, F. M. Comparative teratogenicity of six antiepileptic drugs in the mouse. *Br. J. Pharmacol.* 59:494, 1977.

42. Meyer, J. G. The teratological effects of anticonvulsants and the effects on pregnancy and birth. *Eur. Neurol.* 10:179, 1973.

43. Monaco, F. et al. Free amino acid plasma levels in epileptic patients treated with carbamazepine: Preliminary results. (Italian) *Acta Neurol.* 30:608, 1975.

44. Morselli, P. L., and Bossi, L. Carbamazepine: Absorption, Distribution, and Excretion. In D. M. Woodbury, J. K. Penry, and C. E. Pippenger (Eds.), *Antiepileptic Drugs.* New York: Raven Press, 1982.

45. Morselli, P. L. Clinical pharmacokinetics in neonates. *Clin. Pharmacokinet.* 1:81, 1976.

46. Morselli, P. L., Penry, J. K., and Pippenger, C. E. *Antiepileptic Drug Therapy in Pediatrics.* New York: Raven Press, 1982.

47. Mullally, W. J. Carbamazepine-induced opthalmoplegia. *Arch. Neurol.* 39:64, 1982.

48. Niebyl, J. R. et al. Carbamazepine levels in pregnancy and lactation. *Obstet. Gynecol.* 53:139, 1979.

49. Paulson, R. B., Paulson, G. W., and Jreissaty, S. Phenytoin and carbamazepine in production of cleft palates in mice: Comparison of teratogenic effects. *Arch. Neurol.* 36:832, 1979.

50. Penry, J. K., and Daly, D. D. (Eds.). *Advances in Neurology,* Vol. 11, *Complex Partial Seizures and Their Treatment.* New York: Raven Press, 1975.

51. Penry, J. K. (Ed.). *Epilepsy: The Eighth International Symposium.* New York: Raven Press, 1977.

52. Perucca, E., and Richens, A. Water intoxication produced by carbamazepine and its reversal by phenytoin. *Br. J. Clin. Pharmacol.* 9:302P, 1980.

53. Pippenger, C. E., Penry, J. K., and Kutt, H. (Eds.), *Antiepileptic Drugs: Quantitative Analysis and Interpretation.* New York: Raven Press, 1978.

54. Pisciotta, A. V. Carbamazepine: Hematological Toxicity. In D. M. Woodbury, J. K. Penry, and C. E. Pippenger (Eds.), *Antiepileptic Drugs.* New York: Raven Press, 1982.

55. Puente, R. M. The Use of Carbamazepine in the Treatment of Behavioral Disorders in Children. In W. Birkmayer (Ed.), *Epileptic Seizures—Behaviour—Pain.* Berne: Hans Huber, 1976. Pp. 243–247.

56. Phynnonen, S. et al. Elimination of Carbamazepine in Children After Single and Multiple Doses. In J. K. Penry (Ed.), *Epilepsy: The Eighth International Symposium.* New York: Raven Press, 1977.

57. Rane, A., Bertilsson, L., and Palmer, L. Disposition of placentally transferred carbamazepine (Tegretol) in the newborn. *Eur. J. Clin. Pharmacol.* 8:283, 1975.

58. Reynolds, E. H. Neurotoxicity of Carbamazepine. In J. K. Penry, and D. D. Daly (Eds.), *Advances in Neurology,* Vol. 11, *Complex Partial Seizures and Their Treatment.* New York: Raven Press, 1975.

59. Rodin, E. A., Rim, C. S., and Rennick, P. M. The effects of carbamazepine on patients with psychomotor epilepsy: Results of a double-blind study. *Epilepsia* 15:547, 1974.

60. Rodin, E. A. Psychosocial Management of Patients with Complex Partial Seizures. In J. K. Penry, and D. D. Daly (Eds.), *Advances in Neurology,* Vol. 11, *Complex Partial Seizures and Their Treatment.* New York: Raven Press, 1975.

61. Rodin, E. A. et al. A comparison of the effectiveness of primidone versus carbamazepine in epileptic outpatients. *J. Nerv. Ment. Dis.* 163:41, 1976.

62. Schneider, H. Carbamazepine: An Attempt to Correlate Serum Levels with Anti-epileptic and Side Effects. In H. Schneider et al. (Eds.), *Clinical Pharmacology of Antiepileptic Drugs.* Berlin-Heidelberg: Springer Verlag, 1975.

63. Schneider, H. et al. (Eds.). *Clinical Pharmacology of Antiepileptic Drugs.* Berlin-Heidelberg: Springer Verlag, 1975.

64. Simonsen, N. et al. A comparative controlled study between carbamazepine and diphenylhydantoin in psychomotor epilepsy. *Epilepsia* 17:169, 1976.

65. Singh, A. N., Saxena, B. M., and Germain, M. Anticonvulsive and Psychotropic Effects of Carbamazepine in Hospitalized Epileptic Patients: A Long-

ETHOSUXIMIDE (ZARONTIN) AND OTHER SUCCINIMIDES

19

Thomas R. Browne

Chemistry and Mechanism of Action of Succinimides

There are three marketed succinimide antiepileptic drugs—ethosuximide (Zarontin), methsuximide (Celontin), and phensuximide (Milontin). These drugs are all derivatives of a five-membered succinimide ring (see Table 19-1).

Numerous succinimide derivatives have undergone animal screening tests for antiepileptic activity [11, 12, 19]. The following results have emerged: (1) methyl and ethyl substitutions at the 2 and 3 positions produce drugs that are more effective against pentylenetetrazol seizures than against maximal electroshock seizures; (2) methylation at the 5 position results in increased activity against pentylenetetrazol seizures; (3) activity against pentylenetetrazol seizures decreases with increasing length of alkyl chain substitutions at the 2, 3, and 5 positions; and (4) phenyl substitution at the 2 and 3 positions decreases activity against pentylenetetrazol seizures and increases activity against maximal electroshock seizures.

Effectiveness against pentylenetetrazol seizures in animals is thought to correlate with clinical efficacy against absence seizures in humans, and activity against maximal electroshock seizures in animals is thought to correlate with activity against tonic-clonic and complex partial seizures in humans. The rank order of therapeutic index of succinimides against pentylenetetrazol seizures in animals is (from most to least effective): (1) ethosuximide; (2) methsuximide; (3) phensuximide [12]. Clinical experience indicates that ethosuximide is the most effective succinimide against absence seizures. The rank order of therapeutic index of succinimides against maximal electroshock seizures in animals is (from most to least effective): (1) methsuximide; (2) phensuximide; (3) ethosuximide [12]. Clinical experience indicates that methsuximide has some efficacy against tonic-clonic and complex partial seizures, whereas ethosuximide has almost none.

The ultimate mechanism of action of succinimides is unknown. One attractive hypothesis, for which

Karen Olsen, R. EEG T., assisted in the preparation of this manuscript. This work was supported in part by the Veterans Administration.

Table 19-1. Succinimides

R₁	R₂	R₃	Generic Name	Trade Name
C_2H_5	CH_3	H	Ethosuximide	Zarontin
C_6H_5[a]	CH_3	CH_3	Methsuximide	Celontin
C_6H_5[a]	CH_3	H	N-desmethyl-methsuximide[b]	None
C_6H_5[a]	H	CH_3	Phensuximide	Milontin

[a]Phenyl ring.
[b]Active metabolite of methsuximide.

there is some experimental evidence, is that absence seizures are due to paroxysmal activity of inhibitory pathways and that succinimides inhibit cortical and subcortical inhibitory pathways [23, 24]. Other hypothesized mechanisms of action for which experimental evidence exists are: (1) depression of repetitive transmission; (2) differential modulation of the ability of thalamocortical pathways to excite cerebral cortex; (3) enhancement of inhibitory processes in the brain, perhaps by affecting dopamine or GABA neurotransmission; and (4) inhibition of sodium-potassium–ATPase activity of the presynaptic membrane of brain synapses [19].

Ethosuximide

CLINICAL PHARMACOLOGY

Absorption

Peak serum concentrations of ethosuximide are reached 1 to 7 hours after oral administration [8, 30, 32, 61]. The drug has high bioavailability by the oral route [8]. The capsule and oral suspension forms have similar absorption and bioavailability characteristics [8]. Steady state serum concentrations of ethosuximide are reached after 8 to 10 days of chronic administration [27, 30].

Distribution

Animal studies indicate that ethosuximide is fairly uniformly distributed to most body tissues (including brain) except fat, which has a lower concentration than other tissues [27]. In humans, ethosuximide is detectable in cerebrospinal fluid (CSF) 30 to 60 minutes after an oral dose, and peak CSF ethosuximide concentrations occur almost simultaneously with peak serum concentrations [61]. Ethosuximide has almost no protein binding capability in humans [2, 27, 51]. It readily crosses the placenta in experimental animals [27]. The ratio of ethosuximide plasma concentration to ethosuximide breast milk concentration in nursing mothers is 1:1 [36].

Biotransformation, Excretion, and Clinical Pharmacokinetics

The elimination half-life of ethosuximide varies from 20 to 60 hours [1, 2, 5, 8, 9, 27, 30, 51]. The half-life tends to be shorter in children and longer in adolescents and adults; however, elimination half-lives of as long as 68 hours have been reported in children under 10 years of age [5].

Approximately 20 percent of a dose of ethosuximide is excreted unchanged in the urine [10, 27, 30]. Over 50 percent is excreted as 2-(1-hydroxyethyl)-2-methyl-succinimide [30], which is the major metabolite of ethosuximide and has little antiepileptic effect [10]. Other urinary metabolites identified in humans include 2-(2-hydroxyethyl)-2-methylsuccinimide, 2-ethyl-2-methyl-3-hydroxysuccinimide, 2-acetyl-2-methylsuccinimide, and 2-ethyl-2-hydroxymethylsuccinimide [10, 20, 45]. Thus ethosuximide produces few if any active metabolites, and measurement of ethosuximide serum concentrations measures most, or all, of the active drug in serum.

Drug Interactions

Addition of phenytoin, phenobarbital, or primidone to ethosuximide does little to change the serum concentration of ethosuximide [2, 53]. Addition of carbamazepine may decrease ethosuximide serum concentration [60]. Addition of valproic acid results in no change or an increase in ethosuximide serum concentration [1, 2]. Addition of methylphenobarbital to ethosuximide results in increased ethosuximide serum concentration [53]. Addition of ethosuximide to phenytoin, primidone, or valproic acid does not change the serum concentration of these three drugs [2]. The relative lack of drug interactions of ethosuximide with other antiepileptic drugs may be due in part to the fact that ethosuximide is metabolized by hydroxylation of an ethyl group, whereas most antiepileptic drugs are metabolized by hydroxylation of a phenyl group.

Blood Levels
Ethosuximide serum concentration can be determined by gas-liquid chromatography, high-performance liquid chromatography, or enzyme multiplied immunoassay technique (EMIT; see Chap. 15). There is a general correlation of increasing ethosuximide serum concentration with increasing dosage for patients of a given age [5, 51, 53]. However, the relationship between ethosuximide dosage and serum concentration has a high degree of interpatient variability and may be subject to nonlinear elimination kinetics at higher doses [2, 5]. Furthermore, the ratio of dose to serum concentration varies with age. Children require a higher dose in milligrams per kilogram to produce a given serum concentration than do adolescents or adults, perhaps because children eliminate the drug more rapidly, as described above [5, 51]. There is so much variability in the serum concentration produced by a given dose that it is impossible to predict a given patient's serum concentration from the dose. Serum ethosuximide concentration can be known with accuracy only if it is determined by a laboratory.

The therapeutic range of ethosuximide serum concentration is 40 to 120 µg/ml [5, 51]. Serum concentrations of less than 40 µg/ml do not produce good control of absence seizures in a majority of patients [5, 51]. Increasing the serum concentration of the drug from low therapeutic to high therapeutic levels in patients whose absence seizures are not controlled with low therapeutic levels will result in good control of absence seizures in some patients [51].

Dosage and Administration
Ethosuximide is available in capsule form and syrup form (easier for small children to swallow). The initial dose is 250 mg/day for children 3 to 6 years of age and 500 mg/day for patients 6 years of age or older. The dosage is then increased by 250 mg/day at weekly intervals until seizure control is obtained, side effects preclude further increases, or a high therapeutic serum level is reached. During the first weeks of administration it may be necessary to decrease temporarily the dosage or the rate of increase of dosage because of gastrointestinal side effects or drowsiness. However, full therapeutic doses and serum concentrations can be achieved in most patients if one waits a few weeks for tolerance to side effects to develop. The usual maximum daily dosage is 1500

mg/day. Larger doses should be administered only under strict supervision by a physician. Therapeutic blood levels can be maintained with once daily administration, although the peak levels produced by this regimen sometimes cause nausea or drowsiness [9]. Administration in two divided doses per day is better tolerated by some patients. There is seldom a need to give the drug in three or more divided doses, and such regimens often result in poor compliance (see Chap. 15).

INDICATIONS

Absence Seizures
Treatment of absence seizures is the only indication for ethosuximide approved by the FDA. Most clinical studies of ethosuximide for absence seizures consisted of addition of ethosuximide to the regimens of a group of patients whose absence seizures were not adequately controlled by other medications. In 5 such studies with 50 or more patients, 42 to 54 percent (median, 48 percent) of patients had complete control of absence seizures, and 54 to 80 percent (median, 77 percent) had a 50 percent or greater reduction in the frequency of absence seizures [21, 29, 33, 35, 67]. In 2 studies in which ethosuximide was the first and only antiabsence drug given to patients with newly diagnosed absence seizures, 18 percent and 54 percent of patients had complete control of absence seizures, and 77 percent and 90 percent of patients had a 50 percent or greater reduction in seizure frequency [5, 62].

Measuring the number of 3-Hz spike-wave bursts on prolonged electroencephalographic (EEG) recordings before and after treatment is probably a more accurate way of determining the efficacy of antiabsence drugs than clinical methods utilizing the seizures counts by mothers or hospital personnel [4, 44]. In two studies in which 12-hour EEGs were performed before and during ethosuximide therapy, 44 and 55 percent of patients showed complete suppression of spike-wave bursts while taking ethosuximide, and 89 and 100 percent of patients had a 50 percent or greater reduction in the number of spike-wave bursts [44, 49].

Ethosuximide is thus extremely effective for the treatment of absence seizures and is the drug of first choice for most patients. It offers the following advantages over the other two currently available succinimides (methsuximide, phensuximide): (1) ethosuximide controls absence seizures in a higher percentage of cases; (2) the common side effects of succinimides (drowsiness, gastrointestinal upset) are less severe and less persistent with ethosuximide; (3) the therapeutic range of serum concentrations for ethosuximide is better established; (4) ethosuximide serum concentration determinations are more generally available; and (5) ethosuximide probably has fewer drug interactions with other antiepileptic drugs. The reasons for selecting ethosuximide in preference to other nonsuccinimide antiabsence drugs are reviewed in Chapter 7.

Other Seizure Types

Clinical studies of ethosuximide for myoclonic seizures have produced highly variable results ranging from good control in a high percentage of patients to little effect on any patient [35, 38, 42, 54, 62]. Scattered studies with small numbers of patients indicate that the majority of patients with atypical absence or atonic seizures, or both, do not respond favorably to ethosuximide, and a few become worse. However, a minority of such patients have a very favorable response. Studies of ethosuximide for infantile myoclonic and complex partial seizures report generally unfavorable results.

Most studies report that ethosuximide has no effect upon the frequency of tonic-clonic seizures. A few report a decrease in tonic-clonic seizure frequency, and a few note an increased frequency of tonic-clonic seizures or precipitation of such seizures in patients who previously had never had them [18]. It is difficult to ascertain whether ethosuximide can exacerbate tonic-clonic seizures or precipitate them *de novo* because of the variability of tonic-clonic seizure frequency and because a certain percentage of patients with absence seizures spontaneously develop tonic-clonic seizures (see Chap. 7).

TOXICITY

Common Side Effects

Large series report the presence of side effects due to ethosuximide in 24 to 46 percent (median, 37 percent) of patients (see Table 19-2). The common side effects are gastrointestinal disturbance (nausea, vomiting, anorexia, abdominal pain) and drowsiness. These side effects have no obvious relationship to ethosuximide plasma concentration. Rather they tend to occur early in ethosuximide therapy and diminish as tolerance to the drug develops. It is seldom necessary to discontinue ethosuximide because of gastrointestinal disturbances or drowsiness. These side effects can usually be managed by either continuing ethosuximide therapy at the same dose until tolerance develops or temporarily decreasing the dosage. Other occasional side effects of ethosuximide are dizziness, headache, and hiccoughs.

Idiosyncratic Reactions

There are at least 16 reported cases of leukopenia in association with ethosuximide therapy [5, 7, 25, 35, 40, 62]. The incidence of leukopenia among patients receiving ethosuximide is 0 to 7 percent. It is an idiosyncratic reaction that occurs in sporadic cases. Most patients have no change in white blood cell count while taking ethosuximide [5], and leukopenia is usually transient when it does occur. The white blood cell count usually returns to normal when the drug is discontinued and often returns to normal even if the drug is not discontinued [5, 7, 18, 35, 62]. However, a small percentage of patients receiving ethosuximide develops serious pancytopenia, and there is no way of determining which patient with leukopenia has the benign transient variety and which patient is developing serious bone marrow depression.

There are 8 reported cases of pancytopenia in association with ethosuximide therapy [7, 57], 3 of which ended fatally. Pancytopenia may develop many months after beginning therapy [7, 18]. It is thus necessary to perform blood cell counts periodically as long as a patient continues to take ethosuximide.

Rashes occasionally occur with ethosuximide therapy (see Table 19-2), and eosinophilia is also occasionally detected [7, 18]. Nine cases of systemic lupus erythematosus [7, 52, 57] have been reported in association with ethosuximide therapy. A single patient with nephrotic syndrome, thrombocytopenia, and decreased complement but negative tests for lupus erythematosus has been reported [41]. Extrapyramidal reactions (parkinsonian symptoms, akasthesia, dyskinesia) and erythema multiforme bullosa (Stevens-Johnson syndrome) are rare complications of ethosuximide therapy [7, 18]. Serious hepatic or endocrine side effects have not been noted [7, 18].

Behavioral Toxicity

Drowsiness, usually transient, is not uncommon with ethosuximide. Irritability and unruly behavior are rare side effects and are much more common with methsuximide, barbiturates, and clonazepam.

Reports of the effect of ethosuximide on psychometric performance are conflicting. Some reports indicate that intellectual deterioration, manifest by memory disorders, speech disturbances, and emotional disturbances, may occur [7, 18]. Other reports note intellectual improvement shown by improved full scale IQ, improved verbal IQ, and improved performance on a modified Halstead-Reitan battery [3, 5, 18]. The studies reporting intellectual deterioration contained many patients with baseline mental retardation who were taking other medications (usually

Table 19-2. Reported Incidence of Side Effects of Ethosuximide and Methsuximide in Series With 50 or More Patients

Side Effect	Ethosuximide[a]		Methsuximide[b]	
	Range (%)	Median (%)	Range (%)	Median (%)
Drowsiness	0–16	7	0–28	16
Gastrointestinal disturbances (anorexia, nausea, vomiting, or abdominal pain)	4–29	13	2–30	6
Hiccoughs	0–5	0	0–6	0
Ataxia	0–1	0	0–13	6
Dizziness	0–4	1	0–13	0
Irritability	0	0	0–6	0
Rash	0–6	0	0–17	6
Leukopenia	0–7	0	0–2	0
Any side effect	26–46	37	11–57	35

[a]See references [14, 16, 21, 29, 33, 35, 40, 42, 54, 59, 62, 67].
[b]See references [17, 22, 39, 47, 50, 55, 58, 65].

barbiturates). It is thus impossible to determine whether the intellectual deterioration was due to the underlying cause of mental retardation, seizures, other medications, or ethosuximide.

Probably the most definitive study of the psychometric effects of ethosuximide was a collaborative study coordinated by the National Institutes of Health [3, 5]. Thirty-seven children with typical absence seizures, normal intelligence, and minimal or no evidence of structural nervous system abnormalities were tested with a modified Halstead-Reitan battery before ethosuximide therapy began and during the eighth week of treatment. Matched controls were obtained for each patient, and they underwent the same testing with the same time interval between tests. Results were interpreted "blindly" in that the interpreter did not know which patients received ethosuximide and which were controls. The scores of 1 patient were slightly worse, 19 were the same, and 17 improved on ethosuximide. All the scores of the control subjects were the same on the 8-week reexamination as on the original examination. The difference between the distribution of the reexamination test scores for the control group and the ethosuximide group was significant ($p < 0.001$). It thus appears that ethosuximide has a positive effect on psychometric testing of otherwise normal children who are taking the drug for absence seizures.

There are at least 25 reported cases of psychotic episodes in association with ethosuximide therapy [7, 16, 18, 21]. These episodes typically consist of delu-

sions and hallucinations, anxiety and depression, and depersonalization [7, 18]. Most patients experiencing psychotic episodes are in their teens or twenties and have a prior history of psychiatric disturbances [7, 18]. The psychotic symptoms usually diminish when ethosuximide is discontinued, and the patient's psychiatric disorder returns to its preethosuximide state. Psychotic episodes seldom occur in young children taking ethosuximide for typical absence seizures who have no previous history of psychiatric disease, but the drug should be administered with care to adolescents and to young adults with a history of borderline or overtly psychotic psychiatric disease.

Methsuximide

CLINICAL PHARMACOLOGY

Absorption and Distribution
Peak serum levels of methsuximide occur 1 to 4 hours after an oral dose in humans [28]. Animal work indicates that methsuximide rapidly crosses the blood-brain barrier.

Biotransformation, Excretion, and Clinical Pharmacokinetics
Methsuximide is rapidly converted to N-desmethyl-methsuximide (NDM) with an elimination half-life of 1.0 to 2.6 hours [28, 46]. NDM is then slowly metabolized, with an apparent elimination half-life of 34 to 48 hours [6, 26, 46]. It accumulates to steady state serum concentrations that are, on the average, about

600 to 800 times higher than the concentration of the parent drug methsuximide [37, 56]. Based on the following observations, NDM is probably the major antiepileptic substance in the serum of patients receiving methsuximide: (1) NDM serum levels are much higher than methsuximide serum levels [37, 46, 56]; (2) methsuximide and NDM have similar effectiveness against pentylenetetrazol and maximal electroshock seizures in animals [11]; and (3) a small clinical trial has shown that methsuximide and NDM have similar clinical effectiveness against absence seizures [64].

The major urinary metabolites of methsuximide are hydroxylated at the 3 and 4 positions of the phenyl ring [34]. Unfortunately, the metabolic study just quoted used an analytical method involving methylation, and therefore the relative proportions of hydroxylated methsuximide and hydroxylated NDM in the urine were not determined. The following substances are lesser urinary metabolites of methsuximide: unmetabolized methsuximide, N-methyl-2-hydroxy-methyl-2-phenylsuccinimide; N,2-dimethyl-3-hydroxy-2-phenylsuccinimide; and a dihydrodiol derivative [28, 34, 46]. Steady state NDM plasma concentration is reached after 6 to 12 days of chronic administration [6].

Drug Interactions

The addition of methsuximide to a regimen of phenytoin or phenobarbital causes an appreciable increase in the steady state plasma concentrations of the latter two drugs in most patients [6, 48, 55]. There is also some evidence that patients taking methsuximide in addition to phenytoin or phenobarbital (or both) have higher NDM plasma concentrations than patients taking methsuximide alone [48]. These interactions are presumably due to competitive inhibition of hydroxylation of the phenyl ring, the principal route of metabolism of all three drugs.

Blood Levels

The serum concentration of methsuximide in patients taking the usual doses of the drug is so small that it can be measured accurately only by gas chromatography–mass spectroscopy [56]. There is no apparent correlation between the administered dose of methsuximide and the antiepileptic effect or the serum concentration of methsuximide, presumably because methsuximide is so rapidly converted to NDM.

There is significant correlation between the administered dose of methsuximide and the serum concentration of NDM [6, 56]. On the average, the serum concentration of NDM in $\mu g/ml$ is 1.6 to 2.0 times the daily dose of methsuximide in milligrams per kilogram [6, 56]. Preliminary results indicate that the range of therapeutic serum concentrations of NDM is 10 to 30 $\mu g/ml$ [6, 56, 63]. Serum concentrations of NDM can be determined using conventional gas-liquid chromatography or high-performance liquid chromatography techniques (see Chap. 15).

Dosage and Administration

The usual starting dose of methsuximide is 300 mg/day. The daily dose may be increased at weekly intervals by 300 mg/day until seizures are controlled, toxicity develops, or a maximum dose of 1200 mg/day is reached. Weekly increases in dosage of 150 mg rather than 300 mg/day may decrease the incidence of side effects, especially in young children and in patients of all ages taking other antiepileptic drugs [6].

INDICATIONS

Absence Seizures

Treatment of absence seizures is the only indication for methsuximide approved by the FDA. In four reported series with 20 or more patients in which methsuximide was used as an adjunctive drug for absence seizures, the seizures were completely controlled in 0 to 31 percent of cases, and the frequency of absence seizures was reduced by 50 percent or more in 13 to 66 percent of cases [17, 22, 39, 65]. In the one reported study in which methsuximide was used as the first drug for previously untreated absence seizures, only 20 percent of the patients had a 50 percent or greater reduction in frequency of seizures, and none were completely controlled [39]. For reasons outlined above, ethosuximide is the succinimide of choice for absence seizures. Methsuximide is indicated for absence seizures only when other less toxic drugs fail to produce adequate control.

Other Seizure Types

Stenzel et al. [55] have reported some success with methsuximide in patients with "complex atypical absences" and "slow spike-wave, polyspike-wave, or sharp and slow" EEG patterns. In six reported series with 18 or more patients in which methsuximide was used as an adjunctive antiepileptic drug for complex partial seizures, complete seizure control was obtained in 4 to 38 percent of patients, and a 50 percent or greater reduction in seizure frequency was obtained in 25 to 80 percent of patients [6, 15, 22, 50, 63, 66]. In the one reported study in which methsuximide was used as the first antiepileptic drug in previously untreated patients with complex partial seizures, a 50 percent or greater reduction in seizure frequency occurred in 27 percent of patients, and 18 percent of patients experienced complete control of seizures [39]. Trials of methsuximide for tonic-clonic and simple partial seizures have been generally discouraging.

TOXICITY

Common Side Effects
Large series report side effects from methsuximide in 11 to 57 percent (median, 35 percent) of patients taking the drug. The frequency of common side effects with methsuximide is outlined in Table 19-2. Because patients are less apt to develop tolerance to the common side effects of methsuximide than with ethosuximide, methsuximide has to be discontinued more often than ethosuximide. Some of the drowsiness, irritability, and ataxia reported in association with methsuximide therapy may be due to interference with the elimination of phenobarbital or phenytoin caused by methsuximide rather than to a direct toxic effect of methsuximide or its metabolites.

Idiosyncratic Reactions
Extensive toxicity testing of methsuximide in animals showed no abnormalities on hematologic and chemical tests of blood [12]. Autopsy studies of mice, rats, dogs, and monkeys showed no abnormalities except for "mild centrilobular hepatic necrosis" in rats receiving 600 mg/kg/day of the drug [12]. These changes were felt to be reversible and of no functional consequence.

No serious hepatic damage has ever been reported in humans taking methsuximide. Dow et al. [17] reported an increase in cephalin flocculation in 2 of 62 patients taking methsuximide. Both patients were taking other antiepileptic drugs as well.

Trolle et al. [58] reported 1 case of transient leukopenia in which blood cell counts returned to normal while the patient was still taking methsuximide. Stenzel et al. [55] reported another case of apparently transient leukopenia. Trolle et al. [58] reported 1 patient with multiple small bruises in which a platelet count was not performed.

The only reported fatal blood dyscrasia associated with methsuximide was a case of pancytopenia occurring in a middle-aged woman 3 months after beginning methsuximide [31]. It is not certain that methsuximide was the cause of the pancytopenia because the woman had breast carcinoma and was taking four other medications as well.

Rashes can occur with methsuximide (see Table 19-2).

Overdosage
Four reported patients with methsuximide overdose all recovered without sequellae. Methsuximide overdosage is characterized by stupor and coma, which may develop slowly or which may have a biphasic (coma–more alert–coma) course. The late worsening may be due to conversion of methsuximide to NDM or to interference with metabolism of other antiepileptic drugs caused by methsuximide. Other clinical features reported with methsuximide overdosage include respiratory depression, central neurogenic hyperventilation, increased reflexes, decreased reflexes, myoclonus, and second-degree heart block. A single case of massive combined overdosage of methsuximide and primidone resulted in flaccid coma, respiratory arrest, hypotension, and death.

Uncommon Side Effects
Rare reported complications of methsuximide include behavior changes, confusion, diplopia, blurred vision, headache, periorbital edema, porphyria, and extrapyramidal reactions.

Phensuximide

CLINICAL PHARMACOLOGY

Pharmacokinetics
Peak serum levels occur 1 to 4 hours after an oral dose [28]. The elimination half-life of phensuximide is 4 to 8 hours [28, 46]. The elimination half-life of N-desmethyl-phensuximide, the major active metabolite of phensuximide, has a similar range [28,46]. Because of this rapid elimination, only small concentrations of the drug and its metabolite accumulate during chronic administration. With a dosage of 3000 mg/day, the average fasting serum concentration of phensuximide is 5.7 µg/ml, and the average fasting concentration of N-desmethyl-phensuximide is only 1.7 µg/ml [46]. The failure of phensuximide or its major active metabolite to accumulate at reasonable levels may account for the relatively weak antiepileptic properties of the drug.

Dosage and Administration
The dosage of phensuximide is 1000 to 3000 mg/day in two or three divided doses. The average dose is 1500 mg/day. The drug is available in capsule and oral suspension forms.

INDICATIONS
Absence seizures are the only FDA-approved indication for phensuximide. Four of five clinical trials of the drug for absence seizures reported that a majority of

patients had a 50 percent or greater reduction in frequency of seizures [13]. Nevertheless, phensuximide is seldom used for absence seizures because (1) the incidence of serious idiosyncratic reactions (especially renal toxicity) is much higher with phensuximide than with methsuximide or ethosuximide [43]; (2) the incidence of dose-dependent side effects with phensuximide is at least as great (and probably greater) than with other succinimides; (3) methsuximide proved superior to phensuximide for absence seizures in the only trial in which both drugs were given to the same patients [58], and ethosuximide is probably even more effective than methsuximide; and (4) it is the anecdotal experience of many authorities that phensuximide is the least effective of the marketed succinimides for absence seizures.

TOXICITY

Drowsiness, nausea and vomiting, and dizziness, the usual side effects of succinimides, are at least as common with phensuximide as with ethosuximide and methsuximide [43]. At high doses phensuximide can produce a dreamlike state, something other succinimides rarely do [43]. Moreover, phensuximide has a much higher incidence of serious idiosyncratic reactions than other succinimides.

Millchap [43] reported evidence of renal damage (proteinuria, microscopic hematuria, granular casts) in 10 of 21 patients started on phensuximide. Most patients were receiving the usual therapeutic doses of the drug. Other serious idiosyncratic reactions reported in association with phensuximide include fever, rash, erythema multiforme, and leukopenia.

References

1. Bauer, L. A. et al. Ethosuximide kinetics: Possible interaction with valproic acid. *Clin. Pharmacol. Ther.* 31:741, 1982.
2. Browne, T. R. Clinical pharmacology of antiepileptic drugs. *Drug Ther. Rev.* 2:469, 1979.
3. Browne, T. R. Antiepileptic Drugs and Psychosocial Development: Ethosuximide. In P. L. Morselli, C. E. Pippenger, and J. K. Penry (Eds.), *Antiepileptic Drug Therapy in Pediatrics.* New York: Raven Press, 1983.
4. Browne, T. R. et al. Clinical and electroencephalographic estimates of absence seizure frequency. *Arch. Neurol.* In press, 1983.
5. Browne, T. R. et al. Ethosuximide in the treatment of absence (petit mal) seizures. *Neurology* (Minneap.) 25:515, 1975.
6. Browne, T. R. et al. Methsuximide (Celontin) for complex partial seizures: Efficacy, toxicity, clinical pharmacology, and drug interactions. *Neurology* (N.Y.) In press, 1983.
7. Buchanan, R. A. Ethosuximide: Toxicity. In D. M. Woodbury, J. K. Penry, and R. P. Schmidt (Eds.), *Antiepileptic Drugs.* New York: Raven Press, 1972.
8. Buchanan, R. A., Fernandez, L., and Kinkel, A. W. Absorption and elimination of ethosuximide in children. *J. Clin. Pharmacol.* 9:393, 1969.
9. Buchanan, R. A., Kinkel, A. W., and Turner, J. L. Ethosuximide dosage regimens. *Clin. Pharmacol. Ther.* 19:143, 1976.
10. Chang, T., and Glazko, A. J. Ethosuximide: Biotransformation. In D. M. Woodbury, J. K. Penry, and C. E. Pippenger (Eds.), *Antiepileptic Drugs.* New York: Raven Press, 1982.
11. Chen, G. et al. The anticonvulsant activity of α-phenylsuccinimides. *J. Pharmacol. Exp. Ther.* 103:54, 1951.
12. Chen, G., Weston, J. K., and Bratton, A. C. Anticonvulsant activity and toxicity of phensuximide, methsuximide, and ethosuximide. *Epilepsia* 4:66, 1963.
13. Coatsworth, J. J. *Studies on the Clinical Efficacy of Marketed Antiepileptic Drugs.* Washington, D.C.: U.S. Government Printing Office, 1971.
14. Cohardon, R., Loiseau, P., and Cohardon, S. Results of treatment of certain forms of epilepsy of the petit mal type by ethosuximide. *Rev. Neurol.* 110:201, 1964.
15. Cordoba, E. F., and Strobos, R. R. J. N-methyl-α,α-methyl-phenylsuccinimide in psychomotor epilepsy. *Dis. Nerv. Syst.* 17:383, 1956.
16. Dongier, M. S., Gastaut, H., and Roger, J. Essai d'un nouvel anti-épileptique (PM 671, α-éthyl-α-méthyl-succinimide) chez l-enfant. *Rev. Neurol.* (Paris) 104:441, 1961.
17. Dow, R. S., McFarlane, J. P., and Stevens, J. R. Celontin in patients with refractory epilepsy. *Neurology* (Minneap.) 8:201, 1958.
18. Dreifuss, F. E. Ethosuximide: Toxicity. In D. M. Woodbury, J. K. Penry, and C. E. Pippenger (Eds.), *Antiepileptic Drugs.* New York: Raven Press, 1982.
19. Ferrendelli, J. A., and Klunk, W. A. Ethosuximide: Mechanisms of Action. In D. M. Woodbury, J. K. Penry, and C. E. Pippenger (Eds.), *Antiepileptic Drugs.* New York: Raven Press, 1982.
20. Ferrendelli, J. A., and Kupferberg, H. J. Succinimides. *Adv. Neurol.* 27:587, 1980.
21. Fischer, M., Korskjaer, G., and Pedersen, E. Psychotic episodes in Zarontin treatment: Effects and side-effects in 105 patients. *Epilepsia* 6:325, 1965.
22. French, E. G., Rey-Bellet, J., and Lennox, W. G.

Methsuximide in psychomotor and petit-mal seizures. *N. Engl. J. Med.* 258:892, 1958.

23. Fromm, G. H. et al. Effect of sodium valproate and of ethosuximide on cortical and subcortical inhibitory pathways. *Neurology* (Minneap.) 28:373, 1978.

24. Fromm, G. H. et al. Effect of anticonvulsant drugs on inhibitory and excitatory pathways. *Epilepsia* 22:56, 1981.

25. Gautier, E. Erfahrungen mit PM671 (αethyl-αmethyl-succinimide) in der Behandlung der Kindlichen Epilepsien. *Ther. Umsch.* 17:132, 1960.

26. Gibbs, E. L., Gibbs, T. J., and Appell, M. R. Subtle side effects caused by Dilantin and Celontin: A report of two pilot volunteer studies. *Clin. Electroencephalogr.* 5:192, 1974.

27. Glazko, A. J., and Chang, T. Ethosuximide: Absorption, Distribution, and Excretion. In D. M. Woodbury, J. K. Penry, and C. E. Pippenger (Eds.), *Antiepileptic Drugs.* New York: Raven Press, 1982.

28. Glazko, A. J., and Dill, W. A. Other Succinimides: Methsuximide and Phensuximide. In D. M. Woodbury, J. K. Penry, and R. P. Schmidt (Eds.), *Antiepileptic Drugs.* New York: Raven Press, 1972.

29. Goldensohn, E. S., Hardie, J., and Borca, E. Ethosuximide in the treatment of epilepsy. *J.A.M.A.* 180: 840, 1962.

30. Goulet, J. R., Kinkel, A. W., and Smith, T. C. Metabolism of ethosuximide. *Clin. Pharmacol. Ther.* 20:213, 1976.

31. Green, R. A., and Gilbert, M. G. Fatal bone marrow aplasia associated with Celontin therapy. *Minn. Med.* 42:130, 1959.

32. Hansen, S. E., and Feldberg, L. Absorption and elimination of Zarontin. *Dan. Med. Bull.* 11:54, 1964.

33. Heathfield, K. W. G., and Jewesbury, E. C. O. Treatment of petit mal with ethosuximide. *Br. Med. J.* 2:565, 1961.

34. Horning, M. G. et al. Metabolism of N,2-dimethyl-2-phenylsuccinimide (methsuximide) by epoxide-diol pathway in rat, guinea pig, and human. *Res. Commun. Chem. Pathol. Pharmacol.* 6:565, 1973.

35. Kiørboe, E. et al. Zarontin (ethosuximide) in the treatment of petit mal and related disorders. *Epilepsia* 5:83, 1964.

36. Koup, J. R., Rose, J. Q., and Cohen, M. E. Ethosuximide pharmacokinetics in a pregnant patient and her newborn. *Epilepsia* 19:535, 1978.

37. Kupferberg, H. J. et al. Comparison of Methsuximide and Phensuximide Metabolism in Epileptic Patients. In C. Gardner-Thorpe et al. (Eds.), *Anti-*

epileptic Drug Monitoring. Kent: Pitman Medical, 1977.

38. Lanternier, J. A propos d'un nouvel anticonvulsant l' alpha-ethyl-alpha-methyl succinimide. *Pediatrie* 17:173, 1962.

39. Livingston, S., and Pauli, L. Celontin in the treatment of epilepsy. *Pediatrics* 19:614, 1957.

40. Lorentz de Haas, A. M., and Stoel, L. M. K. Experiences with α-ethyl-α-methyl succinimide in the treatment of epilepsy. *Epilepsia* 1:501, 1960.

41. Mann, L. B., and Habenicht, H. A. Fatal bone marrow aplasia associated with administration of ethosuximide (Zarontin) for petit mal. *Bull. Los Angeles Neurol. Soc.* 27:173, 1962.

42. Matthes, A., and Mallman-Muhlberger, E. Erfahrungen bei der Behandlung kleiner epileptische Anfälle in Kindersalter mit Methyl-äthyl-succinimid (MAS). *Münch. Med. Wochenschr.* 104:1095, 1962.

43. Millichap, J. G. Milontin: A new drug in the treatment of petit mal. *Lancet* 2:907, 1952.

44. Penry, J. K. Correlation of Serum Ethosuximide Levels with Clinical Effect. In H. Schneider et al. (Eds.), *Clinical Pharmacology of Antiepileptic Drugs.* New York: Springer-Verlag, 1975.

45. Pettersen, J. E. Urinary metabolites of 2-ethyl-2-methyl-succinimide (ethosuximide) studied by combined gas chromatography–mass spectrometry. *Biomed. Mass Spectrom.* 5:601, 1978.

46. Porter, R. J., and Kupferberg, H. J. Other Succinimides: Methsuximide and Phensuximide. In D. M. Woodbury, J. K. Penry, and C. E. Pippenger (Eds.), *Antiepileptic Drugs.* New York: Raven Press, 1982.

47. Rabe, F. Celontin (Petinutin): Ein Beitrag zur differenzierten Epilepsiebehandlung. *Nervenarzt* 31:306, 1960.

48. Rambeck, B. Pharmacological interactions of methsuximide with phenobarbital and phenytoin in hospitalized epileptic patients. *Epilepsia* 20:147, 1979.

49. Sato, S. et al. Valproic acid versus ethosuximide in the treatment of absence seizures. *Neurology* (N.Y.) 32:157, 1982.

50. Scholl, M. L., Abbott, J. A., and Schwab, R. S. Celontin: A new anticonvulsant. *Epilepsia* 1:105, 1960.

51. Sherwin, A. L. Ethosuximide: Relation of Plasma Concentration to Seizure Control. In D. M. Woodbury, J. K. Penry, and C. E. Pippenger (Eds.), *Antiepileptic Drugs.* New York: Raven Press, 1982.

52. Silverman, S. H., Gribetz, D., and Rausen, A. R. Nephrotic syndrome associated with ethosuximide. *Am. J. Dis. Child.* 132:99, 1978.

53. Smith, G. A. et al. Factors influencing plasma concentrations of ethosuximide. *Clin. Pharmacokinet.* 4:38, 1979.

54. Spinner, A. Indikation und Wirkung von Suxinutin bei Petit-mal-Epilepsien. *Münch. Med. Wochenschr.* 103:1110, 1961.

55. Stenzel, E., Boenigk, H. E., and Rambeck, B. Methsuximid in der Epilepsiebehandlung. *Nervenarzt.* 48:377, 1977.

56. Strong, J. M. et al. Plasma levels of methsuximide and *N*-desmethylmethsuximide during methsuximide therapy. *Neurology* (Minneap.) 24:250, 1974.

57. Teoh, P. C., and Chan, H. L. Lupus-scleroderma syndrome induced by ethosuximide. *Arch. Dis. Child.* 50:658, 1975.

58. Trolle, E., and Kiørboe, E. Treatment of petit mal epilepsy with the new succinimides: PM 60 and Celontin (a clinical comparative study). *Epilepsia* 1:587, 1960.

59. Vossen, R. Über die antikonvulsive Wirkung von Succinimiden. *Dtsch. Med. Wochenschr.* 29:1227, 1958.

60. Warren, J. W. et al. Kinetics of carbamazepine-ethosuximide interaction. *Clin. Pharmacol. Ther.* 28:646, 1980.

61. Wechselberg, K., and Hubel, G. Zur Resorption und Verteilung von Methyl-äthyl-succinimid (MAS) im Serum und Liquor bei Kinderen. *Z. Kinderheilkd.* 100:10, 1967.

62. Weinstein, A. W., and Allen, R. J. Ethosuximide treatment of petit mal seizures. *Am. J. Dis. Child.* 111:63, 1966.

63. Wilder, B. J., and Buchanan, R. B. Methsuximide for refractory complex partial seizures. *Neurology* (N.Y.) 31:741, 1981.

64. Zimmerman, F. T. New drugs in the treatment of petit mal epilepsy. *Am. J. Psychiatry* 109:767, 1953.

65. Zimmerman, F. T. Evaluation of *N*-methyl-α,α-methylphenylsuccinimide in the treatment of petit mal epilepsy. *N.Y. State J. Med.* 56:1460, 1956.

66. Zimmerman, F. T. *N*-methyl-α,α-methylphenylsuccinimide in psychomotor epilepsy therapy. *Arch. Neurol. Psychiat.* 76:65, 1956.

67. Zimmerman, F. T., and Bergemeister, B. B. A new drug for petit mal epilepsy. *Neurology* (Minneap.) 8:769, 1958.

68. Zimmerman, F. T., and Burgemeister, B. B. Drugs used in treatment of patients with petit mal epilepsy. *J.A.M.A.* 157:1194, 1955.

VALPROIC ACID (DEPAKENE, VALONTIN)

20

Richard H. Mattson
Joyce A. Cramer

Valproic acid (VPA, sodium valproate, 2-propyl penta-noic acid, Depakene, Valontin) is the most important antiepileptic drug introduced for treatment of seizures in the past decade. VPA was synthesized a century ago and used as an organic solvent [6]. Only in the early 1960s were its antiepileptic properties recognized and reported by Meunier, et al. [40]. Using VPA as the solvent in testing a number of drugs for effects on seizure threshold, they observed antiepileptic proper-ties for each drug and recognized that these effects were derived from the solvent rather than from the test drugs. Animal studies and later clinical trials supported the initial evidence of antiepileptic efficacy. The drug has been used extensively throughout the world dur-ing the past decade. VPA is highly effective in control of absence, myoclonic, and tonic-clonic seizures of the primarily generalized type. Efficacy for other sei-zure types is less impressive. Failures often result from use in the wrong seizure type or suboptimal treatment regimens. For those seizures responsive to VPA ther-apy, sufficient dosage should be given to obtain maximal benefit. Coadministration with other anti-epileptic drugs should be avoided, if possible, due to frequent drug interactions that diminish VPA efficacy and/or increase the toxicity of coadministered drugs. Side effects are common at initiation of therapy but infrequent with chronic use [22]. Very rare fatal hepatotoxicity requires a careful consideration of risk-benefit factors before selecting VPA for therapy [65].

Chemistry
VPA is a branched chain carboxylic or fatty acid (pKa 4.8), which is only slightly soluble in water, whereas the sodium salt is freely soluble in water [27]. Unlike most other antiepileptic drugs, which have five- or six-member ring structures, VPA is a simple molecule and contains no nitrogen (Fig. 20-1).

Mechanism of Action
Animal studies of the mechanism of action of VPA sug-gest that the antiseizure effect may be mediated

This chapter was based in part on research supported by the Vet-erans Administration, Abbott Laboratories, and NIH Grant USPHS 5 P01NS06208-12.

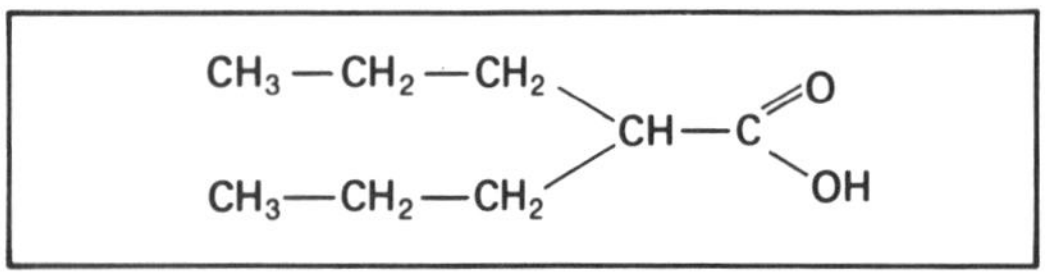

Figure 20-1. Structural formula of valproic acid (VPA).

through changes in gamma-aminobutyric acid (GABA) metabolism. Increases in brain GABA, a known inhibitory neurotransmitter, have been observed following high doses of VPA [27]. The time of elevations of GABA correlated closely with antiseizure effect [15, 27, 52]. VPA has also been effective in blocking convulsive effects of the putative GABA antagonists, picrotoxin and bicuculline [14]. Some evidence suggests that the antiepileptic action of VPA may not be the result of changes in brain GABA. Anlezark, et al. [1] have found antiepileptic effects after VPA administration even in animals not showing increased brain GABA. In addition, doses of VPA causing GABA elevation in animals are five- to tenfold greater than doses administered to patients for treatment. The metabolic pathway by which VPA may alter GABA metabolism is unknown, but animal studies suggest several possibilities acting singly or in combination: (a) inhibition of GABA deamination by gamma-aminobutyric acid transaminase, (b) inhibition of succinic semialdehyde dehydrogenase, (c) inhibition of reuptake of GABA by nerve terminals, and (d) stimulation of the GABA synthesizing enzyme glutamic acid decarboxylase [17, 46]. An independent or alternative antiepileptic mechanism may have a direct CNS depressant action on cell membranes. Such effects have been observed following administration of fatty acids with a chemical structure similar to VPA [27].

Clinical Pharmacology

ABSORPTION
VPA absorption is rapid, peaking within 1 to 2 hours during a fasting state or somewhat more slowly (in 4 to 5 hours) if taken during or after meals (Table 20-1) [34]. The syrup formulation is absorbed immediately if ingested in a fasting state and may produce peak levels in as soon as 15 minutes. Peak levels may vary markedly in different persons taking similar milligram-per-kilogram doses, raising the probability of variations in VPA pharmacokinetics between individuals [28].

DISTRIBUTION
VPA has a small volume of distribution of approximately 0.13 to 0.23 liters/kilogram [28], indicating

that VPA distributes primarily into the extracellular space. Autoradiographic studies of brain concentrations in animals indicate that the drug initially penetrates the gray matter and later the white matter [48]. VPA exhibits very little binding to brain tissue, including proteins and phospholipids, suggesting that the long duration of antiepileptic action after a single dose is due to some mechanism other than binding to brain tissue and that membrane stabilizing effects are not important mechanisms of action for VPA [16].

VPA is 80 to 95 percent bound to plasma protein at usual total VPA concentrations [8, 34]. When the plasma VPA concentration exceeds 80 μg/ml, the percentage of free VPA increases as protein-binding sites become saturated [8]. Increases in free VPA are nonlinear. Thus, doubling the total VPA concentration from 60 μg/ml to 120 μg/ml increases the free VPA from 3 μg/ml to 24 μg/ml, an eightfold rise in the pharmacologically active fraction of the drug.

BIOTRANSFORMATION, EXCRETION, AND CLINICAL PHARMACOKINETICS
Metabolism of VPA is rapid and complete (93 to 99%) [26]. Formation of the conjugated VPA glucuronide and beta oxidation appear to be the major pathways of metabolism prior to excretion [50]. Omega oxidation also occurs [13, 21, 31]. Animal experiments indicate that none of these metabolites have significant antiepileptic activity [31]. Unchanged VPA appears to be responsible for more than 90 percent of the drug's antiepileptic action in humans [31].

The relatively rapid absorption, distribution, biotransformation, and excretion of valproic acid result in a short half-life, averaging 8 to 9 hours for patients taking multiple antiepileptic drugs [34]. If the drug is administered every 8 hours, there is approximately a twofold difference between the maximum and minimum serum concentrations after each dose (Table 20-2). Although seizure control and epileptiform spike-wave activity have not yet been shown to correlate closely with serum levels during a 24-hour period, it is advisable to administer VPA in at least three divided doses to minimize variations in serum levels. When VPA is used as the sole antiepileptic drug, the elimination half-life is longer, and twice daily doses may be adequate. At similar dosage, patients receiving VPA monotherapy have significantly higher serum drug concentrations than patients taking VPA together with one or more other antiepileptic drugs [9, 39]. Some patients may achieve high therapeutic levels (100 μg/ml) only when given very large (and expensive) amounts of VPA (4 gms/day) if they are taking VPA with other enzyme inducing comedication.

Table 20-1. Absorption and Half-Life of Sodium Valproate and Valproic Acid

Absorption and Half-Life	Sodium Valproate (syrup)	Valproic Acid (capsule)
T max[a]	15–60 min	60–120 min
Mean serum half-life[b]	8.73 hr	8.67 hr
Range of serum half-life[b]	6–10.5 hr	6–10.5 hr
Number of patients	13	6

[a]Interval between administration of the oral dose and point of maximum serum concentration.
[b]Mean and range of serum half-life show no important difference between the two formulations.
Source: From R. H. Mattson and J. A. Cramer [34].

Table 20-2. Valproic Acid—Average Dose and Serum Concentrations

Age of Patient		Average Maximum Dose (mg/kg)	Serum Concentration* (μg/ml)	
			Minimum	Maximum
Children	≤ 12 yr	50.0	47.0	96.7
Teenagers	13–19 yr	42.5	64.7	95.3
Adults	≥ 20 yr	21.2	50.5	69.3
Average for all		38.0	54.6	87.1

*Several samples were obtained over approximately 8 hours after the dose was given to determine the minimum and maximum level for each patient on a tid dosing schedule.

DRUG INTERACTIONS

Interactions with other antiepileptic drugs have been observed frequently and may cause clinically important changes in serum concentration of VPA and co-administered drugs [39]. Several investigators have reported increases in phenobarbital serum concentration with addition of VPA therapy [44, 49]. Recent studies indicate that this effect results from a decrease in formation of para-hydroxyphenobarbital [24, 30]. In addition, Mattson and Cramer have documented that the total serum phenytoin concentration declines after addition of VPA secondary to displacement of phenytoin from plasma protein binding sites (Table 20-3) [8, 34]. There is a considerable increase in the percentage of free phenytoin when VPA is administered, beginning during the first week and becoming more pronounced with VPA dose increments (Table 20-3). However, pharmacologically active (free) phenytoin remains unchanged after equilibrium, indicating that the phenytoin dose may not need to be increased.

Several studies indicate that the addition of carbamazepine (CBZ) reduces the plasma concentration and increases the clearance of VPA [3, 10]. Conversely, VPA can decrease CBZ protein binding, yielding higher free CBZ levels, especially at times of peak serum concentrations [38].

Antipyretic doses of aspirin in children resulted in an increase in VPA free fraction from 12 percent to 43 percent in the study of Orr, et al. [42]. The metabolism of VPA also appeared to be inhibited by aspirin in this study.

BLOOD LEVELS

There are reliable methods for determining VPA in serum using gas chromatography and an enzyme multiplied immunoassay technique [27, 34] (Chapter 15). When high doses (50 mg/kg) of VPA are given as the sole antiepileptic drug, the mean peak serum concentration frequently exceeds 100 μg/ml. Much higher levels (200 μg/ml) may be found in some patients, often without evidence of side effects. Equivalent VPA doses coadministered with other antiepileptic drugs result in lower steady state VPA serum concentrations [9]. Although the literature is replete with suggested therapeutic ranges for VPA, minimum effective and maximum tolerable serum concentrations have not yet been determined. Reviews of the literature and clinical experience at this center suggest that the therapeutic range of VPA is between 40μg/ml (mini-

Table 20-3. Protein Binding of Phenytoin Following Valproic Acid Administration

Phenytoin Characteristics	Valproic Acid Dose (mg/day)		
	0	900	1,350[a]
Mean total phenytoin serum concentration (μg/ml)	16.5	13.3	10.2
Mean free phenytoin serum concentration (μg/ml)	1.74	1.94	2.08
Mean percent free phenytoin[b]	10.9	16.1	20.0
Number of patients	25	11	9

[a]The increase in percentage of free phenytoin is dose-dependent.
[b]Protein binding of phenytoin is decreased in the presence of VPA ($p < 0.001$).
Source: From R. H. Mattson and J. A. Cramer [34].

mum) and 150 μg/ml (peak) [4, 5, 26, 30, 31, 34, 35, 43, 44, 48, 49, 53].

Timing is critical in obtaining the blood sample because the VPA serum concentration can be almost twice as high at peak levels as it is immediately before the next dose (8 hours since last dose). Interdose fluctuations are less pronounced for patients receiving the extended release formulation or when taking only VPA.

DOSAGE AND ADMINISTRATION

In the United States VPA is marketed by Abbott Laboratories as 250 mg VPA capsules (Depakene), as sodium valproate syrup containing the equivalent of 250 mg of VPA per teaspoon (Depakene), and as an enteric-coated tablet of sodium divalproex containing the equivalent of 250 mg of VPA per tablet (Depacoat). VPA is also marketed in the United States by Parke-Davis as a tablet of calcium valproate containing the equivalent of 250 mg of VPA (Valontin) and as a chewable tablet of calcium valproate containing the equivalent of 125 mg of VPA (Valontin). Clinical experience indicates that enteric-coated tablets and tablets or capsules formulated with a salt of VPA (sodium, calcium, magnesium) have fewer gastrointestinal side effects than tablets or capsules of unmodified VPA [61]. The cost of equivalent preparations of VPA may vary considerably, and comparison shopping may save the patient money when taking this expensive drug.

Tablets of magnesium valproate and sodium valproate are available in other countries. An amide form (Depamide) has been developed in Europe to obtain a longer half-life of active drug by prolonging the drug's metabolism. No parenteral preparation of VPA is commercially available.

Cautious initiation of treatment will minimize side effects. The recommended starting dose of 15 mg/kg/

day (i.e., 750 to 1000 mg in an adult) of VPA may be too large. In patients weighing more than 30 kg, a single 250 mg dose taken after a meal the first day serves as a simple trial. Gradually increasing the amount to 250 mg three times daily should be attempted over the next few days if the trial dose is well tolerated. If nausea, vomiting, or sedation appear, the next dose should be withheld and a lower daily dose of VPA should be restarted. A few patients will have gastrointestinal side effects even with this cautious startup but can tolerate a smaller dose of 125 mg VPA.

Most children with absence seizures weigh 15 to 30 kg. Initiating treatment with 125 mg of VPA serves as a trial dose. The dosage can be increased as tolerated to 125 mg after each meal and at bedtime during the next several days.

Although many patients will experience a decrease in seizures within a few days or a week of beginning VPA, increased effectiveness occurs as dosage is raised up to 60 mg/kg [60]. In the treatment of absence seizures, the clinical attacks and spike-wave discharges on the electroencephalogram (EEG) are so frequent that evidence of efficacy is readily apparent. VPA blood levels are valuable in recognizing problems that might be explained by poor compliance, atypical absorption, insufficient or excessive dosage, and, in particular, variable rates of metabolism and elimination.

Indications

ABSENCE SEIZURES

Experimental studies in animal models suggest that VPA has a broad spectrum of antiepileptic activity [56]. Clinical studies have confirmed the antiseizure efficacy and the favorable therapeutic index predicted by these animal studies [4, 5, 35, 43, 45, 53]. Controlled studies have shown consistently that VPA is at least as

Table 20-4. Absence Seizure and Spike-Wave Frequency Before Treatment, on Placebo and After 10 Weeks of VPA Therapy in Nine Patients With Intractable Absence Seizures

Seizure and Spike-Wave Frequency	Preplacebo	Placebo	VPA
Mean number of seizures per week	82	60	4*
Mean number of spike-wave discharges per 6-hr recording	179.4	120.4	17.7*

*$p < 0.05$ for both the preplacebo and placebo periods compared to VPA treatment.

effective as ethosuximide [11, 36, 45, 55] in the treatment of absence seizures. VPA may provide excellent control for patients who have not responded to ethosuximide therapy [45]. Some uncertainty about the relative efficacy of VPA remains because the dosage has not always been increased to maximally tolerated levels. Indeed, in the absence of side effects, discontinuation of VPA when blood levels are less than 100 μg/ml peak might be considered an inadequate trial for seizure control. In some patients the combination of ethosuximide and VPA may be more effective than either drug alone [47].

The results of a multicenter, single-blind study of VPA treatment in 97 patients with intractable absence seizures illustrated the dramatic efficacy of the drug [12, 35, 58]. An initial 2-week trial of placebo therapy had minimal effect on seizures or EEG spike-wave discharges, whereas seizures decreased promptly after initiation of VPA. Accompanying the clinical response was a significant decrease in spike-wave discharges recorded on an EEG during a 6-hour period after 12 weeks of treatment compared with the pretreatment EEG record (Table 20-4) [12, 58]. There was a marked increase in the efficacy of VPA (i.e., control of absence seizures) when the dose was raised to more than 30 mg/kg/day. This experience emphasizes the importance of giving each patient an adequate trial of VPA at high doses in order to achieve full efficacy.

MYOCLONIC SEIZURES

Myoclonic seizures have proved to be very responsive to treatment with VPA. Jeavons, et al. [23] specifically subdivided this seizure type for analysis of efficacy. They found that if patients with Lennox-Gastaut syndrome were excluded, 35 of 40 patients with myoclonic seizures obtained 80 to 100 percent seizure control. Several other groups have reported considerable efficacy of VPA for myoclonic seizures [4, 5, 35, 60].

OTHER SEIZURE TYPES

Tonic-clonic attacks often decrease with VPA especially in patients with concomitant absence seizures. Al-

though the data are limited, a careful review of the available studies suggests that 75 percent of patients with primarily generalized tonic-clonic seizures characterized by spike-wave EEG discharges or photic sensitivity have good-to-excellent seizure control when VPA is administered as monotherapy or in combination with other antiepileptic drugs [18, 35].

The efficacy of VPA in treatment of other seizure types is less impressive (Table 20-5). Only about 30 percent of patients with secondarily generalized tonic-clonic attacks have good seizure control with VPA therapy [35].

A variable and less consistent improvement has been reported in the treatment of partial seizures [4, 5, 30, 34, 43, 44, 53]. However, VPA dose was restricted to less than 30 mg/kg, and potential efficacy was not fully tested in many studies of tonic-clonic and partial seizures. In general, atonic, tonic, and akinetic attacks as seen in the Lennox-Gastaut syndrome have been less responsive to VPA therapy [57]. Preliminary trials in the treatment of febrile seizures [7] and alcohol withdrawal seizures [20] hold promise of some value.

VPA may prove to be the drug of choice for patients with coexisting absence and tonic-clonic seizures. Although equivalent control of absence attacks may be obtained with the use of ethosuximide, administration of phenobarbital, primidone, carbamazepine, or phenytoin is usually required to prevent tonic-clonic seizures. The attendant sedative, behavioral, and cosmetic side effects of these additional drugs can be avoided if VPA is used as the sole antiepileptic drug. Furthermore, pharmacokinetic studies indicate that VPA is more effective when used as sole drug therapy; higher serum VPA concentrations are achieved and problems of drug interactions with comedications are avoided [9, 39].

Toxicity

COMMON SIDE EFFECTS

Minor side effects are common at initiation of treatment [22]. Although Pinder, et al. [43] reported that

230

Table 20-5. Treatment of Seizures With Valproic Acid

Seizure Type	No. of Patients*	Reduction in Seizure Frequency		
		100–75%	74–33%	<33%
Simple partial	48	22	17	9
Complex partial	127	44	37	46
Partial seizures secondarily generalized	17	3	7	7
Absence (simple and complex)	218	140	51	27
Atypical absence	67	32	12	23
Myoclonic epilepsy	35	21	7	7
Infantile spasms	19	7	2	10
Tonic seizures	5	1	2	2
Tonic-clonic seizures	279	147	58	74
Atonic/akinetic seizures	39	10	9	20
Combinations of above	236	79	76	81
Others (not classified above)	26	3	6	17
Total	1,116	509 (45.7%)	284 (25.4%)	323 (28.9%)

*1,020 patients: 96 patients with two seizure types considered twice.
Source: From D. Simon, and J. K. Penry, Sodium di-*n*-propylacetate (DPA) in the treatment of epilepsy: A review. *Epilepsia* 16:549, 1975. By permission of Raven Press, New York.

16 to 22 percent of patients had side effects, the incidence was found to be much higher (80%) in a multicenter study of VPA [35] and a large trial of VPA monotherapy in children [19].

Gastrointestinal Side Effects
Nausea and vomiting are common and may be decidedly distressing to the patient. However, these effects are almost always transient and only infrequently require permanent abandonment of VPA therapy. Although the acid may exert a direct irritating effect on the gastrointestinal tract, nausea and vomiting most commonly occur 1 to 2 hours after a dose when peak serum levels are achieved, suggesting a central nervous system effect. In either event, administration of the drug with or after a meal, during initiation of treatment, minimizes this side effect. Alternatively, use of the enteric coated sodium divalproex tablets should reduce chronic gastrointestinal problems [61].

Sedation
Sedative effects occur in about 50 percent of patients [19, 22, 35, 43]. Although these effects are more common when other antiepileptic drugs (especially phenobarbital) are being taken concomitantly, VPA has independent hypnotic properties [51]. Sedation is most common at the onset of VPA therapy and tends to

decrease during chronic therapy even though the VPA blood level is rising. This side effect is rarely an indication for discontinuation of the drug because gradual increments in the VPA dosage, coupled with cautious decrease in phenobarbital levels as necessary, are accompanied by development of tolerance within several weeks. Indeed, the relative freedom from sedative side effects during long-term use constitutes a major advantage of VPA therapy.

SYSTEMIC TOXICITY

Hepatic Toxicity
Two types of hepatic toxicity may occur during VPA therapy. The first is a transient, dose-dependent, asymptomatic rise in serum transaminase (SGOT and SGPT) concentrations, occurring in 15 to 30 percent of patients, which is most likely to be maximal during the first 3 months of therapy [54, 63, 65, 67]. Hyperammonemia also has been reported in patients receiving VPA [41, 66]. Early nausea, sedation, and perhaps tremor may be due in part to elevated blood ammonia [41, 66]. The hyperammonemia may be found in asymptomatic patients having no elevation of other liver function tests. VPA dose reduction produces a lowering of the ammonia levels [41, 66].

The second type of hepatic toxicity is a rare, idiosyncratic, severe, symptomatic hepatitis that may be fatal [32, 54, 63, 65, 67]. As of January 1982, there have been 57 reports from around the world of deaths of patients who had received VPA and in whom there was evidence of hepatic dysfunction [65]. Based on the worldwide use of VPA over this period, fatal liver damage has occurred in one of every 20–40,000 patients who have used VPA. Fifty-four cases of fatal VPA hepatotoxicity were critically reviewed in two recent reports [65, 67]. Most but not all fatal cases began during the first 6 months of VPA therapy. Most but not all of these cases occurred in patients under 15 years of age. Histologic examinations of involved livers have reported centrilobular necrosis and inflammation, cholestasis, and microvesicular fat patterns [65].

Unfortunately, there is no way of distinguishing the benign transient variety of hepatic toxicity from early progressive hepatitis on the basis of any laboratory study [65]. All patients should have baseline liver function tests prior to VPA therapy and at frequent intervals thereafter, especially during the first 6 months of therapy. Two reports have suggested guidelines for monitoring liver function after starting VPA [63, 65]. Since most minor elevations of liver enzymes are not warnings of impending severe hepatic injury, using a decreased dose until transaminase values return to normal would allow continuation of the drug.

Two deaths from VPA-associated hepatic failure have occurred in one family [11]. This raises the question of a genetic factor and suggests that VPA should not be administered to a patient if a family member has had serious hepatic dysfunction associated with VPA use.

Pancreatitis
Pancreatitis is a rare side effect associated with VPA therapy [22]. It usually occurs after 1 to 6 months on VPA and may be fatal [22].

Alopecia
Transient hair loss has also been observed occasionally but has not been marked nor required discontinuation of the medication [22, 23].

Hematologic Side Effects
VPA can provoke thrombocytopenia or platelet dysfunction with or without hemorrhages [29, 64]. These side effects are probably infrequent or at least have little clinical importance [35]. Patients using VPA who are about to undergo surgery should have a platelet count, fibrinogen level, bleeding time, and specific platelet function tests. These hematologic side effects may be more common in patients on high doses of VPA [29].

Teratogenicity
Teratogenicity has been observed in VPA animal studies about as frequently as in phenytoin-treated animals [62]. Although treatment in humans has not indicated any such problem [22], further experience is needed before conclusions can be drawn.

NEUROTOXICITY
Sedation has been discussed earlier. Adverse behavioral changes are rarely observed. Ataxia and incoordination may appear, usually at high dose levels and when other antiepileptic drugs are being used. Asterixis can occur with therapeutic VPA blood levels in patients with normal hepatic function [2]. Hand tremor is the most common long term neurotoxic side effect [19, 25, 35, 37]. The tremor is similar to the type found in benign essential or familial tremor. Occasionally it may be so severe as to interfere with hand movements used for everyday skills. It may be seen in patients receiving VPA alone as well as multiple drug therapy. The problem is most evident when high doses (and high serum concentrations) of VPA are used. Reduction in dosage diminishes the tremor.

Several dozen cases of stupor, coma, hallucinations, behavioral and affective changes, myoclonic jerks, and automatisms in association with therapeutic VPA serum concentrations have been reported [33]. This syndrome may occur when VPA is used alone or in combination with other drugs and is accompanied by increased slowing and/or paroxysmal activity on the EEG [33].

References
1. Anlezark, G. et al. Anticonvulsant action of ethanolamine-O-sulphate and di-n-propylacetate and the metabolism of γ-aminobutyric acid (GABA) in mice with audiogenic seizures. *Biochem. Pharmacol.* 25:413, 1976.
2. Bodensteiner, J. B., Morris, H. H., and Golden, G. S. Asterixis associated with sodium valproate. *Neurology* (N.Y.) 31:194, 1981.
3. Bowdle, T. A., Levy, R. H., and Cutler, R. E. Effects of carbamazepine on valproic acid kinetics in normal subjects. *Clin. Pharmacol. Ther.* 26:629, 1979.
4. Browne, T. R. Medical intelligence: Valproic acid. *N. Engl. J. Med.* 302:661, 1980.
5. Bruni, J., and Wilder, B. J. Valproic acid: Review of a new antiepileptic drug. *Arch. Neurol.* 36:393, 1980.
6. Burton, B. S. Ethyl acetoacetate. *Am. Chem. J.* 3:385, 1882.

232

7. Cavazzuti, G. B., Cappella, L., and Gatti, G. L'acido dipropilacetico (Depakene) nel trattamento della epilessia infantile. *Neuropsichiatr. Infant* 126: 650, 1971.

8. Cramer, J. A., and Mattson, R. H. Valproic acid: In vitro plasma protein binding and interactions with phenytoin. *Ther. Drug. Monit.* 1:105, 1979.

9. Cramer, J. A. et al. Variable free and total valproic acid concentration in sole and multi-drug therapy. In R. H. Levy et al. (Eds.), *Proceedings of the Workshop on the Metabolism of Antiepileptic Drugs.* New York: Raven Press, 1983.

10. Dalby, M. A. Interaction carbamazepine-dipropylacetate. *Acta Neurol. Scand.* 62 (Suppl. 79): 101, 1980.

11. Dreifuss, F. E. How to Use Valproate. In P. L. Morselli, J. K. Penry, and C. E. Pippenger (Eds.), *Antiepileptic Drug Therapy in Pediatrics.* New York: Raven Press, 1982.

12. Erenberg, J. et al. Valproic acid in the treatment of intractable absence seizures in children. *Am. J. Dis. Child.* 136:526, 1982.

13. Ferrandes, B. et al. Metabolism of valproate sodium in rabbit, rat, dog, and man. *Epilepsia* 18:169, 1977.

14. Frey, H. H., and Loscher, W. Di-*n*-propylacetic acid: Profile of anticonvulsant activity in mice. *Arzneimittel-Forschung* 26:299, 1976.

15. Godin, Y. et al. Effects of di-*n*-propylacetate, an anticonvulsive compound, on GABA metabolism. *J. Neurochem.* 16:869, 1969.

16. Goldberg, M. A., and Todoroff, T. Brain binding of anticonvulsants: Carbamazepine and valproic acid. *Neurology* (N.Y.) 30:820, 1980.

17. Harvey, P. K. P., Bradford, H. G., and Davison, A. N. The inhibitory effect of sodium *n*-dipropylacetate on the degradative enzymes of the GABA shunt. *FEBS Lett.* 52:521, 1975.

18. Henriksen, O., and Johannessen, S. I. Clinical and pharmacokinetic observations on sodium valproate: A 5 year follow up. *Acta Neurol. Scand.* 65:504–523, 1982.

19. Herranz, J. L., Artega, R., and Armijo, J. A. Side effects of sodium valproate in monotherapy controlled by plasma levels: A study in 88 pediatric patients. *Epilepsia* 23:203, 1982.

20. Hillbom, M. E. The prevention of ethanol withdrawal seizures in rats by dipropylacetate. *Neuropharmacology* 14:755, 1975.

21. Jacobs, C., and Loescher, W. Identification of metabolites of valproic acid in serum of humans, dog, rat, and mouse. *Epilepsia* 19:591, 1978.

22. Jeavons, P. M. Valproate: Toxicity. In D. M. Woodbury, J. K. Penry, and C. E. Pippenger (Eds.), *Antiepileptic Drugs.* New York: Raven Press, 1982.

23. Jeavons, P. M., Clark, J. E., and Maheshwari, M. D. Treatment of generalized epilepsies of childhood and adolescence with sodium valproate (Epilim). *Dev. Med. Child. Neurol.* 19:9, 1977.

24. Kapetanovic, I. M. et al. Mechanism of valproate-phenobarbital interaction in epileptic patients. *Clin. Pharmacol. Ther.* 29:480, 1981.

25. Karas, B. J. et al. Valproate tremors. *Neurology* (N.Y.) 32:428, 1982.

26. Klotz, U. Pharmacokinetic studies with valproic acid in man. *Arzneimittel-Forschung.* 27:1085, 1977.

27. Kupferberg, H. J. Sodium Valproate. In G. H. Glaser, J. K. Penry, and D. M. Woodbury (Eds.), *Antiepileptic Drugs: Mechanisms of Action.* New York: Raven Press, 1980.

28. Levy, R. H., and Lai, A. A. Valproate: Absorption, Distribution and Excretion. In D. M. Woodbury, J. K. Penry, C. E. Pippenger (Eds.), *Antiepileptic Drugs.* New York: Raven Press, 1982.

29. Loiseau, P. Sodium valproate, platelet dysfunction, and bleeding. *Epilepsia* 22:141, 1981.

30. Loiseau, P. et al. Further pharmacokinetic observations on the interaction between phenobarbital and valproic acid in epileptic patients. Epilepsy International Symposium. Vancouver, Canada, September 10–14, 1978.

31. Loscher, W. Concentration of metabolites of valproic acid in plasma of epileptic patients. *Epilepsia* 22:169, 1981.

32. Madsen, J. A., and Gay, P. E. Valproic acid hepatotoxicity: A clinical assessment. *Epilepsia* 22:241, 1981.

33. Marescaux, C. et al. Stuporous episodes during treatment with sodium valproate: Report of seven cases. *Epilepsia* 23:297, 1982.

34. Mattson, R. H., Cramer, J. A., and Williamson, P. D. Valproic acid in epilepsy—Clinical and pharmacologic effects. *Ann. Neurol.* 3:20, 1978.

35. Mattson, R. H. Valproic Acid and Management of Seizures. In H. R. Tyler, and D. M. Dawson (Eds.), *Current Neurology,* Vol. 2. Boston: Houghton Mifflin, 1979.

36. Mattson, R. H., and Cramer, J. A. Valproic acid and ethosuximide interaction. *Ann. Neurol.* 7:583, 1980.

37. Mattson, R. H., and Cramer, J. A. Tremor due to sodium valproate. *Neurology* (N.Y.) 31:114, 1981.

38. Mattson, G. F., Mattson, R. H., and Cramer, J. A. Interaction between valproic acid and carba-

mazapine: An in vitro study of protein binding. *Therap. Drug. Monitor.* 4:181, 1982.

39. Mattson, R. H. Valproate: Interactions with Other Drugs. In D. M. Woodbury, J. K. Penry, and C. E. Pippenger (Eds.), *Antiepileptic Drugs.* New York: Raven Press, 1982.

40. Meunier, G. et al. Proprieties pharmacodynamiques de l'acide *n*-dipropylacetique. *Therapie* 18:435, 1963.

41. Murphy, J. V., Marquardt, K., and Swick, M. Hyperammonia in children receiving valproic acid. *Neurology* (N.Y.) 31:142, 1981.

42. Orr, J. M. et al. Interaction between valproic acid and aspirin in epileptic children: Serum protein binding and metabolic effects. *Clin. Pharmacol. Ther.* 31:642, 1982.

43. Pinder, R. M. et al. Sodium valproate: A review of its pharmacological properties and therapeutic efficacy in epilepsy. *Drugs* 13:81, 1977.

44. Richens, A., and Ahmad, S. Controlled trial of sodium valproate in severe epilepsy. *Br. Med. J.* 4:255, 1975.

45. Sato, S. et al. Valproic acid versus ethosuximide in the treatment of absence seizures. *Neurology* (N.Y.) 32:157, 1982.

46. Sawaya, M. C. B., Horton, R. W., and Meldrum, B. S. Effects of anticonvulsant drugs on the cerebral enzymes metabolizing GABA. *Epilepsia* 16:649, 1975.

47. Schneble, H. Treatment of atypical absences with a combination of succinimide and dipropylacetate. *Dtsch. Med. Wochenschr.* 100:1564, 1975.

48. Schobben, F., and Van Der Kleijn, E. Pharmacokinetics of distribution and elimination of sodium di-*n*-propylacetate in mouse and dog. *Pharm. Weekbl.* 109:33, 1974.

49. Schobben, F. et al. Pharmacokinetics of di-*n*-propylacetate in epileptic patients. *Eur. J. Clin. Pharmacol.* 8:97, 1975.

50. Schobben, F., and Van Der Kleijn, E. Valproate: Biotransformation. In D. M. Woodbury, J. K. Penry, and C. E. Pippenger (Eds.), *Antiepileptic Drugs.* New York: Raven Press, 1982.

51. Scott, D. F. et al. A Study of the Hypnotic Effects of Epilim and Its Possible Interaction with Phenobarbitone. In J. J. Legg (Ed.), *Clinical and Pharmacological Aspects of Sodium Valproate (Epilim) in the Treatment of Epilepsy.* Tunbridge Wells: MCS Consultants, 1975.

52. Simler, S. et al. Effect of sodium *n*-dipropylacetate on audiogenic seizures and brain gamma-aminobutyric acid level. *Biochem. Pharmacol.* 22:1701, 1973.

53. Simon, D., and Penry, J. K. Sodium di-*n*-propylacetate (DPA) in the treatment of epilepsy: A review. *Epilepsia* 16:549, 1975.

54. Sussman, N. M., and McLain, L. W. A direct hepatotoxic effect of valproic acid. *J.A.M.A.* 242:1173, 1979.

55. Suzuki, J. et al. A double-blind comparative trial of sodium dipropylacetate and ethosuximide in epilepsy in children: With special emphasis on pure petit mal seizures (in Japanese). *Med. Prog.* 82:470, 1972.

56. Swinyard, E. A. et al. The pharmacology of dipropylacetic acid sodium with special emphasis on its effects on the central nervous system. Salt Lake City: University of Utah College of Pharmacy, 1964.

57. Vassella, F. et al. Double-blind trial of the anticonvulsant effect of phenobarbital and valproate on Lennox syndrome. *Schweiz. Med. Wochenschr.* 108:713, 1978.

58. Villarreal, H. J. et al. Effect of valproic acid on spike and wave discharges in patients with absence seizures. *Neurology* (N.Y.) 28:886, 1978.

59. Von Voss, H. et al. Sodium valproate and platelet function. *Br. Med. J.* 2:179, 1976.

60. Wilder, B. J., and Karas, B. J. Valproate: Relation of Plasma Concentration to Seizure Control. In D. M. Woodbury, J. K. Penry, and C. E. Pippenger (Eds.), *Antiepileptic Drugs.* New York: Raven Press, 1982.

61. Wilder, B. J. et al. Gastrointestinal side effects of valproic acid versus a new enteric coated drug, sodium hydrogen divalproate. *Neurology* (N.Y.) 32:A225, 1982.

62. Whittle, B. A. Pre-clinical Teratological Studies on Sodium Valproate (Epilim) and Other Anticonvulsants. In J. J. Legg (Ed.), *Clinical and Pharmacological Aspects of Sodium Valproate (Epilim) in the Treatment of Epilepsy.* Tunbridge Wells: MCS Consultants, 1975.

63. Willmore, L. J. et al. Effect of valproic acid on hepatic function. *Neurology* (N.Y.) 28:961, 1978.

64. Winfield, D. A. et al. Sodium valproate and thrombocytopenia. *Br. Med. J.* 2:981, 1976.

65. Zafrani, E. S., and Berthelot, P. Sodium valproate in the induction of unusual hepatotoxicity. *Hepatology* 2:648, 1982.

66. Zaret, B. S. et al. Sodium valproate induced hyperammonemia without clinical hepatic dysfunction. *Neurology* (N.Y.) 32:206, 1982.

67. Zimmerman, H. J., and Ishak, K. G. Valproate-induced hepatic injury: Analyses of 23 fatal cases. *Hepatology* 2:591, 1982.

BENZODIAZEPINES

21

Thomas R. Browne

A large number of benzodiazepine drugs are marketed in this country and abroad, and many of these drugs have antiepileptic properties. At the present time, diazepam (Valium), clonazepam (Clonopin), and clorazepate dipotassium (Tranxene) are approved by the United States Food and Drug Administration (FDA) as antiepileptic drugs. Lorazepam (Ativan), nitrazepam (Mogadon), and oxazepam (Serax) have all undergone some testing as antiepileptic drugs but are not currently FDA-approved for this indication.

Chemistry of Benzodiazepines

The structural formulas, generic names, and brand names of the six benzodiazepines demonstrated to possess antiepileptic activity in humans are given in Fig. 21-1. It is evident that the six drugs are all variations of the same basic benzodiazepine structure. The six drugs are all qualitatively similar in their antiepileptic and toxic activities, although there are important quantitative differences in these activities.

Mechanism of Action of Benzodiazepines

NEUROPHYSIOLOGIC STUDIES

In humans, benzodiazepines have been shown to suppress most forms of paroxysmal activity on electroencephalograms (EEGs) [11, 13]. Generalized EEG abnormalities are more readily suppressed than focal EEG abnormalities [11, 13]. Benzodiazepines often limit the spread of discharge from a focal lesion while not suppressing the primary focus [11, 13]. In animals, benzodiazepines increase presynaptic and postsynaptic inhibition, increase recurrent inhibition, and decrease the firing rate of normal and epileptic neurons [29].

BENZODIAZEPINE RECEPTORS AND
FACILITATION OF GABA EFFECTS

The preponderance of evidence now indicates that the pharmacologic effects of benzodiazepines are due to facilitation of the effects of the inhibitory neurotransmitter gamma-aminobutyric acid (GABA) and that such facilitation is accomplished through the action of benzodiazepine receptors [24, 28, 29, 49, 59, 60, 62].

This work was supported in part by the Veterans Administration.

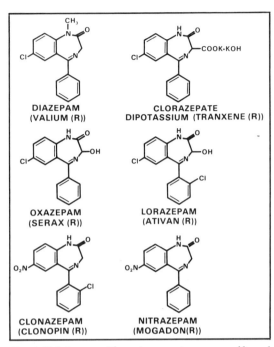

DIAZEPAM
(VALIUM (R))

CLORAZEPATE
DIPOTASSIUM (TRANXENE (R))

OXAZEPAM
(SERAX (R))

LORAZEPAM
(ATIVAN (R))

CLONAZEPAM
(CLONOPIN (R))

NITRAZEPAM
(MOGADON(R))

Figure 21-1. Structural formulas, generic names, and brand names of benzodiazepines shown to have an antiepileptic effect.

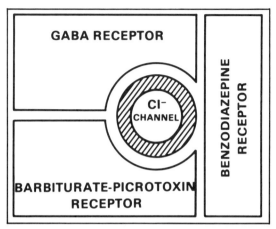

Figure 21-2. Theoretical model of the GABA-ionophore complex. The complex contains a chloride ion channel and three drug binding sites: (1) the GABA receptor, (2) the benzodiazepine receptor, and (3) the barbiturate-picrotoxin receptor. GABA function (opening of the chloride channel) can be modulated by drugs binding to either of the other receptor sites. Drugs (endogenous or exogenous) can be agonists or antagonists of GABA-ionophore function. (Modified from R. Olsen et al. [49].

Benzodiazepine receptors are high-affinity, saturable, and stereospecific binding sites for benzodiazepines that have been found in the mammalian central nervous system. The high correlations obtained between the relative affinities of a series of benzodiazepines for this receptor and their clinical potencies as antiepileptics, anxiolytics, and muscle relaxants suggest that these binding sites may be pharmacologic receptors mediating the therapeutic effects of benzodiazepines.

The most attractive hypothesis explaining the mechanism of action of benzodiazepines is that they interact with postsynaptic benzodiazepine receptors, which in turn enhance the postsynaptic effects of GABA. It appears that in the postsynaptic membrane there is a supramolecular complex consisting of (1) a GABA receptor, (2) a benzodiazepine receptor, (3) a barbiturate receptor, and (4) a chloride channel (see Fig. 21-2) [28, 29, 49, 59, 60, 62]. The postulated sequence of events begins with the attachment of benzodiazepine to a benzodiazepine receptor, which leads to (in turn) increased binding of GABA to GABA receptor, greater inward flux of chloride through a chloride pore, and greater inhibition of the postsynaptic neuron (see Chap. 2). Occupation of the barbiturate receptor site by a barbiturate appears to enhance the binding of GABA to GABA receptors and benzodiazepines to benzodiazepine receptors, thus producing enhanced GABA-ergic activity [49].

The presence of benzodiazepine receptors suggests that endogenous ligands (agonists or antagonists) for these receptors must also be present. This is an area of intensive investigation at present [28, 29, 59, 60, 62].

The benzodiazepine receptor theory also provides attractive hypotheses to explain the phenomena of tolerance and withdrawal hyperexcitability associated with chronic benzodiazepine therapy [24, 60, 62]. Continued exposure to benzodiazepines may affect feedback mechanisms, resulting in an increase in the number of benzodiazepine receptors or a decrease in the production or release of GABA. Either of these changes would result in a need for more benzodiazepine to produce the inhibitory effect previously obtained by the combination of benzodiazepine and GABA. Tolerance may thus develop. If benzodiazepine is rapidly withdrawn and little GABA is available, the resulting loss of inhibition may lead to excitatory withdrawal symptoms.

OTHER POSSIBLE MECHANISMS OF ACTION
There is some data suggesting that each of the following may be mechanisms of action of benzodiazepines: (1) enhancement of adenosine-modulated presynaptic inhibition [52], (2) increased serotonin activity at presynaptic sites [12, 16], (3) mimicking of the effects

of glycine [11], and (4) depression of dopaminergic presynaptic mechanisms [64].

Clonazepam (Clonopin)

CLINICAL PHARMACOLOGY

Methods for Determining Concentration
Methods reported for determining the concentration of clonazepam in biologic fluids include gas chromatography with electron-capture detection, high-performance liquid chromatography, and radioimmunoassay [11, 12, 21, 51].

Absorption and Distribution
Clonazepam is largely nonionized throughout the range of physiologic pH. It is thus relatively insoluble in water (19 μg/ml at pH 7.4) but readily crosses biologic membranes [11]. Preparation of clonazepam as a micronized tablet aids its dissolution in the gastrointestinal tract. Clonazepam passes rapidly from blood into brain in experimental animals [37, 50] and probably does so in humans also. Clonazepam is 47 percent protein bound in humans [45].

Biotransformation and Excretion
The major metabolic pathway of clonazepam is reduction of the nitro group to form a 7-amino derivative [11, 34]. This is the major metabolite in human plasma, and its plasma concentration at steady state is usually equal to or greater than the concentration of clonazepam [11, 34, 44]. Preliminary results indicate that the 7-amino derivative has little antiepileptic activity [11]. An acetamide derivative (from acetylation of the 7-amino derivative) and hydroxylated derivatives (from hydroxylation at the C3 position) are minor metabolites of clonazepam. Less than 5 percent of clonazepam is excreted unchanged in the urine [11, 34]. About 30 percent of clonazepam is excreted as unconjugated metabolites and the remainder as conjugated metabolites [11, 34].

Clinical Pharmacokinetics
Peak serum concentrations of clonazepam occur 1 to 3 hours after oral administration [7, 11, 34, 44]. The elimination half-life of clonazepam is 20 to 40 hours in most people [7, 11, 21, 34, 37, 44]. The serum concentration produced by a given dose of clonazepam is quite variable, and serum clonazepam concentration cannot be accurately predicted from the dosage [3, 12, 14, 21, 34].

Therapeutic and Toxic Serum Concentrations
Most patients whose seizures are controlled with clonazepam have serum concentrations of 5 to 70 nanograms (ng) per ml [3, 11, 21, 41, 42]. Unfortunately, the serum concentrations of patients who do not respond to clonazepam or who have side effects with clonazepam also usually fall in the same range [3, 11, 21, 58]. Thus there is no clear-cut minimum therapeutic serum concentration or a usual toxic serum concentration.

Enzyme Induction and Drug Interactions
Values for the elimination half-life of clonazepam measured during chronic administration are similar to values measured after single doses [7, 21], indicating that clonazepam does not induce its own metabolism. Addition of clonazepam to already existing regimens does not appear to alter the steady state serum concentrations of phenytoin [31, 36, 46], primidone [11, 46], or carbamazepine [36]. There is, however, evidence that the addition of phenytoin [34] or phenobarbital [3, 46] may lower the steady state serum concentration of clonazepam.

Tolerance
Tolerance to the antiepileptic effect of clonazepam occurs in approximately one third of patients who have an initial good response to the drug [11, 39, 46, 47]. Reemergence of seizures has been reported to occur with clonazepam therapy for almost every type of seizure [11]. Tolerance to the antiepileptic effects of clonazepam usually develops after 1 to 6 months of administration [11, 39, 47]. Among patients who develop tolerance, approximately two thirds will continue to receive some beneficial effects with increased dosage of clonazepam, whereas one third will no longer respond to clonazepam at any dosage [11]. The mechanism of action of tolerance probably involves changes in the benzodiazepine receptor–GABA function (see above). Other possible mechanisms of action are reviewed elsewhere [11, 12, 21].

Dosage and Administration
The initial dose for infants and children (up to 10 years of age, or 30 kg of body weight) is 0.01 to 0.03 mg/kg/day but not in excess of 0.05 mg/kg/day given in two or three divided doses. Daily dosage should be increased by no more than 0.25 to 0.5 mg every 3 to 7 days until a daily maintenance dose of 0.1 to 0.2 mg/kg of body weight has been reached, unless seizures are controlled or side effects preclude further increase. The initial dose for adults should not exceed 1.5 mg/day in three divided doses. Daily dosage may be increased in increments of 0.5 mg every 3 to 7 days until seizures are adequately controlled or side effects preclude any further increase. The maximum recommended daily dose in adults is 20 mg. It is usually best

to wait at least 7 days between increases in dosage of clonazepam in order to allow steady state serum concentrations to be reached and the full therapeutic and toxic effects of the increase to be appreciated. More rapid increases in dosage are possible in emergency situations but carry a greater risk of side effects. Tonic-clonic status epilepticus can occur when clonazepam is abruptly discontinued [11, 21], and it is prudent to withdraw the drug slowly.

INDICATIONS

Clonazepam is currently approved by the FDA for use alone or as an adjunctive antiepileptic drug for the following types of seizures—absence (typical petit mal), infantile spasms (infantile myoclonic, massive spasms, salaam), atypical absence (atypical petit mal), myoclonic, and atonic (akinetic, drop attack) (see Table 21-1). The drug is not approved by the FDA for treatment of tonic-clonic (grand mal), complex partial (psychomotor, temporal lobe), or simple partial (focal) seizures; however, it is being tested for these seizure types. Clonazepam has also been tried for a variety of other neurologic disorders.

Absence (Petit Mal) Seizures

Clonazepam is extremely effective in controlling animal models of absence seizures and in stopping 3-Hz spike-wave discharges when injected parenterally in humans [11]. In a large double-blind, randomized collaborative study coordinated by the National Institutes of Health, clonazepam was compared with ethosuximide (Zarontin) for the long-term treatment of absence seizures [21, 54]. Both drugs were found to be extremely effective, but side effects and development of tolerance were more common with clonazepam. In another double-blind study, Chandra [17] randomly assigned 39 patients to receive clonazepam or diazepam as the sole antiepileptic drug for absence seizures. The clonazepam group had significantly ($p < 0.0001$) greater reductions in seizure frequency and in 3-Hz spike-wave discharges on follow up EEGs. A single-blind crossover study with sequential analysis comparing clonazepam with placebo showed clonazepam to be significantly ($p < 0.05$) better than placebo in 10 trials [41]. In addition, there are at least 34 published uncontrolled studies of clonazepam for absence seizures, and they almost invariably report a favorable response.

Although clonazepam and ethosuximide are both very effective for absence seizures, ethosuximide is still the drug of choice for the disorder because clonazepam has higher incidences of side effects and of tolerance to antiepileptic effect [21, 54].

Table 21-1. Effectiveness of Clonazepam in the Treatment of Seizure Disorders

Seizure Type	Effectiveness of Clonazepam*
FDA-approved indications	
Absence	+++
Infantile spasms	++
Atypical absence	++
Myoclonic	+++
Atonic	++
Indications not approved by FDA	
Tonic-clonic	±
Simple partial	++
Complex partial	++

*Key: +++, Proven effective in controlled trials; ++, uncontrolled studies strongly suggest effectiveness; +, uncontrolled studies indicate possible effectiveness; ±, controlled and uncontrolled studies have produced conflicting results.
Source: From T. R. Browne [12]. Reprinted by permission, from The New England Journal of Medicine 299:812, 1978.

Clonazepam is an effective second choice drug for patients whose absence seizures cannot be controlled with ethosuximide. Other drugs that are effective against absence seizures are discussed in Chapter 7.

Infantile Spasms (Infantile Myoclonic Seizures, Massive Spasms, Salaam Seizures)

Five uncontrolled studies with 12 or more patients taking clonazepam as an adjunct to other antiepileptic therapy reported that infantile spasms were completely controlled in 12 to 37 percent of patients and that a 50 percent or greater reduction in seizure frequency was obtained in 21 to 75 percent of patients [11, 55]. In a study of 6 patients whose other antiepileptic drugs were withdrawn except those required to control major seizures, only 2 patients had a 50 percent or greater reduction in infantile spasms, and none had complete control [30]. A direct comparison of clonazepam with corticosteroids and other therapies for infantile spasms has not been performed.

Atypical Absence (Atypical Petit Mal) Seizures

In two small double-blind studies and a large (21 patients) uncontrolled study in which clonazepam was used as an adjunct to other antiepileptic drugs, atypical absence seizures were completely controlled in 38 to 100 percent of patients and were reduced in frequency by 50 percent or more in 75 to 100 percent of patients [5, 15, 46]. In a study in which clonazepam was used as the only drug for a group of 12 patients, 7 patients obtained complete control of atypical absence seizures, and all 12 patients had a 50 percent or greater reduction in seizure frequency [30].

Myoclonic Seizures

In a double-blind crossover study of clonazepam versus placebo as adjunctive antiepileptic drugs, myoclonic seizures were completely abolished in 12 of 15 patients receiving clonazepam, and some improvement occurred in the other 3 [46]. None of the 15 patients improved while taking the placebo. Four uncontrolled studies of clonazepam as an adjunctive antiepileptic drug with 9 or more patients reported that myoclonic seizures were completely controlled in 20 to 33 percent of patients and were reduced in frequency by 50 percent or more in 57 to 100 percent of patients [11, 30, 38, 47]. Clonazepam has been effective in treating a variety of subtypes of myoclonic seizures including photosensitive myoclonic seizures, progressive myoclonic epilepsy with and without Laford bodies, Ramsay Hunt syndrome, and posthypoxic intention myoclonus [11, 35].

Atonic (Akinetic, Drop Attack) Seizures

Three uncontrolled studies with 10 or more patients taking clonazepam as an adjunctive antiepileptic drug reported that atonic seizures were completely controlled in 0 to 30 percent of patients and were reduced in frequency by 50 percent or more in 49 to 90 percent of patients [11, 15, 38]. In a study of 16 patients who took no other antiepileptic drugs except those necessary to control major seizures, atonic seizures were completely suppressed in 31 percent of patients and were reduced in frequency by 50 percent or more in 81 percent of patients [30].

Tonic-Clonic (Grand Mal) Seizures

Studies of the efficacy of clonazepam for tonic-clonic seizures have yielded conflicting results. In two double-blind comparisons of clonazepam with placebo as adjunctive antiepileptic drugs, the clonazepam group had a greater reduction in seizure frequency in one study [46], and the placebo group had a greater reduction in the other study [23]. In 16 uncontrolled studies involving 10 or more patients using clonazepam as an adjunctive antiepileptic drug, tonic-clonic seizures were completely controlled in 10 to 70 percent (median, 38 percent) of patients and were reduced in frequency by 50 percent or more in 10 to 96 percent (median, 56 percent) of patients [2, 11, 15, 20, 38, 55, 57]. In a study in which clonazepam was used as the only drug for tonic-clonic seizures, 10 of 14 patients had no change or an increase in seizure frequency [48].

At least 31 patients whose tonic-clonic seizures became worse during clonazepam therapy have been reported from 14 series. Not all investigators report that clonazepam made some patients with tonic-clonic seizures worse, and some authors specifically state that this did not happen in their series. In series with 10 or more patients that did report this phenomenon, increased frequency of tonic-clonic seizures occurred in 4 to 27 percent of patients. Possible explanations of this phenomenon include (1) the natural variability of seizure frequency, (2) aggravation of the tonic-clonic seizure disorder by clonazepam (possibly by inhibiting inhibition), and (3) reduction in serum concentration of other antiepileptic drugs by clonazepam.

Simple Partial (Focal Motor) Seizures

In a single-blind study using sequential analysis, clonazepam proved to be significantly ($p < 0.05$) more effective than placebo for treatment of simple partial seizures [42]. In seven uncontrolled studies with 10 or more patients who took clonazepam as an adjunctive antiepileptic drug, simple partial seizures were completely controlled in 9 to 100 percent of patients and were reduced in frequency by 50 percent or more in 63 to 100 percent of patients [11, 20, 38, 61].

Complex Partial (Psychomotor, Temporal Lobe) Seizures

In a double-blind comparison of clonazepam with carbamazepine as initial therapy for complex partial seizures, both drugs significantly reduced seizure frequency [40]. There was a tendency (not statistically significant) toward more side effects and less complete seizure control in the clonazepam group.

In a small (7 patients) double-blind study of clonazepam versus placebo as adjunctive antiepileptic drugs for complex partial seizures [5], 3 patients had 100 percent seizure control, and 5 patients had 50 percent or greater seizure control while taking clonazepam. Two patients had complete seizure control, and 5 patients had no significant improvement while taking a placebo. In a single-blind crossover study with sequential analysis, clonazepam proved preferable to placebo ($p < 0.05$) as an adjunctive therapy for complex partial seizures in 21 patients [8]. Seven large (17 or more patients) uncontrolled studies of clonazepam as an antiepileptic adjunct have reported complete suppression of complex partial seizures in 26 to 47 percent (median, 34 percent) of patients, and a 50 percent or greater reduction in seizure frequency in 35 to 89 percent (median, 65 percent) of patients [11].

Status Epilepticus

Experience abroad indicates that intravenous clonazepam is effective for all types of status epilepticus [11]. However, intravenous clonazepam has not been tested in the United States because (1) diazepam is an extremely effective drug for status epilepticus [13], and (2) the major toxic complications of intravenously administered diazepam and clonazepam are sedation and cardiorespiratory depression, and clonazepam appears to have a greater depressant effect than diazepam.

Miscellaneous Disorders

Anecdotal reports indicate that clonazepam may be effective for epilepsia partialis continua, focal sensory seizures, reading seizures, gelastic seizures, trigeminal neuralgia, other cranial neuralgias, lightning pain of lower extremities, Gilles de la Tourette's syndrome, tardive dyskinesia, and Huntington's and other choreas [11, 12, 21].

TOXICITY

Common Side Effects

Six studies [11, 17, 20] with 50 or more patients report side effects with clonazepam in 13 to 91 percent (median, 46 percent) of patients, requiring discontinuance of the drug in 9 to 26 percent. The three most common side effects are drowsiness, ataxia, and behavioral changes. Twelve studies with 50 or more patients report drowsiness in 3 to 85 percent (median, 33 percent) of patients and ataxia in 4 to 79 percent (median, 13 percent) of patients [11, 17, 20, 27, 38, 46, 55]. Coadministration of a barbiturate may increase drowsiness [11]. The drowsiness and ataxia caused by clonazepam tend to be dose-related. They occur early in the course of administration and tend to subside with chronic administration. Drowsiness and ataxia can usually be reduced to tolerable levels by decreasing either the dosage of clonazepam or the rate at which the dosage is increased. In some patients, however, these side effects cannot be reduced to tolerable levels, and the drug must be discontinued [8, 11, 21].

Behavioral disturbances caused by clonazepam occur in a minority of patients, usually children, but can be very disturbing. Affected children are described as hyperactive, irritable, aggressive, violent, or disobedient [11]. These disturbances may represent an exacerbation of a previous disorder or arise de novo. In 21 studies reporting this complication, the frequency ranged from 2 to 52 percent (median, 15 percent) of patients. Behavioral disturbances can be reduced to tolerable levels in some patients by reduc-

ing the dosage of clonazepam. In others the drug must be discontinued. Clonazepam is a potent sedative drug that can cause depression in some patients (especially teenagers) or improved behavior in other patients [11, 15, 27].

Other, not uncommon side effects of clonazepam include hypotonia, dizziness, and thick speech. Hypersalivation and bronchial hypersecretion occur in some patients and can create respiratory difficulties in children [11]. Both anorexia and increased appetite have been reported in association with clonazepam therapy [11, 13].

Increased Seizure Frequency

Increased seizure frequency has been reported in a minority of patients receiving clonazepam for tonic-clonic [1] (see above), absence [1, 20], myoclonic [1, 53], tonic [1, 11, 55], atonic [1], complex partial [1, 2, 11, 20, 39], and simple partial [1, 11] seizures.

Other Reactions

Several small, inconclusive studies indicating that clonazepam may cause thrombocytopenia have been discussed elsewhere [6]. In testing done in the United States, Hoffmann-LaRoche, Inc. found that only 2 of 85 patients taking clonazepam ever had platelet counts below $100,000/mm^3$ [18]. The first patient had a count of $90,000/mm^3$, which returned to normal while the patient was still taking clonazepam. The second patient, reported in detail by Masland [39], developed thrombocytopenic purpura while taking clonazepam. This improved when clonazepam was discontinued, and then returned 1 year after the drug was stopped. No anticlonazepam antibodies were found. No cases of serious hepatic or renal toxicity have been reported in association with clonazepam therapy. Rashes apparently caused by clonazepam occasionally occur [11].

Overdosage

Clonazepam overdosage can cause drowsiness, ataxia, and cyclic coma [11, 12]. To date, all patients with clonazepam overdosage have recovered without sequelae.

Effects on Fetus

The safety of clonazepam during pregnancy has not yet been established.

Diazepam (Valium)

INTRAVENOUS, INTRAMUSCULAR, AND RECTAL DIAZEPAM

At present the major use of diazepam in the management of epilepsy is as an adjunctive drug for the management of status epilepticus. The clinical pharmacology, indications, and toxicity of intravenous, intramuscular, and rectal diazepam are discussed in detail in Chapter 30.

ORAL DIAZEPAM

Clinical Pharmacology
Peak serum concentrations of diazepam are reached 1 to 3 hours after oral administration [13, 56], and steady state serum concentrations are reached after 4 to 10 days of chronic administration [13, 56]. Serum diazepam concentrations of 0.2 to 0.8 μg/ml are needed to control clinical seizures and paroxysmal activity on the EEG [10, 43, 56]. The manufacturer recommends a daily dose of 4 to 40 mg when the drug is used as an adjunctive antiepileptic drug. Adults taking even 30 to 40 mg of diazepam per day by mouth seldom achieve serum diazepam concentrations of 0.2 to 0.8 μg/ml [10]. High serum diazepam concentrations can be consistently achieved by the intravenous route (see Chap. 30) but not by the oral route. This may account for the frequent success of intravenous diazepam in stopping status epilepticus and the frequent failure of oral diazepam as a chronic antiepileptic drug.

Diazepam is demethylated to form desmethyldiazepam and demethylated and oxidized to form oxazepam [26, 56]. Both these metabolic products possess antiepileptic activity [26, 56]. They are inactivated and then excreted when they are conjugated in the liver to form glucuronides and sulfates [26, 56].

The distribution and elimination half-lives of diazepam are discussed in Chapter 30.

Indications
Oral diazepam is approved by the FDA as an adjunctive antiepileptic drug but not as a primary antiepileptic drug. Modest success has been reported when diazepam is used as an adjunctive drug for the treatment of infantile spasms, and for atypical absence, myoclonic, atonic, and photosensitive seizures [13, 56]. However, diazepam is now seldom used when a benzodiazepine antiepileptic drug is chosen for these indications because clonazepam appears to be more consistently effective as a chronic oral antiepileptic drug [11, 12, 17], and because clonazepam is FDA-approved as a primary antiepileptic drug for these seizure types. Diazepam may be useful in managing one of the above-named seizure types in a patient who develops intolerable side effects with clonazepam.

Toxicity
Common side effects with oral diazepam include drowsiness, fatigue, and ataxia [13, 26, 56]. Not un-

common side effects are: dysarthria, diplopia, blurred vision, hypotonia, confusion, agitation, and paradoxical excitement. Most of these side effects are dose-dependent, and some patients develop tolerance to them [13, 26, 56]. Uncommon side effects of diazepam include constipation, depression, headache, hypotension, incontinence, bronchial hypersecretion, rash, jaundice, and neutropenia [13, 26, 56]. The combination of hypotonia and bronchial hypersecretion can create respiratory difficulty in children. Physical dependence and a withdrawal syndrome can occur with chronic diazepam administration, especially at high doses [13, 26, 56]. A number of rare side effects of diazepam have been reported and are reviewed elsewhere [13, 26, 56].

Clorazepate Dipotassium (Tranxene)

CLINICAL PHARMACOLOGY
Clorazepate dipotassium is a carboxylated salt of *N*-desmethyl diazepam (NDD), the primary active metabolite of diazepam. After absorption, clorazepate dipotassium is rapidly decarboxylated to yield NDD [9, 66].

Peak serum concentrations of NDD occur 0.5 to 1 hour after an oral dose of clorazepate dipotassium [66]. NDD is excreted partly as conjugated NDD and partly as conjugated oxazepam after oxidation to form oxazepam [26]. The elimination half-life of NDD in patients with epilepsy is approximately 40 hours [66]. Serum concentrations of NDD in patients whose seizures are controlled with clorazepate dipotassium range from 0.5 to 1.9 μg/ml, but similar levels are found in patients having no response to the drug [9].

The dosage of clorazepate dipotassium is begun at low levels and increased until seizures are controlled or side effects appear. The usual starting dose is 7.5 mg tid or less in adults and 7.5 mg bid or less in children. Daily doses should be increased by no more than 7.5 mg every week. The maintenance dose is usually 22.5 to 90 mg/day in adults and 15 to 60 mg/day in children.

The rapid oral absorption of clorazepate dipotassium and the resulting high peak serum concentrations may lead to toxic side effects. This is why the drug should be given tid despite its long elimination half-life.

INDICATIONS
Clorazepate dipotassium is FDA-approved as an adjunctive therapy for partial seizures. Evidence of efficacy for this indication includes a double-blind crossover comparison of phenytoin and clorazepate dipotassium versus phenytoin and phenobarbital [65]

and an unpublished double-blind multiclinic study of clorazepate dipotassium versus placebo.

TOXICITY

The toxicity of clorazepate dipotassium is similar to that of other benzodiazepines, with drowsiness and dizziness being the most common complaints. The relative toxicity of clorazepate dipotassium versus clonazepam or diazepam in patients with epilepsy has not been established. Special care must be exercised when clorazepate dipotassium is used as an adjunctive drug in combination with phenytoin, barbiturates, and other antiepileptic agents because the side effects of clorazepate and concomitantly administered antiepileptic drugs are similar and additive. Also, clorazepate dipotassium may precipitate personality changes (depression, irritability, aggression) in patients with complex partial seizures, especially those also receiving primidone [22].

Lorazepam (Ativan)

Lorazepam is not an FDA-approved drug for epilepsy. However, oral lorazepam is approved by the FDA for treatment of anxiety, and parenteral lorazepam is approved as a preoperative medication. Intravenous lorazepam is being evaluated for treatment of status epilepticus in the United States.

One hundred and seventy-nine patients with a variety of types of status epilepticus have received intravenous lorazepam in doses ranging from 2.5 to 10 mg [33]. Of these, 75 patients were children, and 104 were adults. Fifty-five patients with generalized tonic-clonic status epilepticus, 65 patients with simple partial status epilepticus, and 59 patients with absence status, myoclonic seizures, or Lennox-Gastaut syndrome have been treated. The rate of success reported in these studies exceeds 90 percent. Complications of therapy include paradoxical activation of tonic seizures, sedation, agitated confusion, tremors, hallucinations, ataxia, and vomiting. Only 1 case of serious (but transient) respiratory depression occurred. Neither permanent impairment nor death has been reported as attributable to lorazepam.

The pharmacokinetic profile of lorazepam appears to be favorable for the treatment of status epilepticus and to offer possible advantages over diazepam. The "distribution phase" fall in serum concentration of lorazepam after intravenous injection lasts approximately 10 minutes and is associated with a fall in serum concentration of approximately 40 percent [25]. By contrast, the distribution phase fall in serum concentration of diazepam lasts approximately 120 minutes and is associated with a fall in serum concentration of

62 to 72 percent (see Chap. 30). These observations probably account for the relatively high incidence of recurrence of status epilepticus 30 to 120 minutes after an injection of diazepam and the high percentage (80%) of long-lasting control of status epilepticus (12 hours or more) with lorazepam in Homan's [32] series.

Perhaps the greatest potential advantage of lorazepam over diazepam lies in the relative safety of intravenous lorazepam. The incidence of serious cardiorespiratory depression appears to be less than 1 percent when intravenous lorazepam is used to manage status epilepticus [33]. These results are quite favorable when compared with those of diazepam, which has a 6 percent incidence of serious cardiorespiratory depression when given intravenously for status epilepticus [13].

Nitrazepam (Mogadon)

Nitrazepam is not presently marketed in the United States but has been available in other countries since 1965. The drug has been reported to be effective against animal models of epilepsy as well as infantile spasms, absence, myoclonic, and atonic seizures in humans [4, 13]. Nitrazepam is currently being evaluated for therapy of infantile spasms in a multicenter trial in the United States, and epilepsy may soon be an FDA-approved indication for the drug.

Oxazepam (Serax)

Oxazepam has been shown to possess antiepileptic properties in animal models of epilepsy and in patients with epilepsy [13]. However, the drug is not currently being tested in the United States for epilepsy, and it is unlikely that it will ever be an FDA-approved drug for epilepsy.

References

1. Alvarez, N., Hartford, E., and Doubt, C. Epileptic seizures induced by clonazepam. *Clin. Electroencephalogr.* 12:57, 1981.
2. Bang, F., Birket-Smith, E., and Mikkelsen, B. Clonazepam in the treatment of epilepsy: A clinical long-term follow-up study. *Epilepsia* 17:321, 1976.
3. Baruzzi, A. et al. Plasma levels of di-n-propylacetate and clonazepam patients. *Int. J. Clin. Pharmacol. Biopharm.* 15:403, 1977.
4. Baruzzi, A., Michelucci, and Tassinari, C. A. Benzodiazepines: Nitrazepam. In D. M. Woodbury, J. K. Penry, and C. E. Pippenger (Eds.), *Antiepileptic Drugs.* New York: Raven Press, 1982.

5. Bensch, J. et al. A double-blind study of clonazepam in the treatment of therapy-resistant epilepsy in children. *Dev. Med. Child. Neurol.* 19:335, 1977.
6. Benzodiazepine anticonvulsant. *Arch. Neurol.* 33:731, 1976.
7. Berlin, A., and Dahlstrom, H. Pharmacokinetics of the anticonvulsant drug clonazepam evaluated from single oral and intravenous doses and by repeated oral administration. *Eur. J. Clin. Pharmacol.* 9:155, 1975.
8. Birket-Smith, E. et al. A controlled trial of Ro5-4023 (clonazepam) in the treatment of psychomotor epilepsy. *Acta Neurol. Scand. [Suppl.]* 53:18, 1973.
9. Booker, H. E. Clorazepate dipotassium in the treatment of intractable epilepsy. *J.A.M.A.* 229:552, 1974.
10. Booker, H. E., and Celesia, G. G. Serum concentration of diazepam in subjects with epilepsy. *Arch. Neurol.* 29:191, 1973.
11. Browne, T. R. Clonazepam: A review of a new anticonvulsant drug. *Arch. Neurol.* 33:326, 1976.
12. Browne, T. R. Medical intelligence: Clonazepam. *N. Engl. J. Med.* 299:812, 1978.
13. Browne, T. R., and Penry, J. K. Benzodiazepines in the treatment of epilepsy: A review. *Epilepsia* 14:277, 1973.
14. Cano, J. P. et al. Determination of flunitrazepam, desmethylflunitrazepam, and clonazepam in plasma by gas liquid chromatography with an internal standard. *Arzneim. Forsch.* 27:338, 1977.
15. Carson, M. J., and Gilden, C. Treatment of minor motor seizures with clonazepam. *Dev. Med. Child. Neurol.* 17:306, 1975.
16. Chadwick, D. et al. Functional changes in cerebral 5-hydroxytryptamine metabolism in the mouse induced by anticonvulsant drugs. *Br. J. Pharmacol.* 62:115, 1978.
17. Chandra, B. Clonazepam in the treatment of petit mal. *Asian J. Med.* 9:433, 1973.
18. Cohn, P. D. Personal communication, 1976.
19. Costa, E. et al. New concepts on the mechanism of action of benzodiazepines. *Life Sci.* 17:167, 1975.
20. D'Onghia, C. et al. Estudio clinico do Ro5-4023 no tratments de epilepsias. *Arq. Neuropsiquiatr.* 31:21, 1973.
21. Dreifuss, F. E., and Satos, S. Benzodiazepines: Clonazepam. In D. M. Woodbury, J. K. Penry, and C. E. Pippenger (Eds.), *Antiepileptic Drugs.* New York: Raven Press, 1982.
22. Feldman, R. G. Clorazepate in temporal lobe epilepsy. *J.A.M.A.* 236:2603, 1976.
23. Feldman, R. G., Hayes, M. K., and Browne, T. R. A
double-blind comparison of clonazepam with placebo for refractory tonic-clonic seizures. *Neurology* (N.Y.) 31:159, 1981.
24. Gallagher, D. Neurophysiology of Benzodiazepines: GABA-Benzodiazepine Unit. In S. Paul et al. (Eds.), *The Pharmacology of Benzodiazepines.* London: Macmillan. In press, 1983.
25. Greenblatt, D. J. et al. Clinical pharmacokinetics of lorazepam: III. Intravenous injection: Preliminary results. *J. Clin. Pharmacol.* 17:450, 1977.
26. Greenblatt, D. J., and Shader, I. *Benzodiazepines in Clinical Practice.* New York: Raven Press, 1974.
27. Gregoriades, A. D., and Frangos, E. G. Clinical Observations on Clonazepam in Intractable Epilepsy. In J. K. Penry (Ed.), *Epilepsy: The Eighth International Symposium.* New York: Raven Press, 1977.
28. Haefley, W. Benzodiazepines and GABA: Summary and Commentary. In S. Paul et al. (Eds.), *The Pharmacology of Benzodiazepines.* London: Macmillan. In press, 1983.
29. Haefley, W. Neurophysiology of Benzodiazepines: Summary. In S. Paul et al. (Eds.), *The Pharmacology of Benzodiazepines.* London: Macmillan. In press, 1983.
30. Hanson, R. A., and Menkes, J. H. A new anticonvulsant in the management of minor motor seizures. *Dev. Med. Child. Neurol.* 14:3, 1972.
31. Hara, T., Inani, M., and Kaneko, T. The Effect of Clonazepam on Plasma Diphenylhydantoin Level in Epileptic Patients. In D. Janz (Ed.), *Epileptology: Proceedings of the Seventh International Symposium on Epilepsy.* Stuttgart: Thieme, 1976.
32. Homan, R. W. Dose-effect relationships for single dose intravenous lorazepam in the treatment of status epilepticus. Presented at the Veterans Administration Epilepsy Center Workshop, Durham, N. C., March 31, 1978.
33. Homan, R. W. Lorazepam for Status Epilepticus. In A. V. Delgado-Escueta et al. (Eds.), *Status Epilepticus: Mechanisms of Brain Damage and Treatment.* New York: Raven Press, 1982.
34. Hvidberg, E. F., and Sjo, O. Clinical Pharmacokinetic Experiences With Clonazepam. In H. Schneider (Ed.), *Clinical Pharmacology of Antiepileptic Drugs.* Berlin: Springer, 1975. Pp. 242–246.
35. Iivanainen, M., and Himberg, J. J. Valproate and clonazepam in the treatment of severe progressive myoclonus epilepsy. *Arch. Neurol.* 39:236, 1982.
36. Johannessen, S. I., Strandjord, R. E., and Munthe-Kaas, A. W. Lack of effect of clonazepam on serum

levels of diphenylhydantoin, phenobarbital and carbamazepine. *Acta Neurol. Scand.* 55:506, 1977.

37. Knop, H. J., van der Kleijn, E., and Edmunds, L. C. Pharmacokinetics of Clonazepam in Man and Laboratory Animals. In H. Schneider (Ed.), *Clinical Pharmacology of Antiepileptic Drugs.* Berlin: Springer, 1975.

38. Lance, J. W., and Anthony, M. Sodium valproate and clonazepam in the treatment of intractable epilepsy. *Arch. Neurol.* 34:14, 1977.

39. Masland, R. L. A controlled trial of clonazepam in temporal lobe epilepsy. *Acta Neurol. Scand. [Suppl.]* 60:49, 1975.

40. Mikkelsen, B. et al. Clonazepam (Rivotril®) and carbamazepine (Tegretol®) in psychomotor epilepsy: A randomized multicenter trial. *Epilepsia* 22:415, 1981.

41. Mikkelsen, B. et al. Clonazepam in the treatment of epilepsy: A controlled clinical trial in simple absences, bilateral massive epileptic myoclonus, and atonic seizures. *Arch. Neurol.* 33:322, 1976.

42. Mikkelsen, B. et al. A controlled trial of clonazepam (Ro 5-4023, Rivotril®) in the treatment of focal epilepsy and secondarily generalized grand mal epilepsy. *Acta Neurol. Scand. [Suppl.]* 60:55, 1975.

43. Milligan, N. et al. Absorption of diazepam from the rectum and its effect on interictal spikes in the EEG. *Epilepsia* 23:323, 1982.

44. Min, B. H., and Garland, W. A. Determination of clonazepam and its 7-amino metabolite in plasma and blood by gas chromatography-chemical ionization mass spectrometry. *J. Chromatogr.* 139:121, 1977.

45. Muller, W., and Wollert, U. Characterization of binding of benzodiazepines to human serum albumin. *Naunyn-Schmiedebergs Arch. Pharmacol.* 280:229, 1973.

46. Nanda, R. N. et al. Treatment of epilepsy with clonazepam and its effect on other anticonvulsants. *J. Neurol. Neurosurg. Psychiatry* 40:538, 1977.

47. O'Donohoe, N. V., and Paes, B. A. A Trial of Clonazepam in the Treatment of Severe Epilepsy in Infancy and Childhood. In J. K. Penry (Ed.), *Epilepsy: The Eighth International Symposium.* New York: Raven Press,

48. Oller-Daurella, L. Resultados obtenidos con nuevos derivados benzodiazepinicos en el tratamento la epilepsia. *Ciencias Neurol.* 3:3, 1969.

49. Olsen, R., and Leeb-Lundberg, F. Convulsant and Anticonvulsant Drug Binding Sites Regulated to GABA-Regulated Chloride Ion Channels. In E.

Costa, G. Di Chiara, and G. L. Gessa (Eds.), *GABA and Benzodiazepine Receptors.* New York: Raven Press, 1981.

50. Parry, G. J. Concentration of clonazepam in serum and cerebrospinal fluid of the sheep. *Pharmacology* 15:318, 1977.

51. Perchalski, R. J., and Wilder, B. J. Determination of benzodiazepine anticonvulsants in plasma by high-performance liquid chromatography. *Anal. Chem.* 50:554, 1978.

52. Phillis, J. Neurophysiology of Benzodiazepines: Benzodiazepines and Adenosine. In S. Paul et al. (Eds.), *The Pharmacology of Benzodiazepines.* London: Macmillan. In press, 1983.

53. Roussounis, S. H., and de Rudolf, N. Clonazepam in the treatment of children with intractable seizures. *Dev. Med. Child. Neurol.* 19:326, 1977.

54. Sato, S. et al. Clonazepam in the treatment of absence seizures: A double-blind clinical trial. *Neurology* (Minneap.) 27:371, 1977.

55. Schlack, H. G. Erfahrungen mit Clonazepam (Ro 5-4023) in der Therapie kindlicher Epilepsien. *Fortschr. Med.* 92:1176, 1974.

56. Schmidt, D. Benzodiazepines: Diazepam. In D. M. Woodbury, J. K. Penry, and C. E. Pippenger (Eds.), *Antiepileptic Drugs.* New York: Raven Press, 1982.

57. Shakir, R. A. et al. Comparison of sodium valproate (Epilim®) and clonazepam (Rivatril®) in intractable epilepsy. In J. K. Penry (Ed.), *Epilepsy: The Eighth International Symposium.* New York: Raven Press, 1977.

58. Sjo, O. et al. Pharmacokinetics and side-effects of clonazepam and its 7-amino-metabolite in man. *Eur. J. Clin. Pharmacol.* 8:249, 1975.

59. Skolnick, P., Marangons, P., and Paul, S. Benzodiazepine Receptors and Their Endogenous Ligand(s): Regulation and Role in Seizures. In A. V. Delgado-Escueta et al. (Eds.), *Status Epilepticus: Mechanisms of Brain Damage and Treatment.* New York: Raven Press, 1982.

60. Snyder, S. H. Opiate and benzodiazepine receptors. *Psychosomatics* 22:986, 1981.

61. Syz, T., and Spieler, U. Clinical Experience With Clonazepam in the Treatment of Post-traumatic Epilepsy. In J. K. Penry (Ed.), *Epilepsy: The Eighth International Symposium.* New York: Raven Press, 1977.

62. Tallman, J. F. et al. Receptors for the age of anxiety: Pharmacology of the benzodiazepines. *Science* 207:274, 1980.

63. Troupin, A. S. et al. Evaluation of clorazepate (Tranxene®) as an anticonvulsant: A pilot study. *Neurology* (Minneap.) 27:376, 1977.

64. Weiner, W. J. et al. Clonazepam and dopamine-related stereotyped behavior. *Life Sci.* 21:901, 1977.

65. Wilensky, A. J. et al. Clorazepate and pheno-barbital as antiepileptic drugs: A double blind study. *Neurology* (N.Y.) 31:1271, 1981.

66. Wilensky, A. J. et al. Clorazepate kinetics in treated epileptics. *Clin. Pharmacol. Ther.* 24:22, 1978.

PARALDEHYDE, ACETAZOLAMIDE, TRIMETHADIONE, PARAMETHADIONE, AND PHENACEMIDE

22

Thomas R. Browne

Paraldehyde, acetazolamide, trimethadione, paramethadione, and phenacemide are less commonly used antiepileptic drugs. Paraldehyde is sometimes useful as an adjunctive therapy, and in certain selected patients as a primary therapy, for status epilepticus. Acetazolamide is seldom used because its antiepileptic effect is often short-lived. Trimethadione, paramethadione, and phenacemide are seldom used because they are more likely to produce toxic side effects compared with other available agents. Each of these drugs is occasionally useful in selected patients.

Paraldehyde

CHEMISTRY

General Properties
Paraldehyde (PA) is a cyclic polymer of acetaldehyde (Fig. 22-1). It is a colorless liquid with a strong aromatic odor and a burning, disagreeable taste. It is miscible with oils and has a molecular weight of 132.16.

Water Solubility
The water solubility of PA is greatest (12.8%) at 12°C and decreases as the temperature rises above or falls below this point. At 37°C the water solubility of PA is 7.8 percent. Unawareness of these crucial facts has led to the practice of injecting PA intravenously in its pure form or as a 10 percent solution. In either case, the solubility of PA at 37°C would be exceeded, and droplets of pure PA may form in the bloodstream, resulting in pulmonary embolization (see below).

Decomposition
PA has a slight tendency to depolymerize back to acetaldehyde. In the presence of air, acetaldehyde oxidizes to acetic acid, which then acts as a catalyst for further depolymerization of PA to acetaldehyde. Improper storage of PA has resulted in some samples containing 40 to 98 percent acetic acid [36], and as little as 7 ml of such decomposed PA has proved fatal

This work was supported in part by the Veterans Administration.

248

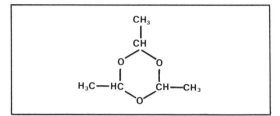

Figure 22-1. Structural formula of paraldehyde.

[2]. A survey of 42 PA samples collected from hospital wards in 1957 revealed that only 11 percent met USP standards [36].

Storage
In 1965 USP specifications were altered to state that PA must be preserved "in well-filled, tight, light-resistant containers...not exceeding 30 ml" and that "the user...discard the unused contents of any container that has been opened more than 24 hours." Such procedures should reduce (but may not completely eliminate) the hazards of decomposed PA.

Methods of Determination
Methods reported for determining the concentration of PA in biologic fluids include gas-liquid chromatography [35], enzymatic analysis [59], spectrophotometry [36], and dichromate titration.

MECHANISM OF ACTION
The mechanism of action of PA is unknown.

CLINICAL PHARMACOLOGY
Absorption
The times to peak plasma concentration of PA by various routes are as follows: IV route, immediately after infusion [29]; IM route, 20 to 60 minutes [59]; oral route (in water), 30 minutes [3]; oral route (in olive oil), 2 to 4 hours [28]; rectal route, 2 to 4 hours [3, 28].

Distribution
PA is rapidly distributed to the brain. Following an intravenous injection, drowsiness ensues within 2 to 5 seconds, and anesthesia occurs within less than 2 minutes [3, 29, 54]. The steady state volume of distribution of PA is 890 ml/kg [3]. PA readily crosses the placental barrier and may cause delayed respirations in neonates.

Biotransformation and Excretion
Seventy to 80 percent of PA is metabolized by the liver, 20 to 30 percent is exhaled by the lungs, and a very small amount is excreted unchanged by the kidney [4]. In patients with liver disease the rate of elimination of PA and the percentage of PA eliminated by the liver decrease, and the percentage of PA eliminated by the lungs increases.

On the basis of indirect evidence it has been widely assumed that PA is depolymerized to acetaldehyde by the liver and that acetaldehyde is then oxidized to acetic acid, which is ultimately metabolized to carbon dioxide and water. Gessner [30] has recently cited indirect evidence that acetaldehyde may not be formed from PA in vivo.

Elimination Half-Life
The elimination half-life of PA is 3.4 to 9.8 (mean, 6.1 to 7.4) hours [3, 59]. The plasma disposition kinetics of PA fit an open two-compartment model after intravenous injection [3].

Plasma Concentration Data
The minimum plasma concentration of PA necessary to control status epilepticus is 300 μg/ml [35]. Plasma concentrations of 120 to 330 μg/ml produce anesthesia [28]. The minimum lethal plasma concentration of PA is 500 μg/ml [36].

Dosage and Administration
This topic is discussed in Chapter 30.

INDICATIONS

Status Epilepticus
PA can be useful as an adjunctive therapy in some patients with status epilepticus and may be the drug of choice for status epilepticus in a few special situations (see Chaps. 26 and 30).

Alcohol Withdrawal Syndrome and Delirium Tremens
There is abundant evidence that PA is effective as a primary therapy for alcohol withdrawal syndrome and for delirium tremens [10, 30].

Other Indications
PA is now seldom used as a hypnotic, as an anesthetic agent, or for treatment of intractable pain because of the availability of safer agents.

TOXICITY

History
Since PA was introduced in 1882, there have been at least 95 reports of death associated with its use [4, 36]. These reports have led to widespread disrepute and infrequent use of PA. However, many (probably most)

of these deaths were due to one of the following factors: (1) suicidal overdosage, (2) use of decomposed drug, (3) use of doses larger than those currently recommended, and (4) use of improperly diluted PA. The incidence of death and serious side effects with USP-quality PA at recommended doses and following recommended administration procedures is unknown but probably is less than is generally supposed.

Overdosage
Overdosage with PA produces coma, right heart failure, and pulmonary edema and hemorrhages [11, 30].

Side Effects by Any Route
PA administered by any route may cause disagreeable breath odor (from exhaled PA), right heart failure, and pulmonary edema and hemorrhage (especially if the drug is used in excessive dosage) [4, 11, 56], rash, irritability, toxic hepatitis, or toxic nephritis. Chronic use of PA may produce a metabolic acidosis [36]. Chronic PA use may produce tolerance and/or physical dependence with a withdrawal syndrome similar to that seen with alcohol withdrawal [36].

Intravenous Route
Three series [5, 29, 54] (totalling 181 patients) in which intravenous PA was used as an anesthetic agent report no serious complications, although many patients experienced coughing, choking, pharyngeal irritation, tachycardia, or pain at the site of infusion. On the other hand, there are case reports of intravenous PA suddenly producing apnea, coughing, cyanosis, hypotension, and clinical and radiographic signs of pulmonary edema [56]. All the above studies involved injection of undiluted or 10 percent solutions of PA, and thus failed to properly dilute PA so that it would remain soluble after intravenous injection (see above). Gessner [30] postulates that the above-cited pulmonary-cardiac complications were the result of pulmonary embolism of precipitated droplets of pure PA in the bloodstream due to improper dilution, and cites two studies [3] in which properly diluted PA (4 to 8% solution) was administered intravenously without complications.

Oral and Rectal Routes
PA can cause irritation and corrosion of the mouth and stomach when given orally and of the rectum and large intestine when given rectally [1]. Rectal administration of decomposed PA has resulted in perforation of the large intestine [1]. The drug should be properly diluted before administration by these routes.

Intramuscular Route
Severe and permanent sciatic nerve damage may result if PA is injected too close to the nerve [36]. Skin sloughing and sterile abscesses have also been caused by intramuscular PA [36].

Decomposed PA
Decomposed PA may contain very high concentrations of acetic acid. Acetic acid is a highly toxic substance, and PA containing acetic acid appears to be considerably more toxic than USP-quality PA [1, 2, 36].

Acetazolamide

CHEMISTRY
Acetazolamide (5-acetamido-1,3,4-thiadiazole-2-sulfonamide; Diamox) is an unsubstituted sulfonamide (Fig. 22-2). The drug inhibits the enzyme carbonic anhydrase in the brain and other tissues, accounting for its antiepileptic properties and side effects.

MECHANISM OF ACTION
Carbonic anhydrase is the enzyme responsible for the synthesis of bicarbonate from carbon dioxide and water. Carbonic anhydrase bound to membranes of glial cells controls extracellular concentrations of bicarbonate in the brain. Because bicarbonate exchanges for chloride, an increase in extracellular bicarbonate results in a decrease in extracellular chloride. This in turn leads to a decreased transneuronal chloride gradient, decreased chloride current, and reduced inhibition. Conversely, carbonic anhydrase inhibitors result in an increased transneuronal chloride gradient, increased chloride current, and increased inhibition (see Chap. 2).

Unlike many other antiepileptic drugs that are effective against absence seizures, acetazolamide does not protect against pentylenetetrazol seizures in mice [47, 68], suggesting that acetazolamide may work by mechanisms that are different from those for ethosuximide.

CLINICAL PHARMACOLOGY
Absorption
Acetazolamide is a weak acid with a pK_a of 7.4 [68]. It is present in gastric juice predominantly in the nonionized form. Because this form is adequately soluble in gastric juice, some absorption takes place in the stomach. However, absorption occurs mainly in the duodenum and upper jejunum where the surface area is larger, the pH higher, and the water solubility of the drug greater.

Peak plasma concentrations are reached 2 to 3 hours after administration of an oral dose [68]. Oral doses

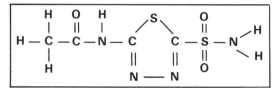

Figure 22-2. Structural formula of acetazolamide.

in the range of 5 to 10 mg/kg appear to be completely absorbed [45]. At higher doses absorption is erratic, resulting in variable plasma concentrations [46].

Distribution

Acetazolamide is 83 to 95 percent protein bound in humans [45, 46, 68]. The extent of protein binding decreases with increasing plasma acetazolamide concentration, indicating saturation of the protein-binding sites [46, 68].

The disappearance of acetazolamide from the plasma has two phases, an initial rapid phase followed by a later slow phase [68]. The rapid component represents movement of unbound acetazolamide into the total body water [46]. After penetrating cells, the drug binds to the carbonic anhydrase present in tissues. The slow component of plasma decay represents the slow dissociation of acetazolamide from carbonic anhydrase in tissues and the renal excretion of the drug [68]. The largest concentrations of acetazolamide are found in erythrocytes, kidney, and stomach, which contain very high concentrations of carbonic anhydrase. The volume of distribution of acetazolamide is 1.8 liter/kg, indicating binding to tissues even during the early phase of distribution [46, 68].

The concentration of acetazolamide in CSF is lower than the free level in plasma [46, 68]. This suggests removal of the drug by either bulk flow or active secretion out of the CSF across the choroid plexus [68].

The concentration of acetazolamide in the brain is higher than the free plasma concentration of the drug [68]. This is to be expected because glial cells contain carbonic anhydrase.

Biotransformation and Excretion

Acetazolamide is secreted by renal tubular cells into the urine completely unchanged [43, 68]. There is no evidence that the drug is metabolized by the liver [43, 68].

Clinical Pharmacokinetics

The half-life of the initial rapid distribution phase of acetazolamide is 95 minutes [46]. The half-life of the slower elimination phase is 10 to 15 hours [68]. The plasma concentration of acetazolamide associated with good antiepileptic effect is 10 to 14 μg/ml [68].

Drug Interactions

Because acetazolamide is not metabolized by the liver, its level cannot be affected by drugs that either induce or inhibit the drug-metabolizing enzymes in the liver [68]. Because acetazolamide is 90 percent protein bound, it is likely (but not proven) that many drugs bound to the same proteins can compete with this drug for binding sites [68]. Acetazolamide is actively excreted into the bile. Drugs that decrease or increase bile flow or inhibit the transport of weak acids into the bile could theoretically alter the plasma concentration of acetazolamide, although such an effect has not been reported in humans [68]. Acetazolamide alters the absorption of certain drugs from the small intestine of experimental animals by inhibiting carbonic anhydrase in the gut wall [55], and such an interaction could also occur in humans.

In rats, acetazolamide has been shown to enhance the degree of CNS depression produced by pentobarbital [53], to increase the duration of pentobarbital-induced sleep time, and to increase the brain pentobarbital space [52]. This last effect probably results from the ability of acetazolamide to decrease CSF flow, thereby decreasing the bulk removal of pentobarbital from the brain [68]. It is likely that this effect occurs in humans for sedative and antiepileptic drugs [68].

Acetazolamide influences the activity of other drugs because of the many effects in the body that result from the inhibition of carbonic anhydrase: alkalinization of urine, saluresis, systemic acidosis, inhibition of CSF production, and decreased secretion of ocular fluids [68]. These effects can alter the penetration of other drugs into fluids and tissues.

Acetazolamide tends to increase the concentration of weak acids in tissues [68]. Because most antiepileptic drugs are weak acids, this tendency results in higher brain levels of the antiepileptic drug with lower doses. This effect provides a partial rationale for using acetazolamide as an adjunctive drug in combination with other antiepileptic drugs in patients with refractory epilepsy.

Dosage and Administration

The usual daily dose of acetazolamide is 10 to 20 mg/kg in three divided doses [68]. Doses higher than 20 mg/kg/day are unnecessary because inhibition of brain carbonic anhydrase is complete at this dosage [68]. When acetazolamide is given in combination with other antiepileptic drugs, the starting dose should be only 250 mg once daily to minimize the tendency of acetazolamide to enhance the sedative and other side effects of other antiepileptic drugs. The dosage of acetazolamide can then be increased as tolerated.

INDICATIONS

The best results with acetazolamide have been obtained in the treatment of absence seizures. The drug is also sometimes useful, principally as an adjunct, in the management of tonic-clonic, myoclonic, and atonic seizures.

Absence Seizures

Several large but uncontrolled studies have shown that acetazolamide is effective as a primary or adjunctive drug for the treatment of absence seizures [16, 37, 42, 48, 68]. Unfortunately, the antiepileptic effect of acetazolamide is often transient, disappearing after 3 months to 2 years of therapy [37, 42, 68]. For this reason, acetazolamide is seldom used as a primary therapy for absence seizures. However, because of its low toxicity and possibly different mechanism of action from other antiabsence drugs, acetazolamide is a worthwhile drug to try when more consistently effective antiabsence drugs (e.g., ethosuximide) have failed.

The use of intravenous acetazolamide for absence status epilepticus is reviewed in Chapter 30.

Tonic-Clonic Seizures

The majority of patients with tonic-clonic seizures initially respond well to this drug [16, 37, 42, 68]. However, as with absence seizures, the therapeutic effect is short-lived [37, 42, 68].

Myoclonic and Atonic Seizures

Only a minority of patients with myoclonic and atonic seizures have a good response to acetazolamide, and the response usually disappears within 1 year of initiation of therapy [16, 42].

Simple and Complex Partial Seizures

Simple and complex partial seizures seldom respond to acetazolamide [16, 42].

TOXICITY

Very large doses of acetazolamide can be tolerated by most patients without important side effects [68]. Approximately 10 percent of patients experience side effects, usually mild, while on acetazolamide [48]. The usual effects of systemic inhibition of carbonic anhydrase have been reviewed above (see under Clinical

Pharmacology—Drug Interactions). Subjective side effects, possibly dose-related, are not uncommon and include drowsiness, paresthesias, loss of appetite, and confusion [16, 48]. As with any sulfonamide, hypersensitivity reactions are possible (fever, rash, thrombocytopenia, leukopenia, hemolytic anemia, and agranulocytosis) [16, 42, 48]. Calculus formation and ureteral colic have been attributed to the marked reduction in urinary citrate produced by acetazolamide [42, 68]. In patients with hepatic cirrhosis, acetazolamide may produce episodes of disorientation, perhaps by interference with renal removal of ammonia [68].

Other occasional side effects of acetazolamide include abdominal distention, polyuria, transient myopia, melena, hematuria, glycosuria, hepatic insufficiency, flaccid paralysis, and convulsions [16].

Studies in rodents have demonstrated teratogenic and embryocidal effects from acetazolamide at high doses [44]. The drug should not be used in pregnancy unless the benefits to be expected outweigh these potential adverse effects.

Trimethadione

CHEMISTRY

Trimethadione (3,5,5-trimethyl 2-4-oxazolidinedione; Tridione; TMO) is an oxazolidinedione with a ring structure similar to that of other classes of antiepileptic drugs (Fig. 22-3). Several other oxazolidinediones also possess antiepileptic properties (Fig. 22-3). Dimethadione (DMO) is of interest because it is the major, and perhaps the only, metabolite of TMO [23]. TMO is a white crystalline powder with a molecular weight of 143.15 [23]. TMO is readily soluble in aqueous and organic solvents [23]. Gas chromatographic methods are available for detection of TMO in plasma [23].

MECHANISM OF ACTION

TMO, like many other antiepileptic drugs, has a heterocyclic (oxazolidinedione) ring with substitutions at various ring sites (Fig. 22-3). As is true with other classes of antiepileptic drugs, substitution of alkyl groups on the oxazolidinedione ring results in efficacy against absence seizures, and phenyl ring substitutions confer the ability to protect against tonic-clonic seizures [23, 47, 58, 67].

TMO, a heterocyclic ring with alkyl substitutions, has a structure similar to that of ethosuximide (see Chap. 19). The mechanism of action of both drugs is unknown but may involve inhibition of paroxysmal activity in the cortical and subcortical inhibitory pathways [26, 67].

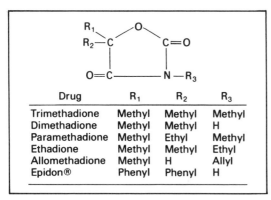

Drug	R_1	R_2	R_3
Trimethadione	Methyl	Methyl	Methyl
Dimethadione	Methyl	Methyl	H
Paramethadione	Methyl	Ethyl	Methyl
Ethadione	Methyl	Methyl	Ethyl
Allomethadione	Methyl	H	Allyl
Epidon®	Phenyl	Phenyl	H

Figure 22-3. Structural formulas of axazolidine-2, 4-diones. (From H. E. Booker [6].)

CLINICAL PHARMACOLOGY

Absorption
TMO is rapidly absorbed by the oral route. Peak plasma TMO concentrations occur 30 minutes after oral administration [7, 8, 64].

Distribution
Neither TMO nor DMO bind to serum proteins [23, 64]. TMO is distributed to the total body water in humans [7, 64], and, in animals, has highest concentrations in brain, kidney, muscle, and liver [64]. Animal work indicates that DMO is rapidly distributed to but not bound by the various body tissues and has a volume of distribution somewhere between extracellular water and total body water volume [64].

Biotransformation and Excretion
TMO is quantitatively demethylated to DMO by hepatic microsomes [12, 25, 65]. DMO is the only important metabolic product of TMO [65] and does not undergo further metabolic change. Of an administered dose of TMO, 96 to 99 percent is excreted in the urine as DMO [7, 61, 64]. TMO and DMO have approximately equal antiepileptic properties [7, 15, 24, 63]. Because TMO is rapidly metabolized to DMO, which is slowly excreted by the kidneys, DMO is the major antiepileptic drug present in the plasma of patients on chronic oral TMO therapy. The ratio of TMO to DMO in the plasma during chronic oral TMO therapy is approximately 1 to 20 [7, 8].

Clinical Pharmacokinetics
The elimination half-life of TMO is approximately 16 hours [7, 8, 25]. DMO is excreted very slowly, with an elimination half-life of approximately 10 days or more [8, 13, 25, 38].

The very slow elimination of DMO has three clinical consequences. First, the time for buildup to steady state DMO level is 30 days or more, and therefore it takes many days before the full therapeutic (and toxic) effects of a given dose of TMO are realized [15, 33, 64]. Second, cessation of TMO therapy does not result in an immediate drop in DMO plasma concentration or in an immediate increase in seizure frequency [33]. Third, DMO plasma levels vary very little during the day, whereas plasma levels of TMO (which is more rapidly eliminated) vary by 30 percent between peak and trough values on a tid or qid regimen [8].

Several studies indicate that 700 μg/ml is the lower limit of the therapeutic range for plasma DMO level [6, 15, 38]. The majority of patients with absence seizures who have DMO levels of above 700 μg/ml have good control of seizures, whereas most patients with DMO levels of below 700 μg/ml do not.

Drug Interactions
Although TMO and DMO have been in clinical use for many years, reports of interactions with other drugs are scarce [66]. The following animal data may have some clinical relevance: (1) TMO and metharbital interfere with demethylation of each other by liver microsomes; (2) DMO inhibits demethylation of TMO and metharbital; (3) drugs causing a distortion of acid-base balance (e.g., NH_4Cl, acetazolamide, and $NaHCO_3$) can affect the distribution or excretion of DMO (a weak acid); (4) TMO does not induce liver enzymes.

Dosage and Administration
The usual starting daily dose is 0.9 g in adults and 0.3 g in children in three or four divided doses. Because of the long elimination half-life of DMO, adequate plasma concentrations should be maintained with doses given once daily, although such a regimen has not been systematically studied to determine the blood levels and side effects of once-daily administration. The dosage of TMO may be increased at weekly intervals by 150 mg/day in children and 300 mg/day in adults. Maintenance dosage should be the least amount of drug required to maintain adequate seizure control. An oral solution form is available for children.

INDICATIONS
TMO is indicated for control of absence seizures that are refractory to less toxic drugs (i.e., ethosuximide, valproic acid, clonazepam, and acetazolamide). Millichap and Aymat [48] collected 431 reported cases of absence seizures treated with TMO from the literature. The absence seizures were reduced in frequency by

75 percent or more in 56 percent of cases and were completely controlled in 18 percent of cases. Coatsworth's review [17] showed similar results. The drug thus possesses considerable antiabsence activity. A trial of TMO may be indicated when absence seizures are not controlled with less toxic drugs and when the potential benefits of TMO outweigh the potential risks (see below—Toxicity). TMO is also sometimes effective for treating the refractory atypical absence, myoclonic, and atonic seizures of the Lennox-Gastaut syndrome [40].

TOXICITY

Hematologic Side Effects
Hematologic side effects are the most frequent and troublesome serious side effects of TMO [27, 62]. Three classes of adverse hematologic responses to TMO have been identified—modified normal response, controlled neutropenia, and pancytopenia [27]. More than 3,000 neutrophils per cu mm constitutes a modified normal response, whereas less than this number is called a controlled neutropenia. The incidence of controlled neutropenia in association with TMO therapy is about 20 percent [19, 62]. Unfortunately, the peripheral blood count is not an accurate reflection of changes in the bone marrow, and agranulocytosis may be established in the bone marrow well before the peripheral count is altered [22]. There are at least 19 reported cases of pancytopenia in association with TMO therapy, and 13 ended fatally [62]. The earliest change in the peripheral blood is a decrease in megakaryocytes, followed by a reduction in the number of platelets; this in turn is followed by a prolonged clot retraction time [22]. Frequent examinations of peripheral blood including megakaryocytes and platelets as well as measurements of clot retraction time are essential in patients taking TMO.

A possible relationship between TMO and lymphadenopathy or tumors of blood-forming organs has been discussed elsewhere [27]. Firm proof of such a relationship has not been established [27].

Hemeralopia
Hemeralopia (day blindness) is a phenomenon in which visual acuity is normal in low illumination but decreased when illumination is normal or brighter than normal. This is thought to be a retinal phenomenon in which the neuronal elements of cones (but not photochemical elements) are affected [57]. There are no external or opthalmoscopic changes [40]. Detailed study reveals that TMO greatly prolongs the time of visual acuity adaptation when illumination changes from low to high or from high to low illumination

[57]. In most patients visual acuity becomes normal after adaptation is complete [57]. Hemeralopia occurs in 30 percent of patients taking TMO [39, 62] and disappears 1 to 10 weeks after TMO is discontinued [27, 39].

Dermatologic Side Effects
Dermatologic side effects include rash, erythema multiforme, and exfoliative dermatitis (including 1 fatal case) [27, 62] and occur in 9 to 14 percent of patients taking TMO [39, 62]. These disorders usually occur early in the course of TMO therapy and may be more frequent in children under the age of 10 years [39]. The more severe dermatologic reactions are rare and are generally nonfatal [27].

CNS Side Effects
Drowsiness occurs in 3 to 6 percent of patients on TMO [39, 62] but often subsides as tolerance to the drug develops [27]. Behavioral disturbances occur in 4 to 8 percent of patients on TMO [39, 62]. Other CNS side effects may include malaise, insomnia, vertigo, headache, paresthesias, and hiccups [27, 39, 62].

Increase in Tonic-Clonic Seizure Frequency
Increased frequency of tonic-clonic seizures has been reported by some workers [39] and denied by others [21, 50].

Gastrointestinal Side Effects
Nausea, vomiting, abdominal pain, or gastric distress occurs in 7 to 8 percent of patients on TMO [39, 62].

Nephrotic Syndrome
At least 9 cases of nephrotic syndrome (albuminuria, decreased serum albumin, hypercholesterolemia) in association with TMO therapy have been reported [27, 62]. Two of these cases ended fatally [62].

Other Side Effects
Myasthenic syndrome, hepatitis, lupus erythematosus, hiccups, anorexia, hair loss, changes in blood pressure, photophobia, and diplopia have been reported to accompany TMO therapy [9, 27].

Teratogenicity and "Fetal Trimethadione Syndrome"
There are numerous reports of fetal malformations in association with TMO therapy [9, 32, 49]. A recent collaborative study reported malformations in 18 of 61 children born to mothers who had taken TMO during the first trimester [49]. In some children a characteristic set of findings has been termed the "fetal trimethadione syndrome" [9, 32]. Malformed or low-set

ears, cleft lip and palate, delayed mental development, speech impairment, urogenital malformations, V-shaped eyebrows, irregular teeth, skeletal malformations, and cardiac defects are the common features [9, 32]. Less common features of the fetal trimethadione syndrome include intrauterine growth retardation, short stature, microcephaly, ocular anomalies, and simian creases [32]. In addition, the spontaneous abortion rate is high [9]. Although the mother was taking other drugs in most of these cases, the evidence suggesting TMO teratogenesis is so strong that TMO should be given during pregnancy only if the potential benefits are great enough to outweigh the considerable potential risks.

Paramethadione

Paramethadione (Paradione, PMO) is structurally similar to TMO, differing only by the substitution of an ethyl group for a methyl group (Fig. 22-3). It is therefore not surprising that the clinical pharmacology, metabolism, dosage, indications, and toxicity of PMO are very similar to those described for TMO [51, 64, 65, 66]. PMO is less widely used than TMO because PMO is less consistently effective against absence seizures [20]. However, the incidence of serious side effects may be less with PMO than with TMO [20, 40]. Perhaps most important, systemic toxicity from one drug does not necessarily carry over to the other, so that either may serve as an alternative medication without cross-sensitivity [51].

Phenacemide

CHEMISTRY
Phenacemide (phenylacetylurea, phenacetylcarbamide, Phenurone, PAC) is a straight chain analog of 5-phenylhydantoin (Fig. 22-4).

MECHANISM OF ACTION
In experimental models of epilepsy, PAC elevates the seizure threshold for minimal electroshock, maximal electroshock, and pentylenetetrazol seizures [47, 51, 58]. In fact, PAC has higher protective indexes against minimal electroshock seizures (a model of complex partial seizures) and maximal electroshock seizures (a model of tonic-clonic seizures) than either phenytoin or phenobarbital [58]. The mechanisms of action of PAC are probably similar to those of phenytoin owing to the similar structural and three-dimensional conformation of PAC and phenytoin [14, 51] (see Chap. 16).

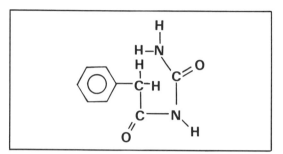

Figure 22-4. Structural formula of phenacemide.

CLINICAL PHARMACOLOGY

Absorption, Distribution, Biotransformation, and Excretion
PAC is well absorbed from the intestine and has a duration of action of many hours [51]. It is degraded ultimately into inactive products by the liver, particularly by para hydroxylation of the phenyl group [51]. Ring closure to form hydantoin does not occur [51]. Unchanged PAC is not found in the urine [51].

Dosage and Administration
For adults the usual starting dose of PAC is 1500 mg/day in three divided doses. The daily dosage may be increased by 500 mg at weekly intervals if seizures are not controlled. The usual daily maintenance dose in adults is 2000 to 3000 mg, although some patients have required as much as 5000 mg/day. In children 5 to 10 years of age, the dosage of PAC is approximately one half the adult dosage, again given in three divided doses. Because of the many side effects of PAC, the maintenance dosage should be the smallest dose that provides adequate seizure control.

INDICATIONS

Complex Partial Seizures
The major indication for PAC is complex partial seizures (CPS) that are refractory to less toxic drugs. Although PAC is moderately effective as a primary drug for CPS [41, 60], it is never used as the first drug for any seizure type because of the high incidence of serious side effects with PAC (see below). Several studies indicate that PAC completely controls or markedly decreases CPS in 30 to 60 percent of patients with CPS refractory to phenytoin and barbiturates [18, 31, 41, 60].

PAC should not be administered to a patient with CPS until it has been documented that maximum tolerated doses of phenytoin, a barbiturate (phenobarbital or primidone), and carbamazepine in combination will not control the seizures. In such a patient temporal lobectomy should probably be considered before therapy with PAC because this surgical procedure has a higher probability of success *and* a lower morbidity than PAC (see Chap. 25). In patients with refractory CPS who refuse surgery or are not surgical candidates, a trial of PAC may be indicated if the potential benefits outweigh the potential risks.

Tonic-Clonic and Simple Partial Seizures
PAC is not especially effective against either tonic-clonic or simple partial seizures, either as a primary or as an adjunctive antiepileptic drug [17, 41, 60]. However, a minority of patients with tonic-clonic seizures refractory to hydantoins and barbiturates have a good response to PAC [18, 31, 41, 60].

Absence Seizures
PAC is effective against absence seizures in only a minority of patients [17, 18, 31, 41, 60]. Given the abundance of less toxic antiabsence drugs available, there is no indication for PAC for this disorder.

TOXICITY
The frequency of the most common and serious side effects of PAC are summarized in Table 22-1.

Psychic Changes
Destructiveness, belligerence, marked irritability, restlessness, and depression are the most commonly observed psychic changes [31, 41, 60]. Suicidal tendencies, paranoia, and acute psychotic states have been reported [60]. Psychic symptoms occur most commonly during the first 4 to 6 weeks of PAC therapy and disappear within a few weeks of stopping the drug [41, 60]. Psychic changes necessitate discontinuing PAC in approximately 10 percent of patients [41]. On the other hand, in some cases of preexisting personality disorders, improvement has been noted with PAC [18, 60].

In patients who have previously had psychiatric disturbances, hospitalization during the first week of PAC therapy may be advisable. The patient and family should be alerted to report changes in behavior such as decreased interest in surroundings, depression, or aggressiveness.

Gastrointestinal Symptoms
Anorexia, nausea, vomiting, weight loss, and vague abdominal pains occur in 8 to 13 percent of patients on PAC [31, 41, 60], requiring discontinuance of the drug in 3 percent of patients on PAC [41].

Table 22-1. Toxicity of Phenacemide

Side Effect	% of Patients
Psychic changes	
All patients	15–20
Patients with preexisting psychiatric problems	27
Patients without preexisting psychiatric problems	5
Gastrointestinal symptoms	8–13
Rash	1–8
Headache	2–6
Drowsiness	4–5
Abnormal urinary findings	1–3
Hepatitis	0.6–2
Blood dyscrasia	0–2

Source: Based on data from Davidson and Lenox [18], Gibbs et al. [31], Livingston and Pauli [41], and Tyler and King [60].

Rashes
Rashes may be of the maculopapular, scarlatiniform, or acneiform type [18, 41, 60]. They commonly appear during the first 3 weeks of PAC therapy and may be accompanied by a fever [18, 41]. The rashes are not dose-related and disappear within a week of stopping the drug [41].

Headache
Headache or a feeling of "fullness in the head" occurs in 2 to 6 percent of patients on PAC [18, 31, 41, 60]. The headache appears during the first few days of PAC therapy and is often severe.

Drowsiness
Drowsiness occurs in up to 5 percent of patients on PAC [60].

Abnormal Urinary Findings
Transient proteinuria without serious renal damage occurs in up to 3 percent of patients during the first week of PAC therapy [31, 41]. Acetonuria and glycosuria may also occur [60]. Nephritis and a fatal case of hepatorenal syndrome have also been reported [41].

Hepatitis
Hepatitis, often reversible, occurs in 0.6 to 2 percent of patients on PAC [18, 31, 41, 60]. At least 10 deaths due to PAC hepatic toxicity have been reported [34, 41]. The histologic picture in these cases was one of zonal (chiefly centrolobular) to submassive toxic necrosis

256

[34]. If the patient survives, postnecrotic cirrhosis may develop [34]. PAC should be used with caution in patients with a history of hepatic disease. Liver function studies should be performed on all patients before and during PAC therapy.

Blood Dyscrasias
Leukopenia, leukocytosis, thrombocytopenia, agranulocytosis, and aplastic anemia occur in 0 to 2 percent of patients on PAC [18, 31, 41, 60]. Two fatal cases of aplastic anemia have been reported [41]. Complete blood counts should be done before starting PAC therapy and at monthly intervals while the patient is on PAC.

Other Side Effects
Other reported side effects of PAC include insomnia, fatigue, fever, dizziness, paresthesias, muscle pain, palpitations, pruritus, and insensitivity to pain [18, 31, 60].

Teratology
The teratogenic potential of PAC in humans is unknown. However, because of PAC's structural similarity to phenytoin and its high incidence of side effects, it must be suspected that PAC is a teratogenic drug and may produce teratogenic effects similar to those of phenytoin (see Chap. 29). PAC should not be given during pregnancy unless the potential benefits outweigh the potential risks.

References

1. Agranat, A. L., and Trubshaw, W. H. D. The danger of decomposed paraldehyde. *S. Afr. Med. J.* 29:1021, 1955.
2. Anonymous. Death from decomposed paraldehyde. *Br. Med. J.* 2:114, 1954.
3. Anthony, R. M. et al. Paraldehyde pharmacokinetics in alcohol abusers. *Fed. Proc.* 36:285, 1977.
4. Baratham, G., and Tinckler, L. F. Paraldehyde poisoning: A little-known hazard of post-operative sedation. *Med. J. Aust.* 2:877, 1964.
5. Beaucheim, J. A., Springer, R. G., and Elliot, G. A. Intravenous anesthesia with paraldehyde. *Med. Times* 63:179, 1935.
6. Booker, H. E. Trimethadone and Other Oxazolidinediones: Chemistry and Methods for Determination. In D. M. Woodbury, J. K. Penry, and R. P. Schmidt (Eds.), *Antiepileptic Drugs.* New York: Raven Press, 1972.
7. Booker, H. E. Trimethadione and Other Oxazolidinediones: Relation of Plasma Levels to Clinical Control. In D. M. Woodbury, J. K. Penry, and R. P. Schmidt (Eds.), *Antiepileptic Drugs.* New York: Raven Press, 1972.
8. Booker, H. E. Trimethadione: Relation of Plasma Concentrations to Seizure Control. In D. M. Woodbury, J. K. Penry, and C. E. Pippenger (Eds.), *Antiepileptic Drugs.* New York: Raven Press, 1982.
9. Booker, H. E. Trimethadione: Toxicity. In D. M. Woodbury, J. K. Penry, and C. E. Pippenger (Eds.), *Antiepileptic Drugs.* New York: Raven Press, 1982.
10. Browne, T. R. Paraldehyde, Chlormethiazole, and Lidocaine. In A. V. Delgado-Escueta, et al. (Eds.), *Status Epilepticus: Mechanisms of Brain Damage and Treatment.* New York: Raven Press, 1982.
11. Burstein, C. L. The hazard of paraldehyde administration: Clinical and laboratory studies. *J.A.M.A.* 121:187, 1943.
12. Butler, T. C. Quantitative studies of the demethylation of trimethadione (Tridione®). *J. Pharmacol. Exp. Ther.* 180:11, 1953.
13. Butler, T. C., and Waddell, W. J. N-Methylated derivatives of barbituric acid, hydantoin, and oxazolidinedione used in the treatment of epilepsy. *Neurology* (Minneap.) 8:106, 1958.
14. Cameron, A., and Cameron, N. Ethylphenacemide and phenacemide: Conformational similarities to diphenylhydantoin and stereochemical basis of anticonvulsant activity. *Pro. Natl. Acad. Sci. USA* 74:1264, 1977.
15. Chamberlin, H. R., Waddell, W. J., and Butler, T. C. A study of the product of demethylation of trimethadione in control of petit mal epilepsy. *Neurology* (Minneap.) 15:449, 1965.
16. Chao, D. H. C., and Plum, R. L. Diamox® in epilepsy: A critical review of 178 cases. *J. Pediatr.* 58:211, 1961.
17. Coatsworth, J. J. *Studies on the Critical Efficacy of Marketed Antiepileptic Drugs* (NINDS Monograph No. 1L). Washington, D.C.: U.S. Government Printing Office, 1971.
18. Davidson, D. T., and Lennox, W. G. Phenacetylurea (Phenurone) in epilepsy. *Dis. Nerv. Syst.* 11:167, 1950.
19. Davis, J. P., and Lennox, W. G. Effect of trimethyloxazolidine dione and of dimethyloxazolidine on seizures and on blood. *Res. Publ. Assoc. Res. Nerv. Ment. Dis.* 26:423, 1947.
20. Davis, J. P., and Lennox, W. G. A comparison of Paradione and Tridione in the treatment of epilepsy. *J. Pediatr.* 34:273, 1949.
21. De Jong, R. N. Effect of Tridione® in control of psychomotor attacks. *J.A.M.A.* 130:565, 1946.

22. Denhoff, E., and Laufer, M. W. Clinical studies of the effect of 3,5,5-trimethyloxazolidine-2-4-dione (Tridone®) on the hematopoietic system, liver, and kidney. *Pediatrics* 5:595, 1950.

23. Dudley, K. H., Buis, D. L., and King, B. T. Trimethadione: Chemistry and Methods of Determination. In D. M. Woodbury, J. K. Penry, and C. E. Pippenger (Eds.), *Antiepileptic Drugs*. New York: Raven Press, 1982.

24. Frey, H. H. Determination of the anti-convulsant potency of unmetabolized trimethadione. *Acta Pharmacol. Toxicol.* (Kbh.) 27:295, 1969.

25. Frey, H. H., and Schulz, R. Time course of the demethylation of trimethadione. *Acta Pharmacol. Toxicol.* (Kbh.) 28:477, 1970.

26. Fromm, G. H. et al. Antiabsence drugs and inhibitory pathways. *Neurology* (N.Y.) 30:126, 1980.

27. Gallagher, B. B. Trimethadione and Other Oxazolidinediones: Toxicity. In D. M. Woodbury, J. K. Penry, and R. P. Schmidt (Eds.), *Antiepileptic Drugs*. New York: Raven Press, 1972.

28. Gardner, H. L., Levine, J., and Bodansky, M. Concentrations of paraldehyde in the blood following its administration during labor. *Am. J. Obstet. Gynecol.* 40:435, 1940.

29. Gardner, H. L., and Sage, E. C. The intravenous administration of paraldehyde during labor. *Am. J. Obstet. Gynecol.* 42:467, 1941.

30. Gessner, P. K. Drug therapy of alcohol withdrawal syndrome. In E. Majchrowicz, and E. Nobel (Eds.), *The Biochemistry and Pharmacology of Ethanol*. New York: Plenum, 1979.

31. Gibbs, F. A., Evert, G. M., and Richards, R. K. Phenurone in epilepsy. *Dis. Nerv. Syst.* 10:47, 1949.

32. Goldman, A. S., and Yaffe, S. J. Fetal trimethadione syndrome. *Teratology* 17:103, 1978.

33. Goodman, L. S., Toman, J. E. P., and Swinyard, E. A. The anticonvulsant properties of Tridione®: Laboratory and clinical investigations. *Am. J. Med.* 1:213, 1946.

34. Gunzel, H. et al. Further clinical, pharmacologic, pathologic, and biochemical observations with phenacemide (German). *Dtsch. Gesundh: Wes.* 19:1877, 1964.

35. Guterman, A. et al. Paraldehyde pharmacokinetics and its use in status epilepticus. *Epilepsia*. In press, 1983.

36. Hayward, J. W. and Boshell, B. R. Paraldehyde intoxication with metabolic acidosis. *Am. J. Med.* 23:965, 1957.

37. Holowach, J., and Thurton, D. L. A clinical evaluation of acetazolamide (Diamox) in the treatment of epilepsy in children. *J. Pediatr.* 53:160, 1958.

38. Jensen, B. N. Trimethadione in serum of patients with petit mal epilepsy. *Dan. Med. Bull.* 9:74, 1962.

39. Lennox, W. G. Tridione in the treatment of epilepsy. *J.A.M.A.* 134:138, 1947.

40. Lennox, W. G., and Lennox, M. A. *Epilepsy and Related Disorders*. Boston: Little, Brown, 1960.

41. Livingston, S., and Pauli, L. L. Phenacemide in the treatment of epilepsy: Results of treatment of 411 patients and review of literature. *N. Engl. J. Med.* 256:588, 1957.

42. Lombroso, C. T., and Forsythe, I. A longterm followup of acetazolamide (Diamox) in the treatment of epilepsy. *Epilepsia* 1:493, 1960.

43. Maren, T. J. Carbonic anhydrase: Chemistry, physiology and inhibition. *Physiol. Rev.* 47:595, 1967.

44. Maren, T. H. Teratology and carbonic anhydrase inhibition. *Arch. Ophthalmol.* 85:1, 1971.

45. Maren, T. H., Mayer, E., and Wadsworth, B. C. Carbonic anhydrase inhibition. I. The pharmacology of Diamox® (2-acetylamino-1,3,4-thiadiazole-5-sulfonamide). *Bull. Johns Hopkins Hosp.* 95:199, 1954.

46. Maren, T. H., and Robinson, B. The pharmacology of acetazolamide as related to cerebrospinal fluid in the treatment of hydrocephalus. *Bull. Johns Hopkins Hosp.* 106:1, 1960.

47. Millichap, J. G. Relation of laboratory evaluation to clinical effectiveness of antiepileptic drugs. *Epilepsia* 10:315, 1967.

48. Millichap, J. F., and Aymat, F. The treatment and prognosis of petit mal epilepsy. *Pediatr. Clin. North Am.* 14:905, 1969.

49. Nakane, Y. et al. Multi-institutional study of the teratogenicity and fetal toxicity of antiepileptic drugs: A report of a collaborative study group in Japan. *Epilepsia* 21:663, 1980.

50. Perlstein, M. A., and Andelman, M. B. Tridione®: Its use in convulsive and related disorders. *J. Pediatr.* 29:20, 1946.

51. Rall, T. W., and Schleifer, L. S. Drugs Effective in the Therapies of the Epilepsies. In L. S. Goodman, and A. Gilman (Eds.), *The Pharmacological Basis of Therapeutics*. New York: Macmillan, 1980.

52. Reed, D. J. The effects of acetazolamide on pentobarbital sleep-time and cerebrospinal fluid flow of rats. *Arch. Int. Pharmacodyn. Ther.* 171:206, 1968.

53. Reed, D. J., and Woodbury, D. M. Effect of urea and acetazolamide on the brain volume and cerebrospinal fluid pressure. *J. Physiol.* (Lond.) 164:265, 1962.

54. Robinson, L. J. Intravenous paraldehyde narcosis for pneumoencephalography. *N. Engl. J. Med.* 219:114, 1938.

55. Schnell, R. C., and Miya, T. S. Altered absorption of drugs from the rat small intestine by carbonic anhydrase inhibition. *J. Pharmacol. Exp. Ther.* 174:177, 1970.

56. Sinal, S. H., and Crowe, J. E. Cyanosis, cough, and hypotension following intravenous administration of paraldehyde. *Pediatrics* 57:158, 1976.

57. Sloan, L. L., and Gilger, A. P. Visual effects of Tridione®. *Am. J. Ophthalmol.* 30:1387, 1947.

58. Swinyard, E. A. Laboratory evaluation of antiepileptic drugs: Review of laboratory methods. *Epilepsia* 10:107, 1969.

59. Thurston, J. H. et al. New enzymatic method for measurement of paraldehyde: Correlation of effects with serum and CSF levels. *J. Lab. Clin. Med.* 72:699, 1968.

60. Tyler, M. W., and King, E. Q. Phenacemide in the treatment of epilepsy. *J.A.M.A.* 147:17, 1951.

61. Waddell, W. J., and Butler, T. C. Renal excretion of 5,5-dimethyl-2, 4-oxazolidione (product of demethylation of trimethadione). *Proc. Soc. Exp. Biol. Med.* 96:563, 1957.

62. Wells, C. E. Trimethadione: Its dosage and toxicity. *Arch. Neurol. Psychiatr.* 77:140, 1957.

63. Withrow, C. D. et al. Anticonvulsant effects of 5,5-dimethyl-2,4-oxazolidinedione (DMO). *J. Pharmacol. Exp. Ther.* 161:335, 1968.

64. Withrow, C. D. Trimethadione: Absorption, Distribution, and Excretion. In D. M. Woodbury, J. K. Penry, and C. E. Pippenger (Eds.), *Antiepileptic Drugs.* New York: Raven Press, 1982.

65. Withrow, C. D. Trimethadione: Biotransformation. In D. M. Woodbury, J. K. Penry, and C. E. Pippenger (Eds.), *Antiepileptic Drugs.* New York: Raven Press, 1982.

66. Withrow, C. D. Trimethadione: Interactions with Other Drugs. In D. M. Woodbury, J. K. Penry, and C. E. Pippenger (Eds.), *Antiepileptic Drugs.* New York: Raven Press, 1982.

67. Withrow, C. D. Trimethadione: Mechanisms of Action. In D. M. Woodbury, J. K. Penry, and C. E. Pippenger (Eds.), *Antiepileptic Drugs.* New York: Raven Press, 1982.

68. Woodbury, D. M., and Kemp, J. W. Other Antiepileptic Drugs: Sulfonamides and Derivatives: Acetazolamide. In D. M. Woodbury, J. K. Penry, and C. E. Pippenger (Eds.), *Antiepileptic Drugs.* New York: Raven Press, 1982.

NURSING MANAGEMENT AND PATIENT EDUCATION

23

Susan E. Norman
Thomas R. Browne

Successful management of patients with epilepsy includes adequate medical intervention, proper patient education, and adjustment to the psychosocial aspects of the disease. Early nursing intervention can set the foundation for successful management and can both complement and supplement the physician in many areas.

The two major aspects of nursing management of patients with epilepsy are (1) care during and immediately after the actual seizure, and (2) long-term planning and management [6]. The first aspect requires the nurse to know what to do and what to observe during the seizure, and what to ask the patient or witnesses in taking the seizure history. The second facet of nursing management is equally important and includes educating the patient about the disorder itself, the medications and their side effects, the importance of compliance, and the anticipated psychosocial consequences of having epilepsy.

Nursing Care During Inpatient Hospitalization

DIAGNOSTIC EVALUATION

Seizure Classification
It is important to establish first whether or not the patient does have epilepsy. If the patient does have epilepsy, it should be determined precisely what type or types of seizure the patient has. The needs of the patient and the plan for medical and nursing intervention will vary with different types of seizures. The classification and clinical manifestations of the various types of epilepsy are reviewed in Chapters 3 to 10.

Diagnostic Tests
The usual diagnostic evaluation for a first seizure includes (1) a complete neurologic examination to look for evidence of a focal neurologic deficit suggesting a focus of origin for seizures, (2) an electroencephalogram (EEG) to help confirm the diagnosis and localize the lesion, (3) skull radiographs to rule out skull fracture, (4) computed axial tomography

This work was supported in part by the Veterans Administration.

(CT scan) to look for a tumor, congenital lesion, infarct, hemorrhage, or arteriovenous malformation, (5) lumbar puncture to look for infection, increased intracranial pressure, and increased protein level, and (6) several blood studies to rule out infectious and metabolic causes of seizures (see Chaps. 1 and 12).

Sources of Anxiety

The two most common sources of anxiety that the nurse can anticipate during the patient's admission are fear and mistrust [20]. Fear is most often observed in the patient who has just had his first seizure and has been admitted for an initial diagnosis. Mistrust is often demonstrated by the patient who has had at least one other seizure and has been seen by other doctors in the past.

The first seizure patient is afraid of the disease itself and all its mysterious connotations. He is afraid of the expected procedures and tests, especially invasive procedures such as a lumbar puncture. He may never have been in a hospital before and may be frightened by the unfamiliar setting. Most of all, he may be terrified of having another seizure. Often the patient will ask (1) Why did I have a seizure? (2) Does this mean that I'm an "epileptic"? (3) Will I have to take pills the rest of my life? (4) Does this mean I have a brain tumor?

The nurse can alleviate many of these fears by explaining the procedures and usual work-up in detail before the tests are done. It is important to allow the patient opportunities to ventilate his concerns. Often a simple explanation is sufficient.

The patient who experiences mistrust has often been to several doctors in the past and enters the hospital with confusing and often conflicting information about his seizure disorder. By allowing the patient to share in some of the decisions concerning his care the nurse is usually able to decrease some of this mistrust. Find out what time the patient took medications at home and if possible set up a similar schedule during the hospital stay. See that the test results are transmitted promptly and accurately to the patient. A delay in feedback can increase mistrust and may lead the patient to think that the doctors and nurses are withholding information. Again, detailed explanations of procedures (do not assume that the patient understands why certain tests are being done because he has had them before) and opportunities to discuss concerns will help to increase the patient's trust in the health team.

Both the fearful and the mistrustful patient must wait until a definitive diagnosis is made before prognosis and management plans are discussed. There is no reason to plan for future life adjustments before the seizure type and etiology have been determined. The information given the patient about the seizure work-up should be consistent so that the patient is not confused by misinformation. The nurse should discuss the test results, the plan for medical treatment, and nursing intervention with the primary physician before approaching the patient.

SEIZURE PRECAUTIONS

Padded Bedrails

Rubber pads are available, made specifically for railing coverage. If such pads are unavailable, rails can be covered with heavy blankets that are thick enough to provide an adequate cushion effect. Bedrail padding can be embarrassing to the patient and calls attention to the fact that there is something unusual about his illness. Explaining the rationale for padding the bedrails and why the rails are raised at night can help to decrease worries of how it looks to others.

Oral Airway

A plastic airway should be taped to the bed in an easily accessible place. There should be one place designated for placement of the airway that is known by all staff members so the airway can be found immediately in an emergency.

Do Not Let the Patient Take a Bath Alone

Instruct the patient not to bathe alone. Patients can and do drown in the bathtub during a seizure. Showers are preferred. If the patient must bathe, observation is required.

Smoking

Instruct the patient not to smoke while in bed or alone in the room. If the patient's seizures are well controlled, permission may be obtained (depending on hospital policy) for the patient to smoke in the hall outside the room.

Temperature Taking

Rectal or axillary thermometers should be used when checking the seizure patient's temperature. There is a risk of biting and breaking an oral thermometer during a seizure.

SEIZURE FIRST AID

Regardless of seizure type, the three major responsibilities of the nurse during a seizure are (1) to prevent physical injury and ensure safety, (2) to observe accurately, and (3) to allay the anxiety of onlookers after the patient has received adequate attention [11].

Prevention of Physical Injury
During Tonic-Clonic Seizures
This is the seizure type that requires the most attention. Once the seizure begins the patient should never be left alone (i.e., *do not* run for help) [6]. The chief dangers to be aware of are physical injury, aspiration, and tongue biting [1].

Physical injuries to the head or bones may result if the patient falls while sitting or standing. The violent muscle contractions of the seizure can result in bruises, lacerations, muscle strains, and broken bones. The patient should usually be left where he has fallen (unless there is some danger, such as an explosion from an auto accident [21]). Roll the patient on to his side to prevent aspiration. Place a pillow under the head (or use any soft material such as a towel or your lap) to prevent the head from banging against the floor. Move objects such as furniture which the patient might strike with his movements out of the way. Gently restrain the extremities to prevent them from striking hard objects. Vigorous restraint may result in orthopedic injuries as the muscles contract against great resistance. After tonic-clonic movements have ceased, move the patient to a bed or couch.

Aspiration can result if pooled secretions flow into the trachea, and on rare occasions the tongue can be "swallowed," resulting in obstruction of the airway. Placement of a soft oral airway will aid in allowing secretions to drain out the side of the mouth. Loosen the patient's collar.

Tongue biting should be prevented, if possible, by placing a soft oral airway between the patient's teeth. *Never* force an object into the patient's mouth, especially a metal spoon or wooden object. Hard objects can cause teeth to break, resulting in aspiration of teeth, and wood can splinter easily. If the tonic stage begins before an object has been placed to prevent tongue biting, it is useless to attempt to do so because the jaws are firmly fixed. Remember that a bitten tongue can heal but not a broken tooth [11].

Do not place a tongue blade wrapped in gauze and tape or the folded edge of a towel in the patient's mouth. The primary reason for placing a soft oral airway is to facilitate breathing and suctioning. Gauze or a towel may impede respiration and removal of secretions.

Protection of Patients with Other Seizure Types
Patients with other seizure types also require attention to possible injuries and ensurance of safety. For example, a patient who is having a complex partial seizure and is wandering about the ward should be followed and prevented from wandering accidentally into a dangerous situation, such as falling down the stairs. If possible, do not attempt to restrain a patient demonstrating complex automatisms because this may cause the patient to become violent. Stay with the patient to ensure safety.

Accurate Observation of the Seizure
The single most important information in establishing a diagnosis of epilepsy and in differentiating the specific type or types of seizure a patient has is what was observed by witnesses and experienced by the patient before, during, and after the actual seizure [24]. The nurse's observations of a seizure may be the most important information available in arriving at a seizure diagnosis because the nurse may be the only professional to observe a seizure [6]. Specific items to be observed are outlined in Table 23-1.

After the Seizure
It is important not to crowd the patient. Speak calmly and slowly. The content of what is said should be aimed at helping the patient to become reoriented and at reassurance that everything is all right. Identify who you are, where you both are, and what has just occurred.

After the patient has received adequate attention the nurse is then responsible for allaying the anxiety of onlookers [1]. The observers should be reassured that the patient will not die and is not injured. Prevent panic. The degree to which the nurse remains calm during the seizure will be reflected in the attitudes of the observers.

If the nurse did not witness the seizure, a history obtained from the onlookers will be essential in determining the seizure type. Listen to the story of those who saw the event, asking them questions about the details that you would have observed yourself (see Table 23-1).

Learn the fears prevalent among the patient's family members or peers. Reassure them that the patient is all right. If appropriate, take the time to instruct them in seizure first aid. By teaching them what to do during and after a seizure their fears and misconceptions can be replaced with helpful activity.

Is a Seizure an Emergency?
Unless there is a succession of attacks there is no need for immediate medical attention. If the nurse determines that the patient is in status epilepticus the doctor should be notified (by a second person) immediately. Status epilepticus is defined as a rapid succession of seizures occurring so frequently that the patient does not fully recover from one before having

Table 23-1. Observations To Be Made During a Seizure

1. Was the patient awake or asleep before the attack?
2. What was the patient doing just prior to the attack? Standing? Sitting? Was the patient excited? Angry?
3. In what part of the body did the seizure begin? Face, arm, or leg? Right or left side?
4. How did the patient attract your attention? Was there an initial cry?
5. Was the onset of movements sudden or gradual?
6. Were any automatisms observed, such as eyelid fluttering, chewing, or swallowing?
7. Was there twitching or jerking of any particular body part? Which part? Which side? Was there a progression of the movement to involve one or more muscle groups (i.e., Jacksonian march)? Where did it spread? What was the duration of these movements? Did the character of these movements change?
8. Did the patient lose consciousness? At what point? For how long? Did the level of consciousness seem altered although the patient was not fully unconscious? Could he respond verbally? Accurately?
9. Did the patient become rigid (tonic phase)? Was the rigidity followed by jerking of limbs (clonic phase)? Which side? Was it equal on both sides? How long did these movements last?
10. Did the head turn to one side? Which side?
11. Did the eyes deviate up, down, or to one side? Which side? Did the pupils change in size? Were they equal and reactive? Were these responses different during the movements compared with after the movements ceased?
12. Did the patient fall?
13. Did the patient hurt himself?
14. Was the patient's head hit during the fall or during the seizure activity?
15. Was there "frothing" or "foaming" from the mouth?
16. Did the face or lips change color? Were they flushed? Ashen? Cyanotic?
17. Did the skin become clammy, cold, or warm?
18. Were lips or tongue bitten? Any bleeding?
19. Was there urinary or fecal incontinence?
20. Describe the respirations. Was there apnea or stertor?
21. Did the patient sleep after the seizure? How long?
22. Was there postictal confusion? Headache? Gastrointestinal upset? Muscle soreness? Impaired speech or comprehension?
23. Were there alterations in motor power after the seizure? Asymmetrically? Transient hemiplegia (Todd's paralysis)?
24. Did the patient know that an attack had occurred?
25. Can the patient describe an aura or other subjective sensations before, during, or immediately after the seizure?

another [4, 19, 23] (see Chap. 30). In addition to the standard precautions, special attention should be paid to the following: (1) maintenance of a clear airway, including pharyngeal suctioning, (2) maintenance of a patent intravenous line for antiepileptic therapy and fluid and electrolyte balance, (3) frequent monitoring of vital signs, (4) use of antipyretics and sponge baths if the patient is febrile, and (5) provision for adequate respiratory exchange and cardiovascular supportive measures as necessary [4, 19, 23].

PATIENT EDUCATION
This topic is reviewed in the following section.

Nursing Care: Outpatient
The nurse's role should include the following tasks: obtaining a seizure history; performing a medication compliance check (sometimes including blood level determinations); checking on drug side effects (sometimes including laboratory tests); assessing the psycho-social status of the patient; explaining in detail changes in medication regime (if ordered); and deciding on a method of telephone contact.

SEIZURE HISTORY
Record any seizure activity experienced by the patient or witnessed by observers. Check that the patient is keeping a seizure calendar. If not, work with the patient to establish a convenient method of recording seizure activity.

MEDICATION COMPLIANCE
Noncompliance with an antiepileptic drug regime is the most frequent cause of recurrent seizures [22] (see Chap. 15). What appears to be a lack of cooperation may be due to a lack of information about the medications before the patient was discharged.

Patients who have not been compliant often feel embarrassed and will deny noncompliance. After the nurse and the patient explore the possible reasons for "forgetting a pill" the patient may admit to "sometimes" missing a pill or two. Once the blood levels have been obtained the nurse will have a better idea of what "sometimes" means. If the level is subtherapeutic there is a very good chance that the patient has missed several doses or is simply taking the wrong dose. Explore with the patient (or the person responsible for giving the patient the medication) when and how the medication is taken.

Other factors causing low blood levels must be investigated before a conclusion about noncompliance is drawn (see Chap. 15). It is usually in poor taste to confront the noncomplier directly with an accusation. Rather than focusing on the noncompliance, explore and identify why the patient is noncompliant.

Sometimes a patient who has had previous excellent seizure control will come to the hospital emergency room in status epilepticus. After the patient is treated the nurse will often discover that the patient has abruptly stopped some or all of his medications. Why? Answers will include "I wanted to see how I'd do without them," "I ran out of medicine," "I thought my seizures were cured." If the patient understands the risks of stopping medication, he will not stop [20].

Sometimes the medication schedule is inconvenient, especially if the person is on a tid or qid schedule. Many patients do not like to take medications at school or work. Phenytoin or phenobarbital can usually be taken in a single dose, preferably at bedtime, or in two divided doses without adverse effects. Ethosuximide can be given in two divided doses. Carbamazepine, primidone, and valproic acid must be taken in divided doses (3 or 4 times) during the day. The timing can be arranged to suit the individual's daily schedule (e.g., at mealtime and at bedtime). Weekly, pocket-sized plastic pill dispensers are a convenient method of helping the patient remember his pills. Whatever schedule is decided upon, a daily routine should be established.

Another factor that plays a significant role in noncompliance is "unconscious forgetting" [20]. An unconscious denial of the illness or a refusal to be dependent on medication may be an important source of poor seizure control. This possibility must be considered and discussed openly with the patient and family.

Fear of being "seizure-free" may be another unconscious motivation for drug noncompliance [20]. A person who has grown used to staying at home, not working, and perhaps collecting a disability pension may want to continue to stay at home.

On the other hand, the patient may present on follow-up visit with unusually high drug blood levels.

Possible causes of high blood levels are outlined in Chapter 15 and must be investigated before adjusting the dose. Because the blood level fluctuates during the day, determining when the patient last took the medication is important in interpreting drug blood level data.

SIDE EFFECTS
Determine if the patient is experiencing adverse side effects from the medications and if the side effects are interfering with the patient's daily activities.

LABORATORY TESTS
The best time to obtain blood levels of a drug is at the end of the longest interval between doses (usually first thing in the morning). If the level is adequate then, it should be adequate throughout the day. Other blood tests include a complete blood count with differential and platelet count (especially when the patient is taking carbamazepine, ethosuximide, or valproic acid). Liver function studies should be checked in patients receiving valproic acid.

CHANGES IN MEDICATION REGIME
Any changes in medication regime should be reviewed thoroughly before the patient leaves the office. Write out the adjusted time and dosage schedule as well as the name of the new medication. This can be done conveniently on a card such as that shown in Figure 23-1.

PSYCHOSOCIAL ASSESSMENT
Have new problems developed at home or at work? Are recurrent seizures perhaps associated with increased stress or altered sleep patterns? Explore problems in adjusting to new routines and try to determine more productive means of coping. Utilize psychiatric and social service consultations as indicated.

TELEPHONE CONTACT
The patient should have the doctor's and the nurse's office telephone numbers as well as their home telephone numbers (or answering service). The three main reasons for a patient to make telephone contact are (1) to ask for a prescription renewal, (2) to report a seizure, or (3) to report drug toxicity.

If the patient telephones to report a seizure, first determine whether there is a problem with noncompliance. If not, find out whether a fever or some other precipitating factor is present (see Fig. 23-2 and Chap. 12). Is the patient drug toxic (i.e., complaining of drowsiness, ataxia, diplopia, or dysarthria)? Adjustment in medication dose, if indicated, can often be·

264

given over the telephone. Often the patient simply needs to be reassured that the symptom he is feeling is not serious.

BEFORE PATIENT LEAVES OFFICE

The nurse should make sure that the patient has all the necessary items—(1) follow-up appointment, (2) prescriptions, (3) medication instructions, (4) laboratory slips, and (5) contact telephone numbers.

Patient Education

Once the diagnosis of epilepsy is confirmed, it is crucial for the patient to understand the disease process. An ongoing coordinated teaching plan is essential throughout the patient's hospital stay. Don't wait until the patient's discharge day to begin!

MEDICAL EDUCATION

Often the patient does not understand what a seizure is and therefore does not understand the rationale for drug management [8]. A thorough explanation of what happens during a seizure and why certain medications have been prescribed is essential. A written medication schedule will help the patient remember when and how to take medications. An example of a medication schedule form that can be stamped onto a 3- × 5-inch index card with an inexpensive rubber stamp is shown in Figure 23-1. A simple explanation of blood levels and why blood samples are important should be given. Explain that the physician or nurse must check the blood level of the antiepileptic drug as well as determine if there are blood dyscrasias.

A list of potential seizure triggers should be given to the patient (see Fig. 23-2 and Chap. 12). The most common precipitating events include fever, emotional upset (anxiety, increased stress), sleep loss, hormonal imbalance (menstruation, pregnancy), alcohol, hyperventilation, trauma, illness, infection, fluid and electrolyte imbalance, sensory stimuli, and drugs.

Side effects of the patient's antiepileptic drug or drugs should be reviewed. Patients taking drugs that may cause bone marrow depression (carbamazepine, ethosuximide, valproic acid) should be warned to watch for fever, persistent infection, easy bruising, bleeding, or hematuria. If the patient notices serious side effects he should contact the doctor or nurse or go to the hospital emergency department. It is imperative that the patient know how to contact the primary clinician.

These measures serve to provide a sense of trust between the patient and the health team. Just knowing that the doctor or nurse is available can serve to allay the patient's anxiety upon discharge. One of the great-

Figure 23-1. Sample patient medication card.

est fears of the newly diagnosed seizure patient at discharge is the fear of a recurrent seizure ("Who will I call?"). At first, patients may be overly dependent on the primary clinician and may call often. As time goes on and the seizures abate, trust in the treatment will increase and the need to check with the clinician will lessen.

It is important to include the family (especially the spouse) in the teaching process. Remind the family that the patient is rarely in any danger when having a seizure and review with them what to observe and what to do when a seizure occurs. Printed information is very helpful. The patient should be instructed that medications must be taken daily in the prescribed dose. Attacks can occur at any time, so continued coverage is essential for maximal protection.

DRIVING

For many patients the loss (or fear of loss) of their driver's license is the worst consequence of having epilepsy. In a few states, physicians are required by law to report the names of patients with epilepsy to the Department of Motor Vehicles [7, 15]. In most states, however, the patient is responsible and the physician cannot report the patient's condition unless a written release is signed by the patient. Mandatory reporting by physicians is undesirable because it may discourage patients from seeking needed medical care and from reporting truthfully about seizure frequency to their physician [15].

The Commission for Control of Epilepsy and Its Consequences [7, 14] recommends that the primary responsibility for reporting must reside with the afflicted person, but that the person needs to be informed of his responsibilities. The Commission recommends that physicians should be required to notify all patients subject to lapses of consciousness

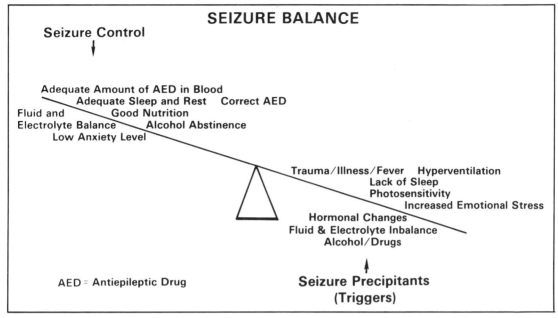

Figure 23-2. Factors promoting seizure control and factors precipitating seizures. (Modified from R. G. Feldman [9].)

of their obligation to report themselves to the motor vehicle department. The patient should be notified in writing, and the notification should be recorded in the patient's record.

The mandatory period of suspension of a driver's license following a seizure varies from state to state. Regardless of legal considerations, a seizure-free period of 6 months to 2 years is probably required before one can be certain that a patient's seizures are completely controlled with medication. The duration of the trial is dictated in part by the patient's risk factors for recurrent seizures (see Chap. 14). Some states have now adopted more flexible regulations that allow a medical panel to authorize driving restrictions based on the medical facts of a given patient's case.

Commercial licenses for driving buses and trucks and airplane pilots' licenses (private or commercial) are usually permanently revoked after a person has had a seizure.

EMPLOYMENT

Specific factual information on employment is contained in Chapter 13. For many patients, concern about loss or potential loss of a job is a severe consequence of having epilepsy. The professional should anticipate that the patient will have both factual questions and emotional responses to the potential loss of employment.

BATHING AND SHOWERS

Bathing and showering are potentially very dangerous to the patient with epilepsy [2, 12, 13, 18]. Patients who have a seizure in a full bathtub can drown. Patients experiencing a seizure while standing in the shower may injure themselves through the impact of the fall, by falling through a glass or plastic shower door, or by striking the faucet handle that regulates the hot water flow and suffering extensive burns. Livingston et al. [13] recommend procedures for minimizing these risks. Children with seizures should never bathe alone. Adults with seizures should ideally also be accompanied when bathing. If this is not possible, the tub should be filled to a height of no more than 7 cm. When showering the patient should sit on the bathtub floor (with the drain open) and use a hand-held showering instrument that will turn off when finger or hand pressure is released. In facilities that offer only wall showers or when the person insists on washing in a shower stall rather than in a bathtub, the patient should be instructed to sit on an appropriate bench throughout the shower.

SWIMMING

Fatalities associated with swimming are rare in persons with epilepsy but may occur [12, 13, 18]. Livingston et al. [12] have never had a swimming fatality in their large population of patients with epilepsy adhering to the following rules. Patients whose seizures are controlled and those who have an occasional seizure may swim in a pool with an informed lifeguard or a competent swimming companion. Swimming under water and diving into deep water should be forbidden. Patients with rare seizures should not swim in large bodies of water, even with a lifeguard present. Patients with frequent seizures should be prohibited from swimming.

SPORTS AND RECREATION
The use of power tools should be avoided. Bicycle riding should be postponed until the patient has been seizure-free for at least 6 months.

PREGNANCY
Harm can be done to the fetus by either seizure activity or antiepileptic drugs. A physician should be consulted before the person becomes pregnant in order to advise the patient of the risks and to help determine how they can be minimized (see Chap. 29).

ALCOHOL CONSUMPTION
Alcohol and most antiepileptic drugs cause sedation and cardiorespiratory depression. When taken together, the combined depressant effects can result in coma or even death. Furthermore, there is good evidence that even moderate consumption of alcohol aggravates seizure disorders in some people [16] (see Chap. 28). The patient with epilepsy is best advised to abstain from alcohol. For many this is a difficult sacrifice and a pleasure that is not easily given up. Careful instruction about the risks involved in drinking may make it easier for the patient to change his lifestyle. Support is crucial, and repeated explanations are usually indicated. Caution patients about over-the-counter and prescription drugs that contain alcohol such as cough syrups and cold remedies (elixir-alcohol).

IDENTIFICATION
The patient with epilepsy should be advised to obtain a medic-alert bracelet, charm, or necklace. The patient should always carry identifying information in a wallet or purse containing the following details: (1) seizure diagnosis, (2) name of primary clinician and hospital for emergency treatment and telephone numbers, (3) medication schedule, (4) name and number of person to be notified in case of an emergency, and (5) allergies, if any [6].

SEIZURE RECORDS
A system of recording seizure activity, auras, and drug side effects should also be established before discharge. Pocket-sized calendars for seizure records are useful, but some people feel awkward writing in them

because it is obvious to others that they are "different." A more inconspicuous method for an executive, for instance, would be to record seizure activity on a personal appointment calendar by developing a symbol that represents seizure activity.

PSYCHOSOCIAL ADJUSTMENTS
The psychosocial problems of the patient with epilepsy are often more devastating than the seizures themselves. Family dynamics are often altered. If the patient was in the role of "breadwinner" a shift in earning responsibility may occur (temporarily or permanently). This shift is often accompanied by a concurrent loss in power and a feeling of lowered self-esteem.

The social stigma and lifestyle restrictions imposed on a person with newly diagnosed epilepsy will prompt many to hide their disease from employers and friends. They may refuse to wear any sort of identification. The fear of social rejection and unemployment, combined with the decision to keep the disease a secret, can create a terrible emotional burden. The anxiety associated with the timing of the next seizure is often intense and can in fact trigger seizures.

The patient who has lost his job will naturally be under great stress. The need for social service intervention should be recognized early. Patients should also be made aware of their regional epilepsy society and various other support programs offered in their region (see Chap. 13).

Within the hospital setting the nurse can anticipate the patient's problems, help work through fears, and work with the social worker for appropriate discharge planning. The more plans made before discharge, the greater the probability of successful adaptation after discharge.

References
1. Abbott, J. A. Epilepsy and the public health nurse. *Public Health Nurs.* 37:595, 1945.
2. Bachman, D. S. Physicians' responsibility for patients with epilepsy. *Ann. Neurol.* 6:279, 1979.
3. Browne, T. R. Clinical pharmacology of antiepileptic drugs. *Drug Ther. Rev.* 2:469, 1979.
4. Browne, T. R. Therapy of status epilepticus. *Comprehensive Therapy* 8:25, 1982.
5. Conway, B. L. *Pediatric Neurologic Nursing.* St. Louis: Mosby, 1977.
6. Conway, B. L. *Neurological and Neurosurgical Nursing.* St. Louis: Mosby, 1978.
7. *Commission for the Control of Epilepsy and Its Consequences: Plan for Nationwide Action on Epilepsy,* Vol. 2. Washington, D.C.: U.S. Department

of Health, Education, and Welfare, 1978. Pp. 569–593.

8. Doolittle, G. J., Greene, V. S., and Vallone, S. V. Epilepsy: Medical and nursing care of epileptic patients. *Am. J. Nurs.* 42:1357, 1942.

9. Feldman, R. G. Neurological Diseases: A Symptomatic Approach. In R. W. Wilkins, and N. G. Levinski (Eds.), *Medicine: Essentials of Clinical Practice.* Boston: Little, Brown, 1978.

10. Hawkon, M., and Ozuna, T. Practical aspects of anticonvulsant therapy. *Am. J. Nurs.* 79:1062, 1979.

11. Lennox, W. G. The epileptic patients and the nurse. *Am. J. Nurs.* 46:219, 1946.

12. Livingston, S. et al. Drowning in epilepsy. *Ann. Neurol.* 7:495, 1980.

13. Livingston, S. et al. Bathing instructions for patients with epilepsy. *J.A.M.A.* 245:702, 1981.

14. Masland, R. L. *Commission for the Control of Epilepsy and Its Consequences: Plan for Nationwide Action on Epilepsy,* Vol. 1. Washington, D.C.: U.S. Department of Health, Education, and Welfare, 1978. Pp. 15–59.

15. Masland, R. L. The physician's responsibility for epileptic drivers. *Ann. Neurol.* 4:485, 1978.

16. Mattson, R. H. et al. Effect of alcohol intake in nonalcoholic epileptics. *Neurology* (N.Y.) 25:361, 1975.

17. Norman, S. E., and Browne, T. R. Seizure disorders. *Am. J. Nurs.* 81:984, 1981.

18. Pern, J. H. Epilepsy and drowning in childhood. *Br. Med. J.* 1:1510, 1977.

19. Roger, J., Lob, H., and Tassinari, C. Status Epilepticus. In O. Magnus, and A. M. L. DeHass (Eds.), *Handbook of Clinical Neurology,* Vol. 15. Amsterdam: North-Holland, 1974.

20. Shope, J. T. The clinical specialist in epilepsy. *Nurs. Clin. North Am.* 9:761, 1974.

21. Skeet, M. Principles and practice of first aid. *Nurs. Mirror* 8:i, 1978.

22. Swift, N. Helping patients live with seizures. *Nursing* 78(8):24, 1978.

23. Waddell, G. H. Status Epilepticus: Nursing Care Management. In A. V. Delgado-Escueta et al. (Eds.), *Status Epilepticus: Mechanisms of Brain Damage and Treatment.* New York: Raven Press, 1982.

24. Williams, A. Classification and diagnosis of epilepsy. *Nurs. Clin. North Am.* 9:747, 1974.

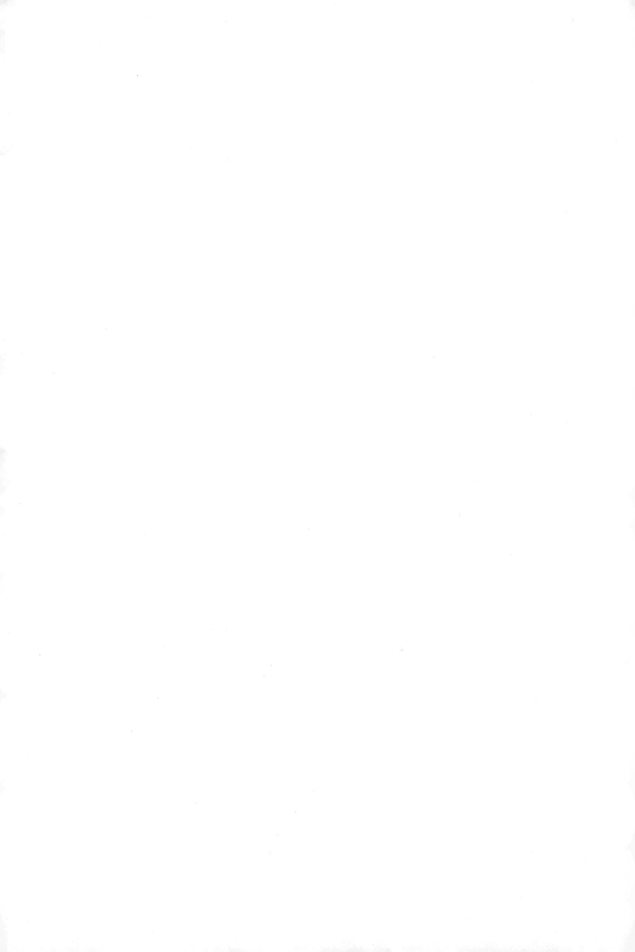

BEHAVIORAL METHODS OF SEIZURE CONTROL

24

Robert G. Feldman
Nancy L. Ricks
Merle M. Orren

Behavioral methods of seizure control have usually been used as adjuncts to pharmacologic treatment. Whether the method is drawn from learning theory, conditioning, psychodynamic process, or various biofeedback techniques, its success can be measured accurately only when variables such as the blood levels of prescribed drugs and intercurrent factors affecting seizure threshold are considered. Evidence suggests that some behavioral methods may be useful in treating selected patients with seizure disorders. The specificity and efficacy of each method for a given type of seizure disorder must be carefully evaluated. What may be an effective behavioral therapy for one seizure type may exacerbate another.

Behavioral therapies for epilepsy have three theoretical targets: (1) the seizure as a response to specific environmental triggers (internal and external); (2) the seizure as a reinforced behavior; and (3) the seizure as a symptom of the emotional state of the patient. Feldman and Ricks [11] used the paradigm stimulus-organism-response (S-O-R) for systematically reviewing the behavioral techniques used in treating patients with epilepsy. Treatment programs can be directed toward antecedent events (stimulus (S)) and toward postictal events or postictal behavior and responses (R). When seizures occur as a symptom of underlying emotional conflicts or psychosocial maladaptations, the personality structure of the organism (O) requires attention as a cause of poor seizure control.

The Seizure as a Response to a Specific Stimulus (S-o-r)

In considering a seizure as a response to a specific stimulus, emphasis is placed on identification of a seizure's antecedents or precipitating events. The relationship between the occurrence of the stimulus or trigger and the seizure is determined by the close timing of antecedent events and seizure occurrence. Often the triggering stimulus is highly specific although not necessarily simple. The aim of behavioral therapies is to alter the seizure threshold by manipulating the presentation of the stimulus.

DESENSITIZATION THERAPY FOR
SENSORY OR REFLEX EPILEPSIES

The clinical and electroencephalographic (EEG) features of sensory and reflex epilepsies are reviewed in Chapter 12. Therapies using classical conditioning models are of interest in stimulus-induced epilepsy. Forster et al. [14, 15, 17, 18] use controlled presentations of noxious stimuli to treat some cases. Two types of stimulus presentation are common. The first involves modification of the noxious stimulus and its repeated presentation. This approach takes two forms—(1) systematic desensitization, a method in which the stimulus is initially too weak to elicit seizures and then increases by increments in intensity; (2) monocular or monaural presentations. With the second type of stimulus presentation the stimulus is presented, and when a seizure occurs, the stimulus is repeated 10 or 15 times during the seizure and postictal period. Several examples of desensitization therapies for specific types of stimulus-induced seizures follow.

Visual Stimulus-Induced Seizures

Most of Forster's patients with photic-induced seizures were treated with a modification of the systematic desensitization method in which the ambient light was varied while stroboscopic intensity was constant. This presentation has the effect of altering the intensity of the stimulus. In addition, these patients were trained while wearing glasses that produced clicks when the ambient lighting changed suddenly. The clicks served to maintain the effect outside the laboratory as reinforcing stimuli [18]. Pattern-induced seizures have been treated with variable success with the methods used for photic-induced seizures.

Auditory Stimulus-Induced Seizures

Startle epilepsy occurs rarely. The usual precipitant is a noise. Bickford and Klass [2] developed a model of startle epilepsy that suggests that the startle threshold is determined by multiple factors and is under the influence of complex regulatory mechanisms. In the presence of an epileptic lesion, the activation of the startle threshold produces a seizure. Booker et al. [3] reported successful treatment of this type of epilepsy using successive presentations of auditory stimuli monaurally, keeping the stimuli below 60 decibels to prevent bone conduction to the opposite ear. The effect seen may be the result of alteration of the startle threshold through habituation.

Musicogenic Seizures

The seizures in Forster's [16] 5 cases of music-induced epilepsy were all of the complex partial type, and 4

patients had EEG dysrhythmia on the left side. In these patients the theme of the music appeared to be the precipitating stimulus rather than the loudness, type, or meaning of the music. Altering the stimulus threshold by playing the music during the seizure and postictal period for approximately 1 hour has been effective in treating these patients. The same procedure was used to treat a 53-year-old woman who developed seizures that were precipitated when she heard a particular person's voice [17].

Sensory-precipitated seizures occur in only a very small proportion of patients with epilepsy. Hence, although desensitization methods appear to be effective in the treatment of sensory-induced seizures, their application to other, more common types of seizure disorders is open to question.

OTHER S-O-R TECHNIQUES FOR OTHER SEIZURE TYPES

Relaxation Techniques

Relaxation techniques are often combined with desensitization methods in treating patients in whom the antecedent event is associated with anxiety or tension. Rarely is the relaxation method used alone.

The most extensive study of the use of relaxation to desensitize patients to the effects of anxiety was reported by Cabral and Scott [4]. Relaxation was one of the two methods used in a study with a crossover design in 3 patients with intractable epilepsy associated with anxiety and phobic symptoms. Training in alpha feedback was given for 3 months before the relaxation procedure was begun in 2 patients, 1 with a long history of both tonic-clonic and absence seizures and the other with complex partial seizures. Three months of relaxation training was the initial treatment for a third patient with absence seizures of long duration and more recent tonic-clonic seizures. During both relaxation and biofeedback training the patients were presented with specific anxiety-provoking stimuli.

The duration of alpha activity was found to increase (by seconds) in patients exposed to the anxiety-provoking stimuli during the period of biofeedback. The number of clinical seizures decreased in all 3 patients by the end of the 6-month treatment period. In the 2 patients treated first with biofeedback, the major reduction in seizure frequency occurred during the biofeedback treatment, with further reduction after relaxation treatment was begun. Clinical seizure frequency was reduced in the third patient during relaxation which was given first, with further reduction during biofeedback. On follow-up examination after 15 months, seizure frequency for all patients was greater than that noted at the end of the treatment period. However, in none did the number of seizures return to pretreatment levels. The fact that both forms of treatment were effective suggests that there was at least a partial influence of the placebo effect.

Aversive Techniques
The use of aversive conditioning in modifying antecedents to seizures was first reported by Efron [8], who treated a patient with uncinate seizures by presenting a noxious smell before the seizures. The smell was later paired with a bracelet so that the patient could prevent seizures by simply looking at it. Seizure frequency did not decrease, but the patient was able to stop seizures once they began. Other successes have been reported with the use of shock administered to stop specific motor behavior such as handwaving or closing the eyes in self-induced seizures in retarded children [14, 45].

Aversive conditioning characterized by shouting "No" and shaking the patient's shoulders was used by Zlutnick et al. [50] in 4 children in an effort to interrupt behavioral chains leading to seizures. The types of disorders were identified as "minor motor seizures" in 3 children, and no seizure type was specified for the fourth. Seizures had begun at least 2 years prior to aversive therapy and were poorly controlled with medication. All 4 children had impaired mental function; 3 had unspecified or undetermined brain damage or were mentally retarded, and the fourth was unable to attend school. Each child had observable seizures (with 90 percent agreement among independent observers) and a minimum of one seizure per day.

In each case, a target behavior was selected for modification after observation and analysis of preseizure behavior. Target behaviors included a fixed gaze, lowered activity level, a subtle behavior change most apparent to the child's mother (which preceded about half of the seizures), and the raising of an arm. Reduction in seizure frequency was reported in 3 cases, the most impressive result occurring in the child with the unspecified seizure type who had no seizures after 7 weeks of treatment. Medications were reduced during the treatment period and discontinued at the end. Six months of follow-up revealed only one questionable seizure involving a fall at the playground. Generally, fairly rapid reduction in the numbers of seizures was seen after treatment was started, followed by a more gradual decline in seizure frequency later in therapy.

The use of stimuli presented at the beginning of electrographic evidence of seizure activity may be viewed as a type of aversive method. Some evidence of reduced duration of spike-and-wave activity with presentation of photic, auditory, or somatosensory stimulation has been observed in several patients with absence seizures [32], but this is by no means a reliable phenomenon. Further, results suggest that to be effective a stimulus must be presented in the first 3 seconds of spike-and-wave activity. Stevens et al. [42] were unable to reduce seizures by a similar method.

Biofeedback
Therapeutic approaches aimed at reducing seizure frequency through modification of the EEG fall under the heading of biofeedback. In biofeedback, EEG information is conveyed to the patient through electronic detection and sensory feedback in the form of auditory, visual or, less frequently, somatic cues. Apart from this common operational requirement, the type of EEG pattern regulating feedback and the specific feedback contingencies have varied from study to study.

The feedback system may simply signal the occurrence of paroxysmal discharge in the EEG, as for example, when a spike triggers the delivery of a feedback stimulus. The possible mechanisms by which such seizure-contingent feedback might suppress paroxysmal discharges and reduce the frequency of clinical seizures are several. The feedback stimulus may allow the patient to undertake abortive maneuvers. Alternatively, the feedback stimulus could directly intervene in the further generation and propagation of seizure discharge by eliciting EEG desynchronization. Finally, if the feedback is perceived as unpleasant, it might serve as an aversive consequence or "punishment" for the preceding paroxysmal EEG discharge.

Seizure-contingent feedback was used in a study [44] of 13 patients with epilepsy who had focal and lateralized spike discharges in the EEG. The relative effectiveness of feedback stimuli in different sensory modalities was assessed for individual patients in preliminary testing sessions. Depending on their lateralization, spike discharges triggered auditory or somatosensory stimuli to the opposite ear or limb to prevent the further cortical spread of epileptic activity. Eight of the patients produced lower rates of focal discharge during spike-triggered feedback and 5 patients showed reduced incidence of clinical seizures over the course of training. However, other studies utilizing feedback triggered by EEG paroxysmal discharge have produced conflicting results [30, 32, 42].

In addition to simple seizure-contingent feedback, more complex feedback systems regulated by sophisticated filters, inhibitory circuits, and discriminators deliver differential cues for desired and undesired EEG patterns. Such a system may be used, at least theoretically, to shape the characteristics of the EEG in a desired direction. In the pioneering work of Sterman and his colleagues [35, 41], feedback contingencies were designed to enhance the occurrence of 12 to 14 Hz EEG activity recorded over the Rolandic region in epileptic patients whose seizures were not well controlled by medication. The choice of this particular sensorimotor rhythm (SMR) was based on Sterman's experimental work with cats and monkeys [34, 36, 37, 39, 49] suggesting that SMR was associated with motor inhibition and that its enhancement through conditioning or physical immobilization increased animals' resistance to drug-induced seizures.

Patients with epilepsy received feedback consisting of chimes, lights, and slide presentations, contingent on the presence of 12 to 14 Hz EEG activity recorded from the scalp over Rolandic regions, provided these frequencies occurred in the absence of electromyogram (EMG) activity, movement artifact, and paroxysmal discharges. The patients underwent three 20 to 40 minute SMR training sessions per week for 6 to 18 months. EEGs were carried out before and at one to six month intervals during training. Medication schedules were kept constant or reduced if warranted by the patient's clinical condition. After several months of training, various signs of improvement were noted. Except for transient increases during training breaks, all of the patients showed a reduction in the rate of tonic-clonic seizures compared to a 2-year period preceding biofeedback. An increase in the occurrence of the reinforced 12 to 14 Hz activity; attenuation of slow frequencies, and a decrease in paroxysmal discharges were also reported. Although one subsequent study failed to find a definite relationship between SMR training and seizure reduction [22], numerous other investigations [12, 13, 25, 33] replicated Sterman's findings and reported substantial clinical improvement during and following SMR training.

Subsequent research, however, suggests that SMR training is not uniquely associated with favorable clinical outcomes. A reduction in seizures has also been reported among epileptic patients receiving feedback for desynchronized EEG patterns recorded over the site of their epileptic foci [46, 48]. In another investigation, positive feedback triggered by a broad band of Rolandic EEG frequencies, including but not limited to Sterman's SMR, resulted in lower seizure rates in 3 of 5 patients [24]. Sterman and Macdonald [40] demonstrated the effectiveness of various programs of differential reinforcement in reducing sei-

zures from baseline rates in 6 of 8 patients. Negative feedback for slow Rolandic frequencies (6 to 9 Hz), concurrent with positive feedback for either 12 to 15 Hz or 18 to 23 Hz activity produced the maximal therapeutic effect, although other combinations of positively and negatively cued EEG frequencies also resulted in significant improvement in seizure rate. More recent work by Sterman [38] has also been aimed at enhancing a range of intermediate Rolandic rhythms, while at the same time minimizing the occurrence of very low and high EEG frequencies, with favorable outcomes in 13 of 15 patients. Finally, Cott and colleagues [6] have demonstrated that feedback for high amplitude slow wave activity in the 4 to 7 Hz band with instructions to minimize these signals was as effective in reducing seizures and EEG abnormalities as training utilizing positive feedback for SMR.

Although the specific feedback contingencies yielding the maximal therapeutic effect are still largely unknown or controversial, a number of factors are clearly important in planning, implementing, and evaluating biofeedback treatment. In terms of instrumentation, the performance properties of the filtering, discriminating and feedback apparatus are critical in ensuring that positive feedback is not inadvertently triggered by epileptiform or other abnormal EEG activity and also that the frequency bands that are nominally reinforced according to the treatment design are, in fact, the frequencies generating positive feedback.

Since the goal of treatment is to reduce the frequency of seizures, the most important variable in evaluating biofeedback is the incidence of seizures before, during, and after biofeedback training. The incidence of seizures should be recorded over pre-treatment, treatment, and post-treatment intervals sufficiently long to span spontaneous variations in seizure frequency. Ideally, continuous monitoring of the patient's EEG and behavior would provide the most accurate information about the occurrence of seizures. Because this is unfeasible, most investigators have relied on self-reported seizure incidence or on seizure logs kept by relatives and professionals (e.g., nurses, teachers), who are in frequent contact with the patient. For this reason, it is important that the patients selected for biofeedback training have recognizable and highly visible seizures. Such patients include those with focal motor, myoclonic, tonic-clonic, or atonic or complex partial seizures with well-defined automatisms. Brief complex partial and absence seizures may not be recognizable (or remembered) by the patient; the paucity of the seizure signs in these disorders makes them difficult for others to detect as well.

Finally, in evaluating the effectiveness of biofeedback, it is important that, wherever possible, the antiepileptic regimen be kept constant throughout the pre-treatment baseline period and for the full duration of EEG training. Patient compliance with the prescribed medication can be estimated by monitoring blood levels as often as possible. A reduction in seizure incidence during EEG training can be attributed to biofeedback procedures only if there are no correlated increases in antiepileptic drug blood levels.

Approximately 50 to 60 percent of patients with epilepsy participating in EEG biofeedback studies have reported reduced seizure frequency. The proportion of patients showing clinical improvement is fairly constant in all studies utilizing different EEG targets and different feedback contingencies, indicating that no single program of positive and/or negative feedback and no particular EEG change, other than idiosyncratic patterns of normalization, are associated with this effect. Because there is no single pathophysiology known to account for all varieties of epilepsy (and no single pharmacologic antidote for all types of seizures), it would be surprising indeed if a single method of behavioral intervention was found to be effective in managing all types of epilepsy.

In seeking an explanation for the results of biofeedback and a more adequate rationale for its implementation, the functional importance of EEG seizure patterns must be taken into account. Focal EEG discharges, if originating in the cortical region approximating the scalp electrode, may reflect excitatory processes or, if projected from a remote active focus, inhibitory phenomena. Generalized EEG discharges of the spike-and-wave variety reflect recurrent excitatory and inhibitory influences, possibly projected (or initially activated) from a distance. When biofeedback is successful in suppressing the occurrence of focal spikes, focal slowing, or generalized spike-wave discharges, the mechanism in each case is likely to be different according to whether the discharge is local or projected, or primarily excitatory or inhibitory. It follows that the most effective method in each instance will be the one that addresses the fundamental disturbance in a particular epileptic disorder.

Even in seizure disorders that are similarly classified according to gross symptomatology and EEG correlates, pathways of propagation are probably not identical in all patients. In a study of 4 patients with similar 3 Hz spike-wave bursts and clinical absences, diverse patterns of seizure-related ocular activity were reported [28]. Although absence attacks were described in all patients, individualized patterns of responses to stimuli presented in different sensory modalities were observed during seizures when the patients were tested on discriminative tasks [29]. This *idiosyncratic* expression of seizures in patients with a common diagnosis implies that a slightly different route is taken by the propagated discharge in each case. To the extent that biofeedback is successful because it engages seizure-susceptible brain regions in normal activity and perhaps "teaches" normal functioning in these pathways with continued training, patients with different or even nominally the same types of seizure disorder may not benefit equally by a given biofeedback procedure.

It is assumed in biofeedback research that by altering the EEG one is effecting a favorable change in critical regions of the nervous system that will result in reduced seizure incidence. However, EEG discharges and clinical seizures are related but somewhat independent manifestations of the pathologic process and may not be referable to the same neural substrate [27]. Thus, instances have been reported in which training resulted in reduced seizure discharge without affecting seizure frequency [44] and in reduced seizure frequency without correlated decreases in paroxysmal EEG activity [22].

Although biofeedback may continue to be used as a therapeutic tool, a specific description of its mechanisms requires a more thorough scientific understanding of the seizure process itself. We need to know, for example, more about the role of inhibitory mechanisms in disrupting neural synchrony and epileptic manifestations and how to activate such mechanisms behaviorally. At the same time, the development of accurate methods of determining the origin and propagation pattern of seizure discharge in individual patients would permit more effective kinds of behavioral intervention.

Other variables may limit the effectiveness of biofeedback. The plasticity of the neural events responsible for seizures may depend on the anatomic location of the active focus and the characteristics of the neural discharge. Apparently not all types of abnormal neural activity are amenable to behavioral control [47]. Antiepileptic drugs may attenuate neural lability or plasticity so that feedback procedures are ineffective [12] no matter how sound the rationale. Nonsynaptic mechanisms also play a role in the pathophysiology of seizure disorders [31] and may not be easily manipulated by environmental contingencies.

Critics of biofeedback studies have emphasized the small number of patients studied, the lack of statistically significant results, the possibility of placebo effect, the possibility that the results may be due to providing the patient with a relaxation technique, and the possibility of inadvertently reinforcing other behaviors that may elicit seizures. Recent investigations have begun to address some of these issues [4, 24, 38].

The Seizure as Reinforced Behavior (s-o-R)

Approaches to the seizure as reinforced behavior view seizures as behavioral responses that either increase or decrease in frequency as a consequence of reinforcement. The frequency of some seizures depends on responses from others that tend to reinforce the behavior. This reinforcement often takes the form of oversolicitous attention from parents, teachers, and peers after a seizure. When such attention or favor becomes an end in itself, it can increase the number of seizures the patient, often a child, has. Behavioral methods have been used to attempt to reduce the frequency of seizures by changing their consequences. The consequences of seizures are emphasized—that is, whether they are followed by reinforcement. Behavior that is not reinforced tends to become extinguished. Frequent reinforcement is generally necessary to establish a new behavior. However, once a response is established, less frequent reinforcement is more effective in maintaining it. New behavior repertoires are built by shaping, a method by which successive approximations of a desired behavior are reinforced. These approaches are called contingency changing and are drawn from the technique known as operant conditioning.

CONTINGENCY CHANGING

The methods often used are (1) planned extinction of behavior by ignoring or providing no positive reinforcement of it, (2) reinforcement for not having seizures, or (3) a combination of both methods.

Cautela and Flannery [5] reported the successful treatment by teachers of a 22-year-old mentally retarded man with uncontrolled seizures characterized by tonic spasms, loss of balance, blackened vision, and loss of consciousness. The seizures were of encephalitic origin and began in the third grade. Generalized, symmetrical discharges were evident on EEG, and the pneumoencephalogram showed enlargement of all four ventricles. The estimated frequency of seizures before treatment varied from three to seven per week. The treatment plan consisted of rewarding the patient with social praise and candy during seizure-free days. In addition, he was told that a teacher would spend time with him at the end of those days on which he had no seizures. If a seizure occurred, the staff member did not talk during or immediately after it. These arrangements, which constituted phase I of treatment, continued for 17 weeks. During phase I it was observed that the presence of one particular patient tended to provoke seizures, so in phase II they were separated. The teacher-therapist was also changed in phase II, and an additional reward of being able to go for coffee during class was given the patient if he had been seizure-free for 3 days. In the course of the 28 weeks of treatment he was seizure-free during 13 weeks, and during 6 weeks he had only one seizure per week.

A similar approach was reported by Balaschak [1] in an 11-year-old girl with "atypical" seizures. One type of seizure was characterized by a brief (1 to 2 minutes) fall of her head to the side or forward while she maintained her position in the chair. Other seizures involved falls, usually backward, and were occasionally accompanied by movement of the left arm and leg. The patient usually recovered from these in 5 minutes. During the treatment program, a reduction in frequency of seizures was observed. When the teacher declined to continue the program, seizure frequency returned to its previous level.

A major problem with contingency changing approaches is that the effects do not appear to outlive the duration of the treatment program, and the treatment period tends to be relatively short. Moreover, a therapist who leaves after a brief period may introduce other stresses for patients. To be viable, approaches that treat seizures as a behavioral response must address the problem of the effects of withdrawal of treatment and develop a means of maintaining the beneficial effects once the treatment is discontinued.

The Seizure as a Symptom of Emotional State (s-O-r)

When seizures occur as a symptom of underlying emotional conflicts or psychosocial maladaptations, the personality structure of the patient requires attention as a source of poor seizure control. Although the precipitation of seizures may be related to the psychodynamics in each case, the symbolic meaning of seizure activity varies among patients. The psychodynamic meaning of seizures may be (1) a defense mechanism [23], (2) a means of getting attention, (3) a means of avoiding distasteful tasks [23], (4) a reaction to dependence upon the mother [21], or (5) a means of reducing tension [9]. The meaning of seizures differs not only among patients but also from time to time in the same patient. The psychodynamic meaning of seizures to family members must also be considered [23]. In some families, seizures gratify unconscious parental wishes; in others, they provide a diversionary focus for parental conflict.

The treatment of seizures as a symptom of the psychodynamics of the individual patient focuses on behavior that is generally thought to be learned, although not necessarily conscious. Emphasis is placed on analysis of defenses and on restructuring of the personality in an effort to promote methods of reducing tension and ways of coping with life events that do not involve seizure activity. These treatment methods may also attempt to identify seizure antecedents such as emotional triggers, but they differ from stimulus-induced treatment in that triggers are viewed as behavior that reflects unresolved conflicts. Therefore the triggers are related thematically rather than by specific physical stimulus properties. Moreover, s-O-r approaches can be distinguished from S-o-r approaches by the assumption that modification of a specific behavior without addressing the underlying problem will be of little benefit to the patient. Dynamic psychotherapy and family and group therapies are examples of s-O-r approaches.

Fremont-Smith [19] found a direct relationship between strong emotion and one or more seizures with loss of consciousness in 31 of 42 patients he studied. Moreover, in 8 patients, major or minor seizures directly precipitated by emotion were observed. Steven's study [43] of 100 patients with epilepsy supports these results.

The weight of the evidence suggests that emotional disturbance is more frequent in patients with epilepsy and that increases in stress may result in increased seizure frequency (see Chap. 5). Patients with complex partial seizures may be more vulnerable to the effects of emotional activation because limbic system structures are involved in both complex partial seizures (see Chap. 5). This involvement of the limbic system has two consequences: (1) control of behavior is more problematic, and (2) memory is affected, which in turn influences the way persons cope with the disorder. Because of the retrograde amnesia in these patients, the identification of emotional precipitants is more difficult.

In an effort to assist 5 patients with long-standing complex partial epilepsy, videotape techniques were developed by Feldman and Paul [10] to identify and stimulate recall of emotional triggers of seizures. The treatment approach proceeded in four phases: (1) exploratory interviews, (2) stimulated recall of emotional stresses with concurrent audio and videotape recording of the patient's verbal and facial expressions and seizures, (3) self-confrontation, in which the tape recording of the seizure and its antecedent events were shown to patient. The interview during which self-confrontation occurred was also taped and then presented together with the recording of the seizure on a split screen so that the patient could observe his reactions to seeing his own seizures. The experience was then discussed with the patient to heighten awareness of the stresses that triggered the seizures. Finally, (4) the patient was reminded through a review of the tapes of the relationship between the seizures and the emotional stimuli so that he would avoid responding in the same way in the future.

All 5 patients had seizure disorders of long duration that had been poorly controlled despite psychotherapy and antiepileptic medications. In each case, after outpatient treatment the frequency of seizures decreased from 5 to 25 per week, depending on the patient, to fewer than 8 per year, and the effect has been maintained during 2 to 4 years of follow-up. Feldman and Paul [10] believe that this approach may be particularly advantageous in treating patients with complex partial seizures because it provides a means of dealing with their memory disturbance.

Indications for Specific Types of Behavioral Therapy

All behavioral therapies have certain general effects. However, certain behavioral approaches seem to have specific efficacy for specific types of seizure disorders. These therapies still must be considered trends rather than approaches of proven value.

GENERAL EFFECTS OF BEHAVIORAL THERAPIES

It is evident from the reported success of a variety of treatment methods in controlling several types of seizure disorders that some effects are probably general and may be considered placebo effects or effects generated from the increased attention that these methods necessarily provide. Moreover, in some patients the effects seem to be related to more careful scrutiny of the patient, leading to better compliance in taking antiepileptic medications or to changes in the medication prescribed. Changes in medication are frequently reported in behavioral studies and are not necessarily reductions of medications based on the effects of behavioral treatment. Although the investigators may de-emphasize the role of medication changes or explain the beneficial effects as an interaction between the behavioral treatment and the medication, the basis for such explanations is not substantial.

DESENSITIZATION METHODS

When a specific physical stimulus can be reliably demonstrated to induce seizure activity, the desensitization methods of Forster [14, 15, 16, 17, 18] appear to be effective. However, the antecedents of the seizures must be carefully evaluated, both in terms of their specificity and their close relationships in time to the occurrence of the seizures. Forster notes the need to differentiate specific sensory stimuli from emotional triggers. In addition, to maintain the beneficial effects, training must be continued. The evidence for the effectiveness of desensitization in treating other antecedents of seizures has not been clearly established.

AVERSIVE CONDITIONING

Aversive conditioning has been used primarily to eliminate motor behavior that may induce or otherwise precede seizures. Such conditioning may on occasion be effective, but it can lead to other maladaptive behavior. It is probably not the treatment of choice for elimination of specific motor antecedents in any type of seizure disorder. Differential reinforcement of other behavior incompatible with the motor antecedent may be a more viable substitute for this method.

BIOFEEDBACK

SMR biofeedback may reduce the frequency of seizures in some patients, particularly those with motor accompaniment, but the reasons for this effect are not well understood. It may be "a complex placebo" [22]. Sudden withdrawal from SMR training tends to exacerbate the seizure disorder and should be avoided.

RELAXATION THERAPY

The effectiveness of relaxation therapy has yet to be demonstrated. Some evidence suggests that its use is contraindicated in patients with absence seizures.

CONTINGENCY CHANGING

Some evidence indicates that changing the contingencies associated with the aftermath of seizures serves to reduce their number. As a specific treatment type, its major liability lies in the relatively short time such programs are generally applied. Because this approach is often used with mentally retarded or otherwise functionally impaired persons, the introduction of a therapist who leaves after a relatively brief but intensive period may in itself reinforce feelings of worthlessness in a person who has few friends, few social skills, and minimal ways of coping with distress.

A major contribution of this work, however, is the documentation of the effects of the responses of people who are important in the patient's environment in either reducing or increasing seizure control.

Contingency changing has broader implications for seizure control than its usefulness in a specific program. Careful evaluation of responses by family members, peers, and teachers to the child after seizures occur may help the physician learn why seizures persist in some patients and not in others despite adequate pharmacologic treatment.

STRESS REDUCTION

Stress tends to increase the frequency of seizures in most seizure disorders. However, the manifestations of stress differ, and no direct correlation exists between evidence of stress and clinical seizure manifestations. Identification of different types of stress and their effects on patients to determine the suitability of different treatment methods may be useful.

Chronic Stress

Chronic stress is often associated with enduring life situations, patterns, and problems. Ways of coping with chronic stress usually become relatively structured within the personality and are consequently more difficult to change. An example of chronic stress is a disruptive family pattern, for which family therapy may be necessary. Recurrent seizures that are severe or poorly controlled are another example of chronic stress. Hence, people with these disorders are more likely to develop other personality disturbances for which a variety of programs may be needed, such as assistance in school, vocational training, or social activity groups, to minimize the effects of poor control. In addition, counseling of family members about inappropriate and appropriate limitations, particularly for children, may be valuable in preventing the development of maladaptive behavior.

Situational Stress

Situational stress is usually characterized by some disruptive event or change in the patient's environment, such as loss of job, an illness, or the death of a family member. Its effect may last several weeks or months, but usually it is time-limited and requires no specific change in treatment unless exacerbation of the seizure disorder is severe or the effect is prolonged. A brief period of hospitalization for evaluation may help if severe exacerbation is seen. When effects are prolonged, short-term counseling directed at understanding the stressful situation and the patient's way of coping with it may be helpful.

Periodic Stress

Periodic stresses are commonly physiologic in nature; hormonal variations such as the menstrual cycle are the clearest examples. The effects are relatively short but recur periodically. Changes in the medication regimen may be necessary. It is often helpful to advise the patient that such changes are likely to occur so that the patient is spared the additional burden of surprise.

Episodic Stresses

Episodic stress does not necessarily appear in a predictable pattern but is specific to certain events. Examples include sleep deprivation, arguments, and family fights. In many respects, these events are normal variations that occur in the lives of everyone. They should cause concern only if a frequent pattern develops.

Acute Stress

Acute stress is generally associated with an anxiety-provoking event and usually does not last long. However, its effects are generalized for the time it is present. Such stress should not cause concern unless it becomes frequent or leads to frequent seizure-inducing behavior such as hyperventilation.

Stress Due to Unconscious Emotional Conflicts

Stress due to emotional conflicts may also be accompanied by anxiety, but here the stress arises not so much from the situation as from the meaning of an occurrence, thought, or action to the patient. In such a situation the patient may not appear to be disturbed until a specific subject is mentioned, or an apparently innocuous event may give rise to inappropriate action. Not only is evidence of this type of stress a sufficient indication for therapy (such as the videotape procedure described above, or therapy directed at uncovering the conflict and bringing it to the patient's attention), but also it often influences the patient's role in the doctor-patient relationship and tends to lead to poor compliance. At times, this type of stress can make the job of the physician difficult, not only in the relationship with the patient but also in working with other professionals who may be treating the patient. Increased friction among professionals and other staff about a certain patient is often the primary clue that such a patient has an underlying conflict that may affect seizure control [26].

When a patient endures chronic stress or conflictual stress, the effects of other stresses may be increased, but their expression vis-à-vis seizure manifestations will differ depending on the types of conflicts, personality disturbances, and family patterns.

References

1. Balaschak, B. A. Teacher-implemented behavior modification in a case of organically based epilepsy. *J. Consult. Clin. Psychol.* 44:218, 1976.
2. Bickford, R. G., and Klass, D. W. Sensory Precipitation and Reflex Mechanisms. In H. H. Jasper, A. A. Ward, Jr., and A. Pope (Eds.), *Basic Mechanisms of the Epilepsies.* Boston: Little, Brown, 1969.
3. Booker, H. E., Forster, F. M., and Klive, H. Extinction factors in startle (acousticomotor) seizures. *Neurology* 15:1095, 1965.
4. Cabral, H. E., and Scott, D. F. Effects of two desensitization techniques, biofeedback and relaxation, on intractable epilepsy: Follow-up study. *J. Neurol. Neurosurg. Psychiatr.* 39:504, 1976.
5. Cautela, J. R., and Flannery, R. B. Seizures: Controlling the uncontrollable. *J. Rehabil.* 39:34, 1973.
6. Cott, A., Pavlovski, R. P., and Black, A. H. Reducing epileptic seizures through operant conditioning of central nervous system activity: Procedural variables. *Science* 302:73, 1979.
7. Daube, J. R. Sensory precipitated seizures: A review. *J. Nerv. Ment. Dis.* 141:524, 1966.
8. Efron, R. The conditioned inhibition of uncinate fits. *Brain* 80:251, 1957.
9. Epstein, A. W., and Ervin, F. Psychodynamic significance of seizure content in psychomotor epilepsy. *Psychosom. Med.* 18:43, 1956.
10. Feldman, R. G., and Paul, N. L. Identity of emotional triggers in epilepsy. *J. Nerv. Ment. Dis.* 162:345, 1976.
11. Feldman, R. G., and Ricks, N. L. Nonpharmacological and Behavioral Methods. In G. S. Ferriss (Ed.), *Treatment of Epilepsy Today.* Oradell, N.J.: Medical Economics Co., 1978.
12. Finley, W. W. Operant conditioning of the EEG in two patients with epilepsy: Methodological and clinical considerations. *Pavlov. J. Biol. Sci.* 12:93, 1977.
13. Finley, W. W., Smith, H. A., and Etherton, M. D. Reduction of seizures and normalization of the EEG following sensorimotor feedback training: Preliminary study. *Biol. Psychol.* 2:189, 1975.
14. Forster, F. M. *Reflex Epilepsy, Conditional Reflexes and Behavioral Treatment.* Springfield, Ill.: Thomas, 1975.
15. Forster, F. M. The classification and conditioning treatment of the reflex epilepsies. *Int. J. Epilepsy* 9:73, 1972.
16. Forster, F. M. Reading epilepsy, musicogenic epilepsy, and related disorders. In H. R. Mykleburst (Ed.), *Progress in Learning Disabilities, III.* New York: Grune & Stratton, 1975.
17. Forster, F. M. et al. A case of voice-induced epilepsy treated by conditioning. *Neurology* 19:325, 1969.

18. Forster, F. M. et al. Stroboscopic-induced seizure discharges: Modification by extinction techniques. *Arch. Neurol.* 11:603, 1964.
19. Fremont-Smith, F. The influence of emotion in precipitating convulsions: Preliminary report. *Am. J. Psychiat.* 30:717, 1934.
20. Gastaut, H., and Tassinari, C. A. Triggering mechanisms in epilepsy. *Epilepsia* 7:85, 1966.
21. Heilbrunn, G. Psychodynamic aspects of epilepsy. *Psychoanal. Q.* 19:145, 1950.
22. Kaplan, B. J. Biofeedback in epileptics: Equivocal relationship of reinforced EEG frequency to seizure reduction. *Epilepsia* 16:477, 1975.
23. Kamph, J. P. et al. The emotionally disturbed child with a convulsive disorder. *Psychosom. Med.* 25:411, 1963.
24. Kuhlman, W. N. EEG feedback training of epileptic patients: Clinical and electroencephalographic analysis. *Electroencephalogr. Clin. Neurophysiol.* 45:699, 1978.
25. Lubar, J. F., and Bahler, W. W. Behavioral management of epileptic seizures following EEG biofeedback training of the sensorimotor rhythm. *Biofeedback Self. Regul.* 1:77, 1976.
26. Main, T. F. The ailment. *Br. J. Med. Psychol.* 30:129, 1957.
27. Mirsky, A. F., and Van Buren, J. M. On the nature of the "absence" in centrencephalic epilepsy: A study of some behavioral, electroencephalographic and autonomic factors. *Electroencephalogr. Clin. Neurophysiol.* 18:334, 1965.
28. Orren, M. M., and Mirsky, A. F. Relation between ocular manifestations and onset of spike-and-wave discharges in petit mal epilepsy. *Epilepsia* 16:771, 1975.
29. Orren, M. M., and Mirsky, A. F. Behavioral correlates of spike-wave discharge in petit mal epilepsy. Paper presented at the Society for Neuroscience, Tenth Annual Meeting, Cincinnati, Ohio, November 9–14, 1980.
30. Ounstead, C., Lee, D., and Hutt, S. J. Electroencephalographic and clinical changes in an epileptic child during repeated photic stimulation. *Electroencephalogr. Clin. Neurophysiol.* 21:388, 1966.
31. Prince, D. A. Neurophysiology of epilepsy. *Annu. Rev. Neurosci.* 1:395, 1978.
32. Ricks, N. L., and Mirsky, A. F. Unpublished data.
33. Seifert, A. R., and Lubar, J. F. Reduction of epileptic seizures through EEG biofeedback training. *Biol. Psychol.* 3:81, 1975.
34. Sterman, M. B. Effects of brain surgery and EEG operant conditioning on seizure latency following monomethylhydrazine intoxication in the cat. *Exp. Neurol.* 50:757, 1976.
35. Sterman, M. B., and Friar, L. Suppression of seizures in an epileptic following sensorimotor EEG feedback training. *Electroencephalogr. Clin. Neurophysiol.* 33:89, 1972.
36. Sterman, M. B., Goodman, S. J., and Kovalesky, R. Effects of sensorimotor EEG feedback training on seizure susceptibility in the rhesus monkey. *Exp. Neurol.* 62:735, 1978.
37. Sterman, M. B., and Kovalesky, R. A. Anticonvulsant effects of restraint and pyridoxine on hydrazine seizures in the monkey. *Exp. Neurol.* 65:78, 1979.
38. Sterman, M. B., and Lantz, D. Effects of sensorimotor EEG normalization feedback training on seizure rate in poorly controlled epileptics. Paper presented at the 34th Annual Meeting of the American Electroencephalographic Society, Boston, Mass., September 5–7, 1980.
39. Sterman, M. B., LoPresti, R. W., and Fairchild, M. D. *Electroencephalographic and Behavioral Studies of Monomethylhydrazine Toxicity in the Cat.* Technical Report AMRL-TR-69-3, Air Systems Command, Wright Patterson Air Force Base, Ohio, 1969.
40. Sterman, M. B., and Macdonald, L. R. Effects of central cortical EEG feedback training on incidence of poorly controlled seizures. *Epilepsia* 19:207, 1978.
41. Sterman, M. B., Macdonald, L. R., and Stone, R. K. Biofeedback training of the sensorimotor electroencephalogram rhythm in man: Effects on epilepsy. *Epilepsia* 15:395, 1974.
42. Stevens, J. R. Endogenous conditioning to abnormal cerebral electrical transients in man. *Science* 137:974, 1962.
43. Stevens, J. R. Psychiatric implications of psychomotor epilepsy. *Arch. Gen. Psychiatry* 14:461, 1966.
44. Upton, A. R. M., and Longmire, D. Effects of feedback on focal epileptic discharges in man. *Can. J. Neurol. Sci.* 3:153, 1975.
45. Wright, L. Aversive conditioning of self-induced seizures. *Behav. Ther.* 4:712, 1973.
46. Wyler, A. R. et al. Conditioned EEG desynchronization and seizure occurrence in patients. *Electroencephalogr. Clin. Neurophysiol.* 41:501, 1976.
47. Wyler, A. R., Finch, C. A., and Burchiel, K. J. Epileptic and normal neurons in monkey neocortex: A quantitative study of degree of operant control. *Brain Res.* 151:269, 1978.

48. Wyler, A. R., Robbins, C. A., and Dodrill, C. B. EEG operant conditioning for control of epilepsy. *Epilepsia* 20:279, 1979.
49. Wyrwicka, W., and Sterman, M. B. Instrumental conditioning of sensorimotor cortex EEG spindles in the waking cat. *Physiol. Behav.* 3:703, 1968.
50. Zlutnick, S., Mayville, W. H., and Moffat, S. Modification of seizure disorders: The interruption of behavioral chains. *J. Appl. Behav. Anal.* 8:1, 1975.

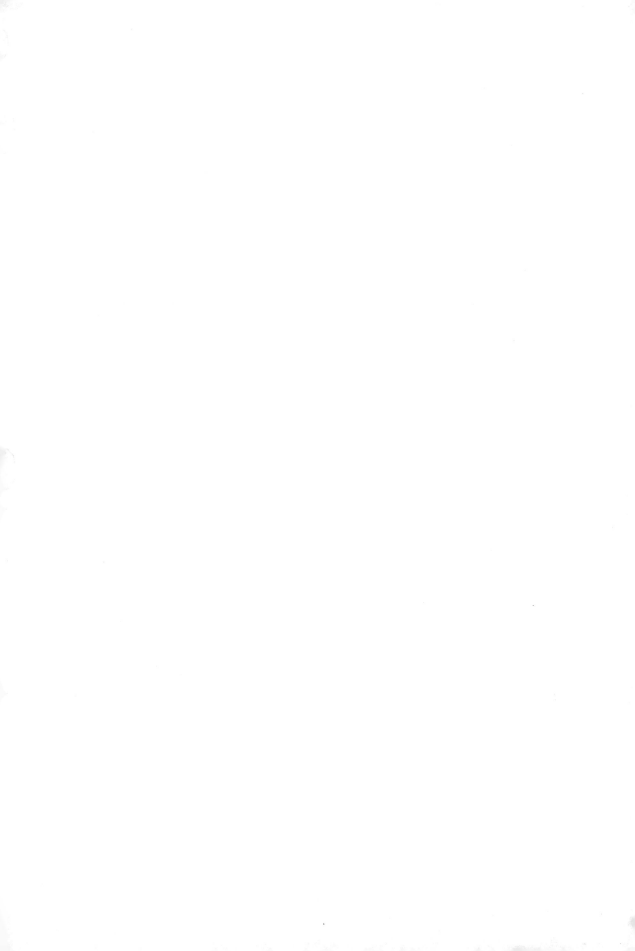

Arthur A. Ward, Jr.

Surgical Treatment of Epilepsy

The role of surgical therapy in the treatment of epilepsy is not widely appreciated. There are many reasons for this. One reason is the usual approach of a physician to a patient who presents with seizures. The common diagnostic strategy is to confirm the diagnosis of epilepsy based on clinical and electroencephalographic (EEG) data and then to assign the patient to one of the traditional classifications of tonic-clonic, absence, or complex partial epilepsy. This empirical approach is not without merit. In many cases it will provide the basis for an empirical decision about which antiepileptic drug to prescribe. However, it does not lead to the next logical step of determining the cause of the symptom called epilepsy. The next question should be: Where is the trouble coming from and what is causing it? If these empirical steps were undertaken in a sophisticated fashion, the cause of the seizures would be determined in a high percentage of adults with seizures. With such information, the physician would then be more inclined to explore other forms of therapy when medication fails to resolve the problem.

In patients with epilepsy, a major diagnostic effort should identify those in whom the cause is a localized structural lesion such as focal atrophy, cicatrix, or, of course, a space-occupying lesion. Clearly, the last requires a different therapeutic approach. In others, however, it should be recognized that the causes of the seizures and the extent of the epileptogenic focus vary widely and represent a spectrum. In some patients the focus may be exquisitely focal; in others the epileptogenic cortex may be widespread, diffuse, bilateral, or multifocal. Many patients with such widespread lesions probably are not candidates for surgical therapy, but those with small, localized foci are excellent candidates for surgical resection. Unfortunately, the majority of patients with epilepsy fall between these two extremes. Judgments about therapy in this group require a broad knowledge of the problem and a flexible and sophisticated approach to diagnosis and management. Such an approach involves multiple disciplines in the neurologic sciences to achieve an

This work was supported by NIH research contract NO1-NS-6-2341 awarded by the National Institute of Neurological and Communicative Disorders and Stroke, PHS/DHEW.

evaluation that is most appropriate for that particular patient.

Goals of Surgical Therapy

SEIZURE CONTROL

The fundamental goal of surgical therapy is seizure elimination or control. The actual clinical seizures represent the handicap that is obvious to both the patient and the doctor. Results of surgical series indicate that good seizure control can be obtained in a high percentage (60 to 80%) of patients who meet strict criteria for such procedures (see Criteria for Operation, below).

FUNCTIONAL AND BEHAVIORAL IMPROVEMENT

Surgical therapy may also relieve subtle neurologic disabilities related to interictal events. The epileptogenic focus is not quiescent between clinical seizures; it is continuously discharging abnormal signals. These vary in degree from abnormal burst firing of individual neurons within the focus that does not propagate outside the focus to more synchronized neuronal events that generate a volley of impulses that may be associated with a gross electrographic event called an epileptic spike. These abnormal signals are propagated over axons of neurons in the focus to more distant circuits to which these axons project. In some circuits, the intermittent input of such interictal discharges can be tolerated with no detectable change in function unless the frequency and magnitude of the volleys are great. The latter state is often reached only during a propagating seizure. However, in other circuits, the presence of such interictal discharges can disrupt normal function. For example, Welch and Penfield [40] first reported a series of 3 patients in whom epileptic foci in the sensorimotor convolutions were excised to free the patients of epileptic attacks. In each case the patient had a preoperative hemiparesis that was not made worse (as had been anticipated) but was actually improved after the surgery. Presumably, the interictal volleys projecting onto neighboring neurons in the motor cortex were blocking their effective action. It may be that the same mechanisms operate in epileptogenic foci in the temporal lobe involving limbic circuits. We and many others have observed considerable improvement in behavior following temporal lobectomy in such cases when the operation has resulted in a major reduction in seizures (see Results Following Cortical Resection, below).

POSSIBLE PREVENTION OF KINDLING

Kindling is a phenomenon, demonstrated in experimental animals, in which repetitive electrical or chemical stimulation to a part of the brain results in spontaneous seizure activity following cessation of the stimulation [34, 38]. This observation suggests that repetitive spontaneous discharges of epileptic foci in humans and the continual exposure of normal neuron pools to this paroxysmal activity may similarly induce ("kindle") seizures in these normal neuron pools. It is uncertain at the present time whether this phenomenon does or does not occur in patients with partial epilepsies.

Criteria for Operation

A patient with epilepsy must meet four criteria if surgical therapy is to be considered: (1) the patient must have intractable seizures that are refractory to adequate medical therapy; (2) the epileptogenic focus generating the seizures must be identified, and confirmation must be obtained from several lines of evidence; (3) this focus must be in dispensable cortex so that it can be surgically removed without major neurologic deficit; and (4) the focus must be located in cortex that is surgically accessible.

These criteria will now be discussed in some detail. In the discussion that follows the general principles, which apply to foci wherever they are located in the cerebral cortex, will be summarized. Nevertheless, the discussion will frequently be centered around foci of temporal lobe origin because of their frequency. It is estimated that, of adult patients with epilepsy, approximately 55 percent have partial complex seizures of temporal lobe origin. In all age groups, partial complex seizures represent 42 percent of all partial seizures [9]. Of those patients who fulfill all the criteria for operation, approximately 70 percent will have foci in one or the other temporal lobe. Of operations for epilepsy, 65 percent were directed at the temporal lobe in our series; the figure is over 70 percent in other published series [25, 28].

FAILURE OF ANTIEPILEPTIC
MEDICATION TO CONTROL SEIZURES

It is obvious that surgical therapy would not be considered if the seizures could be adequately controlled by some other means. However, the definition of "adequate control" is not always clear. In certain occupations and social settings, one or two seizures a year are completely acceptable; in others they are not. For example, many of our social patterns revolve around the capability to drive a car. However, in most states a license to operate a motor vehicle would be denied to people having two or more seizures a year. For such patients, even two seizures a year would constitute a failure of medical therapy. Thus, the determination of what constitutes "medical failure" must be made on an individual basis. Some specific guidelines for determining when a patient has failed a trial of antiepileptic drug therapy are given in Chapter 14.

Clearly, antiepileptic drugs will always be the major form of therapy. The effectiveness of antiepileptic drugs, however, is commonly overestimated. The widely held belief that 70 to 80 percent of patients with epilepsy are controlled by drugs does not agree with the published facts [33]. One finding common to all studies is that the longer the duration of therapy, the worse the seizure control. The consensus that emerges from the literature [31] is that complete seizure control is achieved for 2 years in 37 percent of patients, but this figure falls to 20 percent at 5 years and 10 percent at 10 years. The other discouraging feature of the data [33] is that these figures have not changed appreciably during this century despite the introduction of the drugs that are so universally used at this time. Thus, using the most optimistic of figures, it would appear that 20 to 30 percent of patients with epilepsy have medically intractable seizures.

In recent years there has been increasing awareness that chronic toxicity is a considerable problem associated with the chronic administration of antiepileptic drugs [30]. Although the long-term clinical consequences may not be clear, it is a matter of some concern that a folate deficiency exists in some 50 percent of patients and a vitamin D deficiency in one third [30]. Perhaps the most disabling side effects are the mental changes that have been increasingly documented in recent years. It is unfortunately true that some patients suffer more from chronic drug toxicity · than from their seizure disorder. Thus a satisfactory reduction in seizure frequency achieved by antiepileptic drugs does not remove a patient from the medically intractable category if the reduction is accompanied by disabling neuropsychologic or other deficits.

An important factor to consider is the point when the patient can be considered to have failed medical therapy. There are several reasons for delaying any consideration of surgical therapy. During the early years of development of the epileptic process, particularly in children, and in seizures following trauma, there may be spontaneous remissions lasting several years or longer. The seizures may have varied clinical expression and variable frequencies before a stable pattern of frequency is established. However, once a stable pattern is evident, important changes in seizure frequency are not common. It is often felt that a thorough trial of antiepileptic medication requires many months or even years to determine the optimal

combination and levels of antiepileptic drugs. This time factor is more a matter of custom than biology. There are no factual reasons why an optimal regimen of antiepileptic medication cannot be established relatively rapidly. This is particularly true now that techniques are available for monitoring serum levels of such drugs.

There are other reasons for reaching an early decision. The psychosocial consequences of procrastination and of permitting the patient to continue to have seizures if an alternate form of therapy is available must be considered, particularly in younger patients. During the period of maximal psychosocial maturation, the isolation and disability associated with continuing seizures can modify developing behavior patterns in a fashion that may be irreversible. A young person whose education is compromised because of seizures sustains a loss that cannot be replaced 10 years later. Thus, there is a premium on obtaining effective seizure control in any young patient with epilepsy as soon as possible. The mature patient is not immune to similar problems, although they differ in degree and substance. An adult who has not been able to find gainful employment for many years is not going to be miraculously restored to the mainstream of society in the middle of his life just because he has undergone an operation that may have successfully eradicated his seizures. Motivational, social, and economic patterns become relatively fixed. If an ultimate solution to the problem of recurrent seizures is going to be achieved in a given patient, the sooner it is accomplished the better.

A final important consideration is determining when to make the decision that the seizures are intractable. This decision is related to the biologic consequences of the seizures themselves. At one time it was felt that a single seizure did the brain no harm. It was, of course, recognized that very frequent seizures or status epilepticus are associated with considerable morbidity, especially in children. However, recent evidence indicates that even a single seizure may not be benign. It has been shown that in a primate model of spontaneous epileptic seizures there is unequivocal anatomic evidence of ongoing neuronal degeneration radiating from the epileptogenic focus [8]. Such axonal degeneration is associated with the occurrence of spontaneous seizures and ceases if the seizures are controlled with antiepileptic medication [8]. Similar axonal degeneration has also been reported in human foci in patients with medically intractable epilepsy. There are clues indicating that the magnitude of the neuronal death is related to seizure frequency. This evidence would indicate that the occurrence of occasional seizures is not a benign process. Continuing seizures produce further brain damage. Therefore, vigorous efforts to achieve complete seizure control as quickly as possible are justified. This is the formal policy in the Soviet Union, where the period of conservative therapy has lately been revised and shortened to 1 to 1½ years [36]. An aggressive approach to therapy has been followed by the Russians for some years. Once the diagnosis of epilepsy is established, a very vigorous and intensive effort is made to control the seizures with antiepileptic drugs. They feel that this can be accomplished in 1 year. If seizures are still uncontrolled at the end of 1 year, a determination is made whether or not surgical therapy should be considered.

CONFIRMATION OF THE FOCUS

If surgical therapy is to be considered, the seizures must be arising in a localized region of the cerebral cortex. It is therefore essential that the epileptic focus be identified with as much certainty as possible. The focus should be localized by the clinical pattern of the typical seizure, and this localization should be confirmed by both EEG and evidence of a structural lesion in that locus obtained by some other diagnostic procedure such as computed axial tomography (CT scan), pneumoencephalography, etc.

Clinical Localization

Clinical localization is accomplished by carefully determining the events that occur at the very onset of the seizure. At this time the neurons in the region of the focus are involved in the seizure, and their activity will provide the local sign of the function of that part of the cortex. With adequate knowledge of cortical localization and experience with seizure patterns, a tentative hypothesis about the location of the epileptic focus should be possible [23, 24] (see Chaps. 4 and 5). Once the seizure has propagated and a generalized seizure is under way, the clinical pattern provides little information for purposes of localization. Of course, the aura is really the onset of a local seizure and is of great localizing value.

Surface EEG Studies

The clinical impression should next be confirmed by EEG. EEG studies should be complete and should be carried out by a person experienced in obtaining localizing electrographic data. Such studies may require repeated examinations, sleep recordings, activation techniques, and special electrode arrays including sphenoidal or possibly even implanted electrodes. Perhaps the most reliable information of

all, particularly in confusing or difficult cases, is the recording of spontaneous seizures. This requires facilities for long-term monitoring (see Chap. 11). Because the EEG information is objective, it provides the most definitive data for determining whether or not the seizures are of focal onset in a given patient. It is thus essential to document a focal origin by EEG if surgical therapy is to be considered.

Some of the most difficult decisions arise when the seizure discharge arises in either the frontal or the temporal lobe. In complex partial seizures the clinical pattern may point to the temporal lobe as the origin of the discharge, but it will rarely provide clues to which side is active or whether both temporal lobes are involved. This challenge must be met by the electroencephalographer.

The most common ambiguity arises in patients who have fairly typical seizures assumed to be of temporal lobe origin, but the EEG demonstrates interictal spiking that is nearly equal over the two temporal lobes. Temporal lobectomy should not be considered in these patients unless there is convincing evidence that all or most of the spontaneous seizures arise in one temporal lobe. There are two possible reasons for this EEG ambiguity. The first is that there are epileptic foci in both temporal lobes; the other is that all the discharges are arising in one temporal lobe but are easily projected to the opposite lobe and are recorded bilaterally. There are profuse projections from portions of each temporal lobe to the other. The scalp EEG cannot easily distinguish which side is originating the discharge and which is receiving it. The orientation of the electrical dipoles may be such that the amplitude of the spiking is lower in the scalp EEG record over the temporal lobe containing the focus in the buried hippocampal cortex. It has been shown with continuous surface EEG and depth EEG studies that in patients with bitemporal EEG foci, seizures arise in only one temporal lobe in more than 80 percent.

The final point to be remembered about the EEG is that although all epileptic foci that can be surgically resected must reside in the cortex, only one third of the cortex lies on the surface of the brain. The remaining two thirds are buried. The problem is not confined to temporal lobe foci. A substantial number of foci are located in the frontal lobe, many of them, unfortunately, on the medial or orbital cortex of the frontal lobe. The scalp electrographic correlates of such foci are difficult to resolve. Not only is the discharging focus some distance from the scalp, but the morphology of the electrographic abnormalities may be modified considerably by the neuronal circuits through which they project. At times, the EEG abnormality may resemble a spike-and-wave discharge rather than a focal discharge. Nasoethmoidal electrodes may provide improved localization of orbital frontal EEG foci with surface electrodes (see Chap. 11).

Depth EEG
Use of depth EEG recording may resolve the many problems of lateralization and localization of EEG foci discussed in the preceding section [34, 35].

Depth electrodes are made from sheaves of thin wire covered with a nontoxic and noninflammatory insulating material and exposed at fixed intervals to serve as recording electrodes. Usually several electrode trellises are placed stereotactically for recording up to several days. Long-term recordings using both the indwelling electrodes and those on the scalp and basilar surfaces provide the maximum amount of information. The insertion of depth electrodes may transiently incite local neuronal irritability, producing misleading paroxysmal activity in normal tissue during the first day or two. The most reliable recordings are made several days after implantation. Because depth EEG is used primarily in preparation for surgery, it is important to make recordings during one of the patient's spontaneous seizures. The temporal lobes are the cerebral regions most often studied by intracerebral recording, but the medial surfaces of the cerebral hemispheres and the orbital surfaces of the frontal lobe are also cortical surfaces inaccessible to surface EEG that have been gainfully evaluated by depth electrodes or by subdural strip electrodes.

Spencer [34] performed a comprehensive review of all available data on depth EEGs. She found that the reported surgical success rate is no better at centers employing depth EEG than at those that do not. However, when depth and scalp EEG studies were compared in 178 patients, it was found that use of depth EEG would have enabled 36 percent more patients to be selected for surgery by defining otherwise unidentifiable single epileptogenic foci. Furthermore, depth EEG could have prevented surgery for another 18 percent by demonstrating different or additional epileptogenic foci in patients who were thought to have a single discharging focus amenable to resection. Thus, depth EEG had the potential to alter surgical decisions in more than 50 percent of patients reported. Very recent reports [12, 13, 35] have also presented compelling statistical evidence showing that information obtained from depth EEG recordings can improve the surgical outcome substantially. Spencer [34] postulates that the statistical lack of increased success in centers employing depth electrodes may be due to a more difficult population of patients whose seizure foci are not easily localized by simpler means and who are therefore referred to centers that have depth EEG.

A group at UCLA [2, 12, 13] has made a comprehensive study of the ability of surface and depth EEG recordings made during interictal and ictal periods to predict surgical outcome. Interictal EEG factors that were found to correlate with poor surgical outcome included bilaterally synchronous surface spikes, sharp waves, and diffuse bilateral background slowing. Good surgical outcome was correlated with frequent, deep, or multifocal spikes in the temporal lobe chosen for resection. Ictal EEG factors found to correlate with poor surgical outcome included a high proportion of bilaterally synchronous onsets (on surface or depth recordings or both) and independent left and right onset locations. Good surgical outcome was correlated with a high proportion of seizure onsets (on surface or depth recordings or both) from the chosen side of lobectomy and a high proportion of deep focal onsets. Ictal and interictal EEGs and surface and depth EEGs could all predict surgical outcome at a statistically significant level. The best predictions were made using all four types of data.

Depth EEG recording subjects the patient to the risk of several infrequent complications including bacterial and aseptic meningitis, intracerebral hemorrhage, osteomyelitis, transient amnesia, and gliosis at the site of electrode insertion [11, 34]. Depth EEG procedures should only be performed by teams skilled in the procedure after a careful evaluation of potential risks and benefits.

Radiologic Studies
Once the clinical localization has been confirmed by EEG localization, it is desirable to have information of a structural nature that is consistent with the proposed localization of the focus.

Plain skull films are sometimes of value. They may demonstrate a small temporal fossa, increased skull thickness, or an elevated petrous ridge on the side of a damaged temporal lobe if the damage occurred during early or late childhood [42].

In the past, the pneumoencephalogram was a major source of information for localizing structural lesions. In epilepsy that has been localized to one temporal lobe, it is helpful to identify on the pneumoencephalogram some abnormality of the appropriate temporal horn or of the subarachnoid space in the region of the suspected focus. The diagnostic study may show other changes elsewhere that may be much more dramatic than those in the region under suspicion, but these are irrelevant to the current decision-making process.

What is desired is that there be some evidence of at least a minor anatomic abnormality in the vicinity of the suspected pathological focus. Such radiographic interpretations require experience with studies in patients with epilepsy, and the clinical question to be answered must be clear to those interpreting the films.

With the advent of CT scanning, the desired information can often be obtained by this non-invasive technique. Again, some specialized experience is required because a casual interpretation of the scan may dwell on obvious changes elsewhere in the brain that have no relation to the origin of the seizures and neglect rather subtle changes in the region under suspicion.

Other radiographic studies are usually not required unless special questions arise in the diagnostic workup. The presence or absence of a clinically unrecognized tumor will be uncovered by the CT scan. If there are reasons to suspect the presence of an arteriovenous malformation, a cerebral angiogram will establish the diagnosis.

Positron Emission Tomography
and Cerebral Blood Flow Studies
Positron emission tomography (to localize areas of brain hypofunction), contrast-enhanced CT scan (to localize areas of differential contrast enhancement in the two temporal lobes), and cerebral blood flow studies are new techniques currently under investigation as possible means of identifying seizure foci [3, 4, 10, 16, 17, 34].

FOCUS MUST RESIDE IN DISPENSABLE CORTEX
The third criterion for surgery is that the confirmed focus must lie in cortex that can be surgically removed without major neurologic disability. Assuming that the brain is otherwise intact, such dispensable cortex includes most of the frontal lobes, the anterior temporal lobes, and parts of the posterior parietal lobe in the nondominant hemisphere including, under some circumstances, parts of the parastriate cortex. Thus, surgical therapy is ordinarily not undertaken if the focus lies in the sensorimotor cortex, the speech cortex of the dominant hemisphere, the cortex of the parietal lobe in the nondominant hemisphere subserving processing of spatial information, or the primary visual cortex.

The most important of these constraints relates to speech cortex. The distribution of speech function in the dominant hemisphere is characterized by considerable individual variation [21]. It is often necessary to determine which hemisphere is dominant for speech by diagnostic studies before a final decision about an operation can be made. This is especially important for foci located in the temporal lobe. The cortex of the left temporal lobe anterior to the vein of Labbe is, in general, not involved with speech function in right-handed people. However, disposable cortex of the posterior temporal lobe of the dominant hemisphere may extend posteriorily to varying degrees; it is essential that cerebral dominance for speech be determined before the operation. This can be accomplished by an intracarotid injection of amobarbital sodium (Amytal sodium). As this drug perfuses one hemisphere, it causes a transient blockade of function of the cortex perfused by the anterior and middle cerebral arteries of that hemisphere. This results in a short-lasting contralateral hemiparesis and block of speech function if that hemisphere is dominant. Because less radical temporal lobectomies can be undertaken in the dominant hemisphere, the success of the operation may be somewhat compromised unless the focus is well confined to the anterior or arteromedial temporal cortex. Similar considerations apply if the focus is thought to be located in the frontal operculum close to Broca's area or in the parietal cortex of the dominant hemisphere.

The second cerebral function of concern is memory, and this concern usually arises only in patients with temporal lobe foci. It is well documented that bilateral lesions of the hippocampus result in an incapacitating memory defect in humans. In patients with epilepsy arising in the medial temporal cortex, no deficit will follow temporal lobectomy if the opposite temporal lobe is intact and functioning. Unfortunately, the etiologic factors that result in the damage that causes the epileptic focus in one temporal lobe may also damage the opposite medial temporal cortex. It is essential to have advance knowledge so that the planned surgical procedure will not result in this morbidity. Again, memory function can usually be determined by the injection of intracarotid amobarbital sodium. Tests of memory function are carried out as each hemisphere is perfused by the drug, which produces a transient blockade of function.

Obviously, the determination of which part of the cortex is dispensable is not always straightforward, but this factor must be carefully evaluated. Excising an epileptic focus near the speech cortex may abolish the seizures but only at the price of producing an aphasia. Even a mild aphasia is usually more disabling than the epilepsy. On the other hand, minor neurologic deficits may be tolerable. Temporal lobectomy may not uncommonly produce a partial upper quadrantic hemianopia. Although the visual field loss may be detectable on visual field examination, the patient is unaware of the minor deficit, and it is not a handicap in normal living. In this case the small extra amount of cortex to be removed in order to be sure of removing all the epileptogenic cortex (as demonstrated in the operating room) is justified if the seizures can be abolished. Similar judgments must be made about foci in a variety of cortical areas in which removal might produce a minor loss of neurologic function. Both the surgeon and the patient must weigh the potential benefits against the potential minor disabilities that may result from the procedure.

FOCUS MUST BE IN SURGICALLY ACCESSIBLE CORTEX
Even if diagnostic techniques were available to localize unequivocally all foci in patients with seizures of focal onset, only a percentage of foci would be located in parts of the brain that can be surgically approached with safety. The classic surgical approach involves an open craniotomy and cortical resection. Only certain regions of the cortex are accessible to such an approach. These include the lateral surfaces of the hemispheres, portions of the orbital and medial surfaces of the frontal lobes, and all surfaces of the temporal lobes. It is not usually possible to approach safely the medial portions of the parietal lobes, the cortex of the insula, or the medial occipital lobes. If foci are located in subcortical neuronal masses, they are not accessible to direct surgical attack. The potential role of stereotactically induced lesions in subcortical structures will be discussed in a later section.

The Surgical Procedure—Cortical Resection
The goal of surgical therapy is fundamentally simple: to remove the aggregate of abnormal neurons that are responsible for generating the clinical seizures while sparing vital parts of the brain. Although it is an oversimplification, it can be said that cortical scarring is the cause of focal seizures. Surgical therapy is then directed at removing the cortical scar by techniques that minimize the cortical scarring that must inevitably follow any surgical procedure and that is essential to the healing process. The technique is that of subpial resection. It was originally described some 40 years ago by Penfield [22, 23] and has undergone only minor refinements since then.

PREOPERATIVE PREPARATION
Many surgeons feel that the success of the procedure is closely related to the successful delineation of the extent of the epileptic cortex by electrocorticography. It is thus essential that the electrographic abnormalities be as prominent as possible at the time of operation. It may be necessary to abort the operation if it is not possible to identify any epileptic activity in the

cortical EEG. For this reason, the preoperative antiepileptic medication may often have to be manipulated. If a preoperative scalp EEG shows only minimal abnormalities, it may be necessary to withdraw much or all of the antiepileptic medication. Because the half-life of some antiepileptic drugs is long (e.g., 30 hours for phenytoin), such changes in medication must be carefully planned. However, if the patient is having frequent seizures or if the EEG shows frequent epileptiform discharges, the usual medication should be continued up to the time of operation. The occurrence of one or more spontaneous seizures during the operation is not desirable. In addition to the obvious problems of mechanical restraint of the patient and maintaining sterility of the surgical field, the postictal depression of the cortical EEG will usually make EEG localization of the focus difficult.

Dexamethasone in high doses is started orally a day before the operation, is supplemented during the procedure, and is maintained for 5 days postoperatively. In our experience, as well as in the Montreal series, the use of steroids substantially reduces the incidence of postoperative morbidity.

A final component of the preoperative preparation is establishment of a secure relationship between the patient and the surgeon. The long craniotomy is carried out under local anesthesia, and adequate psychologic preparation of the patient is essential. There must be a close relationship between the patient and the surgeon to generate the necessary confidence on the patient's part that leads to a tranquil operation. This relationship is not established by a simple preoperative discussion the night before the operation.

ANESTHESIA
Whenever possible, the operation is carried out under local anesthesia. Any medication that modifies cortical excitability may modify the cortical EEG to such an extent that precise electrographic localization of the focus is not possible. Drugs that modify the threshold of electrical stimulation of the cortex should not be used. Finally, an alert patient is necessary if it should become necessary to test complex neurologic functions. Because many excisions may be located close to cortex that may potentially mediate speech function, we routinely carry out speech testing utilizing an established protocol. Knowledge of the function of cortex in the vicinity of the resection is essential if the risk of producing a neurologic deficit is to be minimized.

An essential feature of local anesthesia is the role of the anesthetist. Because local anesthesia is rarely used in a modern operating room, most anesthesiologists are unfamiliar with the problems and are unskilled in the psychotherapeutic techniques that are desirable. Although the surgeon plays a role in this effort, a skillful anesthesiologist who has already established a relationship with the patient can avert patient anxieties, thus minimizing any discomfort associated with local anesthesia and considerably reducing the need for supplemental medication.

The choice of local anesthetic and the total amount utilized are important. Because of its longer action, lidocaine 0.5 to 1.0 percent with epinephrine provides a most satisfactory sensory blockade of the scalp. However, lidocaine in low concentrations in the serum is an effective antiepileptic drug and can effectively reduce or block epileptic discharges during corticography. It may be desirable to use another local anesthetic that has less antiepileptic action; we currently use bupivacaine hydrochloride 0.25 percent.

It is important that the patient be positioned in a comfortable fashion. To supplement adequate positioning, we customarily place the patient on an alternating pressure mattress rather than on the usual sponge rubber mattress to minimize local discomfort from pressure areas. Because these surgical procedures take many hours, it is essential to provide as much movement for the patient at periodic intervals as is possible within the limits of a fixed head position. Lying in one position for much more than 20 minutes generates discomfort, and this discomfort grows the longer that position is maintained without movement. The major discomfort experienced by a patient undergoing surgery for epilepsy is generated by his position on the operating table, not by events directly associated with the craniotomy.

CRANIOTOMY

A craniotomy appropriate to the location of the epileptogenic focus is carried out. The exposure of the brain should be planned in such a fashion that there is wide visualization of the region in question. Thus the craniotomy is usually larger than it would be otherwise.

CORTICOGRAPHY

Once the cortex has been exposed, corticography is undertaken utilizing banks of electrodes that can be placed on the cortex. The initial electrode array is so arranged that it covers the area of suspected epileptogenic cortex as well as adjacent cortex. As the 16-channel recording proceeds, judgments are made about the regions of maximal electrographic pathology. Ambiguities regarding the extent of the involved cortex are resolved by replacement of the electrode

arrays until the entire epileptic focus has been mapped. This exercise proceeds most rapidly and with the greatest security if frequent epileptic spiking is encountered. If the spiking is infrequent, the cortical mapping may be tedious. When the degree of cortical spiking is insufficient to permit adequate localization, an attempt may be made to activate the cortex pharmacologically. The intravenous injection of methohexital sodium as a bolus often provides short-term activation of pathologic electrographic activity. However, it ultimately induces sedation, which may prevent subsequent determination of the sensorimotor cortex, speech cortex, or other testing that may be desirable. For this reason, this strategy is not utilized until all other observations have been made. Local electrical stimulation may also be helpful because the threshold of electrically induced afterdischarge is often lower within the focus. Electrical stimulation requires experience with the relevant techniques and careful control of threshold using a constant current stimulator.

ELECTRICAL STIMULATION STUDIES

Once the focus has been mapped electrographically, the function of adjacent cortex is determined by electrical stimulation. In operations upon the temporal lobe, it is useful to determine the foot of the central fissure by eliciting sensory and motor responses from the sensorimotor cortex. The location of the speech cortex is of major importance when undertaking cortical resections adjacent to it in the dominant hemisphere [19].

MICROELECTRODE RECORDING

We often confirm the epileptogenic focus by microelectrode recording. This involves mounting a micromanipulator on the edge of the craniotomy so that a microelectrode can be introduced into the cortex at the presumed focus. Because the tip of the microelectrode has a diameter of less than 10 μ, it does not appreciably damage the cortex, thus permitting the recording of activity of single cortical neurons. The EEG spike activity that can be recorded by cortical electrodes unfortunately does not provide unequivocal evidence for the source of the abnormal discharge. The sharpness of the recorded spike, its amplitude, and other factors may indicate that the discharge is arising locally within the subjacent cortex. However, a synchronous volley of epileptic discharge originating at a distance and transmitted to the cortex under the recording gross electrode may be almost indistinguishable at times. This ambiguity can be resolved by recording the activity of single neurons because spontaneous neuronal activity of epileptic neurons has characteristics that are not shared by normal neurons. This technique, although valuable, is difficult and tedious and requires extensive experience with the problems of microelectrode recording as well as a major investment in electronic instrumentation.

CORTICAL RESECTION

Once all the necessary information has been gathered, a decision must be made about the extent of the cortical resection. Each decision is made on an individual basis according to the findings in that patient. The findings in the operating room, consisting of the visualized gross pathology and the electrographic localization of the focus, should be consistent with the clinical pattern of the spontaneous seizures and the preoperative studies. The limits to the resection are determined by identifying the function of nearby cortex. The area to be resected is then determined and is often identified on the surface of the brain by laying a thread around the limits of cortex to be excised. The abnormal cortex is then removed by subpial resection. The goal is to carefully remove the superficial fibroglial scar or scarred cortex, leaving the white matter and preserving the pial covering of adjacent cortex to minimize subsequent scarring. Scarring of the exposed white matter is of no consequence.

These general principles apply to the surgical attack on a focus wherever it may be located in accessible cortex. The surgical strategy will obviously be modified by the location of the focus. Some foci involve the medial or orbital surfaces of a frontal lobe. The clinical pattern of seizures arising in such foci does not usually provide localizing clues because the attacks often resemble absence seizures. The EEG may reveal a diffuse, atypical spike-and-wave pattern that may be of higher amplitude in the frontal regions and may tend to be more prominent on one side. Implanted electrodes, if fortuitously placed close to the focus, provide the best discrete evidence of a focal electrographic origin for the attacks. If sufficient data are obtained to warrant a surgical procedure, the surgical exposure is inevitably limited, and extensive corticography and other maneuvers, which are usual in most cases, are compromised.

Surgical resections of foci in the temporal lobe also require special techniques. Because patients with temporal lobe foci comprise such a high proportion of patients receiving surgical therapy, it is not surprising that the surgical treatment of epilepsy is often equated with *temporal lobectomy*. This term is somewhat unfortunate because it does not define the procedure. A temporal lobectomy for an infiltrating

glioma is a very different operation from that undertaken for treatment of epilepsy. Even the craniotomy exposure is different. The surgical principles for dealing with temporal lobe foci are no different from those applying to foci elsewhere. The exact location of the focus within the temporal lobe varies from patient to patient, and the cortical resection therefore varies as well. Thus, an obvious area of cortical atrophy and gliosis involving the lateral temporal cortex with associated local EEG abnormalities will not be handled in the same way as a focus involving the medial temporal cortex. However, the majority of foci in seizures of temporal lobe origin involve the medial temporal cortex. Because the amygdala and hippocampus cannot be directly visualized without removing the overlying brain, the cortex of the lateral convexity is removed by subpial resection, exposing the entire insula. The white matter is spared posterior to the anterior tip of the temporal horn of the lateral ventricle to preserve the anterior fibers of the optic radiations. The amygdala and pes hippocampus can then be removed by suction down to the pia overlying the free edge of the tentorium. Again, the extent of the resection is guided by the electrographic data.

In all cases, a postresection cortical EEG is obtained after the initial resection. Not infrequently, continued EEG spiking will be observed at one margin of the resection. If extension of the resection is possible without inducing neurologic deficit, the resection is extended. In cases of temporal lobe epilepsy, the corticography at the completion of the resection may continue to show some EEG abnormalities arising in the cortex of the island of Reil. Since the insula is blanketed by the candelabra of the middle cerebral vessels, a satisfactory resection of the insular cortex is not possible without major risk of inducing infarction in a part of the distribution of the middle cerebral artery. Fortunately, primary foci located in the insula are not common. The occasional spiking recorded from this region after the temporal lobe resection is compatible with an excellent surgical outcome and usually can be ignored.

GENERAL COMMENTS

Surgical procedures used for the treatment of epilepsy are not stereotyped. There are common surgical principles and techniques, but the actual procedure is adapted to the specific needs of each case.

It is apparent that these procedures are complex. The preoperative evaluation requires professional talent and institutional resources that are not widely available. The diagnostic evaluation requires neurologists and neurosurgeons with special interest and experience in epilepsy. A sophisticated electroencephalographer and a well-equipped EEG laboratory, as well as personnel in neuroradiology with experience with these problems, are also required. The operation is not easily undertaken in a standard neurosurgical facility because special instrumentation and physical facilities ae needed. If the operation is to be a streamlined cortical resection that includes little electrical stimulation of the cortex, no special testing of speech or memory function, and no microelectrode recording, the necessary EEG mapping of the focus and cortical resection can be carried out in 4 to 5 hours. If the focus is more complex or less accessible, if additional testing is undertaken during the operation including microelectrode recording (as is usually our custom), the procedure requires 8 to 12 hours.

Prolonged craniotomies carry a higher potential risk of postoperative infection. Thus, all facets of aseptic technique must be unusually meticulous. The most important factor involves the amount of human traffic in the operating room. To minimize such traffic, it is desirable to isolate all recording equipment and the staff operating the equipment from the main floor of the operating room. This is usually accomplished by a somewhat elevated gallery separated from the operating room by glass. Facilities for electronic communication between the recording team in the gallery and the operating team must then be provided. If it is necessary for the operating team also to visualize the recorded data (e.g., cortical EEG), closed circuit TV can be used. If microelectrode recording is to be undertaken, extensive electronic equipment is necessary including special reamplifiers, amplifiers, oscilloscopes, and an FM tape recorder. It is obvious that the capital investment can be considerable. Because these surgical procedures can be so elaborate and expensive, the decision to operate is not made lightly.

Results Following Cortical Resection

IMPROVEMENT IN SEIZURES

Repeated studies have shown that surgical excision of an epileptogenic focus reduces or abolishes seizures in 60 to 80 percent of selected patients with medically refractory focal epilepsy [7, 12, 13, 25, 27, 34, 37]. The surgical results depend upon several variables including the type of pathology, the location of the focus, whether the excision was complete or partial, and the length of follow-up. The best results occur when the epileptogenic focus is due to a meningocerebral scar such as that caused by a penetrating wound of the cortex. A complete or nearly complete eradication of seizures follows operation in 72 percent of patients with birth trauma and anoxia, 68 percent of patients with posttraumatic seizures, 70 percent of patients with postinflammatory lesions, and in only 58 percent of patients with an unknown etiology [27]. Foci in the temporal lobe carry the best prognosis with respect to surgical outcome. In our experience, a complete or nearly complete eradication of seizures occurred in 86 percent of patients following operation upon temporal lobe foci, with lower percentages for foci located elsewhere. In the much larger Montreal series, Rasmussen notes that seizures are abolished or markedly reduced in 71 percent of the temporal lobe group, in 59 percent of the frontal lobe group, in 62 percent of the parietal group, in 61 percent of the central group, in 67 percent of the small occipital group, and in 68 percent of the group with large destructive lesions involving much of one hemisphere [27].

There is no question that the surgical success rate is higher if the procedure includes radical and complete excision of the focus [31, 37]. Van Buren et al. [37] have shown that of patients with seizures of temporal lobe origin who had total excision of the focus, about 33 percent became totally seizure-free; therapeutic failures occurred in only 20 percent. In contrast, in patients who had "partial" excision, failures occurred in more than 50 percent, and total abolition of seizures occurred in less than 5 percent. In our series, we attempted to undertake as complete a resection as possible, and 43 percent of patients were considerably improved. In the temporal lobe group, the success rate is generally slightly less when the operation is carried out on the dominant temporal lobe. In the dominant hemisphere, posterior temporal cortex is usually essential for normal speech function, and therefore the posterior extension of the temporal lobe excision must be conservative to avoid postoperative morbidity. Because this compromises the ability to undertake as large a resection as might otherwise be desirable, the surgical success rate will be slightly less.

Postoperative results cannot be evaluated until some time after the operation. The Montreal data [26] indicate that, like the results of treatment with antiepileptic drugs, the percentage of patients improved by therapy is greatest initially and tends to decrease with time. However, their data show that in patients who have been free of seizures for 5 years after the operation, at least 90 percent have a very high probability of remaining seizure-free. We have not analyzed our data in this way, but it is our impression that, although changes in seizure frequency can occur during the first 3 years after an operation, the results tend to be relatively stable thereafter. The early changes in seizure frequency can be in either direction. Some patients may have an occasional seizure during the first year after operation and then are seizure-free thereafter, whereas others may be seizure-free for 2 years and then start to have rare seizures. There is general agreement that the occurrence of occasional seizures during the immediate postoperative period is of little prognostic significance.

Changes in Behavior

Excluding patients with temporal lobe seizures, changes in behavior or successful socioeconomic rehabilitation are related to the reduction or abolition of clinical seizures. It is generally recognized that the prognosis for successful rehabilitation is greatest in the following groups of patients: (1) those who have had seizures for a relatively short period of time, (2) those who are younger, (3) those whose psychosocial disability was minimal before operation, and (4) those with at least normal intelligence and without other neurologic disability. The prognosis is poorest in those with multiple handicaps (including mental retardation) and in those who have been chronically disabled for many years of their adult life.

Patients with seizures of temporal lobe origin form a somewhat different group. In 36 percent of patients in our series who had temporal lobe resection, behavioral abnormalities of varying degree were noted, confirming the experience in the larger Montreal series [14]. In our series, 95 percent of patients with complex partial seizures and no psychiatric symptoms had a good result, compared with only 70 percent of patients in whom psychiatric problems were diagnosed.

In addition to improving or abolishing the tendency toward seizures, excision of the temporal lobe focus may definitely improve some types of behavioral abnormalities. In a group of children undergoing temporal lobectomy for seizures [7], 40 percent were aggressive and destructive. After operation, 64 percent of this aggressive group showed normal behavior. It is our experience that personality problems in adults are abolished in about one third of patients, a conclusion that agrees with the experience in other series [5, 29, 37].

It is generally accepted that temporal lobectomy does not favorably influence behavior in patients with major psychoses, including schizophrenia [5]. In such patients it can be argued that significant psychiatric problems represent a contraindication to operation. Temporal lobectomy could be justified in such cases if there is reasonable assurance that abolition of the seizures would materially contribute to the psychiatric treatment.

Reasons for Surgical Failure

Little or no improvement occurs in 20 to 40 percent of even optimal cases, and there are a variety of reasons for this [34]. In some, the passage of time may show that the underlying pathology for the presumed focal epilepsy was in fact a progressive brain disease. In most cases, however, the less than satisfactory reduction in seizure frequency is due to four factors. (1) It is sometimes impossible to remove a sufficiently large proportion of the identified epileptogenic cortex, usually because it extends into cortex that is not dispensable, and additional removal would result in an unacceptable neurologic deficit. (2) There is epileptogenicity in the opposite hemisphere. This ambiguity is most prevalent in temporal lobe epilepsy. (3) There is a major subcortical component to the seizure process that was not initially appreciated. (4) There are inherent biologic limitations in the surgical technique. Some cortical scarring will always be induced by the most meticulous and careful procedure. In a certain percentage of cases, this scarring will itself form a new epileptogenic focus.

Refinements in preoperative evaluation as well as localized information obtained in the operating room can reduce instances in which the involvement of either the opposite hemisphere or subcortical circuits would compromise the surgical result. At present, we know least about subcortical mechanisms, and surgical techniques for dealing with this group of patients are the least well established. Little can be done if the focus extends into nondispensable cortex. Finally, there is no way to avoid leaving some scar around the area of cortical resection that may induce continuing epileptic activity. It is clear that with additional advances in understanding the epileptic process, in diagnosis, and in the development of refinements of surgical therapy, future results should be improved.

Risks

The mortality following cortical resection is low. In our series, there has been no mortality in the past 20 years. In larger series from other major centers, the mortality is under 1 percent [25, 27].

Morbidity should also be low, in the range of 5 to 10 percent. The actual figure depends on the definitions employed. A considerable number of patients undergoing temporal lobectomy will have varying degrees of contralateral upper quadrantanopia following operation, but functional visual disability should not occur. There is a low measurable risk of partial hemiparesis, but hemiplegia is very rare. There is always a measurable risk of aphasia when resection is undertaken in the dominant hemisphere, and the risk is determined by the proximity of the focus to speech cortex. This unwanted neurologic deficit occurs in no more than 5 percent of cases at risk and is often transient. The risk of disorders of memory will be high following temporal lobe resections if damage to the contralateral temporal lobe is suspected. Appropriate preoperative evaluation can minimize this risk. Subtle and perhaps functionally insignificant changes in memory or neuropsychologic performance may occur in 5 to 10 percent of patients after temporal lobe resection. All of these complications result from transient or permanent damage to nearby neural circuits. This type of morbidity can be substantially reduced by appropriate use of high doses of dexamethasone and by appropriate maneuvers in the operating room as well as careful postoperative management.

There are other, more general causes of postoperative morbidity. When the resection necessitates amputation of a segment of the ventricular system, the postoperative course may be complicated by hemogenic meningitis. The placement of the incision for temporal lobe resection may compromise the branch of the facial nerve supplying the frontalis muscle, but this should not create any cosmetic disability. Obviously, the potential morbidity in any given case should be discussed with the patient.

Other Surgical Procedures

HEMISPHERECTOMY

At one end of the spectrum of epilepsies of focal origin are those in which the epileptogenic lesion is widely distributed throughout much of one hemisphere. Birth trauma or anoxia and postinflammatory brain scarring are the cause in almost three fourths of these cases. Because the causative events usually occur early in life, and because the seizures and associated neurologic deficit are major handicaps, many of these cases come to operation in childhood. It is feasible to carry out the operation under general anesthesia in these patients because the hemiparesis and other major neurologic deficits so commonly present make it possible to undertake radical cortical excisions without adding to the preoperative deficit.

Clinical seizure patterns vary widely, and all types of focal and generalized seizures may occur. The EEG changes will also be diffuse, but lateralization to one hemisphere is an essential criterion for operation. Because the discharges frequently propagate to the other hemisphere, the intracarotid amobarbital sodium test may be useful in determining the hemisphere of origin. Radiographic studies and CT scans should also verify the presence of major organic pathology in the hemisphere in question. Because the original brain injury often occurs early in life, speech function is often transferred to the opposite intact hemisphere, but this must also be confirmed.

Hemispherectomy requires a large exposure and the removal of large areas of cortex. The amount of cortex removed depends on the extent of the epileptic activity. If epileptogenic activity is confined to the anterior half of the hemisphere, removal of the frontal and temporal lobes may be sufficient. If epileptic spiking involves the posterior half of the hemisphere and if a complete homonymous hemianopsia is present, removal of the occipital and variable amounts of the parietal and posterior temporal lobes may be undertaken. If any element of fine motor activity in the upper extremity is preserved, every effort should be made to preserve the sensorimotor cortex. If epileptogenic activity is widespread and if major neurologic function involving the opposite side of the body is already lost, a complete hemispherectomy may be carried out. Although such a radical procedure is technically possible with low mortality, experience has shown that late morbidity and mortality of significant degree can occur [28]. For this reason, few complete hemispherectomies are currently undertaken. Radical excisions can be performed with safety if a small portion of the hemisphere is preserved. This involves preserving a portion of the least epileptogenic region of the damaged hemisphere. This commonly consists of either the occipital or frontal pole. This modification of the surgical procedure appears to prevent the later development of superficial cerebral hemosiderosis, which is the cause of late morbidity and mortality.

STEREOTACTIC PROCEDURES

The use of the stereotactic technique for producing focal lesions with great accuracy in small subcortical targets in humans is now well established. The possible therapeutic applications of this technique to epilepsy were initiated more than 20 years ago, and since then great experience has been gained and an equally extensive literature has developed. However, a review and analysis of these data by Ojemann and Ward [20] does not provide a clear picture of the therapeutic effectiveness of stereotactic lesions of any specific subcortical target when carried out in a specific type of epilepsy. Part of the difficulty is that many of the reported experiences involve small numbers of patients; the seizure types treated by a given procedure are often not uniformly classified, and there has been no systematic follow-up as is conventional with open operations. The exact clinical classification of the seizure disorder treated by stereotactic operations is often difficult to determine. Patients considered for such treatment are those whose seizures are intractable and complicated and whose EEGs are difficult to unravel. Clearly, no patient is considered for such procedures if the EEG or the clinical pattern indicates a focal onset of the seizures in cortex. Thus the seizures in these patients tend to be those in which the underlying physiology or pathology is least understood. It is not surprising that a clear picture of the potential of this technique for the treatment of epilepsy has not yet emerged.

The general experience appears to be that stereotactic lesions in the fields of Forel may be unusually effective in generalized epilepsy. Pallidal lesions, often in combination with lesions of the amygdala, are reported to be effective in some nonconvulsive generalized seizure conditions. Stereotactic lesions in medial temporal targets including the amygdala, hippocampus, and fornix show some promise for patients with partial complex seizures who are not candidates for open cortical resection [15]. A review of the outcome of various stereotactic lesions for a variety of seizure types shows that about 20 percent of patients are seizure-free and 40 percent are markedly improved if the follow-up is confined to patients who have been evaluated 1 or more years after operation. Treated in the same fashion, the figures for open cortical resection indicate that about 50 to 60 percent of patients are seizure-free. Thus stereotactic surgery does not appear at this time to be as effective as open cortical resection. However, it must be remembered that patients commonly considered for stereotactic surgery are those who not only are medically intractable but also do not meet the criteria for cortical resection. Stereotactic surgery therefore has the potential to salvage patients for whom no other effective therapy is available.

The risks of stereotactic surgery are low, and mortality should be less than 1 percent. Morbidity will vary with the subcortical target and the accuracy of placement of the lesion. Accuracy of lesion placement is not usually a function of the technique but rather a function of anatomical and physiological variability. Stereotactic instruments can place an electrode tip in any desired locus within the brain with great accuracy; the problem is to determine the exact location of the desired subcortical target in that particular brain.

Stereotactic lesions provide a useful therapeutic approach to a very difficult group of seizure types [36]. This is a rapidly developing field, and it can be anticipated that, as knowledge and experience grow, precision of patient selection and determination of the appropriate subcortical target will permit a much broader application of this form of therapy.

CEREBELLAR STIMULATION
Surgical techniques for implanting electrodes onto or into the brain are well established. The electronic tools for stimulation of such electrodes are available, and stimulation can be accomplished safely and without much bother to the patient. What remains to be determined is the therapeutic effectiveness of electrical stimulation of any given neuronal circuits on the frequency of seizures [18].

The impetus for this effort was the report by Cooper [1] that a reduction in seizure frequency could be induced by intermittent stimulation of the anterior vermis of the cerebellum. Modifications of stimulus wave shapes and stimulus trains as well as various loci of implantation have been undertaken since then, and the effect of this therapeutic modality in various seizure types has been studied in several centers. The reports are mixed. Cooper reported a series of 15 cases. Two of six patients with complex partial seizures were seizure-free; 1 of 6 with primarily generalized epilepsy was free of seizures and 3 others were markedly improved; and 1 of 3 patients with myoclonus was free of seizures and the other 2 were markedly improved. Unfortunately, the results in other series are less optimistic. Correl [18] undertook cerebellar stimulation in 7 patients with complex partial seizures and reported that no patient was seizure-free and only 2 showed any degree of improvement in seizure frequency. Van Buren [18] studied 5 patients with various seizure types utilizing a double-blind protocol and trained observers to document seizure frequency. No change in seizure frequency with cerebellar stimulation could be documented. In contrast to objective reports, some patients claim to have a reduced seizure frequency, and many are enthusiastic about their therapy with cerebellar stimulation. It is possible that a reduction in seizure intensity and greater interictal alertness may account for much of this subjective improvement. The difficulty of documenting therapeutic effectiveness in terms of seizure frequency has also characterized studies of the effect of cerebellar stimulation on animal models of chronic epilepsy. Finally, there is evidence from clinical and laboratory studies that chronic cerebellar stimulation may damage the underlying cerebellum [1, 32].

There is no evidence at this time that cerebellar stimulation can be considered a proven form of therapy for epilepsy. Both clinical and experimental research is continuing in this area, and the matter should be clarified in the near future.

COMMISSUROTOMY

Section of the cerebral commissures has been performed by several groups for relief of intractable seizure disorders [6, 39, 41]. The rationale is that section of the projecting pathways should block the spread of the seizure discharge. Clinical experience appears to confirm this expectation. Section of the corpus callosum, anterior commissure, and often the hippocampal commissure may dramatically reduce the frequency of generalized seizures, but the incidence of focal seizures in such patients is not appreciably changed in most cases.

MISCELLANEOUS SURGICAL PROCEDURES

It has been repeatedly noted that, in patients with craniotomy defects in whom cranioplasty is undertaken, lysis of the adhesions may definitely affect the frequency of seizures arising in the underlying cortical focus. In some patients with seizures who also have normal pressure hydrocephalus, shunting procedures for the hydrocephalus may have an unexpected beneficial effect on seizure frequency. It has been known for many years that patients undergoing pneumoencephalography with almost complete replacement of CSF with air may experience a substantial reduction in seizure frequency after such a procedure. This may be a consequence of lysis of dural-pial adhesions by the procedure. Unfortunately, the desirable outcome following pneumoencephalography is rare and can never be predicted. As knowledge grows, it can be anticipated that new therapeutic techniques will be developed.

The Future of Surgical Therapy for Epilepsy

At the current level of knowledge, it is estimated that approximately 10 percent of patients with medically intractable epilepsy are suitable candidates for surgical therapy. This conservative estimate represents less than 5 percent of all patients with epilepsy. Using these conservative figures, it appears that there are some 450,000 patients in North America with seizures that are not controlled by antiepileptic medication. Of these, some 45,000 are presumably candidates for open cortical resection. At the present time, it is estimated that less than 200 surgical procedures for epilepsy are undertaken annually in North America.

This disparity between need and performance is cause for concern. Many factors determine the current practice. It is apparent from this discussion that surgery for treatment of epilepsy is time-consuming, difficult, and expensive. Major resources are necessary to undertake the appropriate studies leading to the surgical decision and to carry out the operation. These involve not only physical facilities and equipment but also teams of specialized personnel at both professional and paraprofessional levels. Current medical care support systems do not encourage the development and maintenance of such resources. Lacking such resources, there is no motivation to train and expand the manpower pool of personnel necessary for such an enterprise. There are no economic motivations to mobilize either medical administrators or health professionals to engage in this therapeutic exercise. For the surgeon, additional training, expertise, and experience are required to undertake a surgical process that is stressful, very time-consuming, and less financially rewarding than equivalent effort expended in delivering care for routine problems. However, it is hoped that recognition of the problem by society will modify the current situation, and there is evidence that this is occurring.

Finally, the underutilization of surgical therapy is due in no small measure to simple ignorance on the part of those charged with the medical care of patients with epilepsy. There is inadequate realization that this therapeutic opportunity exists. Unfortunately, this ignorance is quite understandable. The number of centers engaging in this form of therapy is small, the total number of patients undergoing surgical treatment is small, and little is said in the literature about surgical therapy. If a doctor is not informed about surgical therapy by the literature or by his clinical experiences, it is not surprising that he does not consider this therapeutic modality at the appropriate time for his patients.

References

1. Cooper, I. D. *Cerebellar Stimulation in Man.* New York: Raven Press, 1978.
2. Engel, J., and Crandall, P. H. Comparison of old and new criteria for anterior temporal lobectomy in partial complex epilepsy. *Epilepsia* 23:431, 1982.
3. Engel, J. et al. Pathological correlates of focal temporal lobe hypometabolism in man. *Epilepsia* 22:236, 1981.
4. Engel, J. et al. Re-evaluation of criteria for localizing the epileptic focus in patients considered for surgical therapy of epilepsy. *Epilepsia* 21:184, 1980.

5. Falconer, M. A. Reversibility by temporal-lobe resection of the behavioral abnormalities of temporal lobe epilepsy. *N. Engl. J. Med.* 289:451, 1973.
6. Gates, J. R. et al. Effect of total corpus callosectomy on EEG. *Epilepsia* 23:441, 1982.
7. Green, J. R. Surgical treatment of epilepsy during childhood adolescence. *Surg. Neurol.* 8:71, 1977.
8. Harris, B. A. Degeneration in experimental epileptic foci. *Arch. Neurol.* 26:434, 1972.
9. Hauser, W. A., and Kurland, L. T. The epidemiology of epilepsy in Rochester, Minnesota, 1935 through 1967. *Epilepsia* 16:1, 1975.
10. Homan, R. et al. Xenon tomography in epileptic patients. *Epilepsia* 23:442, 1982.
11. King, D. W. et al. Implantation of depth electrodes in evaluation for ablative epilepsy surgery. *Electroenceph. Clin. Neurophysiol.* In press, 1983.
12. Lieb, J. P. et al. Neuropathological findings following temporal lobectomy related to surface and deep EEG patterns. *Epilepsia* 22:539, 1981.
13. Lieb, J. P. et al. Surface and deep EEG correlates of surgical outcome in temporal lobe epilepsy. *Epilepsia* 22:515, 1981.
14. Milner, B. Psychological Aspects of Focal Epilepsy and Its Neurosurgical Management. In D. P. Purpura, J. K. Penry, and R. D. Walter (Eds.), *Neurosurgical Management of the Epilepsies.* New York: Raven Press, 1975.
15. Narabayashi, H. Long-range Results of Medical Amygdalotomy on Epileptic Traits in Adult Patients. In T. Rasmussen, and R. Marino, Jr. (Eds.), *Functional Neurosurgery.* New York: Raven Press, 1979.
16. Newmark, M. E. et al. Advantages and limitations of ictal and postictal positron emission tomography in partial epilepsy. *Neurology* (N.Y.) 31:109, 1981.
17. Oakley, J. et al. Identifying epileptic foci on contrast-enhanced computerized tomographic scans. *Arch. Neurol.* 36:669, 1979.
18. Ojemann, G. A. The Future Role of Surgery in the Treatment of Epilepsy. In J. A. Wada (Ed.), *Modern Perspectives in Epilepsy.* Montreal: Edem, 1978.
19. Ojemann, G. A. Individual variability in cortical localization of language. *J. Neurosurg.* 50:164, 1979.
20. Ojemann, G. A., and Ward, A. A., Jr. Stereotactic and Other Procedures for Epilepsy. In D. P. Purpura, J. K. Penry, and R. D. Walter (Eds.), *Neurosurgical Management of the Epilepsies.* New York: Raven Press, 1975.
21. Ojemann, G. A., and Whitaker, H. Language localization and variability. *Brain and Language* 6:239, 1978.
22. Penfield, W. Epilepsy and surgical therapy. *Arch. Neurol. Psychiat.* 36:449, 1936.
23. Penfield, W., and Jasper, H. *Epilepsy and the Functional Anatomy of the Human Brain.* Boston: Little, Brown, 1954.
24. Penfield, W., and Rasmussen, T. *The Cerebral Cortex of Man.* New York: Macmillan, 1950.
25. Penry, J. K., and Daly, D. D. *Complex Partial Seizures and Their Treatment.* New York: Raven Press, 1975.
26. Rasmussen, T. Cortical Resection for Medically Refractory Focal Epilepsy: Results, Lessons, and Questions. In T. Rasmussen, and R. Marino, Jr. (Eds.), *Functional Neurosurgery.* New York: Raven Press, 1979.
27. Rasmussen, T. Cortical Resection in the Treatment of Focal Epilepsy. In D. P. Purpura, J. K. Penry, and R. D. Walter (Eds.), *Neurosurgical Management of the Epilepsies.* New York: Raven Press, 1975.
28. Rasmussen, T. Surgery for Epilepsy Arising in Regions Other Than the Temporal and Frontal Lobes. In D. P. Purpura, J. K. Penry, and R. D. Walter (Eds.), *Neurosurgical Management of the Epilepsies.* New York: Raven Press, 1975.
29. Rausen, R., and Crandall, P. H. Psychosocial status related to surgical control of temporal lobe seizures. *Epilepsia* 23:191, 1982.
30. Reynolds, E. H. Chronic antiepileptic toxicity: A review. *Epilepsia* 16:319, 1975.
31. Reynolds, E. H. Unsatisfactory aspects of the drug treatment of epilepsy. *Epilepsia* 17:xiii, 1977.
32. Robertson, L. T. et al. Morphologic changes associated with chronic cerebellar stimulation in the human. *J. Neurosurg.* 51:510, 1979.
33. Rodin, E. A. *Prognosis in Epilepsy.* Springfield, Ill.: Thomas, 1968.
34. Spencer, S. S. Depth electroencephalography in selection of refractory epilepsy for surgery. *Ann. Neurol.* 9:207, 1981.
35. Spencer, S. S. et al. The localizing value of depth electroencephalography in 32 patients with refractory epilepsy. *Ann. Neurol.* 12:248, 1982.
36. Ugrimov, V. et al. Stereotactic treatment of epilepsy in the light of pathophysiological disease concepts. *Acta Neurochir.* [Suppl. 23]:153, 1976.
37. Van Buren, J. M. et al. Surgery of Temporal Lobe Epilepsy. In D. P. Purpura, J. K. Penry, and R. D. Walter (Eds.), *Neurosurgical Management of the Epilepsies.* New York: Raven Press, 1975.
38. Wada, J. A. (Ed.). *Kindling.* New York: Raven Press, 1975.

296

39. Wada, J. A., and Moyes, P. D. Anterior callosal bisection in medically refractory generalized seizure patients. *Electroenceph. Clin. Neurophysiol.* In press, 1983.
40. Welch, K., and Penfield, W. Paradoxical improvement in hemiplegia following cortical excision. *J. Neurosurg.* 7:414, 1950.
41. Wilson, D. H., Reeves, A. G., and Gazzaniga, M. S. "Central" commissurotomy for intractable generalized epilepsy: Series two. *Neurology* (N.Y.) 32:687, 1982.
42. Wyler, A. R., and Ward, A. A. Cranial asymmetry secondary to unilateral hemispheric damage during late childhood. *J. Neurosurg.* 52:423, 1980.

NEONATAL SEIZURES

Cesare T. Lombroso

Convulsive disorders are relatively common during the first 4 weeks of life. They often herald serious problems. Because of immaturities in the morphologic, chemical, and bioelectric connections in and between the neonatal cortical and subcortical structures, seizures in these first weeks differ markedly from those of even slightly older babies. They differ in peripheral manifestations, etiology, correlations with electroencephalographic (EEG) patterns, diagnosis, treatment, and short- and long-term prognosis. Most are symptomatic of prenatal or paranatal lesions or of transient CNS dysfunction.

The amount of research focused on these early convulsive disorders is scant. In fact, because they do not conform to the criteria established by the World Health Organization for "epileptic syndromes," they do not yet have a place in the official classification of the epilepsies. Early research on the subject concerned mainly various aspects of the neonatal EEG [17, 18, 34, 64]. Research began to focus on neonatal ictal phenomena during the 1950s and 1960s [11, 15, 16, 20, 23, 29, 30, 41, 51, 53, 60, 68]. There are still only a few prospective studies of large groups of full-term newborns with seizures that classify seizure patterns, establish etiologies, evaluate correlations with clinical and laboratory findings, and determine short- and long-term prognoses. Such data are even more scarce for premature newborns.

Epidemiologic Observations

The incidence of seizures in newborns is still under debate. Reported figures range from 1.5 per 1,000 for the first 4 days after birth to 3.0 per 1,000 for the first 4 weeks of life [20].

Our research and that of Seay and Bray [60] indicate that the incidence of seizures in preterm babies is comparable to that in full-term infants. Dreyfus-Brisac and Monod [16] found that the "occurrence of convulsions among premature infants is less frequent than among full-term newborns." Their findings, however, were based on a population in which only 10 percent were under 36 weeks of age. In contrast, Fenichel [20] found that the risk of convulsions was "15 times greater in prematures than in term babies" but offered no supporting data. The difficulty of diagnosing these seizures may explain some of the discrepancies. The improving survival rate of very small

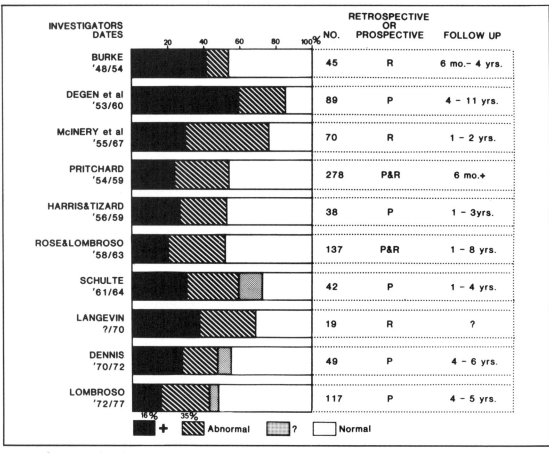

Figure 26-1. Reported morbidity and mortality for neonatal seizures. For original data see references 7, 9, 11, 21, 26, 32, 37, 51, 53, and 59.

premature infants (premies) is likely to increase the incidence of seizures in this population owing to its greater propensity for intracranial hemorrhages, asphyxia, sepsis, and other complications. Seay and Bray [60] report a mortality of 90 percent for premies with seizures, but this figure conflicts with figures obtained in prospective studies of preterm babies with asphyxia [36] or intracranial hemorrhages [8] in whom seizures were present.

There is a striking dichotomy in the clinical outcomes of newborns with seizures. In our 15-year prospective study of 240 full-term babies with seizures, approximately half were "normal" at 5 years of age, whereas the other half had considerable neurologic sequelae or had died early in infancy [30, 53]. Although perinatal practices have improved considerably in the past 15 years, the 50:50 ratio has not changed much. Figure 26-1 compares the results of some of the series investigated during the last few

decades. The more favorable reports [6, 23] reflect the anomalous incidence in these series of "late-onset hypocalcemia," a benign cause of neonatal seizures that has practically disappeared in the United States [30, 33]. Important changes in the percentages of the etiologic factors responsible for neonatal seizures have occurred in the past 20 years (Table 26-1). Survival of previously nonviable newborns has created an increase in neurologic morbidity, but this is countered by a clear decrease in the severity of neurologic sequelae during the past decade [11, 33]. The seizures themselves do not appear to be responsible for the adverse sequelae of this new population of special care babies; they represent but one index of CNS disorder.

Statistically significant differences in seizure occurrence according to gender have not been established for neonatal seizures as a group. Within certain etiologic subgroups sex differences are present. In seizures occurring after intracranial hemorrhages, the male-female ratio is about 2:1.

Table 26-1. Changing Trends in Main Etiologic Factors for Neonatal Seizures

Presumptive Etiologies	1958–1968		1969–1979		
	No.	Percent	No.	Percent	Comparison
Asphyxia[a]	25	11.5	51	24.5	$p<.01$
Intracranial hemorrhage					
Cryptogenic[a]	11	5	25	12	$p<.02$
Direct trauma[a]	22	10	9	4.5	$p<.02$
Infections					
Intrauterine	9	4	6	3	
Perinatal[a]	23	10.5	19	9	NS[c]
CNS dysgenesis (recognized)	14	6.5	18	8.5	NS
Metabolic					
Early-onset hypocalcemia[a]	17	8	29	14	NS
Late-onset hypocalcemia	29	13	6	3	$p<.01$
Hypomagnesemia	4	2	7	3.5	NS
Transient hypoglycemia[a]	13	6	18	8.5	NS
Persistent hypoglycemia[a]	11	5	9	4.5	NS
Hypo- and hypernatremia[a]	7	3	9	4.5	
Inborn errors of metabolism	9	4	12	6	
Postmaturity[a]	10	4.5	5	2.5	NS
Familial neonatal seizures	5	2.5	8	4	
Drug withdrawal	6	3	4	2	
Miscellaneous	9	4	12	5.5	
Cryptogenic	61	27.5	48	23	NS

[a]For each of these categories multiple factors often coexist.
[b]Comparison of 1958–1968 frequency with 1969–1979 frequency using chi-square test.
[c]NS = Not reaching level of significance.

Distribution of the time of onset of seizures is fairly consistent; the onset tends to peak within the first 3 days and again between the first and second weeks after birth. Some correlation with etiologic factors is suggested. The earliest onsets are mainly asociated with severe prenatal asphyxia, acquired CNS infections, systemic sepsis, some congenital CNS malformations, a few congenital metabolic errors, and a variety of probably intrauterine noxae such as small-for-dates or severe dysmaturity. Some infants who have undergone obstetric trauma also fall within this early-onset group; those with cryptogenic intracranial hemorrhage often manifest seizures after 1 to 3 days of uneventful existence. Transient metabolic aberrations such as hypoglycemia or "early-onset hypocalcemia" may be the primary trigger for the seizures in some neonates of the early-onset group.

The group in which seizures begin between the first and third weeks of life used to include mostly the "late-onset hypocalcemia" cases, now almost disappeared. Acquired infections, generalized sepsis with electrolyte disorders, metabolic disorders, and crypto-

genic (genetic) epilepsy often lead to seizures after 1 to 2 weeks of life. Scattered between these two peaks are babies with a variety of etiologic factors, including prenatal infections, sepsis, congenital metabolic disorders, kernicterus, and obstetric trauma. Overlapping occurs between these peaks.

In our experience, the onset of seizures is relatively unpredictable. Neither a history of major disorders of pregnancy or fetal distress nor the value of Apgar scores will reliably predict the incidence of seizures. Whether genetic factors determine the onset of seizures within similar groups at risk is unknown.

Seizure Patterns of the Newborn

The clinical expression of ictal events in the newborn is totally different from that in older children. Typical tonic-clonic convulsions, absences, complex partial seizures, and even organized Jacksonian marches are extremely rare.

During our prospective studies of approximately 300 newborns, a classification of their most common seizure patterns evolved and has been generally ac-

Table 26-2. Common Neonatal Seizure Patterns

Seizure Type	Clinical Signs
Subtle (or minimal)	Abnormal eye movements; mild posturing; oral, lingual, pedaling, rowing movements; brief tremors; apneas
Clonic	
Focal	Rarely implies focal brain lesion
Multifocal (fragmentary, anarchic)	
Hemiconvulsive	
Tonic	Focal or generalized; often accompanied by abnormal eye movements, apnea, cyanosis. More common in preterm newborns
Myoclonic	Often fragments of infantile spasms that are seen in later infancy
Tonic-Clonic	Rare in newborns

cepted. It is summarized in Table 26-2. The prevailing features of several of the patterns described in this table may appear at the same time in a given patient. Analysis of the patterns can provide clues to diagnosis and prognosis.

CLONIC SEIZURE PATTERN

Clonic events are frequently observed, although they are less common now than previously. They can be focal or multifocal. Focal clonic seizures consist of repeated but often irregular clonic movements affecting one or both limbs on the same side; they have a tendency to "wax and wane" and occasionally shift slowly to the opposite side but rarely with any organized march or spread. If they remain localized, even with vigorous or rapid clonus, they seem not to alter the general functions or even change the "state" (see later section, Neurologic Examination) of the baby. If they shift from one hemisphere to the other (especially if there is facial involvement), there may be some interference with respiration and an alteration of "state" or of consciousness. Rarely, one whole side of the baby is affected simultaneously, creating the "hemiconvulsive" pattern that is seen more commonly in later infancy. The clonic movements may be predominantly multifocal. These fragmentary clonic events fleetingly affect one or more limbs or the face, rapidly and unexpectedly shifting at random and following none of the customary rules of "epileptic spread." Thus they are also called migratory or anarchic clonic patterns [29]. If the shifts are very rapid they can create the impression of a generalized seizure or of jitteriness or other nonictal phenomena. Both focal and multifocal clonic patterns may occur in newborns with similar etiologies and in association with otherwise normal or abnormal EEG background patterns and state organizations. *Focal clonic patterns rarely indicate the focal underlying lesions one expects in*

older patients. The most characteristic focal clonic seizures occur in the presence of transient metabolic derangements, classically in benign "late-onset hypocalcemia." Babies with subarachnoid or intraventricular hemorrhages and diffuse encephalopathies following moderate asphyxia also exhibit focal clonic patterns. Babies with intraparenchymal bleeding, porencephaly, or vascular complications of infections are exceptions in that they may show focal EEG patterns. *Multifocal clonic patterns suggest more severe etiological causes* and are more often seen in premature or small-for-dates newborns.

SUBTLE (MINIMAL) SEIZURE PATTERN

The subtle or minimal seizure pattern is now the prevailing one (Table 26-2). It is seen increasingly in full-term and especially in preterm babies. Diagnosis of this pattern is difficult because clonic or tonic manifestations may be lacking and the peripheral phenomena may be few and less dramatic. These phenomena include abnormal eye movements, tonic eye deviations with or without nystagmoid components, chewing and drooling, brief flutter of the eyelids, mild posturing or brief tremor of a limb, and "pedaling" or "rowing" movements. These "soft" peripheral phenomena may be accompanied by apneic episodes of ictal origin, but because they usually occur in isolation or with only a few of the others, they are easily missed without EEG monitoring. The converse may also occur; nonictal phenomena, as described above, may be confused with seizures. The most common problem arises with apneic episodes. Central apnea is common in normal premature and full-term infants during REM states [3]. However, episodes of central apnea occurring in non-REM sleep, lasting from 8 to 20 seconds in term or near-term babies and accompanied by bradycardia and a fall in PO_2, are most often due to some failure in cardiorespiratory control than to seizure events. Ictal apnea is one of the "subtle" seizure patterns. It may occur as an isolated phenomenon but is infrequent [13, 19, 34, 59].

TONIC SEIZURE PATTERN

Tonic patterns occur with either focal or generalized involvement. The former simulates focal posturing, occasionally interrupted by brief clonus or tremors. The latter involves the whole body in extension and may be accompanied by tonic eye movements and apneas with duskiness. This pattern, seen in term and more frequently in preterm babies, is difficult to distinguish from common posturing that occurs normally, especially during REM sleep. Tonic seizure patterns in general are associated with serious CNS problems such as congenital malformations, intracranial hemorrhages, severe asphyxia, and congenital metabolic defects, particularly in term babies. The differential diagnosis includes normal posturing of the preterm infant and true decerebrate episodes accompanied by large and sluggish pupils and arms in pronation. EEG monitoring is often necessary to resolve doubts about whether or not these are ictal events. The accompanying EEG discharge is frequently of the "pseudodelta" type, but other EEG patterns may also occur [34].

MYOCLONIC SEIZURE PATTERN

Myoclonic patterns consist of sudden brief jerking or spasms. Classic infantile spasms rarely occur earlier than the third month of life. The myoclonic seizure pattern can be seen in babies with other seizure patterns, especially the subtle or tonic ones, and is usually an indication of considerable and diffuse CNS disease. They must be distinguished from an exaggerated Moro reflex, from the startles characteristic of normal REM sleep, and from the normal jitteriness or tremulousness seen in babies who are stimulated and aroused from an otherwise rather lethargic state. Myoclonic jerks occur for a few hours or days in babies born to drug-addicted mothers. They also occur in some congenital metabolic disorders. EEG monitoring may be needed for precise diagnosis. Jitteriness can be distinguished from true seizures because it is characteristically elicited or increased by stimulation and, conversely, is abated by manipulation of the limbs through support or gentle flexing. This manipulation will not stop true ictal clonus. The two movement disorders can coexist, especially in babies with metabolic derangements or hypoxic syndromes.

Etiologies

Approximately three quarters of neonatal seizure disorders are "symptomatic." Neonatal seizures have a wide spectrum of etiologies with related short- and long-term implications.

The usual presence of multiple etiologic factors makes it difficult to classify etiologies in neonatal seizures. The case with a single etiologic factor is relatively rare. Some etiologic factors are interdependent; others are not. Cumulative or potentiating noxae that are different in nature and difficult to quantify must be discerned. A typical example is the neonate with seizures and presumed prenatal asphyxia who has an intracranial hemorrhage and is then found to have substantial hypoglycemia, severe respiratory distress, and systemic sepsis. In evaluating possible etiologic factors, we list all the factors that are evident during the acute period and make no effort to establish qualitative or quantitative hierarchies of those dysfunctions. We feel that, for the time being, this strategy encourages specific therapies for specific etiologic factors, including those that might be secondary to the main cause, and will eventually allow classification of clusters of risk factors and their final outcomes.

Significant shifts in etiologic factors have occurred in the past two decades (Table 26-1). Direct birth traumas have decreased significantly. Late-onset hypocalcemia (simple tetany), which has been almost eliminated in the United States, still ranks surprisingly high in series published abroad. Asphyxia and intracranial hemorrhages have increased significantly. Congenital metabolic defects have also increased, probably owing to improved recognition. Congenital CNS malformations and pre- and postnatal infections do not appear to have changed in incidence.

ASPHYXIA

Perinatal asphyxia, defined as a varying combination of hypoxic-ischemic events, has now returned to lead the list of presumptive factors responsible for neonatal convulsions, particularly in intensive care referral units. It accounted for over 24 percent of all cases in our series for the period 1969 to 1979.

Although difficult to make, the diagnosis of asphyxia can be established by evidence of some of the following signs: type 2 deceleration in fetal heart monitoring; loss of beat-to-beat variability; a fetal scalp or umbilical cord pH of less than 7.20; Apgar scores below 5 at 5 minutes with evidence of acidosis; required resuscitation for absent respiration and/or bradycardia. One should then look for continued low Apgar scores at 10 to 15 minutes, a postnatal arterial blood pH of less than 7.20, and the coexistence of positive clinical signs such as abnormalities in sensorium and muscle tone (usually pathologically decreased), and continuing respiratory-cardiac problems without direct organ involvement. In our experience Apgar scores are quite unspecific if considered alone. The presence of meconium is suspicious but again is not diagnostic. Infections, symptoms resulting from maternal drug addiction, and some modalities of accidents of anesthesia may all mimic asphyxia. Any newborn who has experienced any brain insult while still in the uterus may have trouble with CNS respiratory and vascular regulation after birth. In fact, some of these babies may suffer postnatal asphyxic insults after birth [53].

Identification of postnatal hypoxic-ischemic events is easier with documented respiratory or cardiac arrest that requires vigorous resuscitation and with pathologic changes in blood gases, such as a persistent PO_2 below 40 mm Hg. Although the risks of actual brain damage from asphyxia are notoriously hard to quantify, we know that the seizures that occur are difficult to control. Both pre- and full-term neonates usually have such seizures early, 6 to 24 hours after delivery. Metabolic derangements are common; hypoglycemia and "early onset" hypocalcemia occur most frequently and may actually trigger the seizures. Prompt oral or intravenous administration of metabolites may stop them. The seizures may reemerge later, even after the metabolic derangement is under control. In either case these babies are at considerable risk. Perinatal asphyxia may predispose babies to intracranial hemorrhages of various types [8, 45, 67].

The subtle, the tonic, and the multifocal clonic are the seizure patterns most commonly seen in babies with perinatal asphyxia. When the seizures are triggered primarily by the concomitant metabolic derangement, they are predominantly focal clonic.

INTRACRANIAL HEMORRHAGES AND TRAUMAS

Trauma
Direct physical injury such as that caused by labor or "trauma X" should be distinguished from "cryptogenic" hemorrhages [40, 67] because the pathogenesis for the latter has not yet been elucidated. During the past decade there has been a significant increase in the latter group (Table 26-1), partly because of the increased survival of small premature infants, who are particularly prone to cryptogenic subependymal-intraventricular bleeding, and partly because of increased recognition of this condition through computed tomography (CT scans) and sector ultrasonar scanning [22].

Improved obstetric techniques have caused a dramatic decline in birth injuries. Subdural hematomas, however, still occur. Although they rarely cause seizures during the newborn period, they often lead to convulsive states later if left untreated. The usual clinical signs of uncomplicated neonatal subdural hematoma are an enlarging head, bulging fontanelles, lethargy, failure to thrive, retinal hemorrhages, vomiting, and unexplained fever. More acute symptoms

follow laceration of the tentorium cerebelli or falx cerebri owing to compression of the brainstem and severe edema. These emergency situations are rarely associated with convulsive phenomena. Exceptions occur when the trauma has also caused some contusion of the brain parenchyma. In such cases seizures are frequently present, and a skull fracture may be evident on routine roentgenograms. Sonograms, CT scan, and, best of all, angiography will help in the diagnosis of subdural hematoma, which can be confirmed by diagnostic and therapeutic subdural taps.

Subarachnoid Hemorrhage
Except for the common leakage of small amounts of blood during routine delivery, primary subarachnoid hemorrhages (SAH) rank first among types of intracranial bleeding in full-term newborns and are not infrequent in preterm infants. The mechanism by which SAH causes seizures is still unclear. Association of SAH with hypoxic insults and the highly epileptogenic effect of iron byproducts are proposed mechanisms. The seizures begin 1 to 3 days after birth and are often focal or multifocal clonic in pattern. These newborns show little evidence of distress or signs of increased intracranial pressure. Lumbar punctures reveal varying amounts of blood in the CSF, xanthochromia after spinning, and a protein content of 200 mg/100 ml or more. Other constituents remain nearly normal. Recent observations [8] require reexamination of the belief that primary SAH rarely causes late sequelae [20, 53, 68]. The poor outcome in some babies with SAH may correlate with the development of communicating hydrocephalus or with the type of SAH in which blood, instead of seeping freely and diffusely, tends to accumulate over the brain convexity (especially around the temporal lobes), possibly causing focal parenchymal damage [27].

Intraventricular Hemorrhage
The use of ultrasonic and CT scanning techniques has dramatically modified many traditional views about both the incidence and the morbidity of intraventricular hemorrhages (IVH) [40]. Often resulting from a subependymal hemorrhage (SEH), IVH has become the most frequent of all hemorrhagic events in small premature infants [45, 67]. IVH is also found in full-term newborns with seizures [32]. In these babies the bleeding is thought to originate most commonly from the choroid plexus, although in a few cases small arteriovenous malformations may be the source. IVH-SEH in small preterm infants can present clinically in various ways, a few of which are asymptomatic. Babies with large bleedings or extraventricular extension of

the hemorrhage and full-term babies are generally symptomatic and may have either a catastrophic or a saltatory syndrome [24, 25, 45, 67].

In both premies and term babies with IVH one of the most common presenting symptoms is the onset of seizures, usually after a couple of days of uneventful existence. Babies who appear quite ill earlier usually show evidence of asphyxia [25, 32]. Infants with IVH have mixed seizure patterns, but tonic patterns tend to predominate, especially in young premies. Subtle or myoclonic patterns are more common in term babies. A concomitant hypocalcemia or hypoglycemia may produce seizures of more vigorous clonic (usually fragmentary) patterns. Tsiantos et al. [66] concluded that the onset of the hemorrhage correlated to a significant degree with that of the seizures in a study using labeled red blood cells.

Primary Intraparenchymal Hemorrhages
We have seen newborns with seizures who had radiologic or autopsy confirmation of large intracerebral clots that did not appear to be related to IVH-SEH. These clots usually occur in full-term babies who may be asymptomatic at birth but begin to have seizures within 1 to a few days and appear quite ill. These focal seizures and focal EEG findings are one exception to the rule that focal symptoms and signs are usually of little localizing value in newborns.

INFECTIONS OF THE CNS
Infections of the CNS acquired in utero, during birth, or postnatally were the presumptive major cause of neonatal seizures in about 11 percent of our cases (Table 26-1). The main vital organisms causing transplacental CNS infections in the fetus and early seizures in neonates are rubella, cytomegalovirus, coxsackievirus-B, and the protozoan *Toxoplasma.* Syphilis occurs decreasingly as an intrauterine infection and rarely produces paroxysmal symptoms in newborns. Primary vaginal herpes simplex infection results in a usually devastating neonatal encephalitis with severe seizures soon after birth. If maternal vaginal herpetic infection is diagnosed or suspected, cesarean birth is mandatory. The diagnosis of an intrauterine infection in a convulsing newborn is strengthened by evidence of dysmaturity, systemic symptoms and signs (jaundice, rashes, hepatomegaly, chorioretinitis, occasionally cataracts), elevated serum IgM values in the newborn, rising antibody titers, and, when possible, isolation of the agent.

Postnatal CNS infections more commonly result from bacterial invasions (especially *Escherichia coli,* group B beta-*Streptococcus,* and *Haemophilus in-*

fluenzae). Sepsis without evidence of CNS invasion may cause neonatal seizures, possibly owing to electrolyte and other metabolic imbalances.

CONGENITAL CNS MALFORMATIONS
In our series, 7 to 8 percent of neonatal seizures were attributed to dysgenetic CNS conditions. Among these, those related to disorders of neuronal migration and organization are particularly apt to produce early onset of seizures. Polymicrogyria with or without heterotopias of gray matter, failures of normal cortical lamination, lissencephaly, holoprosencephaly, and anencephaly may all exhibit early seizures. Although it is usually expressed in seizures later in infancy, tuberous sclerosis may appear in the neonatal period. Less commonly, neurodermatoses such as incontinentia pigmenti, Sturge-Weber syndrome, and neurofibromatosis may present as early seizures. Hydrocephalus resulting from malformations or secondary to a hemorrhagic event may produce seizures, often tonic in pattern, but usually other paroxysmal events have occurred before. Aicardi's syndrome (see Chap. 9), porencephalic cysts, and congenital heart defects may be associated with early seizures.

METABOLIC FACTORS

Neonatal Hypocalcemic Syndromes
Late-onset hypocalcemia [11, 20, 29, 53, 68] probably results from feeding artificial milk formulas to babies with immature renal phosphate excretion and physiologic hypoparathyroidism, and it occasionally occurs in well babies after the first to second week of life. The seizures are surprisingly focal clonic seizures with normal EEGs interictally, and they respond promptly to calcium gluconate orally or parenterally. Occasionally they are accompanied by hypomagnesemia. The outcome in these infants is almost invariably excellent. Although it has practically disappeared in the United States (Tables 26-1 and 26-3), late-onset hypocalcemia still ranks high in some European series.

Early-onset hypocalcemia [20, 29, 53, 68] occurs in association with either prenatal morbidity (small-for-dates babies, maternal pre-eclampsia, diabetes, or hydramnios) or several perinatal or postnatal insults (e.g., asphyxia, obstetric trauma, intracranial hemorrhages). The seizures occur early, sometimes hours after birth. They are less commonly focal clonic and more often multifocal, subtle, tonic, or myoclonic. Restoring calcium levels to normal may control the seizures, but because there are usually underlying CNS insults, the convulsive state may persist or reemerge. Babies who are also hypoglycemic tend to have a worse prognosis.

Table 26-3. *Correlations Between Etiologic Factors and Outcome at 5 Years in 213 Newborns (1967–1977)*

Presumed Etiology	No. Patients	No. Dead	No. Abnormal	No. Normal	Percent Dead or Abnormal	Percent Normal	Predictive Value[b]
Asphyxia[a]	51	11	29	11	80	20	.01
Intracranial hemorrhage							
Cryptogenic[a]	30	6	15	9	70	30	.025
Traumatic[a]	9	3	3	3	70	30	
Infections							
Intrauterine	7	1	5	1	90	10	
Postnatal	20	5	8	7	65	35	NS[c]
CNS dysgenesis	19	6	12	1	95	5	.005
Metabolic							
Early-onset hypocalcemia[a]	32	8	12	12	66	36	NS
Late-onset hypocalcemia	10	0	1	9	10	90	.025
Transient hypoglycemia[a]	19	1	4	14	27	73	
Persistent (idiopathic) hypoglycemia	10	2	5	3	72	28	
Hypomagnesemia[a]	8	1	2	5	40	60	
Hypo- Hypernatremia[a]	10	2	2	6	40	60	
Inborn errors of metabolism	13	1	9	3	80	20	.05
Postmaturity[a]	6	0	5	1	85	15	
Familial (benign) seizures	9	0	1	8	8	92	.025
Drug-induced							
Iatrogenic	2	0	0	2	0	100	
Withdrawal	5	0	1	4	16	84	
Miscellaneous[a]	18	1	10	7			
Cryptogenic	54	3	14	37	32	68	.01

[a]For each of these categories other factors often coexist.
[b]Ability to predict unfavorable outcome, based on chi-square test.
[c]NS = Not reaching level of significance.

A rare cause of persistent hypocalcemia is DiGeorge's syndrome, which consists of congenital aplasia of the thymus, parathyroid glands, and great vessels and multiple minor congenital facial deformities. This syndrome strikes male babies twice as often as female babies and may cause death from defective cell-mediated immunologic defenses, cardiovascular insufficiency, or untreated persistent severe hypocalcemia.

Hypoglycemia
Transient and asymptomatic hypoglycemic states occur in more than 10 percent of all newborns before they are fed. Their blood glucose levels may be less than 20 to 30 mg/100 ml. In some cases no overt symptoms appear, but in others seizures occur a few hours after birth. These convulsions probably result from the same pre- and perinatal causes described for early-onset hypocalcemia, and they carry similar implications of some cerebral involvement antedating the metabolic disorder.

In our experience transient metabolic aberrations in "stressed" infants differ in outcome from those aberrations associated with anatomic pathologic factors. Babies who have only hypocalcemia appear to fare better than those with hypoglycemia. Furthermore, those who develop late-onset hypoglycemia with seizures (once labeled "idiopathic" hypoglycemia) appear to do poorly even with vigorous treatment. This group of diseases is probably heterogeneous in makeup and in some cases includes various inborn disorders of metabolism as well as hypoglycemia.

Hypernatremia and Hyponatremia
Both hypernatremia and hyponatremia can induce seizures. Hypernatremia is complicated occasionally by hemorrhagic events. Water intoxication is the most common cause of seizures in newborns with hyponatremia.

Inborn Errors of Metabolism
Among the large variety of inborn errors of metabolism, only some induce very early seizures. *Phenyl-*

ketonuria is no longer so important owing to newborn screening. Inborn metabolic errors involving deficiencies in the metabolism of branched-chain ketoacids (*maple-syrup disease*) can trigger neonatal seizures. Within 1 to 3 weeks after birth, these infants develop feeding problems, hypotonia alternating with opisthotonic crises, convulsions, and coma. Because they often have considerable hypoglycemia (often leucine-induced), the seizures may be triggered by the low blood sugar levels. Severe CNS involvement is probably due to the direct toxic effects of accumulating ketoacids, which produce permanent damage to myelination and nerve cells. Other inborn errors of amino acid metabolism that cause early convulsive states and usually irreversible CNS damage are those that induce marked elevation of glycine. *Nonketotic hyperglycinemia* is more common, and babies with this disorder have a fairly similar clinical course—they have no evidence of CNS dysfunction at birth, they develop seizures of early onset (usually myoclonic or tonic in pattern), and they progress through hypotonia and lethargy to coma. Neither the specific enzyme defect nor the severe effect upon the CNS by elevated glycine blood levels has been clarified. All of our cases ended in severe neurologic sequelae or death. The group of congenital episodic acidurias comprises *ketotic hyperglycinemia* (itself represented by different congenital disorders), *propionic acidemia,* and *methylmalonic acidemia.* These tend to induce severe early ketoacidosis, rarely with early seizures, sometimes with hyperammonemia, and often with elevated serum glycine levels. Acute, severe hyperammonemia may cause early convulsive states in the newborn. Some cases are due to primary hepatic disorders and others to congenital enzymatic defects, generally termed urea cycle disorders (e.g., *carbamylphosphate synthetase deficiency, arginosuccinase deficiency, citrullinemia,* and *congenital lysine intolerance*). In all these syndromes the role of elevated NH_3 in triggering convulsions is open to question because elevated serum levels of NH_3 occur in various other conditions without evidence of seizures. *Lipid and glycogen storage* diseases rarely produce seizures in the newborn period. A very rare though dramatic congenital enzyme defect that is responsible for early and intractable seizures with rapid CNS deterioration is *pyridoxine dependency,* which should not be confused with states of pyridoxine deficiency. Inherited as an autosomal recessive trait, its mechanism remains unclear. In contrast to pyridoxine deficiencies, all biochemical processes dependent upon pyridoxal as their coenzyme are not affected. It has been postulated that a specific defect in CNS glutamic decarboxylase leads to a reduction in the inhibitory neurotransmitter gamma-

aminobutyric acid (GABA) and in elevation of the excitatory neurotransmitter glutamic acid. Early recognition and treatment prevents early death and profound neurologic impairment [35, 53].

DRUG-INDUCED SEIZURES
The use of local anesthetics during labor occasionally induces early seizures in the newborn through either transplacental intoxication or accidental direct injection into the fetus [14]. Withdrawal syndromes rarely induce true convulsive states in the newborn unless other factors are present. These other factors result from the greater incidence of uterine and labor complications (small-for-dates babies, asphyxia, obstetric trauma) known to occur in babies of mothers who have been using heroin or propoxyphene [62]. The most common sequelae of neonatal withdrawal from heroin or other narcotic-analgesic drugs and short-acting barbiturates are marked jitteriness, hypermotility, hypertonicity, and autonomic dysfunction. In these cases, EEGs are particularly helpful in diagnosing the rare cases in which true convulsive states are present. For the majority of these newborns Benadryl, chlorpromazine (2–3 mg/kg/day), or paregoric and supportive measures are sufficient. Babies born to ethanol-addicted mothers may have substantial CNS and other organ malformations but commonly do not have neonatal seizures.

DYSMATURITY (OR POSTMATURITY)
In about 4 percent of newborns with seizures no etiologic factors can be established except that they were born 2 to 4 weeks later than expected and show several of the stigmata of postmature newborns [30, 32, 53]. Our experience suggests that if seizures occur early in life, prognosis for these infants should be guarded. Probably these newborns have heterogeneous etiologic factors that cause CNS dysfunction including placental insufficiency, difficult delivery, and asphyxia.

FAMILIAL BENIGN NEONATAL SEIZURES
In a small group of babies with early seizures a familial incidence suggests an autosomal dominant inheritance [52]. These seizures may represent what French authors have called the "seizures of the fifth day of life" [41]. These babies usually have clonic seizures within the first week of life but no evidence of other neurologic problems. Spontaneous remission usually occurs after a few weeks. On follow-up some infants are found to have absences or tonic-clonic seizures.

MISCELLANEOUS GROUP
Between 1958 and 1979 we observed neonatal seizures in 12 babies with systemic sepsis without evidence of

CNS involvement. Other miscellaneous causes of neonatal seizures include Leigh's subacute necrotizing encephalopathy, Alpers' disease, hemorrhagic disease due to Rh factors, idiopathic thrombocytopenia without evidence of gross intracranial bleeding, and fructose intolerance.

Guidelines for Evaluating a Newborn with Seizures

General Approach

First, attempt to discover the underlying cause in order to provide the most specific therapy. Second, as a prerequisite for therapy and prognosis evaluate the condition of the CNS by means of neurologic examination and whatever further tests are necessary.

In seeking the underlying cause(s) and in evaluating the condition of the CNS, the guidelines for handling newborns differ radically from those appropriate for older patients. Terminating a convulsive state in an older patient is the primary emergency goal, with diagnostic procedures coming second, whereas in newborns with seizures prompt discovery of the underlying cause or causes is the first emergency goal. Seizures rarely compromise vital functions in the newborn and are less apt to induce the complications common in older patients in status epilepticus.

Etiologic identification in neonatal seizures is often complicated by the presence of multiple risk factors. Although some risk factors may prove to be secondary or insignificant, the initial evaluation should consider all of them.

The inexact criteria for measuring the severity of conditions before, during, and after birth hamper the clinician severely. Variables such as the multiplicity of secondary metabolic and vascular derangements, the "plasticity" of developing nervous structures, the timing of the insults in relation to specific maturational schedules, and differing genetic predispositions all militate against the early assessment of abnormality on the basis of risk factors alone. Other measures for evaluating neonatal functioning have, therefore, acquired some importance. These include neurologic-behavioral assessments and measures of bioelectric parameters by means of polygraphic and evoked potential tests.

History

To identify promptly as many potentially responsible factors as possible, a complete history of the unusual events of the pregnancy and the labor should be obtained, including types and routes of anesthesia used, fetal heart monitoring, presence of meconium, Apgar scores, time and method of resuscitations, pH values of the umbilical cord blood and of the baby's blood, blood gas measurements, blood pressure, and the occurrence of respiratory and circulatory events and the treatments used for these.

Laboratory Tests

With rare exceptions, serum chemistry tests (calcium, phosphorus, glucose, and sodium), lumbar puncture, and a general sepsis work-up should be performed immediately. Careful assessment of CSF collected in separate tubes and spun promptly to establish the presence and degree of xanthochromia should be a routine test and should include cell counts, cultures, and similar routine procedures. This test will detect promptly a CNS infection or the presence of intracranial bleeding. Routine scanning by ultrasound is also necessary, at least in young premature infants. CT scans should follow as a confirmatory procedure. Both may need to be repeated to check for early signs of posthemorrhagic hydrocephalus.

Neurologic Examination

One would expect the *neurologic examination* to be a most reliable instrument for etiological diagnosis and for prognosis. However, few publications discuss at any length the special aspects of examination in neonatal neurology. By and large, they follow standard neurologic lines, implying that the neonatal CNS is a miniature edition, albeit primitive, of the developed, older CNS. Emphasis is placed on detecting deviations in the functions of cranial nerves, of general motility, of phasic and postural tone, of monosynaptic and polysynaptic reflexes. Observations include presence of malformations, evidence for increased intracranial pressure, deviations in head size, degree of sensorium from lethargy to hyperalertness, aberrations of brainstem functions. What is missing is a discussion of the concepts of *states* in the newborn, their recognition in waking and sleep conditions, and the effects they can have on many of the neurologic signs being examined.

A *state* is defined as a constellation of behavioral, physiologic, and EEG variables that occur together and may recur cyclically [49]. In a full-term infant there are five states: state I (non-REM sleep, "quiet" sleep); state II (REM sleep, "active" sleep); state III (eyes open, alert but inactive); state IV (eyes open, gross movements, no crying); state V (eyes open or closed, high activity, crying). The behavioral, physiologic, and EEG features of each state evolve in such a way that for any given conceptual age there is a characteristic pattern for each state. States are described in more detail elsewhere [5, 34, 47, 49, 50, 72].

As recently as 1979, a pioneer in neonatal neurology, Saint-Anne Dargassies, wrote, "Unfortunately, one cannot always ascertain the location or extent of a lesion, or even its pathology, by clinical examination alone. Thus the goal becomes one of recognizing CNS dysfunction, either transient or permanent" [57]. She emphasizes that serious gestational abnormalities, for instance, may be undetectable, concealed by secondary perinatal impairments. Prechtl, Parmelee, and coworkers [5, 46, 47, 49, 50], strong advocates for specialized neurologic assessment of neonates, recognize the fundamental interdependence in the newborn between behavioral-physiologic states and neurologic performance. This interdependence is significant in evaluating "input" and "output," and in choosing appropriate diagnostic techniques for different gestational ages. The neurologic examination of the newborn is discussed in several publications [1, 2, 54, 55, 56]. These studies exemplify techniques based on classic and careful testing of complex reflex neurophysiology. In general, the writers ignore the dependency of the developing CNS on its rapidly changing *states,* although they do stress the need for age-dependent technique modifications and interpretations. The neurologic techniques developed over the past 15 years primarily by Prechtl, Parmelee and coworkers [5, 46, 47, 49, 50] emphasize first the interdependence between changing states in the newborn, his changing information-processing, and his variable "output" (reflex activities, postural and behavioral responses to stimuli). They also emphasize high interexaminer reliability, detection of "minor" deviations as well as major ones, and long-term predictability. Whether or not these are all attainable, it is a good start in the right direction. These researchers also emphasize recognition of major indications of serious CNS disease (seizures, extreme disorders in muscle tone or sensorium, and lateralized motor defects). Parmalee and Michaelis [47] are less optimistic than Prechtl about long-term prognosis, but both groups stress the importance of serial follow-ups.

BIO-ELECTRIC MEASURES

Polygraphic electroencephalography and evoked potentials have assumed a progressively central role in the field of neonatal seizure diagnosis and treatment [15, 17, 18, 21, 32, 34, 42, 64, 71]. Bio-electric tests can determine whether many uncertain behavioral phenomena are ictal in origin and can suggest such etiological factors as metabolic dysfunctions or intracranial bleeding. Their greatest contribution is their reliability in predictions of short- and long-term outcome. Most information can be obtained from polygraphic EEG by analyzing three main features. The first feature, which we call *ictal patterns,* is the recog-

nition, classification and correlation of ictal EEG phenomena with both diagnostic and prognostic implications. The second, and probably more revealing, feature is *background patterns,* and the third feature is *primary abnormalities affecting states and EEG maturational schedules.* Tables 26-4 and 26-5 summarize the more important of these features and their correlations with clinical outcomes. For more detailed description and discussion of these EEG patterns see Tharp [64, 65], Lombroso [34], Werner et al. [72].

Treatment

Recent laboratory studies of prolonged seizures in adult and immature animal models have elucidated some of the metabolic factors presumed to be responsible for neuropathologic changes resulting from convulsive states [10, 38, 39, 69, 70]. They have demonstrated the presence of serious systemic and CNS complications induced by seizures in the immature animals. Cardiac arrhythmias, anoxia from respiratory embarrassment, decreased autoregulation of CNS cerebral blood flow, failure of blood-brain glucose transport, poor ketone utilization, and less efficient activation of phosphorylase by immature glial cells all contribute to severe depletion of glucose for the brain and interfere with defense against lactic acidosis. Synthesis of DNA, RNA, protein, and cholesterol is affected in the CNS to a marked degree [69, 70].

It is easy to understand how these observations in immature animals undergoing prolonged convulsive states have led to the conclusion that the remarkably poor prognosis for human neonates with seizures is attributable to the effect of the seizures themselves. Although we do not deny that prolonged hypoxia or hypoglycemia may occur in the newborn period and may be of grave concern, we believe that seizures in the neonate differ importantly from those in older babies in that they rarely affect vital functions, either systemically or within the CNS [12, 20, 32, 33]. From our data it appears that the high mortality and morbidity characteristics of neonates with seizures are primarily due to the serious noxae that have already injured the CNS. Hence, the seizures are most frequently epiphenomena of the many insults so apt to occur at this age. Seizures may be short and transient in spite of persistent underlying deficits; they may be dramatic and prolonged with no visible sequelae [32, 33].

With the exception of the urgent need to maintain optimal ventilation and an ample supply of glucose, emergency treatment for neonatal seizures consists of establishing the underlying cause or causes and instituting the appropriate therapies.

Table 26-4. Outcome of Ictal Neonatal EEG Patterns

Neonatal EEG Pattern (Ictal Abnormalities)	Clinical Outcome at 4-7 Years				
	Normal	Abnormal	Dead	Totals	Predictive Value[a]
Focal discharges (spikes or sharp waves) with normal background	38	26	3	67	NS[b]
Multifocal discharges with abnormal background	10	23	8	41	$p < .001$
Beta, alpha, theta, or delta-like discharges	5	14	6	25	$p < .004$
Repeated sharp waves at low frequencies, usually over a low-voltage background	3	8	3	14	$p < .05$
No recordable discharges during clinical ictus	—	2	3	5	NS[c]

[a]Ability to predict unfavorable outcome, based on chi-square test.
[b]NS = Not reaching level of significance.
[c]The chi-square test did not reach a significant level because of the small number of subjects, although none of the children were normal.

VENTILATION AND METABOLITES

Proper ventilation must be ensured immediately and at all times and an intravenous line should be placed for the administration of dextrose immediately following a blood glucose determination. If this determination indicates the presence of hypoglycemia, an infusion of 25 to 30 percent dextrose should be given at a dose of 3 to 5 ml/kg. A slow infusion of dextrose (0.5–1 g/hour) should be given even in the absence of hypoglycemia to obtain above-normal glucose blood levels. Care should be taken to avoid serious hyper- or hypohydration. In general, the baby should be maintained in a mild hypohydrated state. Meanwhile, values of serum calcium and magnesium should be determined. If hypocalcemia is present, a slow infusion of 2.5 to 5 percent calcium gluconate is given at doses of 8 to 10 ml/kg with ECG monitoring. If required, oral calcium preparations can be given for maintenance. With concomitant (or, more rarely, isolated) hypomagnesemia, a solution of 2 to 3 percent $MgSO_4$ is infused in doses of 2 to 8 ml. Some physicians advocate an intramuscular injection of a 50 percent solution in a dose of 0.2 ml/kg. However, care should be exercised in monitoring levels of serum magnesium because it has a curare-like effect and may induce severe hypotonia or even respiratory paralysis. The rare condition of pyridoxine dependency can be diagnosed only empirically through intravenous administration of 25 to 50 mg of pyridoxine. For these potentially diagnostic and therapeutic infusions of metabolites, simultaneous EEG monitoring can be helpful but is not essential. Clinical observations usually suffice. For other rare cases of inborn errors of metabolism, specific therapies (often ineffective) are discussed under Etiologies.

ANTIEPILEPTIC DRUGS

When given a choice, we prefer to postpone antiepileptic drug therapy until the diagnostic profiles are clear. Babies with transient metabolic derangements, mild hypoxic encephalopathies, or sepsis without any CNS invasion may have only mild transient seizures. In these cases effective but short-acting drugs such as diazepam may be preferable.

DIAZEPAM. Intravenous diazepam remains the drug of choice for some patients [4, 29, 32, 61]. It should be injected slowly at doses of 0.08 mg/kg up to 2.70 mg/kg (average, 0.65 mg/kg), preferably diluted in sterile water to obtain a 1 mg/ml solution to be infused at the rate of 1 ml every 2 minutes or until the seizures stop. Another, quicker method is to inject diluted diazepam very slowly intravenously in a total dose of 0.2 to 1 mg for babies weighing about 1,500 to 3,000 g respectively. Care is necessary to avoid accidental intra-arterial infusion, as it may have thrombotic complications. Monitoring of respiration and blood pressure is indicated. At these doses, intravenous diazepam has proved to be a safe drug in infants who have not been given loading doses beforehand of depressant agents such as phenobarbital. Recently, rectally-administered diazepam has been shown to be almost as effective as intravenously-administered diazepam [58].

PARALDEHYDE. Paraldehyde is an older drug now used less frequently. Its indications are similar to those for diazepam for babies in whom seizures may be short-lived. It is also effective and generally safe in cases of true status epilepticus. The dosage is 0.1 to 0.15 mg/kg. An unopened vial should be used because the drug

Table 26-5. Outcome of Interictal Neonatal EEG Patterns in Neonates With Seizures

Neonatal EEG Pattern (Background Abnormalities)	Clinical Outcome at 4–7 Years				
	Normal	Abnormal	Dead	Totals	Predictive Value[a]
Isoelectric	—	4	6	10	$p < .002$
Paroxysmal or "burst-suppression"					
Both awake and asleep	1	12	7	20	$p < .001$
In REM and non-REM sleep only	2	11	4	17	$p < .002$
Low-voltage throughout REM and non-REM sleep	1	7	1	9	$p < .04$
Persistent severe dysmaturity for conceptional age	6	12	—	18	NS[b]
Rolandic positive sharp transient patterns	2	2	2	6	NS
Normal EEGs	92	10	1	103	$p < .001$
Totals	106	131	44	335	

[a]Ability to predict unfavorable outcome, based on chi-square test.
[b]NS = Not reaching level of significance.

decomposes to acetic acid when exposed to light or air. It can be administered rectally, mixed with 2 to 3 ml of mineral oil as a retention enema. Because it is excreted through the lungs, the characteristic odor should be apparent in expired air within minutes to confirm its absorption. For this reason, paraldehyde is not advisable if lung disease is present. Some suggest intravenous administration of a 4 percent paraldehyde solution by slow drip. Paraldehyde administered intramuscularly is rapidly absorbed (peak serum concentrations are reached in 20 to 60 minutes) but in neonates it seems to be particularly apt to cause tissue necrosis, sterile abscesses, or damage to the nerves near the injection site (especially the sciatic nerves). If several doses are needed over a period of time, the rectal route may cause local irritation. It is then preferable to insert a nasogastric tube and administer the drug, possibly with some milk, every 4 to 6 hours for a period of 24 to 64 hours. Longer use of the drug may cause gastric or lung complications. The use of diazepam or paraldehyde is indicated also in babies with familial benign seizures because these tend to disappear in a period of days. Paraldehyde is discussed in more detail in Chapters 22 and 30.

Long-Term Antiepileptic Drug Treatment
Long-term treatment is indicated by a diagnostic profile that suggests the likelihood of continued seizures (e.g., large structural lesions) or by the persistence of frequent seizures after administration of the short-term treatment outlined above. The drugs of choice are still

phenobarbital and phenytoin. Not enough data are available at present on the use and safety of valproic acid in neonatal seizures.

PHENOBARBITAL. In newborns, the blood levels of phenobarbital needed to achieve seizure control are higher than those in children or adults. About 20 μg/ml is the minimum effective level. To achieve these levels, loading doses of 15 to 20 mg/kg, regardless of gestational age, are required [28, 44]. Slightly higher doses (18–22 mg/kg) are necessary if the drug is given intramuscularly. For maintenance, 3 to 5 mg/kg/day should be used parenterally or orally, although the latter route is apt to cause greater fluctuations in blood levels. Blood levels should be monitored closely to avoid toxicity, particularly during the first week of administration. The elimination half-life of phenobarbital in newborns is considerably longer (61 to 173 hours; see Chap. 17) than that in older children owing to immature hepatic enzymes.

PHENYTOIN. Phenytoin may be injected slowly intravenously (20–50 mg/minute) at a dose of 15 to 20 mg/kg [44] to achieve blood levels of 10 to 20 μg/ml. Maintenance levels can be achieved by intravenous doses of 5 mg/kg/day. Oral administration of phenytoin results in very erratic blood levels in the newborn. Intramuscular administration is contraindicated at all ages. Fluctuations in blood levels occur, especially after a few days and particularly when phenytoin is combined with phenobarbital. Because toxicity is hard to assess clinically in infants except by lethargy or vomiting, close blood level monitoring should be maintained.

Refractory Seizures

There will be some neonates who continue to have seizures in spite of adequate blood levels of phenobarbital and phenytoin. It is generally agreed that more harm than good is achieved by increasing these medications above the recommended levels [16, 20, 33].

Duration of Therapy

Still unanswered is the question of how long antiepileptic drug therapy should be continued. Some suggest that drugs should be used only while seizures are present and then discontinued a week or so after they stop. Others suggest that phenobarbital should be continued "until there are no persistent signs of neurological injury, e.g., seizures, motor deficits, or definite developmental delay" [68]. A recent study [63] of 40 neonates with seizures due to perinatal asphyxia reports that 28 had no seizure recurrences after phenobarbital treatment was discontinued after 3 days; 12 required maintenance therapy. More complete data on this issue is desirable. Decisions about starting or stopping antiepileptic drug therapy are not as yet fully resolved.

Effect on Prognosis

It is unknown whether antiepileptic drug therapy, aside from stopping seizures, plays a role in modifying the neurologic outcome in newborns and particularly whether it prevents the emergence of epilepsy years later. Also unknown is the effect on the rapidly developing CNS of the high doses of antiepileptic drugs that are necessary to stop seizures in the newborn.

Prognosis

General prognostic implications have already been mentioned under Epidemiologic Observations. Neonatal seizures should be considered indications of potentially more serious CNS dysfunction than most convulsive syndromes of later childhood. The incidence in past series has varied from 20 to more than 50 percent for mortality and from 40 to 50 percent for severe morbidity (Fig. 26-1). Our latest prospective study [33] shows a mortality rate of 16 percent and a 35 percent incidence of long-term neurologic morbidity (Fig. 26-1), an outlook somewhat improved from past series. These studies have dealt mainly with term or near-term babies. Large prospective investigations of the prognosis of premature infants with seizures are

still unavailable. Retrospective studies report a mortality of 61 to 90 percent and indicate a less favorable prognosis in the premature infant with seizures than in the term infant [60, 65].

In contrast to the dire prognostic implications for about half of the newborns with seizures, the other half appear to escape important sequelae. In the context of such a striking dichotomy in outcome, the clinician must predict how a given infant will fare. Risk factors during pregnancy have proved to be relatively poor indicators both in anticipating neonatal seizures [30] and in predicting later significant neurologic sequelae [15, 41, 43, 57]. Exceptions occur, such as maternal infections at certain periods of pregnancy or CNS malformations that are diagnosed by ultrasound. Events of labor (e.g., dystocia, abnormalities in fetal heart monitoring, low pH from fetal scalp or umbilical cord blood) seem to be better indicators of potential CNS involvement. Very adverse sequelae are fairly accurately ascertained from early signs. The predictability of danger increases with clinical signs such as Apgar scores of 0 to 3 at 1 and 5 minutes or persistent low values at 10 to 15 minutes, multiple apneic episodes with or without bradycardia, feeding problems, lethargy or extreme irritability, marked abnormalities of muscle tone, early onset of seizures, and instability or inability to develop the usual changes in states.

Although neurologic assessment can establish the presence or absence of neonatal CNS dysfunction, it is less helpful in predicting the long-term outcome. There are naturally exceptions, such as marked dysgenetic syndromes, persistent disorders in sensorium or muscle tone, or brainstem dysfunction. Abnormalities observed at a single examination, especially in a newborn who is having a seizure, do not permit reliable prediction.

The prevailing patterns of the seizures (Table 26-2) as well as their time of onset offer some predictive clues. Seizures with minimal or equivocal peripheral manifestations (subtle, myoclonic, and, to a lesser extent, tonic patterns) generally correlate with a worse prognosis than those with focal or multifocal, well-sustained clonic patterns. Seizures that begin in the first few hours or in the first 2 to 3 days postpartum are generally viewed with greater alarm than those beginning after 6 or more days. However, the striking decline in late-onset hypocalcemia may change the more benign prognosis for babies with seizure onset after 6 days.

Predictions are determined to some extent by establishing the underlying presumptive etiologic factors. Our prospective investigations [33, 53] of relatively large numbers of newborns revealed statistically significant correlations between some of these factors and clinical outcomes several years later (Table 26-3). It should be stressed that we made no effort during the follow-up to detect "soft," though possibly important, sequelae such as minor dysfunctions of cognition or attention or minor motor deficits of coordination. Our correlations by and large agree with those of other studies.

Recent studies place the neonatal EEG second in importance only to the etiology in the prognostic profile [16, 17, 34, 42, 64]. Tables 26-4 and 26-5 summarize the correlations found between some features of neonatal EEG polygraphy and the clinical outcome. Large prospective studies of correlations between early EEG features and outcome in very small premies are lacking; reports on small groups suggest that correlations in premature infants are similar to those in full-term infants [8, 34, 42, 65]. Correlations for abnormalities of state organization and duration and correlations for EEG dysmaturity features [17, 31, 71] are still in need of further investigation.

References

1. Amiel-Tison, C. In R. Korobkin, and C. Guilleminault (Eds.), *Advances in Perinatal Neurology,* Vol. I. New York: Spectrum Medical and Scientific Books, 1979.
2. André-Thomas, A., Chesni, Y., Saint-Anne Dergassies, S. Examen Neurologique du Nourrisson. *Vie Médicale* Paris: 1955.
3. Ariagno, R. L. Development of Respiratory Control. In R. Korobkin, and C. Guilleminault (Eds.), *Advances in Perinatal Neurology.* New York: S. P. Medical Aid Scientific Books, 1979.
4. Bailey, D. W., and Fenichel, G. M. The treatment of prolonged seizure activity with intravenous diazepam. *J. Pediatr.* 73:923, 1968.
5. Beintema, D. J. A neurological study of newborn infants. *Clinics in Developmental Medicine,* No. 28. London: Heinemann, 1968.
6. Brown, J. K. Convulsions in the newborn period. *Dev. Med. Child Neurol.* 15:823, 1973.
7. Burke, J. B. The prognostic significance of neonatal convulsions. *Arch. Dis. Child.* 29:342, 1954.
8. Da Costa, J. C., and Lombroso, C. T. Neurophysiological correlates of neonatal intracranial hemorrhages. *Electroencephalogr. Clin. Neurophysiol.* 50:183, 1980.
9. Degen, R., and Koschtial, I. Die Spaetprognose von Kraempfen in der Neurgeborenen-Periode. *Monatsschr. Kinderheilkd.* 116:133, 1968.
10. Delgado-Escueta, A. V. et al. (Eds.), *Status Epilep-*

ticus: *Mechanisms of Brain Damage and Treatment.* New York: Raven Press, 1982.
11. Dennis, J. Neonatal convulsions. Aetiology, late neonatal status and long-term outcome. *Dev. Med. Child Neurol.* 20:143, 1978.
12. Dennis, J. The Implications of Neonatal Seizures. In R. Korobkin, and C. Guilleminault (Eds.), *Advances in Perinatal Neurology.* New York: S. P. Medical Scientific Books, 1979.
13. Deuel, R. K. Polygraphic monitoring of apneic spells. *Arch. Neurol.* 28:71, 1973.
14. Dodson, W. E. Neonatal drug intoxication: Local anesthesia. *Pediatr. Clin. North Am.* 23:399, 1976.
15. Dreyfus-Brisac, C., and Monod, N. Electroclinical Studies of Status Epilepticus and Convulsions in the Newborn. In P. Kellaway, and I. Peterson (Eds.), *Neurological and Electroencephalographic Correlative Studies in Infancy.* New York: Grune & Stratton, 1964.
16. Dreyfus-Brisac, C., and Monod, N. Neonatal Status Epilepticus. In A. Remond (Ed.), *Handbook of Electroencephalography and Clinical Neurophysiology,* Vol. 15-B. Amsterdam: Elsevier, 1972.
17. Ellingson, R. J. EEG of Premature and Full-Term Newborns. In D. W. Klass, and D. D. Daly (Eds.), *Current Practice of Clinical Electroencephalography.* New York: Raven Press, 1979.
18. Engel, R. C. H. *Abnormal Electroencephalograms in the Neonatal Period.* Springfield, Ill.: Thomas, 1975.
19. Fenichel, G. M., Olsen, B. J., and Fitzpatrick, J. E. Heart rate changes in convulsive and nonconvulsive apnea. *Ann. Neurology* 6:171, 1979.
20. Fenichel, G. M. Convulsions. In G. M. Fenichel (Ed.), *Neonatal Neurology.* New York: Livingstone, 1980.
21. Harris, R., and Tizard, J. P. M. The electroencephalogram in neonatal convulsions. *J. Pediatr.* 57:501, 1960.
22. Johnson, M. L., and Rumak, C. M. Ultrasonic evaluation of the neonatal brain. *Radiol. Clin. North Am.* 18:117, 1980.
23. Keen, J. H., and Lee, D. Sequelae of neonatal convulsions, study of 112 infants. *Arch. Dis. Child.* 48:542, 1973.
24. Korobkin, R. The Prognosis for Survivors of Perinatal Intraventricular Hemorrhage. In R. Korobkin and C. Guilleminault (Eds.), *Advances in Perinatal Neurology.* New York: S. P. Medical and Scientific Books, 1979.
25. Krishnamoorthy, D. S. et al. Neurological sequelae in the survivors of neonatal intraventricular hemorrhage. *J. Pediatr.* 64:233, 1979.

312

26. Langevin, P. Les convulsions en période neo-natale. Évaluations de 21 cas. *Union Med. Can.* 103:465, 1974.

27. Larroche, J. C. *Developmental Pathology of the Neonate.* Amsterdam: Excerpta Medica, 1977.

28. Lockman, L. A. et al. Phenobarbital dosage for control of neonatal seizures. *Neurology* 29:1445, 1979.

29. Lombroso, C. T. Neonatal seizure states. In *Proceedings of XI International Congress of Pediatrics.* Tokyo: University of Tokyo Press, 1965.

30. Lombroso, C. T. Seizures in the Newborn Period. In P. J. Vinklen, and G. W. Bruyn (Eds.), *Handbook of Clinical Neurology,* Vol. 15, *The Epilepsies.* Amsterdam: Elsevier, 1974.

31. Lombroso, C. T. Neurophysiological observations in diseased newborns. *Biological Psychiatry* 10:527, 1975.

32. Lombroso, C. T. Convulsive Disorders in Newborns. In R. A. Thompson, and J. R. Green (Eds.), *Pediatric Neurology and Neurosurgery.* New York: Spectrum Publications, 1978.

33. Lombroso, C. T. Prognosis of Neonatal Seizures. In A. V. Delgado-Escueta et al. (Eds.), *Status Epilepticus: Mechanisms of Brain Damage and Treatment.* New York: Raven Press, 1982.

34. Lombroso, C. T. Neonatal Electroencephalography. In E. Neidermeyer, and P. Lopes de Silva (Eds.), *Electroencephalography—Basic Principles, Clinical Application and Related Fields.* Baltimore: Urban and Schwatzenburg, 1982.

35. Lott, I. T. et al. Vitamin B_6 dependent seizures: Pathology and clinical findings in brain. *Neurology* 28:47, 1978.

36. Lutschg, J. et al. Brainstem auditory evoked potentials in asphyxiated and neurologically abnormal newborns. *Electroencephalogr. Clin. Neurophysiol.* 49:27, 1980.

37. McInery, T. K., and Schubert, W. K. Prognosis of neonatal seizures. *Am. Ann. J. Dis. Child.* 117:261, 1969.

38. Meldrum, B. S., and Horton, R. W. Physiology of status epilepticus in primates. *Arch. Neurol.* 28:1, 1973.

39. Meldrum, B. S., Horton, R. W., and Brierly, J. B. Epileptic brain damage in adolescent baboons following seizures induced by allyl glycine. *Brain* 97:407, 1974.

40. Mitchell, W., and O'Tuama, L. Cerebral intra-ventricular hemorrhages in infants: A widening age spectrum. *Pediatrics* 65:35, 1980.

41. Monod, N., Dreyfus-Brisac, C., and Saello, Z. Dépistage et prognostic de l'état de mal neonatal. *Arch. Fr. Pediatr.* 26:1085, 1969.

42. Monod, R., Pajot, N., and Guidasci, S. The neonatal EEG. Statistical studies and prognostic value in full-term and pre-term babies. *Electroencephalogr. Clin. Neurophysiol.* 32:529, 1972.

43. Nelson, K. B., and Broman, S. H. Perinatal risk factors in children with serious motor and mental handicaps. *Ann. Neurol.* 2:371, 1979.

44. Painter, M. J. et al. Phenobarbital and diphenyl-hydantoin levels in neonates with seizures. *J. Pediatr.* 92:315, 1978.

45. Papile, L. A. et al. Incidence and evolution of subependymal and intraventricular hemorrhage. A study of infants with birthweight of less than 1,550 gm. *Neurology* 92:529, 1978.

46. Parmelee, A. H., and Haber, A. Who is the "risk infant?" *Clin. Obstet. Gynecol.* 16:376, 1973.

47. Parmelee, A. H., and Michaelis, R. Neurological Examination of the Newborn. In J. Hellmuth (Ed.), *Exceptional Infant,* Vol. 2, *Studies in Abnormalities.* London: Butterworth, 1971.

48. Plum, F., House, D. C., and Duffy, T. F. Metabolic Aspects of Seizures. In F. Plum (Ed.), *Brain Dysfunction in Metabolic Disorders.* New York: Raven Press, 1974.

49. Prechtl, H. F. R. The behavioral status of the newborn infant (a review). *Brain Res.* 76:185, 1974.

50. Prechtl, H. F. R., and Beintema, D. J. The neurological examination of the full-term newborn infant. *Clinics in Developmental Medicine,* No. 12. London: Heinemann, 1964.

51. Prichard, J. S. The Character and Significance of Seizures in Infancy. In P. Kellaway, and I. Petersen (Eds.), *Neurological and Electroencephalographic Correlative Studies in Infancy.* New York: Grune & Stratton, 1964.

52. Quattelbaum, T. G. Benign familial convulsions in the neonatal period and early infancy. *J. Pediatr.* 95:257, 1979.

53. Rose, A. L., and Lombroso, C. T. Neonatal seizure states: A study of clinical, pathological and electroencephalographic features in 137 full-term babies with long-term follow-up. *Pediatrics* 45:404, 1970.

54. Saint-Anne Dargassies, S. La naturation neurologique des prématurés. *Études neonatales* 3:101, 1954.

55. Saint-Anne Dargassies, S. *Le Développement Neurologique du Nouveau-Né à Terme et Prematuré.* Paris: Masson, 1974.

56. Saint-Anne Dargassies, S. *Neurological Development in the Full-Term and Premature Neonate.* Amsterdam: Elsevier, 1977.

57. Saint-Anne Dargassies, S. The Normal and Abnormal Neurological Examination of the Neonate: Silent Neurological Abnormalities. In R. Korobkin, and C. Guilleminault (Eds.), *Advances in Perinatal Neurology.* New York: S. P. Medical and Scientific Books, 1979.

58. Schmidt, D. Benzodiazepines: Diazepam. In D. M. Woodbury, J. K. Penry, and C. E. Pippenger (Eds.), *Antiepileptic Drugs.* New York: Raven Press, 1982.

59. Schulte, F. J. Apnea. *Clin. Perinatol.* 4:65, 1977.

60. Seay, A. R., and Bray, P. F. Significance of seizures in infants weighing less than 2,500 grams. *Arch. Neurol.* 34:381, 1977.

61. Smith, B. T., and Masotti, R. E. Intravenous diazepam in the treatment of prolonged seizure activity in neonates and infants. *Dev. Med. Child Neurol.* 13:630, 1971.

62. Stone, M. L. et al. Narcotic addiction in pregnancy. *Ann. J. Obstet. Gynecol.* 109:715, 1971.

63. Sun, S. et al. Long-term follow-up of neonatal seizures due to perinatal asphyxia. *Pediatr. Res.* 15:712, 1981.

64. Tharp, B. R. Pediatric Electroencephalography. In M. Aminoff (Ed.), *Electrodiagnosis in Clinical Neurology.* New York: Livingstone, 1980.

65. Tharp, B. R., Cukier, F., and Monod, N. The prognostic value of the electroencephalogram in premature infants. *Electroencephalogr. Clin. Neurophysiol.* 51:219, 1980.

66. Tsiantos, A. et al. Intracranial hemorrhage in the prematurely born infants; timing of clots and evaluation of clinical signs and symptoms. *J. Pediatr.* 85:854, 1974.

67. Volpe, J. J. Intracranial hemorrhage in the newborn: Current understanding and dilemmas. *Neurology* 29:632, 1979.

68. Volpe, J. J. Neonatal seizures. *Clin. Perinatol.* 4:43, 1977.

69. Wasterlain, C. G. Effects of neonatal status epilepticus on cat brain development. *Neurology* 26:975, 1976.

70. Wasterlain, C. G., and Duffy, T. E. Status epilepticus in immature cats. *Arch. Neurol.* 33:821, 1976.

71. Watanabe, K., and Iwase, K. Spindle-like fast rhythms in the EEGs of low birth-weight infants. *Devel. Med. Child Neurol.* 14:378, 1972.

72. Werner, S. S., Stockard, J. E., and Bickford, R. *Atlas of Neonatal Electroencephalography.* New York: Raven Press, 1977.

FEBRILE SEIZURES

27

Eileen M. Ouellette

Definition

Febrile seizures are an age-related form of epilepsy that occur within the context of a febrile illness. They are among the most common of pediatric medical problems, affecting in 3 to 5 percent of young children [18, 23, 30, 37, 38, 56, 58]. Their definition, management, and prognosis continue to be a source of disagreement among physicians. Management and outcome data differ dramatically depending on the definition used.

Four seizure types are currently termed febrile seizures by different investigators:

1. *Simple febrile seizures* are associated with a fever of 38°C or higher in a child between the ages of 3 months and 5 years who has been previously normal. The seizure lasts less than 15 minutes and has no focal component. The source of the fever lies outside the central nervous system [25, 26, 27, 47].
2. *Complex febrile seizures* are focal or prolonged. The previous neurologic state of the child is unspecified. The source of the fever is not neurologic in origin [10, 37].
3. *Febrile status epilepticus* is a continuous tonic-clonic seizure or a series of such seizures lasting more than 30 minutes during which there is no return to consciousness. The prior status of the child is not addressed. The source of fever lies outside the central nervous system [1, 2, 7, 24, 37, 40].
4. *Any seizure with fever* is one that occurs in the context of a febrile illness, regardless of its type, duration, or complexity or whether the child has had any prior neurologic abnormality or seizures. It includes symptomatic seizures associated with acute neurologic illness such as meningitis, lead poisoning, or infantile hemiplegia [37, 41, 42, 43, 44].

Etiology

GENETICS

Among the close relatives of patients with the first three types of febrile seizures, there is a higher than expected prevalence of epilepsy (10 to 40%) and of febrile seizures (8 to 18%) [18, 39]. Autosomal dominant inheritance appears to be the most common pattern, but there is evidence that autosomal recessive or polygenetic mechanisms may also be involved [18, 39].

AGE

One to 2 percent of the first three seizure types occur in patients under 6 months of age, and 1 to 6 percent occur in children more than 5 years of age [16, 24, 32, 58]. The great majority occur within the first 3 years [17, 31, 40]. In boys the rate of occurrence declines gradually during the first 4 years. In girls there is a marked drop in frequency after 2 years of age [40, 56].

SEX

Females appear to have an increased frequency of complex febrile seizures, febrile status epilepticus, and their sequelae [40, 56]. When all types of febrile seizures are considered together, however, they appear to be more common in males than in females. The male-female ratio of febrile seizures ranges from 1.4:1 to 4:1 [32, 40]. The more rapid rate of cerebral maturation and myelination in females may be the cause of the rapid decline in incidence of febrile seizures in girls after the age of 2 years [40, 56].

PREDISPOSING FACTORS

Some data suggest that children with previous neurologic impairment are more vulnerable to complex febrile seizures, febrile status epilepticus, and any seizure associated with a fever [60, 61, 62]. The same relationship is not found in simple febrile seizures [37].

Most febrile seizures are associated with tonsillitis, otitis, pharyngitis, and gastrointestinal disorders [24, 32, 40, 62]. Roseola and *Shigella* infections are associated with an increased number of seizures. The very high fevers generally seen with roseola probably account for this association with seizures, and it is believed that a *Shigella* endotoxin is responsible for the seizures seen in this disorder. Some infections of the central nervous system, such as meningitis, cause febrile seizures in children without any apparent genetic predisposition.

Pathophysiology

REGULATION OF BODY TEMPERATURE

Fever does not result from the inactivation or alteration of the normal mechanisms for controlling body temperature [28]; the regulatory mechanism continues to function but at a higher temperature. Control of body heat depends on the integrity of the anterior hypothalamus and the preoptic area (AH/POA) [46]. This region contains clusters of temperature-sensitive neurons.

There is evidence that exogenous pyrogens, bacterial products known to be lipopolysaccharides, interact with phagocytic leukocytes, causing them to

become activated [8]. This phase is followed by a period of mRNA and protein synthesis, from which endogenous pyrogen (EP) is released. EPs enter the bloodstream and are excreted into the cerebral ventricular system, exerting an effect on the hypothalamus that results in fever [9]. Additional evidence indicates that interaction between viruses and monocytes also results in the release of EPs (Fig. 27-1). EPs are regarded as mediator substances of all fevers regardless of their source. They comprise a variety of chemicals with the common ability to produce fever and are not thought to be normal products of thermal regulation.

There is a site in the AH/POA close to the wall of the third ventricle where microinjection of EP causes fever after a minimal latency period [8]. The central action of the leukocyte pyrogen is such that the thermoregulatory mechanism appears to work at a new high level but retains its usual sensitivity. The sensitivity of the central warm receptors in the hypothalamus is not altered.

ROLE OF NEUROTRANSMITTERS

In monkeys and rabbits a cholinergic mechanism has been shown to be important in both the production and lysis of fever [55]. Both nicotinic and muscarinic receptors are present in the hypothalamus. A hypothalamic nicotinic receptor is concerned with heat production, and muscarinic agents produce an initial thermal response followed by hypothermia.

Cholinergic and monoaminergic systems interact in the hypothalamus. Dopamine, 5-hydroxytryptamine (5-HT), norepinephrine, and epinephrine have important roles in regulating body temperature [55]. Norepinephrine injected into the cerebral ventricles of monkeys produces hyperthermia, whereas 5-HT causes the temperature to fall. In other studies, release of these substances in the AH/POA produces an opposite effect. It may be that the neurotransmitters influence both temperature-raising and temperature-lowering mechanisms depending on environmental circumstances.

The fever process is also mediated in part by release of a prostaglandin of the E series into the tissue of the brain [33]. Neurons in the area of the AH/POA are sensitive to this substance, and injections of minute amounts of prostaglandins into the ventricular system or the AH/POA cause fever. Prostaglandins do not appear to be involved in normal thermoregulation.

ROLE OF ANTIPYRETICS

There is no evidence that antipyretics administered in therapeutic doses exert any bactericidal or bacteriostatic effect that interferes with the synthesis of EPs, nor

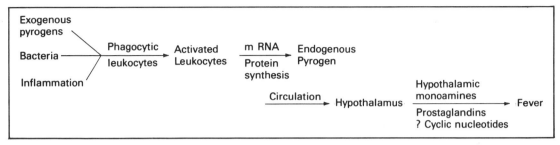

Figure 27-1. Pathogenesis of fever.

do these drugs affect the release of EPs from leukocytes [71]. Antipyretics do not appear to affect the end organs responsible for fever. Antipyretic drugs such as acetylsalicylic acid, 4-acetamidophenol, and indomethacin inhibit the enzyme system concerned with prostaglandin synthesis and consequently interfere with the action of EP on the thermoregulatory centers in the hypothalamus [33].

PRODUCTION OF SEIZURES
It is hypothesized that neurochemicals involved in the production of fever, acting on other parts of the brain, produce seizures. Experimental evidence for this hypothesis is currently lacking.

Seizure Phenomena

TYPES OF SEIZURE
Most seizures seen with a febrile illness are generalized; about 15 percent are focal. Approximately 80 percent of seizures are clonic, 14 percent are tonic, and 6 percent are atonic [32, 40].

DURATION OF SEIZURES
Most febrile seizures are brief, lasting less than 10 to 15 minutes [32]. Forty percent last less than 5 minutes, and 75 percent less than 30 minutes. Only 2 percent last 1 hour or more. Most episodes of febrile status epilepticus occur in infants less than 18 months of age, peaking at 12 to 13 months. This type of seizure is more common in girls [40].

Electroencephalographic Phenomena

At the time of any febrile seizure the electroencephalogram (EEG) is inevitably abnormal. Either fever or seizures alone cause slowing of the EEG. Marked slowing is usually seen after febrile seizures [23, 27]. Slowing may be asymmetric or focal in the absence of any focal component to the seizure [15]. Asymmetric slowing has little diagnostic or prognostic significance in the first 10 days after a febrile seizure. Only 1.4 percent of

patients with the first three types of febrile seizures have paroxysmal EEG activity on tracings performed soon after a seizure. One third remain abnormal (because of slowing) at 7 days. By 10 days the EEG has reverted to normal in patients with simple febrile seizures [26, 27]. Continued slowing on the EEG 10 days after the seizure may be of some help in delineating a simple febrile seizure from other types when the history is not clear or the seizure was not witnessed.

Evaluation of a First Febrile Seizure

CAUSE OF FEVER
It is of utmost importance to *determine the cause of the fever* [40]. An acute disorder of the central nervous system must be ruled out. Included in this category are bacterial and viral meningitis, encephalitis, Reye's syndrome, acute toxic encephalopathy, infantile hemiparesis, and dehydration with cortical venous thrombosis. Chronic diseases of the central nervous system may first become manifest with a febrile seizure. These disorders include lead poisoning, tuberous sclerosis, subdural hematoma, vascular malformations, neonatal hypoxia, and other developmental defects of the brain.

HISTORY
A history should be elicited that stresses the type and duration of the seizures, any antecedent history of infection or trauma, changes in alertness, exposure to toxins, and family history of seizures.

PHYSICAL EXAMINATION
A thorough physical examination should be carried out that specifically excludes signs of trauma, increased intracranial pressure, central nervous infection, and other neurologic disease. When appropriate, the fontanelle should be examined to determine whether it is soft and pulsatile. Fundi should be well seen, nuchal rigidity should be evaluated, and focal neurologic signs should be noted. A Woods lamp examination of the skin should be carried out to search for the congenitally present "ash-leaf spots" seen with tuberous

318

sclerosis [40]. Transillumination of the skull should be performed in young children. Auscultation of the skull for bruits is also necessary.

EXAMINATION OF CEREBROSPINAL FLUID
The cerebrospinal fluid should be examined in all children with a first febrile seizure and in all children under the age of 2 years who may be having a repeat febrile seizure. In children under 2 years of age with meningitis nuchal rigidity may be absent, and other clinical signs of meningitis may be absent. Older children with repeat febrile seizures should have a lumbar puncture when a central nervous system infection is suspected. In one study, 13 percent of 325 children with meningitis had seizures [48]. A third of these lacked meningeal signs, and 50 percent of those children had bacterial meningitis. Some children were over 2 years of age.

A pressure recording of the cerebrospinal fluid should be made. The fluid should be examined for the number and types of cells and for protein and glucose concentrations. Bacterial cultures should be obtained.

LABORATORY EVALUATIONS
Blood sugar and calcium determinations are often carried out. In addition, serum transaminases and ammonia should be determined if Reye's syndrome is suspected. Recent studies indicate that radiographs of the skull are inevitably normal in simple febrile seizures [21, 34]. Skull films and CT scans need not be ordered routinely. They are, however, indicated in the following situations: evidence of trauma or increased intracranial pressure, focal seizure, abnormal neurologic examination, persistent seizures despite antiepileptic drug therapy, and deteriorating clinical condition [21, 34].

Management

ACUTE TREATMENT OF FEBRILE SEIZURES

Reduction of Fever
Reduction of the patient's temperature with antipyretics and sponging is of primary importance [40, 65]. Acetaminophen (Tylenol) or aspirin may be given by mouth in a dose of 60 mg per year of age or 120 mg by rectum. Medication may be repeated every 4 hours for a temperature higher than 38°C. Vigorous sponging all over the child's body with tepid water for 10 to 15 minutes is a very effective means of reducing temperatures. Sponging should be interrupted after a 15-minute period for 15 minutes and resumed if the fever is still above 39°C.

Antiepileptic Drug Therapy
If the seizure has continued for more than 10 or 15 minutes, the child should be placed in a semiprone position to minimize the risk of aspiration. Intravenous antiepileptic medication is indicated [40, 45]. Phenobarbital in a loading dose of up to 10 to 15 mg/kg of body weight can be given slowly intravenously [47]. Oral phenobarbital in a dose of 3 to 6 mg/kg/24 hours may then be continued while the child remains febrile. Giving oral phenobarbital without an intravenous loading dose is useless because it takes days to achieve therapeutic blood levels by this route alone (see Chap. 14) [4, 23, 45, 53].

An alternative regimen consists of diazepam, 0.3 mg/kg intravenously at a rate of 1 mg/minute [40]. Both drugs are effective in stopping seizures. Phenobarbital has the added advantage of having an antipyretic action and can also be used as a maintenance therapeutic drug. Diazepam is not useful orally for treating these seizures, and its duration of action is brief (see Chap. 30). Recurrence of seizures may occur.

Diazepam and phenobarbital should not be given parenterally together because respiratory arrest may occur (see Chap. 30).

FEBRILE STATUS EPILEPTICUS
Status epilepticus is a continuous tonic-clonic seizure or series of seizures lasting more than 30 minutes without an intervening period of consciousness. It should be considered a medical emergency whether fever is present or absent. Mortality and risk of serious sequelae remain high (see Chap. 30). Adequate oxygenation must be maintained. Overmedication with resultant respiratory arrest must be avoided.

The usual therapy consists of administration of an intravenous loading dose of phenobarbital or a dose of intravenous diazepam (see above). If a single dose of diazepam is ineffective in stopping the seizure, the same dose may be repeated in 30 minutes [29, 40]. If seizures persist for more than 1 hour, paraldehyde, 1 ml per year of age up to a total dose of 10 ml, may be mixed with an equal amount of mineral oil and given rectally (see Chap. 22).

PROPHYLACTIC ANTIEPILEPTIC DRUG THERAPY

Intermittent versus Continuous Antiepileptic Drug Therapy
Excellent data now exist indicating that intermittent oral phenobarbital therapy given early in the febrile episode is useless for managing febrile seizures [45, 47, 67, 68, 70]. Unless an intravenous loading dose is given, steady state blood levels of phenobarbital are

not attained until 14 to 21 days after the initiation of oral therapy [4, 11, 12, 40, 45, 53]. Oral phenobarbital is therefore not helpful in the management of such seizures, many of which occur at the onset of the febrile illness as the temperature is rising. There is evidence that rectal diazepam preparations (not yet available in the United States) are absorbed rapidly enough to provide immediate protection from seizures induced by rising temperatures [47, 50, 57].

Continuous antiepileptic therapy is sometimes advised (see below). Phenytoin and carbamazepine have been shown to be ineffective in the management of such seizures [6, 31, 69]; when indicated, phenobarbital is the drug of choice [31, 47, 69]. Serum concentrations of 15 to 30 μg/ml must be maintained to ensure an adequate therapeutic effect [23, 24, 47, 69].

Complex Febrile Seizures, Febrile Status Epilepticus, and Seizures Occurring in the Context of an Acute Neurologic Illness

These types of seizures should be considered serious epileptic events, and every attempt should be made to prevent a recurrence. Such children should be placed on long-term phenobarbital therapy.

Simple Febrile Seizures

There is controversy about the advisability of treating simple febrile seizures with long-term antiepileptic therapy. Recent studies indicate that when continuous phenobarbital prophylaxis with serum concentrations of more than 15 μg/ml were maintained, recurrent febrile seizures were significantly decreased in febrile seizures of all types, including simple febrile seizures in previously normal children [47, 67, 68, 69, 70]. Recurrent complex febrile seizures did not occur in any children taking daily phenobarbital therapy but did occur in 4.4 percent of children receiving either intermittent phenobarbital, or none.

There is no evidence that prolonged therapy with antiepileptic drugs prevents the later development of chronic epilepsy or significant neurologic defects [36, 47].

Side effects and toxic reactions occur in 10 to 40 percent of infants and children receiving phenobarbital [37, 47, 69]. These reactions are usually of the following types: (1) behavioral changes (irritability, hyperactivity, somnolence); (2) prolonged nocturnal awakenings; (3) interference with higher cognitive or cortical functions (e.g., defects in short-term memory, decreased attention span, defects in general comprehension) [5, 20, 47, 51, 52, 69]. Other known or potential risks associated with chronic antiepileptic drug

administration in children include possible adverse effects on nervous system development [47, 54], allergic reactions [66], effects on vitamin D metabolism [66], drug interactions [66], and compliance failure [66].

Based on the prognosis of simple febrile seizures (see below) and the factors outlined in this section on management, a consensus on the management of simple febrile seizures evolved from a recent National Institutes of Health symposium [47]. Antiepileptic drug prophylaxis is unnecessary and probably undesirable in the majority of patients with simple febrile seizures. However, phenobarbital prophylaxis in therapeutic levels may be considered under any of the following conditions: (1) in the presence of abnormal neurologic development (e.g., cerebral palsy syndromes, mental retardation, microcephaly); (2) when a febrile seizure is (a) longer than 15 minutes or (b) focal, or (c) followed by transient or persistent neurologic abnormalities; and (3) when there is a history of nonfebrile seizures of genetic origin in a parent or sibling. The physician occasionally may elect, in certain selected cases, to provide antiepileptic treatment when a patient has multiple febrile seizures or when seizures occur in an infant under 12 months.

When antiepileptic prophylaxis is instituted, it is usually continued for at least 2 years or 1 year after the last seizure, whichever is the longer period of time. Discontinuation of therapy should be done slowly over a 1- to 2-month period.

Parents and others who are responsible for the care of young children play a key role in the prevention and management of febrile seizures. Family education and counseling should address (1) the relatively benign nature of febrile seizures, (2) the recognition of and management of fever, (3) the use of antipyretic agents, (4) medication and compliance, (5) side effects of medication, (6) first aid for a seizure, and (7) when and how to seek emergency assistance if needed.

Prognosis of Febrile Seizures

RECURRENT FEBRILE SEIZURES

Repeat febrile seizures of all types are common, occurring in 12 to 54 percent of patients [17, 18, 32, 38, 40, 47]. Children less than 13 months old at the time of the first seizure have a 2:1 chance of recurrence compared with a 1:5 risk when the first seizure occurs between 14 and 32 months [15]. Girls are more likely to have recurrent febrile seizures [23]. There is no difference in the recurrence rate between previously "normal" children and those with pre-, peri-, and postnatal abnormalities [68]. Only 1 percent of patients with febrile seizures experience prolonged seizures during a recurrence if the initial seizure was not prolonged.

Some data indicate that the risk of complex febrile seizures or status epilepticus increases with recurrent febrile seizures [24]. Both types are more common in children under 18 months of age. These data are difficult to interpret because the percentage of children known to be neurologically impaired prior to the first febrile seizure has not been given. Recent studies indicate that long-term phenobarbital prophylaxis is effective in preventing recurrent febrile seizures of all types [31, 47, 69].

RECURRENT AFEBRILE SEIZURES

The risk of the occurrence of nonfebrile seizures following one or more febrile seizures has been reported as between 1.4 and 5 percent [18, 19, 37]. This risk is two- to threefold higher than that expected in the general population [3, 18, 38]. The period of greatest risk for the development of epilepsy following febrile seizures is the first 3 years [26, 27, 37], but this increased risk continues at least until the third decade of life [3].

The Collaborative Perinatal Study of the NIH followed from birth to age 7 years a group of 1706 children who experienced one or more febrile seizures [37, 38]. Risk factors associated with the development of chronic epilepsy included a family history of afebrile seizures, a preexisting neurologic abnormality, and a complicated initial seizure. Among children with none of these risk factors, 1 percent developed epilepsy. Among patients with one risk factor, 2 percent developed epilepsy, and among those with two or more of these factors 10 percent developed epilepsy. In a similar cohort study performed by the Mayo Clinic, the risk of developing epilepsy after a febrile seizure was 2.5 percent in children without prior neurologic disorders or atypical or prolonged seizures, and 17 percent in those with such complications [3].

COMPLEX PARTIAL SEIZURES

Some investigators have reported that febrile seizures are a predisposing factor in the development of complex partial seizures [13, 14, 18, 30, 42, 43, 44, 56]. They postulate that hypoxic damage to neurons in the mesial temporal area results in mesial temporal sclerosis and subsequent epilepsy. These data are based primarily on children with febrile status epilepticus including children whose source of fever was acute neurologic illness [24]. There is no current evidence that other types of febrile seizures carry such an increased risk of complex partial seizures [47], and recent epidemiologic studies strongly indicate that they do not [15, 18, 22, 38].

LOWERED INTELLIGENCE

Some investigators have reported relatively high rates of mental retardation in children with febrile seizures [10, 37, 49, 51, 60, 61, 62]. However, inclusion in these studies of children with known neurologic impairment prior to the first febrile seizure and failure to define the types of febrile seizures studied have made it difficult to interpret these data.

Recent analysis of the relationship of febrile seizures not associated with acute neurologic illness to subsequent intellectual and academic performance demonstrated no difference in mean full scale IQ scores on the Wechsler Intelligence Scales for Children between children with febrile seizures and siblings who were seizure-free [10]. Children with prolonged seizures or with two or more febrile seizures did not differ from control siblings in later IQ at age 7 years. The status of the children before the first febrile seizure was significantly related to later IQ, but the occurrence, type, and duration of febrile seizures were not.

There is experimental evidence that repeated or prolonged febrile seizures in immature rats result in reduced brain weight and numbers of brain cells [63, 64]. Simple hyperthermic seizures in young rats have no effect on the acquisition of developmental reflexes but do interfere with maze-solving ability at a later age [35].

NEUROLOGIC ABNORMALITIES

Recent prospective cohort studies have not demonstrated long-term neurologic dysfunction in association with febrile seizures [18, 38].

MORTALITY

In the absence of preexisting neurologic disturbance, there does not appear to be significant mortality associated acutely with febrile seizures, and no long-term alteration in mortality has been demonstrated [18].

References

1. Aicardi, J., and Chevrie, J. J. Febrile Convulsions: Neurological Sequelae and Mental Retardation. In M. A. B. Brazier, and F. Coceani (Eds.), *Brain Dysfunction in Infantile Febrile Convulsions.* New York: Raven Press, 1976.
2. Aicardi, J., and Chevrie, J. J. Convulsive status epilepticus in infants and children. *Epilepsia* 11:87, 1970.

3. Annegers, J. F. et al. The risk of epilepsy following febrile convulsions. *Neurology* 29:297, 1979.

4. Buchthal, F., and Lennox-Buchthal, M. A. Phenobarbital: Relation of Serum Concentration to Control of Seizures. In D. M. Woodbury (Ed.), *Antiepileptic Drugs*. New York: Raven Press, 1972.

5. Camfield, C. S., and Camfield, P. R. Behavioral and Cognitive Effects of Phenobarbital in Toddlers. In K. B. Nelson, and J. H. Ellenberg (Eds.), *Febrile Seizures*. New York: Raven Press, 1981.

6. Camfield, P. R., Camfield, C. S., and Tibbles, J. Carbamazepine does not prevent febrile seizures in phenobarbital failures. *Neurology* (N.Y.) 32:288, 1982.

7. Chevrie, J.-J., and Aicardi, J. Duration and lateralization of febrile convulsions. Etiological factors. *Epilepsia* 16:781, 1975.

8. Cooper, K. E., Veale, W. L., and Pittman, Q. J. Pathogenesis of Fever. In M. A. B. Brazier, and F. Coceani (Eds.), *Brain Dysfunction in Infantile Febrile Convulsions*. New York: Raven Press, 1976.

9. Dinarello, C. A., and Wolf, S. M. Exogenous and Endogenous Pyrogens. In M. A. B. Brazier, and F. Coceani (Eds.), *Brain Dysfunction in Infantile Febrile Convulsions*. New York: Raven Press, 1976.

10. Ellenberg, J. H., and Nelson, K. B. Febrile seizures and later intellectual performance. *Arch. Neurol.* 35:17, 1978.

11. Faero, O. et al. Phenobarbital as prophylaxis for febrile convulsions. *Epilepsia* 12:109, 1971.

12. Faero, O. et al. Successful prophylaxis of febrile convulsions with phenobarbital. *Epilepsia* 13:279, 1972.

13. Falconer, M. A. Febrile convulsions in early childhood. *Br. Med. J.* 2:292, 1972.

14. Falconer, M. A., Serafetinides, E. A., and Corsellis, J. A. N. Etiology and pathogenesis of temporal lobe epilepsy. *Arch. Neurol.* 10:233, 1964.

15. Frantzen, E., Lennox-Buchthal, M., and Nygaard, A. Longitudinal EEG and clinical study of children with febrile convulsions. *Electroencephalogr. Clin. Neurophysiol.* 24:197, 1968.

16. Frantzen, E. et al. A genetic study of febrile convulsions. *Neurology* 20:909, 1970.

17. Friderichsen, C., and Melchior, J. Febrile convulsions in children, their frequency and prognosis. *Acta Paediat. Scand.* [Suppl.] 100:307, 1954.

18. Hauser, W. A. The Natural History of Febrile Seizures. In K. B. Nelson, and J. H. Ellenberg (Eds.), *Febrile Seizures*. New York: Raven Press, 1981.

19. Hauser, W. A. et al. Prognosis of patients with febrile convulsions in Rochester, Minnesota, 1945–1967. *Trans. Am. Neurol. Assoc.* 95:257, 1970.

20. Hirtz, D. G. Effects of Treatment for Prevention of Febrile Seizure Recurrence on Behavioral and Cognitive Function. In K. B. Nelson, and J. H. Ellenberg (Eds.), *Febrile Seizures*. New York: Raven Press, 1981.

21. Kudrjavcev, T. Skull X-rays and Lumbar Puncture in a Young Child Presenting With a Seizure and Fever. In K. B. Nelson, and J. H. Ellenberg (Eds.), *Febrile Seizures*. New York: Raven Press, 1981.

22. Lee, K., Diaz, M., and Melchior, J. C. Temporal lobe epilepsy: Not a consequence of childhood febrile convulsions in Denmark. *Acta Neurol. Scand.* 63:231, 1981.

23. Lennox-Buchthal, M. Febrile convulsions, a reappraisal. *Electroencephalogr. Clin. Neurophysiol.* [Suppl.] 32:138, 1973.

24. Lennox-Buchthal, M. A. A Summing Up: Clinical Session. In M. A. B. Brazier, and F. Coceani (Eds.), *Brain Dysfunction in Infantile Febrile Convulsions*. New York: Raven Press, 1976.

25. Livingston, S., Bridge, E. M., and Kajdi, L. Febrile convulsions: A clinical study with special reference to heredity and prognosis. *J. Pediatr.* 31:509, 1947.

26. Livingston, S. Infantile febrile convulsions. *Devel. Med. Child Neurol.* 10:374, 1968.

27. Livingston, S. Febrile Convulsions. In *Comprehensive Management of Epilepsy in Infancy, Childhood and Adolescence*. Springfield, Ill.: Thomas, 1972.

28. Lomax, P. Temperature Regulation: An Overall View. In M. A. B. Brazier, and F. Coceani (Eds.), *Brain Dysfunction in Infantile Febrile Convulsions*. New York: Raven Press, 1976.

29. Lombroso, C. Treatment of status epilepticus with diazepam. *Neurology* 16:629, 1966.

30. Margerison, J. H., and Corsellis, J. A. N. Epilepsy and the temporal lobes. *Brain* 89:499, 1966.

31. Melchior, J. C., Buchthal, F., and Lennox-Buchthal, M. The ineffectiveness of diphenylhydantoin in preventing febrile convulsions in the age of greatest risk, under three years. *Epilepsia* 12:55, 1971.

32. Millichap, J. G. *Febrile Convulsions*. New York: Macmillan, 1968.

33. Milton, A. S. Prostaglandins in Fever. In M. A. B. Brazier, and F. Coceani (Eds.), *Brain Dysfunction in Infantile Febrile Convulsions*. New York: Raven Press, 1976.

34. Nealis, J. G. T. et al. Routine skull roentgenograms in the management of simple febrile seizures. *J. Pediatr.* 90:595, 1977.

35. Nealis, J. G. T. et al. Neurologic sequelae of experimental febrile convulsions. *Neurology* 28:246, 1978.

36. Nelson, K. B. Can Treatment of Febrile Seizures Prevent Subsequent Epilepsy? In K. B. Nelson, and J. H. Ellenberg (Eds.), *Febrile Seizures.* New York: Raven Press, 1981.

37. Nelson, K. B., and Ellenberg, J. H. Predictors of epilepsy in children who have experienced febrile seizures. *N. Engl. J. Med.* 295:1029, 1976.

38. Nelson, K. B., and Ellenberg, J. H. Prognosis in children with febrile seizures. *Pediatrics* 61:721, 1978.

39. Newmark, M. E., and Penry, J. K. *Genetics of Epilepsy: A Review.* New York: Raven Press, 1980.

40. Ouellette, E. M. The child who convulses with fever. *Pediatr. Clin. North Am.* 21:467, 1974.

41. Ounsted, C. Genetic Messages and Convulsive Behavior in Pyrexia. In M. A. B. Brazier, and F. Coceani (Eds.), *Brain Dysfunction in Infantile Febrile Convulsions.* New York: Raven Press, 1976.

42. Ounsted, C., Lindsay, J., and Norman, R. *Biological Factors in Temporal Lobe Epilepsy.* London: Hinemann Co., 1966.

43. Ounsted, C. Temporal lobe epilepsy: The problem of aetiology and prophylaxis. *J. R. Coll. Physicians Lond.* 1:273, 1967.

44. Ounsted, C. Some Aspects of Seizure Disorders. In D. Hull, and D. Gairdner (Eds.), *Recent Advances in Pediatrics.* London: Churchill, 1970.

45. Porter, R. J. Pharmacokinetic Basis of Intermittent and Chronic Anticonvulsant Drug Therapy in Febrile Seizures. In K. B. Nelson, and J. H. Ellenberg (Eds.), *Febrile Seizures.* New York: Raven Press, 1981.

46. Preston, E., and Schönbaum, E. Monoaminergic Mechanisms in Thermoregulation. In M. A. B. Brazier, and F. Coceani (Eds.), *Brain Dysfunction in Infantile Febrile Convulsions.* New York: Raven Press, 1976.

47. Proceedings of the Consensus Development Conference on Febrile Seizures. *Epilepsia* 22:377, 1981.

48. Ratcliffe, J. C., and Wolf, S. M. Febrile convulsions caused by meningitis in young children. *Ann. Neurol.* 1:285, 1977.

49. Schiottz-Christensen, E., and Bruhn, P. Intelligence, behavior and scholastic achievement subsequent to febrile convulsions: An analysis of discordant twin pairs. *Devel. Med. Child Neurol.* 15:565, 1973.

50. Schmidt, D. Benzodiazepines: Diazepam. In D. M. Woodbury, J. K. Penry, and C. E. Pippenger (Eds.), *Antiepileptic Drugs.* New York: Raven Press, 1982.

51. Smith, J. A., and Walace, S. J. Febrile convulsions: Intellectual progress in relation to anticonvulsant therapy and recurrence of fits. *Arch. Dis. Child.* 57:104, 1982.

52. Stores, G. Behavioral Effects of Antiepileptic Drugs. In K. B. Nelson, and J. H. Ellenberg (Eds.), *Febrile Seizures.* New York: Raven Press, 1981.

53. Svensmark, O., and Buchthal, F. Diphenylhydantoin and phenobarbital serum levels in children. *Am. J. Dis. Childh.* 108:82, 1964.

54. Swaiman, K. F. In Vitro Studies of Antiepileptic Drug Safety. In K. B. Nelson, and J. H. Ellenberg (Eds.), *Febrile Seizures.* New York: Raven Press, 1981.

55. Tangri, K. K., Misra, N., and Bhargava, K. P. Central Cholinergic Mechanism of Pyrexia. In M. A. B. Brazier, and F. Coceani (Eds.), *Brain Dysfunction in Infantile Febrile Convulsions.* New York: Raven Press, 1976.

56. Taylor, D. C., and Ounsted, C. Biological mechanisms influencing the outcome of seizures in response to fever. *Epilepsia* 12:33, 1971.

57. Thorn, I. Prevention of Recurrent Febrile Seizures: Intermittent Prophylaxis With Diazepam Compared With Continuous Treatment With Phenobarbital. In K. B. Nelson, and J. H. Ellenberg (Eds.), *Febrile Seizures.* New York: Raven Prss, 1981.

58. Van den Berg, B. J., and Yerushalmy, J. Studies on convulsive disorders in young children. *Pediatr. Res.* 3:298, 1969.

59. Van den Berg, B. J., and Yerushalmy, J. Studies on convulsive disorders in young children. *J. Pediatr.* 79:1004, 1971.

60. Wallace, S. Aetiological aspects of febrile convulsions. *Arch. Dis. Childh.* 47:171, 1972.

61. Wallace, S. J. Neurological and Intellectual Deficits: Convulsions with Fever Viewed as Acute Indications of Life-Long Developmental Defects. In M. A. B. Brazier, and F. Coceani (Eds.), *Brain Dysfunction in Infantile Febrile Convulsions.* New York: Raven Press, 1976.

62. Wallace, S. J. Treatment of Convulsions with Fever. In M. A. B. Brazier, and F. Coceani (Eds.), *Brain Dysfunction in Infantile Febrile Convulsions.* New York: Raven Press, 1976.

63. Wasterlain, C. G., and Plum, F. Retardation of behavioral landmarks after neonatal seizures in rats. *Trans. Am. Neurol. Assoc.* 98:320, 1973.

64. Wasterlain, C. G., and Plum, F. Vulnerability of developing rat brain to electroconvulsive seizures. *Arch. Neurol.* 29:38, 1973.

65. Wilson, J. T. Antipyretic Management of Febrile Seizures. In K. B. Nelson, and J. H. Ellenberg (Eds.), *Febrile Seizures.* New York: Raven Press, 1981.

66. Wilson, J. T. Observed and Potential Risks of Anti-convulsant Medications in Children. In K. B. Nelson, and J. H. Ellenberg (Eds.), *Febrile Seizures.* New York: Raven Press, 1981.

67. Wolf, S. M. Effectiveness of daily phenobarbital in the prevention of febrile seizure recurrences in "simple" febrile convulsions and "epilepsy triggered by fever." *Epilepsia* 18:95, 1977.

68. Wolf, S. M. The effectiveness of phenobarbital in the prevention of recurrent febrile convulsions in children with and without a history of pre-, peri-, and postnatal abnormalities. *Acta Paediatr. Scand.* 66:585, 1977.

69. Wolf, S. M. Prevention of Recurrent Febrile Seizures With Continuous Drug Therapy: Efficacy and Problems of Phenobarbital or Phenytoin Therapy. In K. B. Nelson, and J. H. Ellenberg (Eds.), *Febrile Seizures.* New York: Raven Press, 1981.

70. Wolf, S. M. et al. The value of phenobarbital in the child who has had a single febrile seizure: A controlled prospective study. *Pediatrics* 59:378, 1977.

71. Ziel, R., and Krupp, P. Mechanisms of Action of Antipyretic Drugs. In M. A. B. Brazier, and F. Coceani (Eds.), *Brain Dysfunction in Infantile Febrile Convulsions.* New York: Raven Press, 1976.

SEIZURES ASSOCIATED WITH ALCOHOL USE AND ALCOHOL WITHDRAWAL

Richard H. Mattson

It has been recognized since ancient times that the abuse of alcohol may be accompanied by seizures [16]. The Romans called this problem "morbus convivialis" [9]. Only in the past few decades has it been demonstrated that most of these seizures are the result of withdrawal from alcohol. Victor and Adams [19] emphasized that the complications associated with alcoholism (including delirium tremens, tremulousness, and seizures) were observed at the time of cessation or decrease in alcohol consumption. These clinical observations were confirmed in important studies by Isbell et al. [7] 20 years ago. They carefully evaluated 10 volunteer patients who consumed large quantities of ethyl alcohol daily for up to 3 months. Tremulousness, seizures, and delirium occurred when alcohol intake decreased or stopped. In 1967, Victor and Brausch [20] reported studies of alcoholic patients presenting with seizures and defined the characteristics of a large group who had so-called "rum-fits" or "alcoholic epilepsy." Recognition of the fact that these seizures were due to a withdrawal phenomenon allowed the appropriate treatment by replacement of alcohol with a cross-tolerant drug such as paraldehyde or a benzodiazepine.

Differential Diagnosis

Although seizures secondary to withdrawal from alcohol constitute the major reason for such attacks in the alcoholic patient, there are many other possible causes for seizures in patients using alcohol. These require specific diagnosis and, at times, quite different treatment (Table 28-1). At the time of initial evaluation, it is often not possible to determine whether the seizures are caused entirely by alcohol withdrawal, by some acute metabolic disturbance in association with alcoholism, by alcoholism associated with a chronic seizure disorder, or by epilepsy aggravated by alcohol intake. Management of the acute problem requires identification of the basic cause of the seizures so that specific therapy can be instituted. Although withdrawal is the most common explanation for seizures occurring in the alcoholic, the patient is susceptible to many other disturbances of brain function that also produce seizures.

Table 28-1. Causes of Seizures Associated With Alcohol Use

Seizure Category	Onset (age)	Seizure Occurrence During Time of			Interictal EEG	Photic Sensitivity	Treatment
		Acute Intoxication	First 48 hr of Withdrawal	Prolonged Abstinence			
Acute seizures (electrolyte, disturbance, hypoglycemia, meningitis)	Any age	Yes	Yes	No	Abnormal (slow)	Absent	Specific correction
Withdrawal seizures ("rum-fits," alcoholic epilepsy)	30+ (90%)	No	Yes	No	90% normal	50% photomyoclonic (photomyogenic) or photoconvulsive	Diazepam or paraldehyde and abstinence
Epilepsy Following alcoholism				Yes	Usually abnormal (epileptiform patterns or slowing)	50% photomyoclonic (photomyogenic) or photoconvulsive	Diazepam or paraldehyde plus maintenance antiepileptic drugs and abstinence
Preexisting alcoholism	Any age	Infrequently	Yes				
Nonalcoholic epilepsy	Any age	Infrequently	Yes	Yes	70% abnormal (epileptiform patterns)	5–10% photoconvulsive	Antiepileptic drugs and alcohol moderation
Latent epilepsy	Any age	No	Yes	No	Often normal*	5–10% photoconvulsive	Alcohol moderation or abstinence

Alcoholic Seizures (Acute seizures, Withdrawal seizures, Epilepsy)

Epileptic Seizures (Nonalcoholic epilepsy, Latent epilepsy)

*Epileptiform EEG abnormality precipitated by ETOH and sleep deprivation.

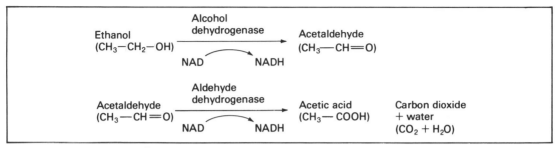

Figure 28-1. The metabolism of alcohol.

ACUTE BRAIN DISORDERS

The chronic alcoholic patient is particularly suscepti-ble to a variety of disturbances of brain function that may lead to seizures. Head trauma, with or without subdural hematoma, must always be considered. A his-tory of headache or injury, as well as the finding of a neurologic deficit, requires further diagnostic tests such as lumbar puncture, CT scan, or contrast radio-logic studies. Alcoholic patients are generally sus-ceptible to infections and may develop meningitis. Typical signs and symptoms include fever, stiff neck, headache, and abnormal cerebral spinal fluid examina-tion. Disturbances of renal or hepatic function are common and must be considered in the differential diagnosis. Electrolyte imbalance may accompany the long-term abuse of alcohol, and both hyponatremia and hypomagnesemia are conditions that predispose the patient to seizures [22]. The appropriate blood tests should readily identify most of these problems and allow specific correction. Hypoglycemia is an in-frequent but readily treatable disorder accompanying chronic alcoholism. The metabolism of alcohol re-quires and may deplete NAD, an enzyme essential for gluconeogenesis (Fig. 28-1). A period of fasting in an alcoholic patient may deplete glycogen stores and allow no alternative pathway for the production of glu-cose. The resultant hypoglycemia can cause seizures and other neurologic deficits, producing a serious and even life-threatening situation [1]. The treatment of these electrolyte and glucose problems can be readily accomplished with the parenteral infusion of elec-trolyte solutions with glucose supplementation even before laboratory reports are available. Intravenous thiamine (50 to 100 mg) should be given before ad-ministering intravenous glucose; otherwise such a glucose infusion might precipitate Wernicke's en-cephalopathy in nutritionally deficient patients by depleting the body's low stores of thiamine [3].

ALCOHOLIC PATIENTS WITH EPILEPSY

Two groups of alcoholic patients may be susceptible to chronic epilepsy in addition to the seizures associated with the acute problems previously mentioned. These two groups are alcoholics with acquired epilepsy and patients with epilepsy who become alcoholics. Epi-lepsy in alcoholics may result from brain disease secondary to head trauma, prior infection, or other causes of adult onset epilepsy that may affect the gen-eral population (e.g., tumors, vascular lesions, or de-generative disorders, among others). These patients have a history of seizures occurring not only at the time of drinking or, more specifically, at the time of with-drawal, but also during periods of prolonged absti-nence. Clues to the presence of associated epilepsy in these patients are an abnormal electroencephalogram (EEG) and focal onset of the seizures. These patients require not only treatment of the withdrawal state but also continued administration of antiepileptic drugs to prevent attacks that may occur over a long period of time regardless of alcohol use.

PATIENTS WITH EPILEPSY WHO BECOME ALCOHOLIC

Patients with long-standing epilepsy may develop alcoholism, although Lennox [9] found that the fre-quency of alcoholism in patients with epilepsy was less than that in the general population. In such patients seizures occur at times independent of alcohol intake but may be accentuated by withdrawal after chronic intake. Both the alcoholic who has developed epilepsy and the patient with epilepsy who has become alco-holic are doubly susceptible to seizures because their alcoholism is often accompanied by poor intake of meals, sleep deprivation, and noncompliance with antiepileptic drug treatment [11]. These patients will usually require treatment of the acute causes of sei-zures, correction of withdrawal effects, and adminis-tration of loading and maintenance doses of usual antiepileptic drugs.

Alcohol-Precipitated Seizures in Patients with Epilepsy

Seizures may also accompany the excessive use of alcohol in the nonalcoholic patient with epilepsy upon occasions of excessive drinking [10]. In studies of 122 nonalcoholic patients with epilepsy we found that one to two drinks had little if any effect on seizures, but 85 percent of patients experienced an exacerbation of seizures when their consumption was moderate to heavy (five to six drinks). Alcohol intake itself does not trigger seizures. In fact, we have found that the immediate effect of alcohol ingestion is suppression of epileptiform EEG activity [10]. However, there is a rebound phenomenon of increased seizure frequency during the period of rapidly falling alcohol blood levels ("morning after effect") [10], which apparently can activate seizures. The occurrence of attacks in these patients is usually self-limited and is best treated by reinstituting their normal antiepileptic drug program coupled with counseling about abstinence or at least moderation in alcohol intake in the future.

LATENT EPILEPSY

A small group of nonalcoholic, nonepileptic patients may experience seizures only on occasions of excessive intake of alcohol and rarely or never at other times. It seems likely that these persons have latent epilepsy that is unmasked by the precipitating factor of excessive alcohol intake and the secondary lowering of seizure threshold as the alcohol disappears from the blood. Giove and Gastaut [5] have termed this phenomenon "activation par la fete" ("activation by celebration"). Quite possibly, such patients need only to avoid excessive alcohol use, and long-term antiepileptic drug therapy may not be necessary.

Withdrawal Seizures

DIAGNOSIS

Seizures associated with heavy use of alcohol are most frequently caused by withdrawal from alcohol [20]. These patients have also been termed "rum-fitters" or "alcoholic epileptics." Seizures that occur in this setting are similar to those that follow chronic use of many sedative addictive drugs such as barbiturates, glutethamide, or other sedatives, and are caused by an increase in cerebral excitability following withdrawal. A number of characteristics have been identified that help to make the diagnosis of alcohol withdrawal seizures. These patients are usually chronic alcoholics, 30 years of age or older. Ninety percent of alcohol withdrawal seizures occur 7 to 48 hours after cessation of drinking, and 50 percent occur 13 to 24 hours after drinking has ceased [20]. Because alcohol withdrawal seizures usually occur relatively soon after cessation of drinking, some alcohol is often still present in the plasma at the time of the seizure, and the patient may have the odor of alcohol on his breath when brought to the hospital. Clinical examination frequently reveals tremulousness and some myoclonic jerks of the ex-

tremities. When seizures occur, they are typically generalized in onset and tonic-clonic or clonic-tonic-clonic in type. Seizures may be single (40%) or multiple (usually two to four seizures) [20]. The time between the first and last seizure is usually less than 6 hours but can be up to 6 days [7, 20]. A small number of these patients (3%) develop status epilepticus [20].

The EEG can be helpful in identifying the patient whose seizures are due to alcohol withdrawal. The interictal EEG recording is normal in 90 percent of these patients and is often characterized by low-voltage fast activity. On the other hand, photic stimulation elicits evidence of abnormal excitability in approximately 50 percent of patients withdrawing from alcohol, regardless of whether or not they have alcohol withdrawal seizures [20]. This heightened excitability to photic stimulation is present for 12 to 130 hours after cessation of drinking [20] and may take the form of either photoconvulsive (Fig. 28-2) or photomyoclonic (photomyogenic) activity (Fig. 28-3). The photoconvulsive response represents spike-and-wave discharge arising from cerebral cortical areas, whereas photomyoclonic activity is a muscle response (see Chap. 11). Although the electrographic potentials are produced by different physiologic mechanisms, both responses are evidence of increased cerebral excitability and are valuable signs of the presence of withdrawal phenomena. The recognition of such abnormal photic sensitivity may be a useful clue to the identification of unrecognized alcohol abusers such as executives or housewives who drink excessively but surreptitiously.

TREATMENT

As described earlier, the patient requires treatment of medical problems including careful management of fluid and electrolyte balance. Specific treatment of seizures is also indicated.

It can be argued that no treatment is needed following a withdrawal seizure because such seizures are often single (40%) in occurrence, and the period of susceptibility is relatively brief [20]. However, subsequent seizures can be expected in 60 percent of these patients. During the seizure the patient is susceptible to many complications including tongue laceration, trauma from falling, compression fracture, or aspiration. The treatment of withdrawal seizures also helps to prevent subsequent delirium tremens, which may develop in one third of patients [20]. For these reasons, drug therapy is recommended even following a single withdrawal seizure.

Specific Seizure Treatment

Treatment of alcohol withdrawal seizures is best accomplished by replacing the substance to which the

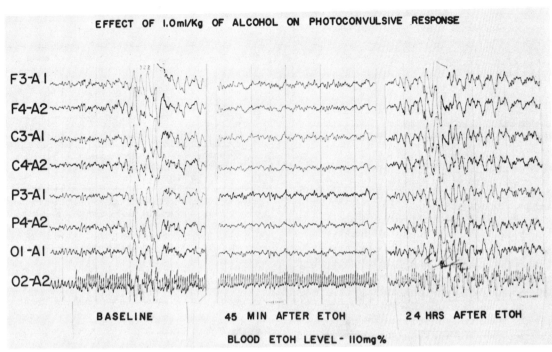

Figure 28-2. Spike-wave (photoconvulsive) discharge is seen in a patient withdrawing from alcohol. The photoconvulsive response is abolished with intake of alcohol.

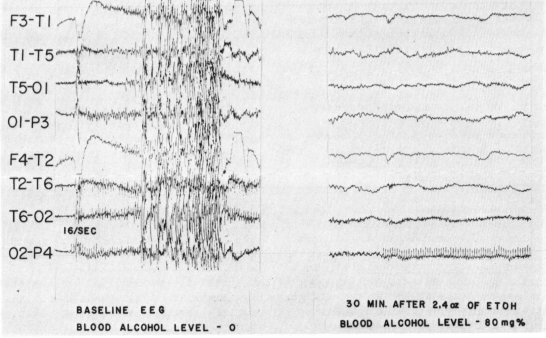

Figure 28-3. The left side of the figure shows a characteristic photomyoclonic (photomyogenic) response to photic stimulation in a patient withdrawing from alcohol. Prompt reversal of this excitability follows intake of alcohol. A similar effect occurs after administration of paraldehyde or diazepam.

330

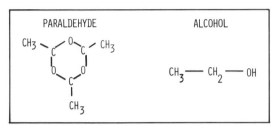

Figure 28-4. Structural formulas of paraldehyde and ethyl alcohol.

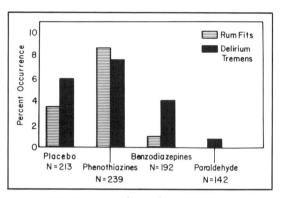

Figure 28-5. Frequency of rum fits and delirium tremens among patients in early alcohol withdrawal treated with placebo, phenothiazines, benzodiazepines, or paraldehyde (in some cases, paraldehyde with chloral hydrate). (From W. L. Thompson [18]. Copyright 1978, American Medical Association.)

patient has become addicted with a drug having cross-tolerance. Because the period of increased cerebral excitability usually lasts only a few days and because the period of seizure occurrence is often present for only a few hours, drug therapy can be tapered and discontinued after a period of a few days to a week. A large number of drugs, some of which have cross-tolerance with alcohol, have been used, and many have been reported to be efficacious in treatment of withdrawal seizures. These drugs include alcohol, paraldehyde, diazepam and other benzodiazepines, magnesium sulfate, phenytoin, barbiturates, valproic acid, and phenothiazines.

ALCOHOL. Replacement with alcohol itself can promptly reverse the increased cerebral excitability (Figs. 28-2 and 28-3). Such treatment has distinct disadvantages. Alcohol therapy perpetuates metabolic problems such as hypoglycemia and may be difficult to administer if associated medical problems, such as gastritis and pancreatitis, prevent oral intake. Additionally, the effect of alcohol is transient, and the therapeutic dose is quite close to the amount that produces undesirable toxic and sedative effects. Because the eventual goal of treatment in this group of patients is reduction of alcohol intake and ultimately long-term abstinence, there is a reluctance to continue administration of alcohol even for temporary therapy.

PARALDEHYDE. Paraldehyde is a cyclic trimer of acetaldehyde and is chemically related to alcohol (Fig. 28-4). In patients able to take the medication by mouth, paraldehyde not only corrects the withdrawal symptoms but produces independent antiepileptic effects. Thompson [18] has summarized a number of clinical studies that have demonstrated the efficacy of paraldehyde in management of "rum-fits" as well as delirium tremens (Fig. 28-5). We have found that paraldehyde reverses EEG photic sensitivity as promptly as alcohol intake. The usual dose of paraldehyde is 5 to 15 ml in fruit juice every 2 to 4 hours. The quantity required to produce modest sedation and symptomatic relief will vary.

Although paraldehyde is very effective in treating alcohol withdrawal seizures, a number of side effects may occur (see Chap. 22). (1) Intravenous paraldehyde can cause pulmonary edema, pulmonary hemorrhage, and circulatory or respiratory collapse. (2) Intramuscular paraldehyde is very painful; it can cause tissue necrosis and damage to nerves (e.g., the sciatic nerve) near the injection site. (3) Oral or rectal paraldehyde can cause corrosion of local mucosa. (4) Paraldehyde by any route has a disagreeable odor and taste and may cause a rash or toxic hepatitis. Despite these limitations, paraldehyde is still considered by many to be the drug of choice.

DIAZEPAM. Intravenous administration of 5 to 10 mg of diazepam promptly terminates acute withdrawal seizures and eliminates evidence of EEG photic sensitivity. It is both effective and safe when given slowly (not more than 5 mg/minute). Diazepam has a short duration of action and requires repeated doses every 15 minutes to several hours. This short duration of action is due to a rapid fall in plasma diazepam concentration as the drug is distributed to other tissues following intravenous administration (see Chap. 30). Because the period of increased excitability in patients with alcohol withdrawal seizures often lasts for only a day, this short duration of action and the development of tolerance is a less serious problem than it is in treating repeated seizures associated with chronic epilepsy. Diazepam must be given intravenously to produce its considerable efficacy. As a result, patients are susceptible to the infrequent complications of hypotension and respiratory depression if the medication is given too rapidly, especially when other sedatives or antiepileptic drugs have also been used.

OTHER BENZODIAZEPINES. Chlordiazepoxide has been demonstrated to be highly effective in treating the alcohol withdrawal state [8] but has no clear advantage over diazepam, which is the more potent of the two benzodiazepines and is more easily used parenterally. Recent reports suggest that parenteral lorazepam, another benzodiazepine, is useful in treating status epilepticus [21]. Lorazepam may prove to be superior to diazepam for a prolonged period of treatment because it has a much smaller decrease in plasma drug concentration during distribution after an intravenous injection (see Chap. 21).

MAGNESIUM SULFATE. Chronic alcoholics may have low serum and CSF magnesium levels, particularly at the time of abstinence. Wolfe and Victor [22] have shown that this fall in magnesium levels, as well as an accompanying respiratory alkalosis, correlates closely with withdrawal seizures and with EEG photic sensitivity. They found that intravenous administration of 2 to 5 g of magnesium sulfate reversed both seizures and photic sensitivity in many patients. Further reports confirming the efficacy of this form of treatment have not appeared. We have found the response to paraldehyde or diazepam to be much quicker and more dependable.

BARBITURATES. Barbiturates such as phenobarbital or amobarbital show cross-tolerance to alcohol and can also be effective in the treatment of withdrawal seizures. Barbiturates are suboptional drugs for acute therapy because they are often associated with sedation, making the recognition of concurrent complicating neurologic disease more difficult to evaluate.

VALPROIC ACID. Valproic acid has shown some promise of being effective in the prevention and treatment of withdrawal seizures [6]. In an animal model of alcohol withdrawal seizures, brain gamma-aminobutyric acid (GABA) levels fell at the time of alcohol withdrawal [15]. The administration of valproic acid prevented this fall in GABA levels, and withdrawal seizures did not occur. Limited experience in humans shows promise of usefulness in patients able to take the medication by mouth [2], but the risk of valproic acid hepatotoxicity may limit its usefulness.

PHENYTOIN. Phenytoin alone or together with paraldehyde or diazepam has been recommended by a number of authors for the treatment of alcohol withdrawal seizures [12, 13]; the dosage recommended is 100 mg tid. However, it is difficult to expect that such treatment would achieve therapeutic concentrations in the blood until long after the period of increased brain excitability associated with alcohol withdrawal seizures has passed, because steady state phenytoin plasma concentrations usually are not reached for at least 7 to 8 days after beginning chronic oral administration (see Chaps. 14 and 16). Furthermore, experimental animal studies indicate that phenytoin is an inferior agent for preventing withdrawal seizures [4] or photic-sensitive seizures [14].

The addition of phenytoin may be useful for some patients with withdrawal seizures if there is evidence that the patient also has a chronic seizure disorder. In such cases, however, a loading dose of 13 to 18 mg/kg must be given intravenously to obtain prompt therapeutic plasma concentrations of phenytoin (see Chaps. 16 and 30). It should be realized that administering a loading dose of phenytoin does not eliminate the need for more appropriate medications for management of the withdrawal seizures (e.g., diazepam or paraldehyde).

PHENOTHIAZINES. Phenothiazines may be effective in controlling hallucinations during alcohol withdrawal but have no place in the treatment of alcohol withdrawal seizures. The rates of occurrence of alcohol withdrawal seizures and of later development of delirium tremens are much higher with phenothiazine therapy than with benzodiazepine or paraldehyde therapy [17, 18]. This is to be expected because phenothiazines have no antiepileptic properties and indeed lower seizure threshold in animal models of epilepsy (see Chap. 12).

References

1. Arky, R. A. The effect of alcohol on carbohydrate metabolism: Carbohydrate metabolism in alcoholics. *The Biology of Alcoholism*. Vol. 1, *Biochemistry*. New York: Plenum, 1971.
2. Bastie, Y. Suppression des crises d'epilepsie du sevrage par la depakine dans les cures de desintoxication ethylique. *Ann. Med. Psychol.* (Paris) 128:400, 1970.
3. Drenick, E. J., Joven, G. B., and Swenseid, M. E. Occurrence of acute Wernicke's encephalopathy during prolonged starvation for the treatment of obesity. *N. Engl. J. Med.* 274:937, 1966.
4. Essig, C. F., and Carter, W. W. Failure of diphenylhydantoin in preventing barbiturate withdrawal seizures in the dog. *Neurology* (Minneap.) 12:481, 1962.
5. Giove, G. G., and Gastaut, H. Epilepsia alcoolique et d'enclinchement alcoolique des crises ches les epileptiques. *Revue Neurol.* 113:347, 1965.
6. Hillbom, M. E. The prevention of ethanol withdrawal seizures in rats by dipropylacetate. *Neuropharmacol.* 14:755, 1975.

332

7. Isbell, H. et al. An experimental study of the etiology of "rum fits" and delirium tremens. *Q. J. Study Alcohol* 16:1, 1967.

8. Kaim, S. C., Klett, C. J., and Rothfeld, B. Treatment of the acute alcohol withdrawal state: A comparison of four drugs. *Am. J. Psychiatr.* 125:1640, 1969.

9. Lennox, G. Alcohol and epilepsy. *Q. J. Study Alcohol* 2:1, 1941.

10. Mattson, R. H. et al. Effect of alcohol intake in nonalcoholic epileptics. *Neurology* (Minneap.) 25:361, 1975.

11. Rodin, E. A. et al. Effects of acute alcohol intoxication on epileptic patients. *Arch. Neurol.* 4:102, 1961.

12. Sampliner, R., and Iber, F. L. Diphenylhydantoin control of alcohol withdrawal seizures: Results of a controlled study. *J.A.M.A.* 230:1430, 1974.

13. Sellers, E. M., and Kalant, H. Medical intelligence: Drug therapy: Alcohol intoxication and withdrawal. *N. Engl. J. Med.* 294:757, 1976.

14. Stark, L. G., Killam, K. F., and Killam, E. K. The anticonvulsant effects of phenobarbital, diphenylhydantoin, and two benzodiazepines in the baboon, *Papio papio. J. Pharmacol. Exp. Ther.* 173:125, 1970.

15. Sytinsky, I. A. et al. The gamma aminobutyric acid (GABA) system in brain during acute and chronic ethanol intoxication. *J. Neurochem.* 25:43, 1975.

16. Temkin, O. *The Falling Sickness* (2nd ed.). Baltimore: Johns Hopkins Press, 1971.

17. Thomas, D. W., and Freedman, D. X. Treatment of the alcohol withdrawal syndrome: Comparison of promazine and paraldehyde. *J.A.M.A.* 188:316, 1964.

18. Thompson, W. L. Management of alcohol withdrawal syndromes. *Arch. Intern. Med.* 138:278, 1978.

19. Victor, M., and Adams, R. D. The effect of alcohol on the nervous system. *Res. Nerv. Ment. Dis.* 34:526, 1953.

20. Victor, M., and Brausch, J. The role of abstinence in the genesis of alcoholic epilepsy. *Epilepsia* 8:1, 1967.

21. Waltrezny, A., and Dargent, J. Preliminary study of parenteral lorazepam in status epilepticus. *Acta Neurol. Belgica* 75:219, 1975.

22. Wolfe, S. M., and Victor, M. *The Relationship of Hypomagnesemia and Alkalosis to Alcohol Withdrawal Symptoms.* New York: New York Academy of Science, 1955.

EPILEPSY, SEXUAL FUNCTION, AND PREGNANCY

29

Thomas R. Browne

Sexual Function

SEX HORMONES

There is considerable animal evidence that estrogen lowers the seizure threshold (i.e., is epileptogenic) and that progesterone raises the seizure threshold (i.e., is antiepileptic) [10, 20, 40, 47, 58, 65]. Several human studies in women have demonstrated an increase in clinical seizure frequency and in paroxysmal activity on the electroencephalogram (EEG) at times of high estrogen levels (prior to and during menses, midcycle, and during anovulatory cycles) and a decrease in seizure frequency and paroxysmal EEG activity at times of high progesterone activity (midluteal phase and during ovulatory cycles) [4, 11, 16, 34, 37, 47, 58]. Clinical trials of progesterone have resulted in decreased seizure frequency in some women with uncontrolled seizures [16, 22, 38, 47].

There is evidence that antiepileptic drugs may alter the metabolism and protein binding of sex hormones and vice versa [47]. The hydroxylation of steroids is enhanced by antiepileptic drugs [55, 67]. For example, phenobarbital increases the conversion of testosterone to polar metabolites [55]. There is also evidence that antiepileptic drug therapy increases sex hormone–binding globulin, leading to decreased amounts of free testosterone [66]. These observations may partly explain the effects of antiepileptic drugs on ovulation, oral contraceptives, and libido (see below).

Herzog et al. [25] investigated the response of 7 patients with complex partial seizures to an intravenous infusion of luteinizing-hormone-releasing hormone. All 4 men had decreased luteinizing hormone response curves, while the 3 women showed a range of responses that extended well above and below the normal range. These findings suggest that hypothalamic-pituitary control of gonadotropin may be altered in patients with complex partial seizures.

MENSTRUATION AND CATAMENIAL EPILEPSY

Several reports indicate that clinical seizures and paroxysmal EEG activity tend to be more frequent just prior to and during menstruation and at ovulation and

This work was supported in part by the Veterans Administration.

less frequent during the midluteal phase [4, 11, 16, 20, 34, 37, 40, 47, 58]. Premenstrual exacerbation of seizures occurs in 50 to 80 percent of women with epilepsy [34, 39, 47]. The most likely mechanism behind these observations is cyclic changes in the epileptogenic hormone estrogen or in the antiepileptic hormone progesterone. Other postulated mechanisms include cyclic fluid changes, changes in antiepileptic drug levels, and stress [47].

Catamenial epilepsy sometimes responds to the administration of acetazolamide 250 or 500 mg daily beginning 5 to 7 days before the expected onset of menses and continuing until cessation of bleeding [16, 47, 51].

MENARCHE AND MENOPAUSE

Menarche appears to have little specific effect on absence or myoclonic seizures [47]. Tonic-clonic and complex partial seizures occasionally begin at menarche, especially in women with catamenial epilepsy [47]. Little is known about the effects of menopause on seizure frequency except that early attempts to control seizures in women by castrating them were unsuccessful [47].

OVULATION

Women with epilepsy who are taking antiepileptic drugs have a larger number of anovulatory cycles (31 percent vs. 5 percent for controls) [36], possibly caused by altered metabolism or protein binding of sex hormones due to antiepileptic drugs (see above).

ORAL CONTRACEPTIVE PILLS

A higher than expected incidence of failure of oral contraceptive pills has been found in women receiving antiepileptic drugs, probably as a result of increased metabolism of contraceptive hormones [17, 60]. The progesterone effect of some oral contraceptive pills may decrease the frequency of catamenial seizures [22, 38, 60]. In other patients, oral contraceptives may exacerbate seizures or provoke a first seizure, possibly because of an estrogenic effect [16, 60].

LIBIDO AND IMPOTENCE

Decreased libido or impotence is a frequent complaint of patients with epilepsy, especially males. In a large prospective study of adult males receiving antiepileptic drugs for the first time, over 15 percent of the patients complained of decreased libido and/or impotence (partial or complete) [36]. This effect is probably partially due to depression, underlying brain disease, associated medical problems (e.g., diabetes), and concomitant medications. There is also evidence

that hyposexuality may be a feature of the "temporal lobe personality" (see Chap. 5). However, it is the anecdotal experience of many neurologists that antiepileptic drugs (especially barbiturates) have a specific, dose-dependent depressant effect on libido and potency. This effect may be related to the ability of antiepileptic drugs to increase the metabolism and binding of testosterone (see above).

SEXUAL SENSATIONS, AFFECT, AND AUTOMATISMS DURING SEIZURES

These topics are discussed in Chapter 5.

Pregnancy

Epilepsy is the most common serious neurologic problem encountered by the obstetrician [16]. It involves 0.3 to 0.5 percent of all pregnancies [27, 46].

EFFECT OF PREGNANCY ON SEIZURE FREQUENCY

Most evidence indicates that pregnancy *per se* has relatively little influence on seizure frequency [52, 59]. Seizure frequency increases in about 25 percent of pregnant women with known seizures, decreases in 25 percent, and remains unchanged in 50 percent [52, 59]. Altered disposition of antiepileptic drugs (see below) and noncompliance seem to be the major reasons for increased seizure frequency in pregnancy, although hormonal, metabolic, respiratory, and psychologic factors may also play a role [52, 59]. There are no reliable data that allow the physician to predict the course of epilepsy during pregnancy in a given individual. There is some evidence that increased seizure frequency during pregnancy may be more likely in patients with frequent seizures, a history of catamenial seizures, or excessive weight gain during pregnancy [16, 33, 47, 65]. Status epilepticus is no more frequent during pregnancy but presents a life-threatening emergency for mother and child when it occurs [59].

EFFECT OF PREGNANCY ON ANTIEPILEPTIC DRUGS

Plasma concentrations of phenytoin, phenobarbital, primidone, carbamazepine, and chlorazepate tend to fall during pregnancy in patients taking unaltered maintenance drug dosages [9, 31, 35, 43, 44, 50, 52, 53, 54, 57]. There is evidence that decreased intestinal absorption is partly responsible for the drop in plasma concentration of phenytoin, phenobarbital, and carbamazepine and that increased metabolism is partly responsible for the drop in plasma concentration of carbamazepine and chlorazepate [50, 53]. Altered renal function, volume of distribution, and protein binding and concomitant folate and iron therapy appear to be of minor importance [50].

TERATOGENICITY OF EPILEPSY

The malformations associated with epilepsy *per se* and with antiepileptic drugs are similar—heart anomalies and facial clefts. The incidence of such malformations is higher in the children of parents (of *either* sex) with epilepsy who take no antiepileptic drugs than in the general population [16, 18, 28, 42, 52]. The incidence of such malformations is also higher in patients with epilepsy and in the relatives of patients with epilepsy [19, 42]. Furthermore, there is an increased incidence of epilepsy among parents of children with facial clefts [18]. These data suggest a genetic predisposition to heart anomalies and facial clefts in the offspring of patients with epilepsy regardless of exposure to antiepileptic drugs.

TERATOGENICITY OF ANTIEPILEPTIC DRUGS

General Comments

Studies of the teratogenicity of antiepileptic drugs are complicated by many confounding variables. The genetic predisposition of the offspring of patients with epilepsy to develop heart anomalies and facial clefts is discussed above. Seizures presumably have a deleterious effect on the fetus, and this increases with seizure frequency. Women with epilepsy who take no antiepileptic drugs during pregnancy usually have "mild" conditions and therefore may have a lesser genetic tendency to produce malformed children and a lesser exposure to the harmful effects of seizures. Conversely, women with epilepsy who take antiepileptic drugs during pregnancy tend to have more severe epilepsy and may have a greater genetic tendency to produce malformed children and a greater exposure to the harmful effects of seizures. Persons with the most severe epilepsy tend to take the largest doses of antiepileptic drugs and to take several antiepileptic medications.

To determine the teratogenicity of a drug definitively it would be necessary to control all of the variables described in the preceding paragraph and to study a large enough group of mothers taking only that drug to determine whether the small risk of producing a child with a malformation while taking that drug was greater than the risk in an appropriate control group. To date such a study has not been performed for even one antiepileptic drug.

The clinician is thus put in the unfortunate position of having to recommend antiepileptic drug therapy to pregnant women without having definitive scientific knowledge of the absolute teratogenicity of any antiepileptic drug or the relative teratogenicity of available agents. For what it is worth, the available data will now be reviewed.

Absolute Teratogenicity of Antiepileptic Drugs

A large number of incompletely controlled studies indicate that the expected incidence of congenital malformations (of all types) is as follows: 2 to 3 percent in the general population, 4 to 5 percent in children born to mothers with epilepsy taking no antiepileptic drugs, and 6 to 11 percent in children born to mothers with epilepsy who are taking antiepileptic drugs (of all types) [2, 3, 23, 42]. For reasons outlined above, one cannot be certain if the high risk in the mothers taking antiepileptic drugs is due to the drugs, to genetic factors, or to high seizure frequency.

Relative Teratogenicity of Antiepileptic Drugs

The relative teratogenicity of antiepileptic drugs is equally confusing. Initial studies indicated that phenytoin might produce a higher incidence of congenital malformations than other antiepileptic drugs [2, 16]. However, recent studies indicate that the incidence of malformation is similar in children born to mothers taking either hydantoins or barbiturates [2, 3] or is even greater with barbiturates [42]. Questionable animal studies and early human studies based on a small number of subjects indicated that carbamazepine may be associated with fewer congenital malformations than hydantoins or barbiturates (see Chap. 18). However, a recent prospective study reported a statistically significant decrease in head circumference of neonates born to mothers taking carbamazepine monotherapy, which was not present in neonates born to mothers taking phenytoin or phenobarbital monotherapy [26].

Although evidence is not definitively established in a controlled study, a considerable body of uncontrolled data indicate very strongly that trimethadione is an extraordinarily teratogenic agent (see Chap. 22). This is the one antiepileptic drug that should be avoided if at all possible in women who might become pregnant or who are already pregnant.

Effects of Antiepileptic Drugs on Later Growth and Development

There have been controversial reports of retarded later growth and/or mental development in children born to mothers taking antiepileptic drugs [1, 16, 24, 26, 29, 46, 52, 64]. There is evidence that carbamazepine, phenobarbital, primidone, and phenytoin given alone and/or in combination during pregnancy may result in decreased head circumference at birth and that phenobarbital or primidone in combination with other drugs may result in decreased birth weight [1, 26]. However, Anderman et al. [1] performed serial Griffith's developmental scales for 3 years to a group of infants born to mothers taking antiepileptic drugs and found mean scores were at or above the average range for all age groups and did not show any significant correlation with reduced neonatal head circumference.

OTHER RISKS TO THE FETUS FROM EPILEPSY
AND/OR FROM ANTIEPILEPTIC DRUGS

There is evidence (not definitive) that epilepsy and/or the taking of antiepileptic drugs during pregnancy may increase the risk of abortion, stillbirth, toxemia, or complicated delivery and may also increase the risks of epilepsy in the child born to these mothers [16, 24, 29, 46, 52, 64]. Chronic exposure to antiepileptic drugs in utero creates a risk of sedation and/or withdrawal symptoms in the neonatal period [8, 43, 45].

MANAGEMENT OF EPILEPSY DURING PREGNANCY

Counseling

The woman with epilepsy who is pregnant or is planning to become pregnant should be counseled about the risks of congenital malformations associated with pregnancy and antiepileptic drugs, the risk that the child might develop epilepsy owing to genetic transmission (see Chaps. 4 to 9 for information on genetic risks associated with specific seizure types), the dangers of antiepileptic drugs in breast milk, and the risk of injury to the fetus or infant if the mother should have a seizure.

General Measures

Excessive weight gain and fluid retention should be prevented because these factors may increase the frequency of seizures during pregnancy [63]. Chronic administration of phenytoin, phenobarbital, or primidone may result in a low plasma folic acid level (see Chaps. 16 and 17). Folic acid deficiency has been correlated with third trimester bleeding [62] and neonatal hemorrhage (see Neonatal Hemorrhage below).

Antiepileptic Drug Therapy for Women With Epilepsy Planning to Become Pregnant in the Near Future

The first step is to determine if the seizures can be controlled with no medication and to do so if possible. If this is not possible, the woman should be managed ideally with the least teratogenic drug that will control her seizures. Unfortunately, the relative teratogenicity of the marketed antiepileptic drugs has not been definitively established at this time (see above). No firm data exist that allow the physician to select the safest drug (except that trimethadione should be avoided if at all possible, see above).

If antiepileptic drug therapy is required for seizure control, an attempt should be made to use only one drug (monotherapy). There is some evidence that the risk of teratogenicity is less with monotherapy than with polytherapy [1, 42].

Seizures should be controlled with the lowest effective plasma concentration of the chosen antiepileptic drug. Animal and human data suggest that the teratogenicity of antiepileptic drugs (especially phenytoin and phenobarbital) may increase with increasing plasma concentrations [13, 49].

Antiepileptic Drug Therapy for the Woman With Epilepsy Who Becomes Pregnant While Taking Antiepileptic Drugs

The major malformations associated with antiepileptic drugs are those related to organ systems that develop within the first 6 to 8 weeks of gestation. By the time pregnancy is diagnosed, it is usually too late to discontinue or alter antiepileptic medication to reduce possible teratogenic effects. At this point a good case can be made for continuing the same antiepileptic drug (except trimethadione, see above) to reduce the danger to the fetus from maternal seizures [28]. Discontinuing or changing antiepileptic medication carries a risk of increased seizure frequency.

The plasma concentration of the patient's antiepileptic drug should be maintained at the lowest level known to be effective for the patient in order to reduce possible teratogenic effects and to minimize the chance that the drug may alter cerebral maturation of the fetus [6, 12, 14, 15]. The dosage required to maintain this plasma concentration may increase during pregnancy (see Effect of Pregnancy on Antiepileptic Drugs above).

Management of New Seizure Disorder Beginning During Pregnancy

The incidence of onset of new seizures during pregnancy does not appear to be greater than that expected due to chance [59]. The pregnant woman should have a work-up similar to that given any patient with newly diagnosed epilepsy (see Chap. 1), except that the risks of exposure to x-rays and to contrast material must be considered before deciding whether to perform roentgenograms and contrast procedures (including CT scans with contrast). The general use of antiepileptic drugs during pregnancy is considered above. If no cause for an isolated seizure during pregnancy is found, antiepileptic drugs are often withheld, especially during the first trimester [16].

Neonatal Hemorrhage

There are at least 14 reported cases of fatal neonatal hemorrhage in infants born to mothers taking hydantoins [7, 56]. The hemorrhage can occur within the cranium, pleural cavity, or abdominal cavity and has its onset 1 to 5 days after birth [7, 56]. The mother's clotting factors are normal, but a depression of vitamin K–dependent clotting factors has been demonstrated in the affected neonates [5, 7, 56]. These considerations have led Bleyer and Skinner [7] to make the following suggestions for managing pregnant mothers taking antiepileptic drugs and their newborns. (1) Avoid other drugs with adverse effects on hemostatic mechanisms in the last trimester (aspirin, indomethacin, thiazides, promethazine). (2) Consider cesarean section if difficult or traumatic delivery is expected. (3) Administer phytonadione to the mother prior to delivery and to the infant (intravenously) immediately after birth. (4) Cord blood should be submitted for immediate clotting studies, and fresh frozen plasma should be given immediately if diminished vitamin K–dependent factors are found. (5) The neonate should be watched carefully and should receive an exchange transfusion at the first sign of development of a hemorrhage.

Lactation and Breast Feeding
The ability to lactate is not impaired by epilepsy or antiepileptic drugs [16]. Breast milk is essentially an ultrafiltrate of plasma, and the concentration of an antiepileptic drug in breast milk is similar to the concentration of unbound drug in plasma [32, 45, 48, 57]. Knowledge of the unbound plasma concentration of drug in the mother and the volume of breast milk delivered enables the physician to estimate the amount of drug received by an infant [32, 48, 57].

The risk to the infant from antiepileptic drugs is controversial. It is the author's opinion that breast feeding is best avoided in most mothers taking antiepileptic drugs because of the risk of sedation, poor feeding, and idiosyncratic reactions to the drug [21, 30, 61], the slow and unpredictable metabolism of antiepileptic drugs by the neonate [30, 43, 45] (see Chap. 14), and the possibility that antiepileptic drugs may interfere with brain maturation [6, 12, 14, 15, 41, 52].

References
1. Anderman, E. et al. Growth and development in offspring of epileptic mothers. *Epilepsia.* In press, 1982.
2. Annegers, J. F. et al. Do anticonvulsants have a teratogenic effect? *Arch. Neurol.* 31:364, 1974.
3. Annegers, J. F. et al. Congenital malformations and seizure disorders in the offspring of parents with epilepsy. *Int. J. Epidemiol.* 7:241, 1978.
4. Backstrom, T. Epileptic seizures in women related to plasma, estrogen, and progesterone during the menstrual cycle. *Acta Neurol. Scand.* 54:321, 1976.
5. Battino, D. et al. Coagulation Function in Newborns Treated in Utero with Antiepileptic Drugs. In D. Janz et al. (Eds.), *Epilepsy, Pregnancy, and the Child.* New York: Raven Press, 1982.
6. Bergey, G. K. et al. Adverse effects of phenobarbital on morphological and biochemical development of fetal mouse spinal cord neurons in culture. *Ann. Neurol.* 9:584, 1981.
7. Bleyer, W. A., and Skinner, A. L. Fatal neonatal hemorrhage after anticonvulsant therapy. *J.A.M.A.* 235:626, 1976.
8. Bossi, L. et al. Pharmacokinetics and Clinical Effects of Antiepileptic Drugs in Newborns of Chronically Treated Epileptic Mothers. In D. Janz et al. (Eds.), *Epilepsy, Pregnancy, and the Child.* New York: Raven Press, 1982.
9. Christiansen, J., and Dam, M. Plasma and Salivary Levels of Carbamazepine and Carbamazepine-10, 11-epoxide During Pregnancy. In D. Janz, M. Meinardi, and C. E. Pippenger (Eds.), *Antiepileptic Drug Monitoring.* Avon: Pitman Press, 1977.
10. Costa, P. J., and Bonnycastle, D. D. Effects of DCS, compound E, testosterone, progesterone and ACTH in modifying "age induced" convulsions in dogs. *Arch. Internat. Pharmacodynam.* 91:330, 1952.
11. Creutzfeldt, O. D. et al. EEG changes during spontaneous and controlled menstrual cycles and their correlation with psychological performance. *Electroencephalogr. Clin. Neurophysiol.* 40:113, 1976.
12. Culver, B., and Vernadakis, B. Effects of anticonvulsant drugs on chick embryonic neurons and glia in cell culture. *Dev. Neurosci.* 2:74, 1979.
13. Dansky, L. et al. Malformations in offsprings of epileptic women: Correlation with maternal anticonvulsant plasma levels during pregnancy. *Epilepsia* 22:235, 1981.
14. Diaz, J., and Schain, R. Chronic phenobarbital administration: Effects upon behavior and brain of artificially reared rats. *Science* 199:90, 1978.
15. Diaz, J., and Shields, W. B. Effects of dipropylacetate on brain development. *Ann. Neurol.* 10:465, 1981.
16. Donaldson, J. O. *Neurology of Pregnancy.* Philadelphia: Saunders, 1978.
17. Espir, M., Walker, M. E., and Lawson, J. P. Epilepsy and oral contraception. *Br. Med. J.* 1:294, 1969.
18. Friis, M. L. Epilepsy among parents of children with facial clefts. *Epilepsia* 20:69, 1979.
19. Friis, M. L. et al. Increased Prevalence of Cleft Lip and/or Palate Among Epileptic Patients. In D. Janz

et al. (Eds.), *Epilepsy, Pregnancy and the Child.* New York: Raven Press, 1982.

20. Glazer, G. H. Metabolic Endocrine, and Toxic Disease. In A. Redmond (Ed.), *Handbook of Electroencephalography and Clinical Neurophysiology,* Vol. 15, *The Epilepsies.* Amsterdam: North-Holland, 1976.

21. Granstrom, M. L., Bardy, A. H., and Hiilesmaa, V. K. Prolonged Feeding Difficulties of Infants of Primidone Mothers During Neonatal Period: Preliminary Results From the Prospective Helsinki Study. In D. Janz et al. (Eds.), *Epilepsy, Pregnancy, and the Child.* New York: Raven Press, 1982.

22. Hall, S. M. Treatment of menstrual epilepsy with a progesterone-only oral contraceptive. *Epilepsia* 18:235, 1977.

23. Hassell, T. M. et al. Summary of an international symposium on phenytoin-induced teratology and gingival pathology. *J. Am. Dent. Assoc.* 99:652, 1979.

24. Helge, H. Physical, Mental, and Social Development, Including Diseases: Review of the Literature. In D. Janz et al. (Eds.), *Epilepsy, Pregnancy, and the Child.* New York: Raven Press, 1982.

25. Herzog, A. G. et al. Neuroendocrine dysfunction in temporal lobe epilepsy. *Arch. Neurol.* 39:133, 1982.

26. Iivanainen, M. Effect of antiepileptic drugs on human body maturation. In P. L. Morselli, J. K. Penry, and C. E. Pippenger (Eds.), *Antiepileptic Drug Therapy in Pediatrics.* New York: Raven Press, 1982.

27. Janz, D. The teratogenic risk of antiepileptic drugs. *Epilepsia* 16:159, 1975.

28. Janz, D. On Major Malformations and Minor Anomalies in the Offspring of Parents With Epilepsy: Review of the Literature. In D. Janz et al. (Eds.), *Epilepsy, Pregnancy, and the Child.* New York: Raven Press, 1982.

29. Janz, D., and Back-Mannagetta, G. Complications of Pregnancy in Women with Epilepsy: Retrospective Study. In D. Janz et al. (Eds.), *Epilepsy, Pregnancy, and the Child.* New York: Raven Press, 1982.

30. Kaneko, S. et al. The Problems of Antiepileptic Medication in the Neonatal Period: Is Breast Feeding Advisable? In D. Janz et al. (Eds.), *Epilepsy, Pregnancy, and the Child.* New York: Raven Press, 1982.

31. Kirsten, K. I., Darn, M., and Christiansen, J. Phenytoin and phenobarbital clearance during pregnancy. *Acta Neurol. Scand.* 54:150, 1974.

32. Koup, J. R., Rose, J. Q., and Cohen, M. E. Ethosuximide pharmacokinetics in a pregnant patient and her newborn. *Epilepsia* 19:535, 1978.

33. Knight, A. H., and Rhind, E. G. Epilepsy and pregnancy: A study of 153 pregnancies in 59 patients. *Epilepsia* 16:99, 1975.

34. Laidlaw, J. Catamenial epilepsy. *Lancet* 271:235, 1956.

35. Lander, C. M. et al. Plasma anticonvulsant concentrations during pregnancy. *Neurology* 27:128, 1977.

36. Mattson, R. H. Unpublished data, 1982.

37. Mattson, R. H., Cramer, J. A., and Caldwell, B. V. Seizure frequency and the menstrual cycle: A clinical study. *Epilepsia* 22:242, 1981.

38. Mattson, R. H. et al. Medroxy progesterone treatment of women with uncontrolled seizures. *Epilepsia* 23:436, 1982.

39. Mattson, R. H., Lerner, E., and Dix, G. Precipitory and inhibitory factors in epilepsy: A statistical study. *Epilepsia* 15:271, 1974.

40. Millichap, J. G. Metabolic and Endocrine Factors. In P. J. Vinken, and G. W. Bruyn (Eds.), *Handbook of Clinical Neurology,* Vol. 15, *The Epilepsies.* Amsterdam: North-Holland, 1974.

41. Morselli, P. L., Penry, J. K., and Pippenger, C. E. (Eds.), *Antiepileptic Drug Therapy in Pediatrics.* New York: Raven Press, 1982.

42. Nakane, Y. et al. Multi-institutional study of the teratogenicity and fetal toxicity of antiepileptic drugs: A report of a collaborative study group in Japan. *Epilepsia* 21:663, 1980.

43. Nau, H. et al. Placental Transfer at Birth and Postnatal Elimination of Primidone and Its Metabolites in Neonates of Epileptic Mothers. In D. Janz et al. (Eds.), *Epilepsy, Pregnancy, and the Child.* New York: Raven Press, 1982.

44. Nau, H. et al. Pharmacokinetics of Primidone and Metabolites During Human Pregnancy. In D. Janz et al. (Eds.), *Epilepsy, Pregnancy, and the Child.* New York: Raven Press, 1982.

45. Nau, H. et al. Anticonvulsants during pregnancy and the lactation period: Pharmacokinetic and clinical studies. *Epilepsia.* In press, 1983.

46. Nelson, K. B., and Ellenberg, J. H. Maternal seizure disorder, outcome of pregnancy, and neurologic abnormalities in the children. *Neurology* (N.Y.) 32:1247, 1982.

47. Newmark, M. E., and Penry, J. K. Catamenial epilepsy: A review. *Epilepsia* 21:281, 1980.

48. Niebyl, J. R. et al. Carbamazepine levels in pregnancy and lactation. *Obstet. Gynecol.* 53:139, 1979.

49. Paulson, R. B., Paulson, G. W., and Jerissatsy, S. Phenytoin and carbamazepine in production of cleft palates in mice: Comparison of teratogenic effects. *Arch. Neurol.* 36:832, 1979.

50. Philbert, A., and Dam, M. Antiepileptic Drug Disposition During Pregnancy: Review of the Literature. In D. Janz et al. (Eds.), *Epilepsy, Pregnancy, and the Child.* New York: Raven Press, 1982.
51. Poser, C. M. Modification of therapy for exacerbation of seizures during menstruation. *J. Pediatr.* 84:799, 1974.
52. Proceedings: Workshop on Epilepsy, Pregnancy, and the Child. In D. Janz et al. (Eds.), *Epilepsy, Pregnancy, and the Child.* New York: Raven Press, 1982.
53. Ramsay, E. R. et al. Status epilepticus in pregnancy: Effect of phenytoin malabsorption on seizure control. *Neurology* 28:85, 1978.
54. Rane, A., Bertilsson, L., and Palmer, L. Disposition of placentally transferred carbamazepine (Tegretol®) in the newborn. *Eur. J. Clin. Pharmacol.* 8:283, 1975.
55. Resan, T. Y., Shahidi, M. T., and Korst, D. R. The effect of phenobarbital on testosterone-induced erythropolesis. *J. Lab. Clin. Med.* 79:187, 1972.
56. Reynolds, E. H. Chronic antiepileptic toxicity: A review. *Epilepsia* 16:319, 1975.
57. Richens, A. Clinical pharmacokinetics of phenytoin. *Clin. Pharmacokinet.* 4:154, 1979.
58. Sanchez, L. P., and Saldana, L. E. Hormones and their influence in epilepsy. *Acta Neurol. Latinoam.* 12:29, 1966.
59. Schmidt, D. The Effect of Pregnancy on the Natural History of Epilepsy: Review of the Literature. In D. Janz et al. (Eds.), *Epilepsy, Pregnancy, and the Child.* New York: Raven Press, 1982.
60. Sonnen, A. E. H. Hormonal contraception anticonvulsant treatment. *Epilepsia* 21:201, 1980.
61. Stirrat, G. M. Prescribing problems in the second half of pregnancy and during lactation. *Obstet. Gynecol. Surv.* 31:1, 1976.
62. Streift, R. R., and Little, B. Folic acid deficiency in pregnancy. *N. Engl. J. Med.* 276:776, 1967.
63. Suter, C., and Klingman, W. O. Seizure states and pregnancy. *Neurology* 7:105, 1957.
64. Teramo, K., and Hiilesmaa, W. Pregnancy and Fetal Complications in Epileptic Pregnancies: Review of the Literature. In D. Janz et al. (Eds.), *Epilepsy, Pregnancy, and the Child.* New York: Raven Press, 1982.
65. Timiras, P. S., and Hill, H. F. Hormones and Epilepsy. In G. H. Glaser, J. K. Penry, and D. M. Woodbury (Eds.), *Antiepileptic Drugs: Mechanism of Action.* New York: Raven Press, 1980.
66. Toone, B. K., Wheeler, M., and Fenwick, P. B. C. Sex hormone changes in male epileptics. *Clin. Endocrinol.* 12:391, 1980.
67. Wesk, E. E., MacGee, J., and Sholiton, L. J. Effect of diphenylhydantoin on cortisol metabolism in man. *J. Clin. Invest.* 43:1824, 1964.

STATUS EPILEPTICUS

30

Thomas R. Browne

Status epilepticus is defined as seizures occurring so frequently that the patient does not fully recover from one seizure before having another. There are several types of status epilepticus including tonic-clonic (grand mal), simple partial (focal motor), absence (petit mal), and complex partial (psychomotor, temporal lobe). In each type of status epilepticus there is continuing seizure activity without full recovery before the next seizure occurs. Tonic-clonic (grand mal) status epilepticus is the most common and most life-threatening form of status epilepticus.

Tonic-Clonic (Grand Mal) Status Epilepticus

DEFINITIONS

A patient is defined as being in tonic-clonic status epilepticus if he is having repeated tonic-clonic seizures without fully recovering from the postictal phase of one seizure before having another. Ongoing tonic-clonic seizure activity lasting longer than 30 minutes is also usually classified as status epilepticus even if the patient is having his first seizure. The seizures consist of a tonic phase followed by a clonic phase. The clonic phase often decreases in duration in a patient with continuing tonic-clonic seizures [54]. The seizures are bilaterally synchronous at onset in 45 percent of cases [54]. In the remainder of cases the seizures are adversive or focal in onset.

INCIDENCE AND SIGNIFICANCE

The reported incidence of tonic-clonic status epilepticus among patients with epilepsy varies from 1 to 5 percent [6, 11, 24, 27, 29, 31, 48]. The mortality of tonic-clonic status epilepticus in the preantiepileptic drug era was 10 to 50 percent [6, 24, 31]. Today the reported mortality is 3 to 20 percent [12, 24, 29, 31, 48, 55]. Death during tonic-clonic status epilepticus may be due to medical complications, overmedication, or the basic disease process causing status epilepticus. Tonic-clonic status epilepticus is responsible for one third of all epilepsy-related deaths [29]. Furthermore, animal studies indicate that prolonged seizure activity, even in paralyzed, respirated animals, may result in irreversible cerebral damage [6, 18, 19, 45, 66].

MANAGEMENT OF PATIENTS WITH
TONIC-CLONIC STATUS EPILEPTICUS

Overall

The overall objectives in managing status epilepticus are (1) to maintain vital functions at all times, (2) to identify and treat precipitating factors of status epilepticus, (3) to prevent or correct medical complications of status epilepticus, and (4) to administer a loading dose of a long-acting antiepileptic drug [6, 16, 49, 61].

Maintain Vital Functions

The vital signs and electrocardiogram (ECG) should be checked immediately and appropriate corrective measures taken when necessary. The patient should be positioned to avoid aspiration, suffocation, or falls. A soft plastic oral airway should be taped in place if it is possible to do so without forcing the teeth apart. Forcing an airway between clenched teeth may result in dental injury and aspiration of teeth. Wooden tongue blades may cause injuries from splinters and cuts, and metal spoons may injure teeth. Intubation may be necessary to maintain respirations. A large intravenous catheter should be placed for administration of medication and fluids. It is always prudent to administer a bolus of intravenous glucose (e.g., 50 ml of a 50% solution) to a patient who presents with altered consciousness as soon as blood for routine laboratory determinations is obtained. Thiamine (e.g., 50 mg intravenously and 50 mg intramuscularly) should be administered before administering glucose if chronic alcoholism or alcohol withdrawal is suspected.

Identify and Treat Underlying Causal Factors

Most cases of tonic-clonic status epilepticus occur in patients with known chronic seizure disorders, but occasionally tonic-clonic status epilepticus is the presenting symptom of a seizure disorder [31]. Over two thirds of cases of tonic-clonic status epilepticus occur in patients with "symptomatic" epilepsy (i.e., epilepsy due to a known structural or metabolic lesion) as opposed to "idiopathic" epilepsy [11, 27, 29, 31, 48, 55]. The symptomatic lesions most commonly associated with tonic-clonic status epilepticus are tumors, post-traumatic injuries, CNS infections, prenatal-perinatal injuries, and cerebrovascular accidents [11, 27, 29, 31, 48, 55]. Occasionally tonic-clonic status epilepticus seems to be precipitated by the massive size of a cerebral lesion without any other identifiable precipitating factor.

Most cases of tonic-clonic status epilepticus do not occur randomly or as a result of a massive cerebral lesion. Rather, there is a specific precipitating factor that causes a patient with a known seizure disorder to develop status epilepticus at a specific time. The most frequent causes of tonic-clonic status epilepticus are withdrawal from antiepileptic drugs and fever activating a seizure disorder [27, 29, 31, 55]. Other precipitating factors include (1) withdrawal from alcohol or sedative drugs, (2) a metabolic disorder (hypocalcemia, hyponatremia, hypoglycemia, hepatic or renal failure), (3) sleep deprivation, (4) acute new CNS insult (meningitis, encephalitis, cerebrovascular accident, or trauma), (5) diagnostic procedures (e.g., pneumoencephalogram, cerebral angiography), (6) drug intoxication (e.g., tricyclics or isoniazid) [6, 12, 29, 31, 55]. The precipitating factors in a case of status epilepticus must always be vigorously sought and treated to facilitate seizure control and to be certain that any reversible cause of cerebral dysfunction is treated before it results in irreversible cerebral damage.

Prevent or Correct Medical Complications of Status Epilepticus

The common pathophysiologic changes occurring during tonic-clonic status epilepticus are summarized in Table 30-1. Severe metabolic acidosis and profound loss of base reserve are generally present in prolonged status epilepticus [70]. Metabolic acidosis may prevent seizure control with antiepileptic drugs by increasing the amount of potassium in the extracellular space and may contribute to irreversible cerebral damage during status epilepticus [66, 70]. Arterial blood gas determination should be performed early in the management of status epilepticus. Sodium bicarbonate (100 mEq intravenously) should be administered if the pH is less than 7.21 or if tonic-clonic status epilepticus has continued for more than 15 minutes and blood gas determination results are not immediately available [70].

Other medical complications of status epilepticus include cardiac arrhythmias, hypertension and hypotension, myoglobinuria, pulmonary edema, hyperthermia, excessive sweating, dehydration, pneumonia, disseminated intravascular coagulation, and orthopedic injuries [6, 15, 20, 21, 70].

Administer a Loading Dose of a Long-Acting Antiepileptic Drug

To control status epilepticus quickly and prevent its recurrence, a high therapeutic serum concentration of a long-acting antiepileptic drug must be immediately obtained and then the serum concentration must be maintained in the therapeutic range. To obtain a high therapeutic serum concentration quickly, an intravenous loading dose of drug must be given. This method avoids the otherwise long delay in achieving a

Table 30-1. Pathophysiologic Changes of Status Epilepticus

Parameter	Early Status (15–30 min)	Late Status ($>$30 min)
Pulse	Rapid	Weak and rapid
Blood pressure	Mildly to moderately hypertensive	Normal to hypotensive
Arterial oxygen tension	Decreased	Decreased
Arterial carbon dioxide tension	Elevated	Elevated
Bicarbonate	Decreased	Severely decreased
Glucose	Normal to elevated[a]	Decreased
Potassium	Elevated	Elevated
Sodium	Normal[b]	Normal to elevated[b]
pH	Depressed (7.0–7.2)	Depressed (6.7–7.1)
Lactic acid	Elevated	Elevated

[a]Hypoglycemia may rarely be a cause of status epilepticus.
[b]Hyponatremia may be a causative factor and should be corrected immediately.
Source: From Wilder and Bruni [70].

therapeutic steady state serum concentration of the drug if it is given in its usual maintenance dosage (7 to 8 days for phenytoin and 14 to 21 days for phenobarbital—see Chaps. 14, 16, and 17).

PHENYTOIN

Indications
Phenytoin is the antiepileptic drug of choice for most patients with tonic-clonic status epilepticus because (1) phenytoin is extremely effective in controlling tonic-clonic status epilepticus [14, 44, 65, 71]; (2) an intravenous loading dose of phenytoin can be rapidly and safely administered; (3) phenytoin does not depress respiration as much as alternative drugs; (4) phenytoin does not depress the level of alertness as much as alternative drugs and therefore allows better evaluation of mental status; (5) if adjunctive therapy with diazepam is required, diazepam probably causes less cardiorespiratory depression in combination with phenytoin than in combination with phenobarbital or paraldehyde; (6) phenytoin has the best efficacy-to-toxicity ratio for the chronic treatment of tonic-clonic seizures in most adult patients.

Contraindications and Warnings
Phenytoin is contraindicated in patients with a history of hypersensitivity to hydantoins. Because of its depressant effect on cardiac conductivity and automaticity, phenytoin is contraindicated in patients with sinus bradycardia, sinoatrial block, second and third degree AV block, hypotension, and severe myocardial insufficiency. In certain situations (see below) it may be decided before treating a patient with tonic-clonic status epilepticus that phenobarbital would be a better

chronic antiepileptic drug than phenytoin. These patients should be treated with a loading dose of phenobarbital rather than with phenytoin.

Pharmacokinetics and Dosage
The pharmacologic objectives in using intravenous phenytoin to treat status epilepticus are to obtain a high therapeutic serum concentration of phenytoin immediately and then to maintain this concentration without any substantial dips. The therapeutic range of phenytoin serum concentration during chronic oral administration for prevention of tonic-clonic seizures is 10 to 20 μg/ml (see Chaps. 14 and 16), and Wallis et al. [65] reported similar serum phenytoin concentrations in patients whose status epilepticus was successfully treated with intravenous phenytoin. Table 30-2 shows that administration of the usual daily dose of phenytoin (4 mg/kg) as a single intravenous injection does not produce a consistently high therapeutic serum concentration, and the serum concentration falls to subtherapeutic levels within 1 hour. An initial dose of 7 mg/kg produces therapeutic serum concentrations of phenytoin, but again the serum concentration often becomes subtherapeutic within 1 hour after administration. A loading dose of 13 to 15 mg/kg of phenytoin will produce therapeutic serum concentrations for 6 hours [13, 65, 71], and therapeutic serum concentrations will be maintained if maintenance doses (100 mg orally or intravenously every 6 to 8 hours) are begun 6 hours after the loading dose [65]. Alternatively, a loading dose of 18 mg/kg can be given, and maintenance doses need not be started until 24 hours after the loading dose [13, 14].

The data in the preceding paragraph were obtained from studies of adults. Work with neonates indicates

Table 30-2. *Serum Concentration (μg/ml) of Phenytoin After Single Intravenous Loading Doses of Sodium Phenytoin in Adults*

Dosage (mg/kg)	Peak		1 Hour		24 Hours	
	Mean	Range	Mean	Range	Mean	Range
3.3	10.5	3.9–17.4	5.2	3.8–6.4	1.9	1.0–2.4
3.4–4.2	12.7	9.9–18.2	7.9	6.9–9.1	2.6	1.6–3.8
7	17	10–24	9	6–11		
12					7.1	
10.9–17.2 (mean 13.0)	31.5	17–59	16.3	8–27	7.9	3–19
14	19	12–32	17	12–30		
18			23.5		15.0	

Source: This table was compiled from various studies reviewed by T. R. Browne. Modified from Browne [6] with the publisher's permission.

that an intravenous loading dose of 15 to 20 mg/kg of phenytoin will produce a serum concentration of 12 to 18 μg/ml [37, 50]. Orally administered phenytoin is not well absorbed in neonates, and both loading and maintenance doses of the drug must be given intravenously to maintain a therapeutic serum concentration [50].

If intravenous phenytoin is administered at the maximum recommended rate of 50 mg/minute it will take approximately 20 minutes to administer a full loading dose to an adult. Peak brain parenchyma and peak cerebrospinal fluid concentrations of phenytoin may not be reached until approximately 1 hour after the intravenous loading dose has been completely administered [51, 71]. Therefore, if a loading dose of phenytoin is infused as the only medication for status epilepticus, the seizures may continue during the infusion and for up to 1 hour after the infusion is completed [71]. Diazepam is often a useful adjunctive drug to control tonic-clonic status epilepticus in the period while phenytoin serum and brain concentrations are being built up (see below—Diazepam, Indications).

There is abundant evidence from human and animal studies that intramuscular phenytoin is very slowly absorbed (Fig. 30-1) [34, 65]. Peak serum phenytoin concentrations occur approximately 24 hours after a single intramuscular injection and are significantly less than the peak concentrations produced by the same dose given intravenously [34]. Intramuscular phenytoin should never be used for the treatment of status epilepticus or any other medical emergency in which a therapeutic phenytoin serum concentration must be rapidly and predictably achieved.

Administration
Intravenous phenytoin should not be given at a rate greater than 50 mg/minute in adults (1 mg/kg/minute

in children) because of the danger of cardiorespiratory depression associated with faster administration [1]. The only FDA-approved method for administering intravenous phenytoin is a direct intravenous push. The drug should not be mixed with intravenous fluids (especially those with glucose) because of the possibility of precipitation of the drug. Pulse, blood pressure, and ECG should be monitored frequently during the administration of a loading dose of phenytoin. Phenytoin sodium for injection is an irritative substance that can cause chemical phlebitis and, if extravasated, tissue damage. Therefore, the following precautions should be observed when administering intravenous phenytoin: (1) use a large infusion catheter in a large vein; (2) follow each injection of phenytoin by an injection of sterile saline (which is less likely to precipitate phenytoin than a glucose solution); and (3) avoid extravasation.

Toxicity
Reported serious complications of intravenous phenytoin include hypotension, atrial and ventricular conduction depression, ventricular fibrillation, cardiovascular collapse, and respiratory arrest. Serious complications are most likely to occur with rapid infusion, in elderly patients, and in the gravely ill [6, 13]. Less serious complications include drowsiness, circumoral tingling, vertigo, nausea, and rarely, vomiting. These side effects usually occur when the serum phenytoin concentration is greater than 20 μg/ml.

The incidence of serious complications with full loading doses of intravenous phenytoin is quite low. Cranford et al. [13] administered loading doses of 10.5 to 25.3 mg/kg of phenytoin with ECG and blood pressure monitoring on 159 occasions for the control of seizures. There were only 4 serious complications (all reversible). These consisted of 1 case each of respira-

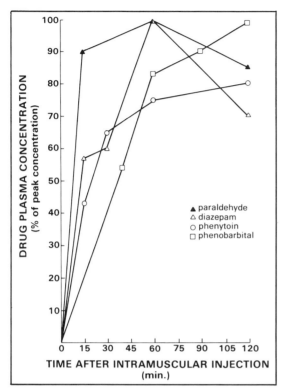

Figure 30-1. Plasma concentration versus time relationships for paraldehyde, diazepam, phenytoin, and phenobarbital following intramuscular injection. (Based on data from L. Hillestad et al. [26], B. Jalling [28], H. B. Kostenbauder et al. [34], and J. H. Thurston et al. [60].)

tory depression, hypotension requiring discontinuation of the phenytoin infusion, atrial fibrillation, and sinus tachycardia. Cranford et al. [13] did, however, report that 25 percent of patients had a fall in blood pressure of more than 10 mm Hg diastolic and/or 20 mm Hg systolic and that the blood pressure usually normalized with a decreased infusion rate. The toxicity of intravenous phenytoin depends chiefly on the rate of administration rather than on the dose administered.

PHENOBARBITAL

Indications
Phenobarbital is indicated for the treatment of tonic-clonic status epilepticus in the following situations: (1) in patients allergic to phenytoin, (2) in patients with evidence of disorders of cardiac conductivity or automaticity on ECG, (3) in patients who continue to have seizures despite a full loading dose of phenytoin, and (4) in patients with tonic-clonic status epilepticus for whom it may be decided before treatment that phenobarbital would be a better chronic antiepileptic

drug than phenytoin. Examples of persons in the last category include (1) those who have taken phenytoin in the past and have discontinued the drug because of unacceptable side effects (e.g., gingival hyperplasia and hirsutism in a young woman), (2) neonates, because they absorb oral maintenance doses of phenobarbital but do not absorb oral maintenance doses of phenytoin [36, 49, 50], and (3) children under 6 years of age, because phenytoin may stimulate rather than inhibit seizure activity in the immature brain [63] and because phenytoin may have deleterious effects on developing connective tissue [53].

Contraindications, Warnings, and Administration
Phenobarbital is contraindicated in patients with hypersensitivity to any barbiturate and in patients with porphyria. Intravenous phenobarbital usually causes sedation and may cause hypotension or respiratory depression. The drug should be used with care in patients with impaired respiratory, cardiac, hepatic, or renal function and in patients with myasthenia gravis and myxedema. The cardiorespiratory depressant effects of phenobarbital and diazepam may be additive [9], and special caution must be used when these two drugs are given in combination. Solutions for intravenous injection should be freshly prepared and administered no faster than 60 mg/minute.

Pharmacokinetics and Dosage
Studies in neonates indicate that repetitive seizures are not controlled until phenobarbital serum concentrations reach 15 to 20 μg/ml [36, 50]. Loading doses of 16 to 20 mg/kg are required to achieve this serum concentration; they do not produce excessive sedation [36, 50]. This loading dose in neonates should be followed by a maintenance dose of 3 to 5 mg/kg/day [36, 50].

In adults, Goldberg et al. [22] recommend an initial loading dose of 3 to 5 mg/kg. This produces a phenobarbital serum concentration of 8 to 9 μg/ml and prolonged sedation in most patients. If seizures persist for 20 to 30 minutes after the first injection, a second 3- to 5-mg/kg dose is given. A third 3- to 5-mg/kg dose is given if necessary after another 20- to 30-minute interval. The initial loading dose is followed by a maintenance dose of 3 mg/kg/day.

Indirect evidence using a double-indicator dilation method strongly indicates that peak phenobarbital brain concentrations do not occur for 60 minutes or longer after an intravenous infusion [51]. The following indirect evidence also suggests that the rate of brain penetration of phenobarbital in humans is slow. (1) In animals, peak brain or CSF concentrations of phenobarbital and appearance of anesthesia do not occur until 20 to 90 minutes after an intravenous injection of phenobarbital. (2) In humans, the peak sedative effect often does not occur until 1 hour or more after an intravenous injection of phenobarbital [8, 41].

Peak serum concentrations occur 1 to 12 hours after intramuscular injections of phenobarbital (Fig. 30-1) [6, 28, 64]. The bioavailability of intramuscular phenobarbital compared with intravenous phenobarbital has never been determined. However, bioavailability is less by the intramuscular route than by the oral route [64], and presumably the difference in bioavailability would be even greater when comparing the intramuscular with the intravenous route. Intramuscular phenobarbital should not be used in the treatment of status epilepticus because (1) peak phenobarbital serum concentrations are not reached quickly; (2) the patient will continue to have seizures until the phenobarbital serum concentration has risen into the therapeutic range; (3) toxic doses of phenobarbital may eventually accumulate if the patient is given multiple intramuscular doses of phenobarbital to control seizures; (4) the unknown, but lower, bioavailability of intramuscular phenobarbital makes it difficult to estimate the proper loading dose based on data from studies using the intravenous route.

DIAZEPAM

Indications

The objectives in treating tonic-clonic status epilepticus, as stated previously, are to support vital functions, to treat the precipitating factors, and to administer a loading dose of a long-acting antiepileptic drug. Intravenous diazepam has a relatively brief duration of action, is not a definitive therapy for status epilepticus, and can cause serious side effects. However, because intravenous diazepam produces transient high serum and brain concentrations of the drug, it can be a helpful adjunct in the treatment of tonic-clonic status epilepticus in some patients. Intravenous diazepam is indicated for tonic-clonic status epilepticus (1) if generalized tonic-clonic activity has been going on without interruption for more than a few minutes, or (2) if a tonic-clonic seizure occurs in a postictal patient who is being evaluated and who is receiving a loading dose of a long-acting antiepileptic drug. (Since status epilepticus may end spontaneously, intravenous diazepam should not be administered to a patient who arrives at the hospital in a postictal state unless he has another seizure.) In practice, many patients with tonic-clonic status epilepticus will meet one or both of these criteria. The effectiveness of diazepam in controlling tonic-clonic status epilepticus is documented in Table 30-3.

In some cases of tonic-clonic status epilepticus the tonic-clonic seizures are brief or the interval between tonic-clonic seizures is long enough to administer a loading dose of a long-acting antiepileptic drug. In these cases diazepam is not necessary and should be avoided because use of the drug exposes the patient to an unnecessary risk.

The use of intravenous diazepam to control tonic-clonic seizure activity after a full loading dose of phenytoin or phenobarbital has been administered requires even more medical judgment. Most cases of status epilepticus that are due to failure to take medication or to fever quickly respond to a loading dose of phenytoin or phenobarbital plus antipyretic measures, if necessary. Cases of refractory tonic-clonic status epilepticus are rare and are usually due to large brain tumors or to large acute cerebral insults (e.g., encephalitis). In these cases judicious use of the smallest effective dose of intravenous diazepam to control the seizures temporarily is indicated if the seizures compromise vital functions. Care must be exercised in using diazepam in this situation because of the additive cardiorespiratory toxicity when diazepam is given to a patient with a high serum concentration of another depressant drug. The major thrust of the management of refractory tonic-clonic status epilepticus should be to treat the precipitating factors and to add appropriate additional long-acting antiepileptic drugs. Management of refractory tonic-clonic status epilepticus with repeated doses of diazepam frequently results in accumulation of toxic concentrations of diazepam and/or active diazepam metabolites.

Contraindications and Warnings

Diazepam is contraindicated in patients with a known hypersensitivity to the drug, acute narrow angle glaucoma, or open angle glaucoma. Because of possible cardiorespiratory depression, extreme care must be taken in administering intravenous diazepam to the elderly, the very ill, patients with limited pulmonary reserve, patients in shock, and patients who have received sedative drugs (including alcohol).

Probably the most common and most dangerous error made in the management of status epilepticus is to treat repeated seizures with repeated doses of intravenous diazepam without treating the precipitating factors definitively and without administering an adequate loading dose of a long-acting antiepileptic drug. In this situation, the patient will continue to have seizures, toxic concentrations of diazepam and/or diazepam metabolites will accumulate, and serious morbidity may result from diazepam overdosage. It is probable that at many hospitals more status epilepticus–related deaths are due to diazepam overdosage than to status epilepticus.

Another frequent error is to administer intravenous diazepam unnecessarily to a patient who is not truly in tonic-clonic status epilepticus. The following are

Table 30-3. Summary of Reported Effectiveness of Diazepam in Various Types of Status Epilepticus

Type of Status Epilepticus	No. of Reports	No. of Patients	Effects on Status Epilepticus		
			No Effect	Temporary Control	Lasting Control
Tonic-clonic	19	188	23 (12%)	37 (20%)	128 (68%)
Secondarily generalized tonic-clonic	6	38	4 (10%)	6 (16%)	28 (74%)
Focal motor (including unilateral and jacksonian)	17	103	13 (13%)	15 (15%)	75 (73%)
Absence (petit mal)	10	30	2 (7%)	3 (10%)	25 (83%)
Myoclonic	9	28	4 (14%)	4 (14%)	20 (71%)
Complex partial (psychomotor, temporal lobe)	4	8	2 (25%)	1 (13%)	5 (62%)
Tonic	4	8	3 (38%)	0	5 (62%)
Clonic	3	9	1 (11%)	0	8 (89%)
Hemiclonic	2	22	2 (9%)	6 (27%)	14 (63%)
Infantile myoclonic	2	5	0	4 (80%)	1 (20%)

Source: This table was compiled from various studies reviewed by T. R. Browne. Reprinted by permission of the publisher from T. R. Browne, Drug therapy of status epilepticus, *Drug Ther. Rev.* 2:449, 1979. Copyright 1979 by Elsevier Science Publishing Co., Inc.

examples of patients who may be given diazepam for nonexistent status epilepticus: (1) a patient who had several tonic-clonic seizures before arrival at the hospital but who arrives at the hospital fully alert; (2) a patient who arrives at the hospital fully alert and then has a single tonic-clonic seizure; (3) a patient who arrives at the hospital in a postictal state after a single tonic-clonic seizure. Administration of intravenous diazepam to these patients exposes them to an unnecessary risk.

Pharmacokinetics

Serum diazepam concentrations of at least 0.3 to 0.7 μg/ml are needed to control status epilepticus and interictal paroxysmal activity on the EEG [5, 57]. Injection of 10 mg of diazepam intravenously in adults produced peak serum concentrations of 0.3 to 2.0 (mean 0.9) μg/ml in the study of Booker and Celesia [5]. Injection of 20 mg of diazepam intravenously in adults produced a mean serum concentration of 1.6 μg/ml in the study of Hillestad et al. [26]. The clearance of diazepam from the serum follows a biphasic curve. Immediately after an intravenous injection of diazepam the distribution phase half-life ($T\frac{1}{2}\alpha$) of the serum concentration is 16 to 90 minutes [5, 32]. The later elimination phase half-life ($T\frac{1}{2}\beta$) of diazepam is much slower [5, 32]. Serum diazepam concentrations decrease by 34 to 50 percent during the first 20 minutes after intravenous injection and decrease by 62 to 72 percent during the first 2 hours after an intravenous injection [5, 26, 30]. This rapid clearance of diazepam from the serum after an intravenous injection during the distribution phase probably accounts for the frequent recurrence of seizure activity when diazepam alone is used to control status epilepticus [9].

After intravenous infusion of diazepam in man half-maximal brain concentration is reached in 1.6 minutes, and maximal brain concentration is reached in 12 minutes [51]. Brain parenchyma concentration of diazepam then falls rapidly at a rate that closely parallels the fall of the serum diazepam concentration [6, 51]. The brain parenchyma concentrations of phenytoin and phenobarbital rise more slowly after an intravenous injection of drug, but the brain concentrations tend to remain relatively constant despite falling serum concentrations [6, 51, 71]. These observations provide a pharmacokinetic basis for a frequently employed therapeutic strategy of initial use of intravenous diazepam to effect immediate seizure control followed by prompt administration of a loading dose of phenytoin or phenobarbital to maintain seizure control when the serum and brain concentrations of diazepam fall below the therapeutic range [6, 71].

Intramuscular diazepam is absorbed relatively slowly. Peak serum diazepam concentrations are reached approximately 60 minutes after an intramuscular injection (Fig. 30-1) [26, 33, 58]. Furthermore, the peak serum diazepam concentration following intramuscular injection is much less than the peak concentration following intravenous injection. In the study of Hillestad et al. [26] the mean peak serum diazepam concentration was 1.6 μg/ml following a 20-mg intravenous injection and 0.3 μg/ml following a 20-

348

mg intramuscular injection. Thus intramuscular diazepam should not be used to treat status epilepticus because the onset of action is too slow, and even large doses may not produce serum concentrations of diazepam that are effective against epilepsy.

Rectal diazepam is not marketed in the United States, but it is marketed in Europe [46, 57]. Rectal diazepam solution in children produces peak serum concentrations in 4 to 60 minutes, produces therapeutic serum concentrations (0.5 μg/ml) in 2 to 6 minutes, and appears suitable for treatment of status epilepticus [57]. Rectal diazepam solution in adults and rectal diazepam suppositories in patients of all ages do not appear suitable for treatment of status epilepticus because of slower time to peak serum concentration and lower peak serum concentration [46, 57].

Dosage and Administration
The usual initial adult dose of diazepam for tonic-clonic status epilepticus is 5 to 10 mg intravenously at a rate of no more than 5 mg/minute. In children 5 years of age or older the recommended dose is 1 mg every 2 to 5 minutes up to a maximum of 10 mg. In infants over 30 days of age and children under 5 years of age the recommended dose is 0.2 to 0.5 mg slowly every 2 to 5 minutes up to a maximum of 5 mg. The efficacy and safety of parenteral diazepam has not been established in infants 30 days of age or less.

Because diazepam for injection is an irritative substance, it should not be administered into small veins, and care should be taken to avoid extravasation or interarterial injection. Diazepam should not be mixed with intravenous fluids.

Toxicity
The most worrisome complications of intravenous diazepam are respiratory depression and hypotension. In an earlier review [9] the author found 26 cases of respiratory depression and/or cardiac depression among 401 cases of various types of status epilepticus treated with diazepam. The incidence of cardiorespiratory depression is probably greater when diazepam is given in combination with other depressant drugs [9]. Animal work indicates that some of the adverse cardiorespiratory effects of intravenous diazepam (and also of intravenous phenytoin) may be due to the propylene glycol solvent used in preparing the drug [56]. Other less serious side effects of intravenous diazepam include drowsiness, ataxia, dysarthria, confusion, paradoxical excitement, and diplopia.

LORAZEPAM
Lorazepam for intravenous administration currently is approved by the FDA as a preoperative medication. It is not approved for status epilepticus. Preliminary results

indicate that lorazepam may have a longer duration of action and less cardiorespiratory depressant effect than diazepam in the management of status epilepticus (see Chap. 21).

PARALDEHYDE
The chemistry, mechanism of action, clinical pharmacology, and toxicity of paraldehyde are discussed in detail in Chapter 22.

Indications
Evidence for the efficacy of paraldehyde (PA) in status epilepticus consists of 52 case reports in three uncontrolled trials [23, 43, 69] and two widely quoted testimonials [17, 67]. These reports contain few details but suggest that (1) PA can probably control status epilepticus in the majority of patients, both adult and pediatric; (2) PA may control status epilepticus when other agents fail; (3) PA may be more effective for tonic-clonic status epilepticus than for partial status epilepticus.

A comparison of PA with other agents for status epilepticus has never been done in a controlled clinical trial. Comparison of the reported evidence for the efficacy and toxicity of antiepileptic drugs leads this reviewer to conclude that for most patients intravenous diazepam is preferable to intravenous PA when immediate control of seizures is necessary and that for most patients a loading dose of phenytoin or phenobarbital followed by maintenance doses is preferable to continued PA therapy for more long-term control of status epilepticus. There are four special situations in which PA may be preferable for control of status epilepticus: (1) when the initial therapy must be given intramuscularly, (2) when status epilepticus is caused by alcohol withdrawal, (3) when other agents fail, (4) when the patient is allergic to safer agents.

When initial therapy must be given intramuscularly (no physician immediately available, suitable vein cannot be found, resuscitation equipment not available, and so on), intramuscular paraldehyde may be the drug of choice for status epilepticus. PA absorption by the intramuscular route produces near peak serum concentrations in 15 to 20 minutes [60]. Diazepam, phenytoin, and phenobarbital require significantly longer times for absorption by the intramuscular route (Fig. 30-1) and do not produce therapeutic serum concentrations within 15 to 20 minutes when given in the usual doses intramuscularly [26, 28, 33, 34, 58, 64, 65].

In status epilepticus thought to be due entirely or chiefly to alcohol withdrawal, PA may be the drug of choice. Such patients include those with no history of seizures except during alcohol withdrawal and patients with true seizure disorders and therapeutic blood levels of antiepileptic drugs who have seizures only when withdrawing from alcohol. Paraldehyde may be the drug of choice because (1) paraldehyde is very effective for control of alcohol withdrawal symptoms and prevention of delirium tremens [7]; PA thus might be administered regardless of the status epilepticus, and use of one drug avoids the dangers of polypharmacy; (2) the preponderance of experimental and clinical evidence suggests that phenytoin is not effective for alcohol withdrawal seizures [7]; (3) barbiturates are not generally used for treatment of alcohol withdrawal symptoms in the United States because of concern about habituation to barbiturates as well as to ethanol [7].

When status epilepticus continues after full loading doses of phenytoin and phenobarbital have been administered, PA will sometimes stop the seizures [7, 67].

When the patient is allergic to safer agents used to treat status epilepticus (diazepam, phenytoin, phenobarbital), PA may be an effective alternative.

Dosage and Administration

The dosage of PA for treatment of status epilepticus is 0.1 to 0.15 ml/kg. This dose may be repeated every 2 to 4 hours if necessary. Before any PA is administered it should be checked for purity and conformity with USP standards for storage (see Chap. 22). The minimum therapeutic serum concentration of PA for control of status epilepticus is approximately 300 μg/ml [23].

The safety of PA by the *intravenous route* is controversial (see Chap. 22). When immediate control of seizures with an intravenous medication is indicated, one should probably use another drug (e.g., diazepam) whose safety by the intravenous route has been better documented. If intravenous PA is given, it must be diluted to a 4% solution and infused slowly.

PA can decompose plastic syringes and tubing within less than 2 minutes [7]. Only glass syringes should be used, and PA should not be infused in plastic tubing.

PA by the *intramuscular route* should be injected deep into the buttocks, taking care to avoid the sciatic nerve, and administering a maximum dose of 5 ml per injection site.

Absorption by way of the *oral route* is slower than by the intramuscular route (see Chap. 22). There is also a risk of aspiration of PA, which is highly noxious to the lungs. The oral route is best avoided in patients with status epilepticus.

The ease of administration of PA by way of the *rectal route* probably accounts for its frequent administration this way. However, absorption of PA by the rectal route is considerably slower than by the intramuscular or

oral route, making the rectal route particularly undesirable for treating status epilepticus (see Chap. 22). Furthermore, the slow absorption of PA by the rectal route can result in administration of very large doses of rectal PA in order to obtain a serum concentration high enough to control seizures. When the large rectal reservoir of PA is eventually absorbed, toxic PA serum concentrations may result [7]. If rectal PA is administered, it should be diluted 2:1 in oil (olive or cottonseed) or diluted in 200 ml of 0.9% sodium chloride.

REFRACTORY TONIC-CLONIC STATUS EPILEPTICUS

Causes

Basic therapy of tonic-clonic status epilepticus is to treat the precipitating factors and to administer a full loading dose of phenytoin (or phenobarbital). If the seizures still are not controlled, a loading dose of phenobarbital (or phenytoin) should be added. Most cases of "refractory" tonic-clonic status epilepticus occur because the precipitating factors are not treated or because the dosage of phenytoin and/or phenobarbital administered is not sufficient to reach or maintain a therapeutic serum concentration. There are a small number of cases of tonic-clonic status epilepticus that do not respond to high therapeutic serum concentrations of phenytoin and phenobarbital. These patients usually have a large brain tumor or a large acute cerebral lesion (e.g., encephalitis) and represent a difficult therapeutic problem. Possible therapies will be considered now.

Paraldehyde

Paraldehyde is sometimes effective in controlling status epilepticus when phenytoin and phenobarbital fail (see above).

Muscle Relaxants (Curarisation)

Curarisation will prevent tonic and clonic movements and physical injury and will allow control of respirations [68]. However, this form of treatment does not prevent ongoing cerebral seizure activity. Animal studies indicate that prolonged seizure activity, even in paralyzed, respirated animals, may result in irreversible cerebral damage [6, 18, 19, 45, 66].

General Anesthesia

General anesthesia prevents tonic and clonic movements and allows control of respirations. General anesthesia also has the advantage of reducing cerebral seizure activity and reducing cerebral metabolic needs. There has never been an extensive study indicating the general anesthetic agent of choice or the proper duration of anesthesia for treating status epilepticus. Goldberg and McIntyre [22] reported excellent results in 5 patients treated with pentobarbital coma (burst suppression on EEG monitor) for 8 to 12 hours. A nonflammable anesthetic should be used if the EEG is going to be monitored.

Lidocaine
The evidence for the efficacy of lidocaine in status epilepticus consists of 148 cases in eight reports [4, 7, 59, 73]. In the only one of these studies that was controlled [59], lidocaine proved superior to placebo in all 3 patients studied. In almost every case, the patients received multiple drugs in addition to lidocaine. Nevertheless, these studies suggest that (1) intravenous lidocaine is effective against tonic-clonic and simple partial status epilepticus; (2) there are too few case reports to judge the efficacy of lidocaine against other types of status epilepticus; (3) lidocaine may sometimes control status epilepticus when varying combinations of diazepam, phenytoin, phenobarbital, and paraldehyde fail; (4) the antiepileptic effect of an intravenous bolus of lidocaine is rapid, with a decrease in seizures often noted in 20 to 30 seconds; (5) the antiepileptic effect of lidocaine is often transient, lasting 20 to 30 minutes; (6) it is sometimes necessary to start a continuous lidocaine infusion in order to keep the seizures under control; (7) lidocaine does not cause drowsiness.

The dosage of lidocaine for status epilepticus is not known precisely. Bernhard and Bohm [4] have the largest experience. They recommend initiating intravenous lidocaine with a single dose of 2 to 3 mg/kg. If the seizures do not stop, they may be refractory to lidocaine. If the seizures stop and then recur, they recommend a lidocaine infusion at a rate of 3 to 10 mg/kg/hour.

Before administering intravenous lidocaine for seizures one should be aware of the following precautions: (1) epilepsy is not an FDA-approved indication for lidocaine; (2) in high doses lidocaine may cause convulsions; (3) constant ECG and blood pressure monitoring is necessary to detect possible cardiovascular complications; (4) lidocaine should not be injected faster than 25 to 50 mg/minute; (5) the dosage recommended by Bernhard and Bohm [4] may exceed the maximum recommended by the manufacturer (200 to 300 mg/hour); and (6) evidence for proper usage in children is limited.

Simple Partial (Focal Motor) Status Epilepticus

CLINICAL PRESENTATION
Simple partial status epilepticus is the second most common form of status epilepticus [31] and may occur in patients with chronic seizure disorders or as a presenting symptom of an acute neurologic event. Focal motor status epilepticus in patients with chronic seizure disorders tends to be localized to the face and eyes or to the face and upper limbs [54]. The facial seizures tend to be more clonic, whereas the seizures affecting the limbs are apt to be tonic-clonic [54]. Even though the motor seizure activity remains localized, there may be some impairment of consciousness and/or autonomic disturbances [54]. The seizure focus on the EEG is usually frontal, central, or anterior temporal [54]. The ictal discharges are variable and may consist of spikes followed by slow waves, "recruiting" rhythm of 8 to 15 Hz, erratic activity, or no apparent abnormality on routine scalp EEG recordings [54]. Electrocorticographic examinations show many more electrical seizures than clinical seizures [54].

Focal motor status epilepticus occurring in the context of an acute neurologic event tends to be associated with serious conditions (vascular, traumatic, metabolic, encephalopathic) [54]. This type of status epilepticus is associated with the following features: altered consciousness, very high frequency of subclinical discharges, erratic seizure discharges on the EEG, and a tendency to develop into secondarily generalized tonic-clonic seizures [54].

MANAGEMENT
In managing focal motor status epilepticus the relative risks and benefits of therapies must be weighed. Intravenous diazepam will usually temporarily halt focal motor status epilepticus (see Table 30-3), and an intravenous loading dose of phenytoin will often completely end the attack [14, 65, 71]. However, there is some risk to administering intravenous diazepam or phenytoin, as mentioned earlier. If the focal motor seizures can be temporarily tolerated, it is less dangerous to administer an oral loading dose of phenytoin or phenobarbital.

In adults, 1000 mg of oral phenytoin can be given during an 8-hour period (400 mg initially, 300 mg after 4 hours, 300 mg 4 hours later), followed by maintenance doses of 300 to 400 mg/day (see Chap. 16). Therapeutic phenytoin serum concentrations will be reached 14 to 20 hours after the first dose. In children, four oral doses of 5 to 6 mg/kg of phenytoin at 8-hour intervals followed by maintenance doses of 3 mg/kg every 12 hours will result in therapeutic serum concentration 16 to 38 hours after the first dose [72]. An oral loading dose of phenobarbital may be administered by giving twice the maintenance dose for 4 days and then maintenance doses. With this regimen a steady phenobarbital serum concentration is reached in 3 days (see Chap. 17).

In patients whose focal motor seizures are not controlled with diazepam, phenytoin, and phenobarbital, a trial of oral carbamazepine or intravenous lidocaine, as previously described, may be helpful.

Complex Partial (Psychomotor, Temporal Lobe) Status Epilepticus

CLINICAL PRESENTATION
This rare form of status epilepticus may take 2 forms: (1) a prolonged twilight state with partial responsiveness, partial speech, and quasipurposeful automatisms; or (2) a series of complex partial seizures with staring, total unresponsiveness, speech arrest, and stereotyped automatisms with a twilight state between seizures [3, 10, 12, 39, 40, 42, 62]. The EEG during complex partial status epilepticus may show continuous slow activity (especially during twilight states) or temporal spike-and-slow-wave activity superimposed on a slow background (especially during actual complex partial seizures) [3, 10, 12, 39, 40, 62].

MANAGEMENT
Therapy of complex partial status epilepticus consists of administering an intravenous loading dose of phenytoin [71] or phenobarbital. Intravenous diazepam may rapidly end an attack (see Table 30-3) but carries some risk. Intravenous diazepam is indicated when the ongoing complex partial seizure activity represents an immediate serious threat to the patient's health and/or makes it impossible to administer a loading dose of a long-acting antiepileptic drug. There is some limited evidence that prolonged complex partial status epilepticus may result in permanent cognitive disability [61, 62], and this type of status epilepticus should be treated rapidly.

Absence (Petit Mal) Status Epilepticus

CLINICAL PRESENTATION
The clinical presentation of absence status epilepticus is altered consciousness often accompanied by mild clonic movements of the eyelids and hands and automatisms of the face and hands [2, 38, 47, 54]. The alteration of consciousness may range from a vague feeling that can be recognized only subjectively to stupor from which the patient can be aroused only with difficulty [2, 38, 47, 52, 54]. Attacks may last 30 minutes to 12 or more hours [2, 54]. Although absence seizures occur chiefly in children, a considerable percentage of cases of absence status epilepticus occurs in adults [2, 35, 54]. Adults who have failed to "outgrow" absence seizures seem particularly prone toward developing absence status epilepticus, and some adults with previously undiagnosed absence seizures may present in absence status epilepticus without a history of a seizure disorder [2]. The differential diagnosis of absence status epilepticus includes drug intoxication, psychosis, metabolic encephalopathy, structural brain lesion, complex partial seizure status epilepticus, and hysteria. The diagnosis of absence status epilepticus is definitively established with an EEG that shows spike-wave activity. The spike-wave activity may be continuous or discontinuous [2, 52, 54]. It may consist of regular 3-Hz spike-wave activity, but more commonly it shows irregular 2- to 3-Hz spike-wave and polyspike-wave activity [2, 38, 52, 54].

MANAGEMENT
Ethosuximide, valproic acid, and clonazepam, the long-acting antiepileptic drugs of choice for absence seizures, are not available in a preparation for intravenous administration and require several days to reach steady state serum concentration when administered orally (see Chaps. 14, 19, 20, and 21). Acetazolamide is a moderately effective antiabsence drug but is seldom used because other drugs are more consistently effective, and the antiabsence effect of acetazolamide is often transient (see Chap. 22). In absence status epilepticus intravenous acetazolamide is usually the first drug to try. It causes fewer side effects than intravenous diazepam, and if it is effective, oral maintenance doses can be begun simultaneously. The dosage of intravenous acetazolamide in absence status epilepticus is 250 mg for children weighing less than 35 kg and 500 mg for persons weighing more than 35 kg.

If acetazolamide fails to control absence status epilepticus, intravenous diazepam is usually very effective (see Table 30-3), although the effect may be transient. The patient may be managed with one or more doses of intravenous diazepam until an effective serum concentration of ethosuximide can be built up by the oral route. In this situation it may be necessary to use higher than usual starting doses of ethosuximide to achieve a therapeutic serum concentration rapidly. A starting dose of 750 mg/day in divided doses has been shown to produce relatively few side effects [6].

Febrile Status Epilepticus
This topic is reviewed in Chapter 25.

Tonic, Myoclonic, and Unilateral Status Epilepticus
These rare forms of status epilepticus have been reviewed by Roger et al. [54].

References

1. Albani, M. How to Use Phenytoin. In P. L. Marselli, J. K. Penry, and C. E. Pippenger (Eds.), *Antiepileptic Drug Therapy in Pediatrics.* New York: Raven Press, 1982.

2. Andermann, F., and Robb, J. P. Absence status: A reappraisal following a review of 38 patients. *Epilepsia* 13:177, 1972.

3. Belaisky, M. A. et al. Prolonged epileptic twilight states: Continuous recordings with nasopharyngeal electrodes and videotape analysis. *Neurology* (Minneap.) 28:239, 1978.

4. Bernhard, C. G., and Bohm, E. *Local Anesthetics as Anticonvulsants.* Uppsala: Almquist and Wiksell, 1965.

5. Booker, H. E., and Celesia, G. G. Serum concentration of diazepam in subjects with epilepsy. *Arch. Neurol.* 29:191, 1973.

6. Browne, T. R. Drug therapy of status epilepticus. *Drug Ther. Rev.* 2:449, 1979.

7. Browne, T. R. Paraldehyde, Chlormethiazole, and Lidocaine. In A. V. Delgado-Escueta et al. (Eds.), *Status Epilepticus: Mechanisms of Brain Damage and Treatment.* New York: Raven Press, 1982.

8. Browne, T. R. Unpublished data, 1982.

9. Browne, T. R., and Penry, J. K. Benzodiazepines in the treatment of epilepsy: A review. *Epilepsia* 14:277, 1973.

10. Celesia, G. G. EEG Monitoring in Status Epilepticus. In D. Janz (Ed.), *Epileptology.* Stuttgart: Thieme, 1976. Pp. 328–337.

11. Celesia, G. G. Modern concepts of status epilepticus. *J.A.M.A.* 235:1571, 1976.

12. Celesia, G. G., Messert, B., and Murphy, M. J. Status epilepticus of late adult onset. *Neurology* (Minneap.) 22:1047, 1972.

13. Cranford, R. E. et al. Intravenous phenytoin: Clinical and pharmacokinetic aspects. *Neurology* (N.Y.) 28:874, 1978.

14. Cranford, R. E. et al. Intravenous phenytoin in acute seizure disorders. *Neurology* (N.Y.) 29:1474, 1979.

15. Darnell, J. C., and Jay, S. J. Recurrent postictal pulmonary edema: A case report and review of the literature. *Epilepsia* 23:71, 1982.

16. Delgado-Escueta, A. V. et al. Current concepts in neurology: Management of status epilepticus. *N. Engl. J. Med.* 306:1337, 1982.

17. De Elio, F. J., De Jalon, P. G., and Obrador, D. Some experimental and clinical observations on the anticonvulsive action of paraldehyde. *J. Neurol. Neurosurg. Psychiatry* 12:19, 1949.

18. Duffy, T. E., Howse, D. C., and Plum, F. Cerebral energy metabolism during experimental status epilepticus. *J. Neurochem.* 24:925, 1975.

19. Epstein, M. H., and O'Connor, J. S. Destructive effects of prolonged status epilepticus. *J. Neurol. Neurosurg. Psychiatry* 29:251, 1966.

20. Fischer, S. P. et al. Disseminated intravascular coagulation in status epilepticus. *Thromb. Haemostas.* 38:909, 1977.

21. Glaser, G. H. Medical Complications of Status Epilepticus. In A. V. Delgado-Escueta et al. (Eds.), *Status Epilepticus: Mechanisms of Brain Damage and Treatment.* New York: Raven Press, 1982.

22. Goldberg, M., and McIntyre, H. Barbiturates in the Treatment of Status Epilepticus. In A. V. Delgado-Escueta et al. (Eds.), *Status Epilepticus: Mechanisms of Brain Damage and Treatment.* New York: Raven Press, 1982.

23. Guterman, A. et al. Paraldehyde pharmacokinetics and its use in status epilepticus. *Epilepsia.* In press, 1983.

24. Hauser, W. A. Epidemiology, Morbidity, and Mortality of Status Epilepticus. In A. V. Delgado-Escueta et al. (Eds.), *Status Epilepticus: Mechanisms of Brain Damage and Treatment.* New York: Raven Press, 1982.

25. Heimann, G., and Gladtke, E. Pharmacokinetics of phenobarbital in childhood. *Eur. J. Clin. Pharmacol.* 12:305, 1977.

26. Hillestad, L. et al. Diazepam metabolism in normal man: 1. Serum concentrations and clinical effects after intravenous, intramuscular, and oral administration. *Clin. Pharmacol. Ther.* 16:479, 1974.

27. Hunter, R. A. Status epilepticus: History, incidence, and problems. *Epilepsia* 1:162, 1959–1960.

28. Jalling, B. Plasma and cerebrospinal fluid concentrations of phenobarbital in infants given single doses. *Dev. Med. Child Neurol.* 16:781, 1974.

29. Janz, D. Conditions and causes of status epilepticus. *Epilepsia* 2:170, 1961.

30. Kaplan, S. A. et al. Pharmacokinetic profile of diazepam following single intravenous and chronic oral administrations. *J. Pharm. Sci.* 62:1789, 1973.

31. Kas, S., and Orszagh, J. Clinical study of status epilepticus: Review of 111 statuses. *Acta Univ. Carol. [Med.] (Praha)* 22:133, 1976.

32. Klotz, V., Antoinin, K. H., and Bieck, P. R. Pharmacokinetics and plasma binding of diazepam in man, dog, rabbit, guinea pig and rat. *J. Pharmacol. Exp. Ther.* 199:67, 1976.

33. Korttila, K., Stohman, A., and Anderson, P. Polyethylene glycol as a solvent for diazepam: Bio-

availability and clinical effects after intramuscular administration, comparison of oral, intramuscular and rectal administration, and precipitation from intravenous solutions. *Acta Pharmacol. Toxicol.* 39:104, 1976.

34. Kostenbauder, H. B. et al. Bioavailability and single-dose pharmacokinetics of intramuscular phenytoin. *Clin. Pharmacol. Ther.* 18:449, 1975.

35. Lipman, I. J., Saacs, E. R., and Suter, C. G. Petit mal status epilepticus. *Electroencephalogr. Clin. Neurophysiol.* 30:162, 1971.

36. Lockman, L. A. Phenobarbital Dosage for Neonatal Seizures. In A. V. Delgado-Escueta et al. (Eds.), *Status Epilepticus: Mechanisms of Brain Damage and Treatment.* New York: Raven Press, 1982.

37. Loughnan, P. M. et al. Pharmacokinetic observations of phenytoin disposition in the newborn and young infant. *Arch. Dis. Child.* 52:302, 1977.

38. Lugaresi, E., Pazzaglia, P., and Tassinari, C. A. Differentiation of absence status and temporal lobe status. *Epilepsia* 12:77, 1971.

39. Markand, O. N., Wheeler, G. L., and Pollack, S. L. Complex partial status epilepticus (psychomotor status). *Neurology* (N.Y.) 28:189, 1978.

40. Mayeux, R., and Lueders, H. Complex partial status epilepticus: A case report and a proposal for diagnostic criteria. *Neurology* (N.Y.) 28:957, 1978.

41. Maynert, E. W. Phenobarbital, Mephobarbital, and Metharbital: Absorption, Distribution, and Excretion. In D. M. Woodbury, J. K. Penry, and R. P. Schmidt (Eds.), *Antiepileptic Drugs.* New York: Raven Press, 1972.

42. McBride, M. C., Dooling, E. C., and Oppenheimer, E. Y. Complex partial status epilepticus in young children. *Ann. Neurol.* 9:526, 1981.

43. McGreal, D. A. The emergency treatment of convulsions in childhood. *Practitioner* 181:719, 1958.

44. McWilliam, P. K. A., and Leeds, M. B. IV phenytoin sodium in continuous convulsions in children. *Lancet* 2:1147, 1958.

45. Meldrum, B. S., Vigouroux, R. A., and Brierly, J. B. Systemic factors and epileptic brain damage: Prolonged seizures in paralyzed, artificially ventilated baboons. *Arch. Neurol.* 28:82, 1973.

46. Milligan, N. et al. Absorption of diazepam from the rectum and its effect on interictal spikes in the EEG. *Epilepsia* 23:323, 1982.

47. Moe, P. G. Spike wave stupor: Petit mal status. *Am. J. Dis. Child.* 121:307, 1971.

48. Oxbury, J. M., and Whitty, C. W. M. Causes and consequences of status epilepticus in adults: A study of 86 cases. *Brain* 94:733, 1971.

49. Painter, M. J. Principles of Treatment: Neonates. In A. V. Delgado-Escueta et al. (Eds.), *Status Epilepticus: Mechanisms of Brain Damage and Treatment.* New York: Raven Press, 1982.

50. Painter, M. J. et al. Phenobarbital and phenytoin in neonatal seizures: Metabolism and tissue distribution. *Neurology* (N.Y.) 31:1107, 1982.

51. Paulson, O. B., Gyory, A., and Hertz, M. H. Blood-brain transfer and uptake of antiepileptic drugs. *Clin. Pharmacol. Ther.* 32:466, 1982.

52. Porter, R. J., and Penry, J. K. Absence Status (Spike-Wave Stupor). In A. V. Delgado-Escueta et al. (Eds.), *Status Epilepticus: Mechanisms of Brain Damage and Treatment.* New York: Raven Press, 1982.

53. Reynolds, E. H. Chronic antiepileptic toxicity: A review. *Epilepsia* 16:319, 1975.

54. Roger, J., Lob, H., and Tassinari, C. A. Status Epilepticus. In O. Magnus, and A. M. Lorentz de Hass (Eds.), *The Epilepsies.* Amsterdam: North-Holland, 1974. Pp. 145–188.

55. Rowan, A. J., and Scott, D. F. Major status epilepticus: A series of 42 patients. *Acta Neurol. Scand.* 46:573, 1970.

56. Sharer, L., and Kutt, H. Intravenous administration of diazepam. *Arch. Neurol.* 24:169, 1971.

57. Schmidt, D. Benzodiazepines: Diazepam. In D. M. Woodbury, J. K. Penry, and C. E. Pippenger (Eds.), *Antiepileptic Drugs.* New York: Raven Press, 1982.

58. Sturdee, D. W. Diazepam: Routes of administration and rate of absorption. *Br. J. Anaesth.* 48:1091, 1976.

59. Taverner, D., and Bain, W. A. Intravenous lignocaine as an anticonvulsant: In status epilepticus and serial epilepsy. *Lancet* 2:1145, 1958.

60. Thurston, J. H. et al. New enzymatic method for measurement of paraldehyde: Correlation of effects with serum and CSF levels. *J. Lab. Clin. Med.* 72:699, 1968.

61. Treiman, D. M. General Principles of Treatment: Responsive and Intractable Status in Adults. In A. V. Delgado-Escueta et al. (Eds.), *Status Epilepticus: Mechanisms of Brain Damage and Treatment.* New York: Raven Press, 1982.

62. Treiman, D. M., and Delgado-Escueta, A. V. Complex Partial Status. In A. V. Delgado-Escueta et al. (Eds.), *Status Epilepticus: Mechanisms of Brain Damage and Treatment.* New York: Raven Press, 1982.

63. Vernadakis, A., and Woodbury, D. M. Maturational Factors in the Development of Seizures. In H. H. Jasper, A. A. Ward, and A. Pope (Eds.), *Basic Mecha-*

nisms of the Epilepsies. Boston: Little, Brown, 1969. Pp. 535–541.

64. Viswanathan, C. T., Booker, H. E., and Welling, P. G. Bioavailability of oral and intramuscular phenobarbital. *J. Clin. Pharmacol.* 18:100, 1978.

65. Wallis, W., Kutt, H., and McDowell, F. Intravenous diphenylhydantoin in treatment of acute repetitive seizures. *Neurology* (Minneap.) 18:513, 1968.

66. Wasterlain, C. G. Consensus on Basic Mechanisms of Status Epilepticus. In A. V. Delgado-Escueta et al. (Eds.), *Status Epilepticus: Mechanisms of Brain Damage and Treatment.* New York: Raven Press, 1982.

67. Wechsler, I. S. Intravenous injection of paraldehyde for the control of convulsions. *J.A.M.A.* 114:2198, 1940.

68. Whitty, C. W. N., and James, J. L. The electroencephalogram as a monitor of status epilepticus suppressed peripherally by curarisation. *Lancet* 2:239, 1961.

69. Whitty, C. W. N., and Taylor, M. Treatment of status epilepticus. *Lancet* 2:591, 1949.

70. Wilder, B. J., and Bruni, J. *Seizure Disorders: A Pharmacological Approach to Treatment.* New York: Raven Press, 1981.

71. Wilder, B. J. et al. Efficacy of intravenous phenytoin in treatment of status epilepticus: Kinetics of central nervous system penetration. *Ann. Neurol.* 1:511, 1977.

72. Wilson, J. T., Hojer, B., and Rane, A. Loading and conventional dose therapy with phenytoin in children: Kinetic profile of parent drug and main metabolites in plasma. *Clin. Pharmacol. Ther.* 20:48, 1976.

73. Ying-K'un, F. et al. The therapeutic effect of intravenous Xylocaine on status epilepticus. *Clin. Med. J.* 82:668, 1963.

INTRACTABLE SEIZURES

31

Roger J. Porter

A considerable and disheartening proportion of patients with epilepsy are subject to seizures that resist even the most vigorous therapeutic efforts. Every seizure type is represented among these patients, but infantile spasms and atonic-myoclonic attacks in children and partial seizures in both children and adults are especially prevalent. The patient with intractable seizures has suffered uncontrolled attacks for years. He has seen numerous physicians, taken many medications, and experienced considerable drug toxicity. His hopes have been raised many times by this regimen or that, only to be followed by frustration when each has failed. He may then become cynical or withdrawn, and his enthusiasm for physicians and their skills is understandably diminished.

The subject of intractable seizures will be discussed in six sections: (1) the general approach to the patient and the recognition of truly intractable cases; (2) the use of newer diagnostic and therapeutic techniques; (3) the use of these techniques in a highly resistant group of patients; (4) nonpharmacologic approaches; (5) the role of institutionalization; and (6) the value of this information to the practitioner. This chapter will concentrate on complex partial seizures, the most common form of intractable seizures in adults, because their control achieves major functional gains in affected patients, most of whom have normal intelligence. The management principles suggested here for complex partial seizures can be applied to other types of seizures as well.

The General Approach

The key to outpatient diagnosis and therapy of patients with intractable seizures is the history. The initial history gives the information needed to make a "seizure diagnosis," and the continuing history provides feedback on the efficacy of therapy. The "seizure diagnosis," usually based on the International Classification of Epileptic Seizures [3], is the name given empirically to the patient's type of attack. Although not necessarily of etiologic importance, the seizure diagnosis is extremely important in the therapeutic effort. Failure to establish a proper seizure diagnosis, either by obtaining and interpreting a history or by special diagnostic techniques, often leads to poor seizure control and medication toxicity from improper drugs.

Furthermore, when the physician is uncertain of the seizure diagnosis, he may use medications in a nonspecific way, resorting to polypharmacy before single drugs have been given an adequate trial. The physician who knows that he is dealing with absence seizures, for example, will utilize ethosuximide or valproic acid with confidence and vigor. When the seizure diagnosis is unknown, however, the usual starting medications are phenytoin or phenobarbital, or both, which are often given in subtherapeutic doses and frequently end in failure and frustration.

The first priority, therefore, is to establish the seizure diagnosis. To accomplish this, a detailed description of the attacks must be obtained. Many patients are not prepared for such a description, and others will give a terminology oriented description, using such terms as *petit mal* or *temporal lobe*. The physician must reorient the patient to more fundamental descriptive terms. I usually begin by asking patients to select a typical seizure (or one that they specifically recall) and then ask, "What is the first thing that happens?" Patients with simple partial seizures, or those with auras only, will be able to describe the entire event by themselves in logical sequence. Patients with complex partial seizures will need assistance, either from persons who have seen the attacks or from a knowledge of what they have been told. I often ask, for example, "What do other people see when you have a seizure? What do they observe?" Finally, it is important to learn whether the attack ends abruptly or whether it tapers into a postictal state. One good question is "Do you feel 'bad' or 'tired' after an attack?" A positive response strongly suggests the presence of an abnormal postictal state, which would generally rule out absence seizures.

It is not usually necessary, except when hysteria is part of the differential diagnosis, to obtain a detailed description of generalized tonic-clonic (grand mal) seizures because these are generally stereotyped and accompany a wide variety of more fundamental seizure types. They are probably secondary to the fundamental type and are relatively easy to control in most patients.

When a seizure diagnosis cannot be made from the history alone, the task becomes more difficult. Routine electroencephalograms (EEGs) will be of some assistance, and activation procedures, such as hyperventilation, photic stimulation, and sleep deprivation, should always be used in recording the EEG (see Chap. 11). Naturally, general and neurologic examinations should be performed, but they are infrequently useful in determining the seizure diagnosis. CT scans are also not particularly useful in this regard but may be very helpful in uncovering unsuspected lesions, especially in this group of chronically affected patients who are not often restudied.

Newer Diagnostic and Therapeutic Techniques

A growing number of centers are beginning to recognize the value of the "seizure diagnosis" and are utilizing advanced techniques to obtain this information when the historical data are inadequate and confirmation by more objective means is desired. Because a maximum degree of observation and control must be exercised for the period of evaluation, these techniques have been grouped under the heading *intensive monitoring* [21]. It is not entirely possible to separate diagnostic and therapeutic efforts, but one approach is shown in Figure 31-1. The techniques employed in these efforts are described below.

The first technique is long-term EEG recording. This is useful for diagnosis when an ictal recording of a seizure is needed to assist in establishing the seizure type [15, 21, 22, 23, 28]. Long-term EEG recording also gives objective information about the severity of the disorder, as in absence seizures, in which the number of spike-wave bursts may be counted; these have a high correlation with decreased mental function [1, 20]. Quantification of abnormal paroxysmal discharges also allows evaluation of the efficacy of therapy, especially with seizures that occur frequently such as absence seizures [14]. Long-term EEG recording is accomplished either by direct recording with the EEG apparatus or by telemetry; the latter technique allows more freedom of movement for the patient and encourages a more normal environment. The various systems have been reviewed elsewhere [18, 24].

Video recording of seizures is the most effective way to establish the "seizure diagnosis" [15, 21, 22, 23, 28]. When the history is inadequate or even, surprisingly, when it appears to be rather good, a video record of an attack can be very revealing. Several methods of combining the televised view of the patient with the simultaneously recorded EEG have been developed [22], and long-term video and EEG recordings are carried out together at many epilepsy centers. Nevertheless, video analysis has not been adequately utilized to define exactly the characteristics of many seizure types. Although this technique has provided an extensive understanding of absence attacks [13], and some data are available on complex partial seizures [4], much work remains to be done on other types of attacks.

The final technique used in intensive monitoring is frequent determinations of antiepileptic drug levels. These should be performed daily and more often when indicated. The blood should be drawn prior to the morning dose of medication; the level obtained reflects the lowest drug concentration of the day. Blood drug levels are easily compared from day to day in the same patient because the morning drug concentration

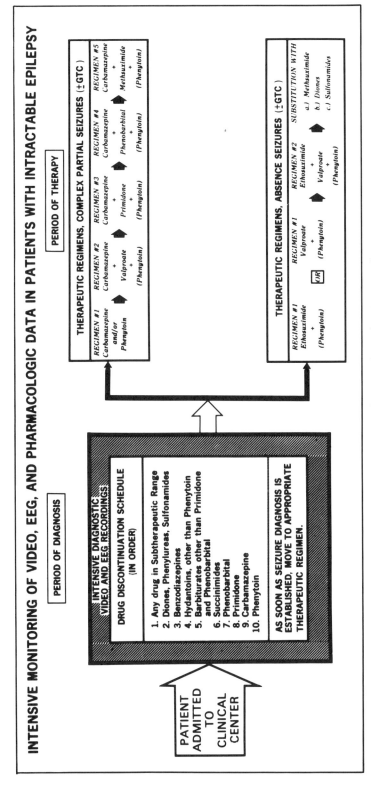

Figure 31-1. Method for evaluation and treatment of in-tractable seizures (suspected complex partial seizures). Each patient undergoes a period of diagnostic evaluation followed by a therapeutic regimen appropriate to the seizure diagnosis. During the diagnostic period, medications are gradually dis-continued in the order listed, although this sequence may not always be rigidly followed. After the seizure diagnosis is estab-lished (see text), the patient is started on the appropriate thera-peutic regimen. Regimen 1 is preferred because there are fewer side effects at therapeutic doses. Each succeeding regi-men is more likely to be associated with medication toxicity.

Regimens 4 and 5 are of questionable value for complex partial seizures. The substitution of other succinimides, diones, or sulfonamides is likewise of questionable value for absence seizures. Clonazepam, despite its considerable toxi-city, may be useful in cases of especially refractory absence seizures. A seizure diagnosis will often be established before the elimination of all unwanted medications; these can be eliminated as appropriate therapy is begun. Patients with concomitant generalized tonic-clonic seizures may require phenytoin, which is included in parenthesis for each regimen. In all cases, single drug therapy is preferred whenever possible.

is the level least affected by peaks of drug absorption that occur during the day. The use of blood drug level determinations in therapeutic decisions has been amply reviewed in Chapter 15 and elsewhere [9, 17] and will be only summarized here. The key elements are: (1) Blood drug levels are a *guide* to changes in therapy; they are not a substitute for clinical judgment; (2) expected therapeutic levels are average values; individual patients will have individual optimal levels; (3) blood drug level determinations assist in achieving the maximal effects of single medications; (4) measurement of blood drug levels is invaluable in the presence of toxic effects, especially in patients taking multiple drugs; (5) noncompliance, malabsorption, and altered metabolism can be identified, but only the first is a common problem.

The critical feature of intensive monitoring in patients with intractable seizures is the combined use of these techniques to obtain improved seizure control with minimal drug toxicity. Figure 31-1 outlines the basic plan employed in the Clinical Epilepsy Section of the National Institutes of Health for patients with intractable seizures suspected to be of the complex partial type. Because a significant number of these patients have absence seizures [21], a therapeutic regimen has been outlined for these two seizure types. Each patient is hospitalized and enters the "period of diagnosis" in which long-term video and EEG recordings are obtained at the same time medications are gradually discontinued. The discontinuation schedule, which is only a general guide, serves two purposes—it allows elimination of drugs that are thought to be inappropriate or unnecessarily toxic, and it causes a gradually increasing seizure frequency. This increased frequency increases the yield of long-term video and EEG recordings, permitting a seizure diagnosis as early as possible. Medications with long half-lives and those that are primarily antiabsence in effect can be stopped abruptly. Primidone and carbamazepine are discontinued more slowly, and phenytoin, when it is the last drug to be removed, is also removed cautiously to avoid excessive generalized tonic-clonic attacks. Patients are permitted a weekend pass only when their medication regimen is stable and not, as a rule, during the drug discontinuation period.

As soon as a seizure diagnosis is established by analysis of the long-term video and EEG recordings, the patient enters the "period of therapy" and begins a series of suggested regimens that are chosen according to the seizure diagnosis. Although the regimens shown in Figure 31-1 are designed for patients who have either complex partial or absence seizures, the concept can be easily applied to other kinds of seizures.

A detailed analysis of which drugs are most appropriate for common seizure types is available [19]. Although barbiturates have long been considered the safest antiepileptic drug, some investigators [6, 8, 11, 26, 27, 28, 29] have urged neurologists to recognize their often subtle cognitive and behavioral toxicity and to consider other nonsedative medications. The regimens recommended here reflect the strong view that physicians no longer need to handicap their patients with sedating agents.

Application of Newer Techniques in a Selected Population

Patients with severe epilepsy are referred to the Clinical Epilepsy Section of the National Institutes of Health for evaluation and for possible participation in research protocols. Twenty-three of 105 such patients were chosen for a study evaluating the hypothesis that intensive monitoring by video recording, long-term telemetered EEGs, and daily antiepileptic drug level determinations could improve seizure control, decrease medication toxicity, and enhance rehabilitation potential. The results of this study have been published [22, 23] and will be summarized here.

The 23 patients were selected according to the following criteria: (1) complex partial seizures were probable, but in many cases the diagnosis was uncertain; (2) attacks were frequent; (3) seizures were intractable to previous therapy; (4) no previous surgical therapy had been tried; and (5) seizures were severely limiting or incapacitating socially. All but 2 patients were referred by neurologists and neurosurgeons. The patients were admitted for baseline evaluation before entering the period of intensive monitoring and drug discontinuation (Fig. 31-1). Most were taking numerous medications. Attacks were recorded and analyzed in all but 1 patient, who had no seizures on camera despite 14 6-hour recordings. Sixteen of the patients were found to have complex partial seizures, and 4 had absence seizures. Following baseline seizure frequency determinations, these patients then entered the appropriate "period of therapy" (Fig. 31-1). Of the remaining 3 patients, 1 had clonic seizures, 1 had hysterical attacks, and 1 remained without a seizure diagnosis. After application of the most efficacious regimen, the patients were discharged; the average total hospitalization time was slightly over 8 weeks. At discharge, seizure frequency was reduced in 61 percent, medication toxicity was decreased in 74 percent, and improvement in job or school rehabilitation was realized in 40 percent. These results were maintained at the time of follow-up 25 months later [23]. This study strongly suggests that patients with intractable epilepsy can benefit from intensive monitoring techniques and that therapy should be specific and appropriate to the seizure diagnosis. Other groups have now applied similar intensive monitoring techniques for managing refractory epilepsy with similar beneficial results [7, 28].

Nonpharmacologic Approaches to the Patient with Intractable Seizures

Although this chapter is concerned primarily with the proper use of antiepileptic drugs in patients with severe seizures, other therapeutic approaches require at least a brief discussion. The most important of these is surgical management, which is reviewed in Chapter 25 and elsewhere [25]. When the lesion can be localized both electrographically and anatomically, extirpation of the focus is relatively straightforward, and the difficulty of removal is related primarily to the proximity of the lesion to such critical brain structures as the speech area or motor strip. When pharmacologic approaches fail, there should be little hesitation in considering surgical intervention in patients with well-localized lesions.

When the lesion is not well localized, different surgical strategies can be tried. Stereotactic lesions have been made in the internal capsule, basal ganglia, thalamus, hypothalamus, cingulate gyrus, and fields of Forel. As Ojemann and Ward [12] point out, these are largely experimental procedures for severely refractory seizures, and no definitive methods have been established. Although some stereotactic methods are used to destroy foci, other methods are designed to interrupt neural pathways of propagation and generalization and are theoretically appropriate for patients with primarily generalized seizures or with multifocal disease. Cerebral commissurotomy has also been used with some success (see Chap. 25). Cerebellar stimulator implants for patients with intractable seizures are reviewed in Chapter 25.

A relatively new approach to seizure disorders is that of behavior modification, which is reviewed in Chapter 24 and elsewhere [5, 10]. The effectiveness of these techniques requires much more study in well-defined and well-controlled populations before serious consideration can be given to their use as a routine alternative to drug therapy in patients with intractable seizures.

Institutionalization

Although the most recent trend in the United States in the management of epilepsy has been toward deinstitutionalization, there are still a number of incapacitated patients who require a sheltered environment. The kind of environment needed is well stated by the Commission for the Control of Epilepsy and Its Consequences [2]:

The ultimate objective is a therapeutic community that breaks down the barrier between the institution and the natural community; provides living arrangements so similar to ordinary ones as not to be distinguished by the casual observer; concentrates on the special medical needs of persons with epilepsy; and preserves the dignity of the individual in spite of the need for supervision.

The commission was not able to identify such institutions in the United States. In Europe, however, several, such as De Cruquiushoeve in the Netherlands and The David Lewis Centre in England, are dedicated to implementing the concepts expressed above. Whether the United States will reverse its trend and begin to provide the needed environment for these patients is uncertain.

Implications for the Practitioner

Although sophisticated techniques have been described here, most patients with seizures do not require such intensive study. The seizure diagnosis can be made in most patients by taking a careful history. The pharmacologic approaches outlined here and in the articles noted in references provide the necessary information for treating seizure disorders as specifically as possible using current understanding of seizure types. Plasma drug levels can now be reliably obtained from a large number of laboratories [16], allowing maximal therapeutic benefit of the most effective and least toxic medications. Drug tapering and removal *can* be accomplished in outpatients, even though many months may be necessary to complete the task.

The patient whose seizure history does not yield a specific seizure diagnosis or in whom various therapeutic regimens, properly delivered and compliantly followed, have been unsuccessful must be referred to a center specializing in the most difficult cases. Intensive monitoring is increasingly available, and surgical expertise can usually be found in the same centers. Such centers often have research protocols for investigational drugs when further trials of conventional medications seem unwarranted. The majority of patients with intractable seizures can attain some seizure control by making use of the expertise now available. Virtually all patients with seizures, barring other physical or mental handicaps, can become participating and productive members of society. This certainly should be the goal of the treating physician.

References

1. Browne, T. R. et al. Responsiveness before, during, and after spike-wave paroxysms. *Neurology* (Minneap.) 24:659–665, 1974.

2. Commission for the Control of Epilepsy and Its Consequences. *Plan for Nationwide Action on Epilepsy*, Vol. 2, Part I (Department of Health, Education and Welfare Publication No. (NIH) 78-312). Bethesda, Md.: National Institutes of Health, 1977.

3. Dreifuss, F. E. Proposal for revised clinical and electroencephalographic classification of epileptic seizures. *Epilepsia* 22:489, 1981.

4. Escueta, A. V. et al. Lapse of consciousness and automatisms in temporal lobe epilepsy: A videotape analysis. *Neurology* (Minneap.) 27:144, 1977.

5. Feldman, R. G., and Ricks, N. L. Nonpharmacologic and Behavioral Methods. In E. S. Ferriss (Ed.), *Treatment of Epilepsy Today*. Dradill, N. J.: Medical Economics Co., 1978.

6. Gamstorp, I. Treatment with Carbamazepine: Children. In J. K. Penry, and D. D. Daly (Eds.), *Complex Partial Seizures and Their Treatment*, Vol. 11, *Advances in Neurology*. New York: Raven Press, 1975.

7. Gumnit, R. J. Treatment of intractable seizures. *Epilepsia*. In press, 1983.

8. Hutt, S. J. et al. Perceptual-motor behavior in relation to blood phenobarbital level: A preliminary report. *Dev. Med. Child Neurol.* 10:626, 1968.

9. Kutt, H., and Penry, J. K. Usefulness of blood levels of antiepileptic drugs. *Arch. Neurol.* 31:283, 1974.

10. Mostofsky, D. I., and Balaschak, B. A. Psychobiological control of seizures. *Psychol. Bull.* 84:723, 1977.

11. Mycek, M. J., and Brezenoff, H. E. Tolerance to centrally administered phenobarbital. *Biochem. Pharmacol.* 25:501, 1976.

12. Ojemann, G. A., and Ward, A. A., Jr. Stereotactic and Other Procedures for Epilepsy. In D. P. Purpura, J. K. Penry, and R. D. Walter (Eds.), *Neurosurgical Management of the Epilepsies,* Vol. 8, *Advances in Neurology*. New York: Raven Press, 1975.

13. Penry, J. K., Porter, R. J., and Dreifuss, F. E. Simultaneous recording of absence seizures with video tape and electroencephalography. A study of 374 seizures in 48 patients. *Brain* 98:427, 1975.

14. Penry, J. K., Porter, R. J., and Dreifuss, F. E. Ethosuximide. Relation of Plasma Levels to Clinical Control. In D. M. Woodbury, J. K. Penry, and R. P. Schmidt (Eds.), *Antiepileptic Drugs*. New York: Raven Press, 1972.

15. Perry, T. R., Gumnit, R. J., and Gates, J. R. A comparison of the effectiveness of routine EEG and intensive monitoring in evaluating of intractable epilepsy. *Epilepsia*. In press, 1983.

16. Pippenger, C. E. et al. Proficiency testing in determinations of antiepileptic drugs. *J. Analyt. Toxicol.* 1:118, 1977.

17. Pippenger, C. E., Penry, J. K., and Kutt, H. *Antiepileptic Drugs: Quantitative Analysis and Interpretation*. New York: Raven Press, 1978.

18. Porter, R. J. Methodology of Continuous Monitoring with Videotape Recording and Electroencephalography. In J. A. Wada, and J. K. Penry (Eds.), *Advances in Epileptology: The Tenth Epilepsy International Symposium*. New York: Raven Press, 1980.

19. Porter, R. J., and Penry, J. K. Efficacy and Choice of Antiepileptic Drugs. In H. Meinardi, and A. J. Rowan (Eds.), *Advances in Epileptology, 1977: Psychology, Pharmacotherapy, and New Diagnostic Approaches*. Proceedings of the Thirteenth Congress of the International League Against Epilepsy and Ninth Symposium of the International Bureau for Epilepsy, Amsterdam, September 1977. Amsterdam: Swets and Zeitlinger, 1978.

20. Porter, R. J., Penry, J. K., and Dreifuss, F. E. Responsiveness at the onset of spike-wave bursts. *Electroencephalogr. Clin. Neurophysiol.* 34:239, 1973.

21. Porter, R. J., Penry, J. K., and Lacy, J. R. Diagnostic and therapeutic reevaluation of patients with intractable epilepsy. *Neurology* (Minneap.) 27:1006, 1977.

22. Porter, R. J., Penry, J. K., and Wolf, A. A., Jr. Simultaneous Documentation of Clinical and Electroencephalographic Manifestations of Epileptic Seizures. In P. Kellaway, and I. Petersen (Eds.), *Quantitative Analytic Studies in Epilepsy*. New York: Raven Press, 1976.

23. Porter, R. J., Theodore, W. H., and Schulman, E. A. Intensive monitoring of intractable epilepsy: A two year follow-up. *Acta Neurol. Scand.* (Suppl. 79) 62:48, 1980.

24. Porter, R. J., Wolf, A. A., Jr., and Penry, J. K. Human electroencephalographic telemetry. A review of systems and their applications and a new receiving system. *Am. J. EEG Technol.* 11:145, 1971.

25. Purpura, D. P., Penry, J. K., and Walter, R. D. (Eds.), *Neurosurgical Management of the Epilepsies,* Vol. 8, *Advances in Neurology*. New York: Raven Press, 1975.

26. Schain, R. J., and Watanabe, K. Effect of chronic phenobarbital administration upon brain growth of the infant rat. *Exp. Neurol.* 47:509, 1975.

27. Schain, R. J., and Watanabe, K. Research note. Origin of brain growth retardation in young rats treated with phenobarbital. *Exp. Neurol.* 50:806, 1976.

28. Sutula, T. P. et al. Intensive monitoring in refractory epilepsy. *Neurology* 31:243, 1981.
29. Trimble, M Effect of antiepileptic drugs on psychosocial development: Phenobarbital and primidone. In P. L Morselli, J. K. Penry, and C. E. Pippenger (Eds.), *Antiepileptic Drug Therapy in Pediatrics.* New York: Raven Press, 1982.

Conversion Table of Units for Antiepileptic Drug Serum Concentration Determinations ("Blood Levels")

Weight-per-Volume Conversions
10 micrograms per milliliter (μg/ml) = 10 milligrams per liter (mg/L) =
1.0 milligrams per 100 milliliters (mg/100 ml) = 1.0 milligrams per deciliter (mg/dl)

Weight per Volume to Molar Conversions

DRUG	CONVERSION FACTOR (μg/ml to micromoles)
Carbamazepine	4.232
Clonazepam	3.168
Diazepam	3.511
Ethosuximide	7.083
Ethotoin	4.896
Mephenytoin	4.581
Metharbital	5.044
Methsuximide	4.920
Methylphenobarbital	4.060
N-Desmethyl-methsuximide	5.285
Paramethadione	6.362
Phenacemide	5.611
Phenobarbital	4.306
Phensuximide	5.285
Phenytoin	3.964
Primidone	4.581
Trimethadione	6.985
Valproic acid	6.934

INDEX

Fetal trimethadione syndrome, 253–254
Fetus. *See* Pregnancy
Fever
    cause of, in febrile seizure evaluation, 317
    reduction of, in febrile seizure management, 318
    seizures and, 135, 315–320. *See also* Febrile seizure(s)
First aid for seizure, 260–262
Flame ionization detector, for gas chromatography, 166
Flexor spasms, 95–106. *See also* Infantile spasms
Focal hypersynchrony in interictal EEGs, 33
Focal motor status epilepticus, 350–351
Focal paroxysmal activity, in interictal EEGs, 56
Focal seizures, 3, 29–37. *See also* Simple partial seizure(s)
Focal slow-wave activity, in interictal EEGs, 33
Focal spikes, in interictal EEGs, 33
Focus(i), epileptogenic
    confirmation of, as criteria for surgical therapy, 284–287
    functional changes in, 13–16
    morphologic changes in, 16
Folate, low serum levels of, from phenytoin, 184–185
Friends, as resource for patient with epilepsy, 139–140

Gamma-aminobutyric acid (GABA)
    and benzodiazepine receptors, 235–236
    disorders of metabolism of, 15–16
Gas chromatographic mass spectrometry, 168
Gas chromatography, 165–168
    applications of, 166–167
    basic principles of, 165–166
    derivitization of antiepileptic drugs in, 166
    detectors for, 166
    extraction of antiepileptic drugs in, 166
    internal standard for, 166
    sources of error in, 167–168
Gastroesophageal reflux, infantile spasms differentiated from, 101
Generalized epilepsies, classification of, 27
Generalized seizure(s)
    classification of, 24–25
    complex partial seizures evolving to, 43
    simple partial seizures evolving to, 32–33
    tonic-clonic, definition of, 51
Generic preparations, oral, effect on absorption, 145
Genetics
    absence seizures and, 62
    febrile seizures and, 315

Genetics—*Continued*
    in infantile spasms, 97
    of tonic-clonic seizures, 51–52
Gestural automatisms, in complex partial seizures, 42
Glia
    amino acid production by, 15
    damage to, symptomatic epilepsy due to, 124
    metabolic stimulation of, 14–15
    potassium regulation and, 14
    transmitter clearance by, 15
Gliomas, seizures and, 131
Gliosis, in epilepsy, 16
Global tonic seizures, 85
Glucose levels, low, seizures and, 133
    in neonate, 304
Glycogen storage diseases, neonatal seizures and, 305
Grand mal seizures, 4, 51–58. *See also* Tonic-clonic seizure(s)
Growth, effects of maternal use of antiepileptic drugs on, 335–336
Gustatory seizures, 32

Hallucinations, simple partial onset of complex partial seizures with, 41
Head, injuries to
    during tonic-clonic seizures, prevention of, 261
    epileptogenic effects of, 130
Hematologic system
    effects of carbamazepine on, 210
    effects of phenytoin on, 184–185
    effects of trimethadione on, 253
    effects of valproic acid on, 231
Hemeralopia, from trimethadione, 253
Hemispherectomy, 292
Hemodialysis, effects of, on antiepileptic drug elimination, 149
Hemorrhage
    intracranial, neonatal seizures and, 302–303
    neonatal, antiepileptic drugs and, 336–337
Hepatic failure
    effects of, on antiepileptic drug biotransformation, 148–149
    epileptic seizures and, 133
Hepatic toxicity
    from phenacemide, 255–256
    from phenytoin, 183
    from valproic acid, 230–231
Heroin, maternal use of, and neonatal seizures, 305
History
    in febrile seizure evaluation, 317
    in intractable seizure diagnosis, 355, 356
    in neonatal seizure evaluation, 306
Hormone(s)
    brain levels of, in infantile spasms, 97
    sex, seizures and, 333
Hospitalization
    nursing care during, 259–262

Hospitalization—*Continued*
    seizures and, 135
Hydantoins, 175–189. *See also specific drug*
Hydrocephalus, shunting for, seizure frequency and, 294
Hyperammonemia, neonatal seizures and, 305
Hyperglycinemia, neonatal seizures and, 305
Hypernatremia
    neonatal seizures and, 304
    seizures and, 132
Hypersynchrony, focal, in interictal EEGs, 33
Hyperventilation
    absence seizures and, 70
    activating effect of, 121
    normal response to, 120–121
    pathophysiology of, 120
    seizures precipitated by, 134
    in study of complex partial seizures, 44
Hypnagogic slowing of EEG, in children, 120
Hypnotics, for tonic seizures, 90
Hypocalcemia
    neonatal seizures and, 299, 303–304
    phenytoin and, 184
    seizures and, 132
Hypoglycemia
    neonatal, infantile spasms and, 97
    neonatal seizures and, 304
    seizures and, 133
Hyponatremia, seizures and, 132
    neonatal, 304
Hypoxic-ischemic insults, infantile spasms and, 97
Hypsarrhythmia, in infantile spasms, 99–101
Hysterical seizures, epilepsy differentiated from, 113–115, 124

Ictal period
    of atonic seizure EEG changes in, 81–82
    of atypical absence seizures, EEG changes in, 76
    in bilateral massive epileptic myoclonus, EEG changes in, 80
    of complex partial seizure, EEG changes in, 43–44
    of infantile spasms, EEG changes in, 101
    of neonatal seizures, EEG in, 307, 308
    of seizure, 2
    of simple partial seizure, EEG in, 33–34
    of tonic seizures, EEG changes in, 86, 87
Identification, patient education on, 266
Illusions, simple partial onset of complex partial seizures with, 41
Immunizations, infantile spasms and, 98